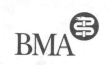

Ovarian Cancer

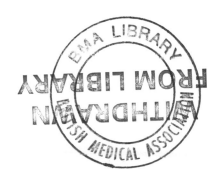

Ovarian Cancer

I. J. Jacobs
J. H. Shepherd
D. H. Oram
A. D. Blackett
D. M. Luesley
A. Berchuck
C. N. Hudson

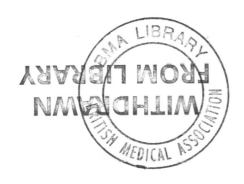

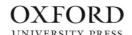

OXFORD
UNIVERSITY PRESS

OXFORD
UNIVERSITY PRESS

Great Clarendon Street, Oxford OX2 6DP

Oxford University Press is a department of the University of Oxford.
It furthers the University's objective of excellence in research, scholarship,
and education by publishing worldwide in

Oxford New York

Auckland Bangkok Buenos Aires Cape Town Chennai Dar es Salaam
Delhi Hong Kong Istanbul Karachi Kolkata Kuala Lumpur Madrid
Melbourne Mexico City Mumbai Nairobi São Paulo Shanghai
Taipei Tokyo Toronto

and an associated company in Berlin

Oxford is a registered trade mark of Oxford University Press
in the UK and in certain other countries

Published in the United States
by Oxford University Press Inc., New York

A catalogue record for this title is available from the British Library.

Library of Congress Cataloging in Publication Data

Textbook of ovarian cancer/C.N. Hudson ... [et al.].–2nd ed.
Rev. ed. of: Ovarian cancer/edited by C.N. Hudson. 1985.
Includes bibliographical references and index.
1. Ovaries–Cancer   I. Hudson, Christopher N.   II. Ovarian cancer
[DNLM: 1. Ovarian Neoplasms. WP 322 O9621 2001]
RC280.O8 O88 2001   616.99'465–dc21   2001031171

ISBN 0 19 850826 3 (Hbk.alk. paper)

10 9 8 7 6 5 4 3 2 1

Typeset by EXPO Holdings, Malaysia
Printed in Great Britain
on acid-free paper by Butler and Tanner Ltd, Frome

Foreword

The Helene Harris Memorial Trust

The Helene Harris Memorial Trust was founded in 1986 with the aim of encouraging the global interchange between scientists and clinicians of the latest information on research and treatment of ovarian cancer. To achieve its aims the HHMT has organized biennial 4-day meetings, which have been attended by many of the foremost international researchers and clinicians. So far these meetings have taken place in London, Graz, Charleston, Toronto, Glasgow, Los Angeles, Stockholm and Houston. The proceedings of the Stockholm meeting, carried out in conjunction with the Karolinska Institute, are included in this book.

Also included are chapters prepared following a recent addition to the work of the HHMT—the establishment of Travelling Fellowships, designed to provide an opportunity for the best and the brightest of the younger generation to present their work to their peers. This innovation was a tremendous success in Stockholm, where the finalists presented papers of the highest quality.

The meetings held by the HHMT, have brought it to the forefront for information interchange on the latest research and techniques in ovarian cancer. Readers will find in this book key information and data on developments that have been presented and discussed at the HHMT meeting.

John Harris

Preface

Ovarian cancer is intended to provide a comprehensive synthesis of clinical management and research progress in the field of ovarian malignancy. The book is now a combination of two separate but complementary initiatives. One initiative was a series of reviews commissioned to cover the spectrum of clinical management of ovarian cancer from prevention, screening, and diagnosis, to surgery, chemotherapy, and palliative care. The second initiative has been coordinated by the Helene Harris Memorial Trust (HHMT) which has organized key biennial meetings on ovarian cancer for the past 12 years. Attendance at the meetings on research aspects of ovarian cancer is by invitation to a small group of international authorities. The participants at the Stockholm HHMT meeting were asked to prepare a chapter based upon their contribution.

Setting clinically focused reviews alongside the HHMT research-focused chapters has created a unique book. First, it presents recent advances not readily available elsewhere, such as on 'tumour biology' and 'novel therapies'. The review chapters are set alongside detailed coverage of recent clinical and basic science research developments. Examples of this are the coverage of familial cancer, prevention, screening, and current therapy, which are consequently much more topical and exciting. Finally, the contributions are from a representative spectrum of authors from both research and clinical backgrounds and with a truly international perspective.

The book is aimed at both clinicians and researchers who require access to a comprehensive resource in this field but may not have the time, to find and read original publications outside their key area of expertise. This will include trainees and practitioners in general gynaecology, medical and radiation oncology, pathology, and palliative care, whose main focus is clinical expertise but who are expected to remain up to date regarding research and therapeutic developments. It will also include researchers who wish to obtain a broader and balanced view of both clinical and research progress outside their focused research field. Readers of this book can be confident that they have access to the state of the art and exciting new areas of progress in ovarian cancer.

Contents

Contributors

Abbas Abdollahi
Ovarian Cancer Program, Fox Chase Cancer Center, 7701
Burholme Ave, Philadelphia, PA 19111, USA

Nigel Acheson
CRC Institute for Cancer Studies, University of Birmingham,
Birmingham B15 2TA, UK

Mansour S. Al-Moundhri
Department of Medicine, The Royal Marsden NHS Trust, Fulham
Road, London SW3 6JJ, UK

Angeles Alvarez
Department of Obstetrics and Gynecology, Division of
Gynecologic Oncology, Duke University Medical Center,
Durham, NC 27710, USA

Garnet Anderson
Cancer Prevention Research Program, Fred Hutchinson Cancer
Research Center, Seattle, Washington, USA

Kenneth Anderson
Department of Poultry Science, Box 7608, College of Agriculture
and Life Science, North Carolina State University, Raleigh,
NC 27695, USA

Marianne Andresen
Department of Tumorbiology, The Norwegian Radium Hospital,
Oslo, Norway

Caroline Arnott
ICRF Translational Oncology Laboratory, Barts and the London
Queen Mary's Medical School, Charterhouse Square, London
EC1M 6BQ, UK

Rudi Bao
Ovarian Cancer Program, Fox Chase Cancer Center, 7701
Burholme Ave, Philadelphia, PA 19111, USA

Russ Baldocchi
University of California San Francisco, Cancer Research Center,
San Francisco, California, USA

Fran Balkwill
ICRF Translational Oncology Laboratory, Barts and the London
Queen Mary's Medical School, Charterhouse Square, London
EC1M 6BQ, UK

John Barnes
College of Veterinary Medicine, Department of Animal Health
and Resource Management, Box 8401, North Carolina State
University, Raleigh, NC 27695, USA

Robert C. Bast
Division of Medicine, University of Texas M.D. Anderson Cancer
Center, 1515 Holcombe Boulevard, Box 092, Houston, TX 77030,
USA

Debra A. Bell
Massachusetts General Hospital, Harvard Medical School, MA
02114, USA

Uziel Beller
Division of Gynecologic Oncology, Shaare Zedek Medical Center,
PO Box 3235, Jerusalem 91031, Israel

Andrew Berchuck
Department of Obstetrics and Gynecology, Division of
Gynecologic Oncology, Duke University Medical Center,
PO Box 3079, Durham, NC 27710, USA

Jonathan S. Berek
Department of Obstetrics and Gynecology, University of
California, Los Angeles School of Medicine and UCLA Women's
Reproductive Cancer Program, Jonsson Comprehensive Cancer
Center, Los Angeles, California, USA

Ross S. Berkowitz
Brigham and Women's Hospital, Harvard Medical School,
Boston, MA 02115, USA

George R.P. Blackledge
AstraZeneca Pharmaceuticals, Alderly House, Alderly Park,
Macclesfield, Cheshire, SE10 4TF, UK

Guido Hoctin Boes
EORTC Data Center, Brussels, Belgium

Keith E. Britton
St. Bartholomew's and the Royal London School of Medicine and
Dentistry, Queen Mary Westfield, University of London, London
EC1M 6BQ, UK

Monica R. Brown
Laboratory of Pathology, National Cancer Institute, Bethesda,
MD 20892, USA

T.E. Buekers
University of Iowa Hospitals and Clinics, Iowa City, IA 52242-1009, USA

R.E. Buller
Division of Gynecologic Oncology, University of Iowa Hospitals and Clinics, 200 Hawkins Drive—#4630 JCP, Iowa City, IA 52242-1009, USA

Joy Burchell
ICRF Breast Cancer Biology Laboratory, Thomas Guy House, Guys Hospital, London SE1 9RT, UK

Frances Burke
ICRF Translational Oncology Laboratory, Barts and the London Queen Mary's Medical School, Charterhouse Square, London EC1M 6BQ, UK

Ian G. Campbell

VBCRC Cancer Genetics Laboratory, Peter MacCallum Cancer Institute, Melbourne, Victoria, Australia

Silvana Canevari
Unit of Molecular Therapies, Department of Experimental Oncology, Istituto Nazionale per lo Studio e la Cura dei Tumori, 20133, Milan, Italy

Donna Carver
Department of Poultry Science, Box 7608, College of Agriculture and Life Science, North Carolina State University, Raleigh, NC 27695, USA

Raphael Catane
Oncology Institute, Shaare Zedek Medical Center, PO Box 3235, Jerusalem 91031, Israel

Angela Chetrit
Department of Clinical Epidemiology, Sheba Medical Center, Tel-Hashomer, Israel

Lauren Clarke
Cancer Prevention Research Program, Fred Hutchinson Cancer Research Center, Seattle, Washington, USA

Mark Cline
Comparative Medicine Research Center, Wake Forest University School of Medicine, Winston-Salem, NC 27157, USA

Maria I. Colnaghi
Unit of Molecular Therapies, Department of Experimental Oncology, Istituto Nazionale per lo Studio e la Cura dei Tumori, 20133, Milan, Italy

Isabel Correa
ICRF Breast Cancer Biology Laboratory, Thomas Guy House, Guys Hospital, London SE1 9RT, UK

Daniel W. Cramer
Obstetrics and Gynecology Epidemiology Center, Brigham and Women's Hospital, 221 Longwood Avenue, Boston, MA 02115, USA

Robin A. F. Crawford
Addenbrooke's Hospital NHS Trust, Box 242, Hills Road, Cambridge CB2 2QQ, UK

Bruce Cuevas
Department of Molecular Oncology, The University of Texas, M. D. Anderson Cancer Center, Houston, Texas 77030, USA

O. Marigold Curling
Department of Cytopathology, St Bartholomew's Hospital, West Smithfield, London EC1A 7BE, UK

Steven de Jong
Department of Medical Oncology, University Hospital Groningen, The Netherlands

Paul DePriest
Department of OB/GYN, Division of Gynecologic Oncology, University of Kentucky, 800 Rose Street, Lexington, Kentucky 40536, USA

Elisabeth G.E. de Vries
Department of Medical Oncology, University Hospital Groningen, The Netherlands

Charles Drescher
Marsha Rivkin Center for Ovarian Cancer Research, Seattle, Washington, USA

Astrid Eder
Department of Molecular Oncology, The University of Texas, M.D. Anderson Cancer Center, Houston, Texas 77030, USA

Michael Emmert-Buck
Laboratory of Pathology, National Cancer Institute, Bethesda, MD 20892, USA

Xianjun Fang
Division of Medicine, University of Texas M.D. Anderson Cancer Center, Houston, TX 77030, USA

Guiceppe Favalli
University of Brescia, Brescia, Italy

E. Ferreux
Division of Oncology and Cellular Pathology, University of Sheffield Medical School, Beech Hill Road, Sheffield S10 2RX, UK

Mariangela Figini
Unit of Molecular Therapies, Department of Experimental Oncology, Istituto Nazionale per lo Studio e la Cura dei Tumori, 20133, Milan, Italy

Kerry D. Fisher
CRC Institute for Cancer Studies, University of Birmingham,
Birmingham B15 2TA, UK

Øystein Fodstad
Departments of Gynecologic Oncology and Tumorbiology,
The Norwegian Radium Hospital, Oslo, Norway

Harold Fox
Department of Pathological Sciences, Stopford Building,
University of Manchester, Manchester M13 9PT, UK

Tatsuro Furui
Department of Molecular Oncology, The University of Texas,
M.D. Anderson Cancer Center, Houston, Texas 77030,
USA

P. Andrew Futreal
Departments of Obstetrics and Gynecology/Division of
Gynecologic Oncology, Genetics, and Surgery, Duke University
Medical Center, Box 3079, Durham, NC 27710, USA

David Gibbs
Department of Medicine, Royal Marsden Hospital, Fulham Road,
London SW3 6JJ, UK

Martin Gore
Department of Medicine, Royal Marsden Hospital, Fulham Road,
London SW3 6JJ, UK

Orit Gotfeld
Division of Medical Genetics, Shaare Zedek Medical Center,
PO Box 3235, Jerusalem 91031, Israel

Rosalind Graham
ICRF Breast Cancer Biology Laboratory, Thomas Guy House,
Guys Hospital, London SE1 9RT, UK

Marie Granowska
St. Bartholomew's and the Royal London Schools of Medicine
and Dentistry, Queen Mary Westfield, University of London,
London ECTA 7BE, UK

Joe W. Gray
Department of Laboratory Medicine, University of California,
San Francisco, CA 94143, USA

Thomas C. Hamilton
Division of Medical Science, Fox Chase Cancer Center, 7701
Burholme Ave, Philadelphia, PA 19111, USA

Marco N. Helder
Department of Gynaecology, University Hospital Groningen,
The Netherlands

Lukas Heukamp
ICRF Breast Cancer Biology Laboratory, Thomas Guy House,
Guys Hospital, London SE1 9RT, UK

Galit Hirsh-Yechzkel
Department of Clinical Epidemiology, Sheba Medical Center, Tel-
Hashomer, Israel

Davod Hogg
Department of Medicine, University of Toronto, Toronto,
Ontario, Canada M5G2C4

Hanne Høifødt
Departments of Gynecologic Oncology and Tumorbiology, The
Norwegian Radium Hospital, Oslo, Norway

JoAnn Horowitz
Department of Clinical Oncology, Schering-Plough Research
Institute, Kenilworth, NJ, USA

Stephen B. Howell
Department of Medicine and the Cancer Center, University of
California, San Diego,
9500 Gilman Drive, La Jolla, CA 92093–0058, USA

C.N. Hudson
Department of Gynaecology, St Bartholomew's Hospital, West
Smithfield, London ECTA 7BE, UK

Claude Hughes
Department of Obstetrics and Gynecology, Duke University
Medical Center, Durham, NC 27710, USA

Kelly Hunt
Division of Surgery, University of Texas M. D. Anderson Cancer
Center, Houston, TX 77030, USA

Thomas E.J. Ind
Gynaecological Cancer Centre, St. Bartholomew's Hospital and
the NHS Trust, West Smithfield, London EC1A 7BE, UK

Pamela D. Isner
Division of Gynecologic Oncology, Duke University Medical
Center, Durham, NC 27710, USA

Ian J. Jacobs
Bart's and the London Queen Mary School of Medicine and
Dentistry, Charterhouse Square, London EC1M 6GR

Robert Jaffe
University of California San Francisco, Cancer Research Center,
San Francisco, California, USA

Hikmat Jan
St. Bartholomew's and the Royal London Schools of Medicine
and Dentistry, Queen Mary Westfield, University of London, UK

Stephen R. D. Johnston
Department of Medicine, The Royal Marsden NHS Trust, Fulham
Road, London SW3 6JJ, UK

Janne Kærn
Department of Gynecologic Oncology, The Norwegian Radium Hospital, Oslo, Norway

Beth Karlan
Cedars-Sinai Medical Center, Los Angeles, California, USA, and University of Los Angeles School of Medicine, Los Angeles, California, USA

Bella Kaufman
Oncology Institute, Shaare Zedek Medical Center, PO Box 3235, Jerusalem 91031, Israel

Sean Kehoe
Department of Gynaecological Oncology, The Birmingham Women's Hospital, Edgbaston, Birmingham B15 2TG, UK

Lloyd R. Kelland
Cancer Research Campaign Centre for Cancer Therapeutics 2, The Institute of Cancer Research, 15 Cotswold Road, Belmont, Sutton, Surrey SM2 5NG, UK

Heung-Ki Kim
Department of Medicine and the Cancer Center, University of California, San Diego, 9500 Gilman Drive, La Jolla, CA 92093–0058, USA

H. C. Kitchener
St Mary's Hospital for Women and Children, Department of Obstetrics and Gynaecology, Oxford Road, Manchester, M13 0JH

Andres J. P. Klein-Szanto
Division of Medical Science, Fox Chase Cancer Center, 7701 Burholme Avenue, Philadelphia, PA 19111, USA

Anna Kobierska
Medical Academy, Gdansk, Poland

Elise C. Kohn
Laboratory of Pathology, National Cancer Institute, Bethesda, MD 20892, USA

G. Konecny
Division of Hematology/Oncology, UCLA School of Medicine

R. Kreienberg
University of Ulm, Ulm, Germany

Hannah Krigman
Department of Pathology, Duke University Medical Center, Durham, NC 27710, USA

David B. Krizman
Laboratory of Pathology, National Cancer Institute, Bethesda, MD 20892, USA

Wen-Lin Kuo
Department of Laboratory Medicine, University of California, San Francisco, CA 94143, USA

S. Kupesic
Department of Obstetrics and Gynecology, Medical School, University of Zagreb, Sveti Duh Hospital, Zagreb, Croatia

A. Kurjak
Department of Obstetrics and Gynecology, Medical School, University of Zagreb, Sveti Duh Hospital, Zagreb, Croatia

Angel J. Lacave
Hospital Central de Asturias, Oviedo, Spain

Ruth Lapushin
Department of Molecular Oncology, The University of Texas, M. D. Anderson Cancer Center, Houston, Texas 77030, USA

Ofer Lavie
Division of Gynecologic Oncology, Shaare Zedek Medical Center, PO Box 3235, Jerusalem 91031, Israel

Bruce Lessey
Department of Obstetrics and Gynecology, University of North Carolina at Chapel Hill, Chapel Hill, NC, USA

Ephrat Levy-Lahad
Division of Medical Genetics, Shaare Zedek Medical Center, PO Box 3235, Jerusalem 91031, Israel

C.E. Lewis
Division of Oncology and Cellular Pathology, University of Sheffield Medical School, Beech Hill Road, Sheffield S10 2RX, UK

Xinjian Lin
Department of Medicine and the Cancer Center, University of California, San Diego, 9500 Gilman Drive, La Jolla, CA 92093–0058, USA

Lance A. Liotta
Laboratory of Pathology, National Cancer Institute, Bethesda, MD 20892, USA

David Lowe
Department of Histopathology, St Bartholomew's and Royal London School of Medicine and Dentistry, Queen Mary Westfield, University of London, ECTA 7BE, UK

Karen H. Lu
Brigham and Women's Hospital, Harvard Medical School, Boston, MA 02115, USA

Yiling Lu
Department of Molecular Oncology, The University of Texas, M. D. Anderson Cancer Center, Houston, Texas 77030, USA

David M. Luesley
Department of Obstetrics and Gynaecology, University of Birmingham, Faculty and Medicine and Dentistry, Edgbaston, Birmingham B15 2TT

Andrea Lundell
Yale University School of Medicine, New Haven, CT, USA

James Mackay
CRC Department of Oncology, University of Cambridge, Addenbrooke's Hospital, Cambridge, UK

Christopher Mann
Department of Gynaecological Oncology, City Hospital NHS Trust, Dudley Road, Birmingham B18 7QH, UK

Jeffrey Marks
Division of Surgery, Duke University Medical Center, Durham, NC 27710, USA

Christian Marth
Department of Gynecologic Oncology, The Norwegian Radium Hospital, Oslo, Norway, and Department of Obstetrics and Gynecology, Innsbruck University Hospital, Innsbruck, Austria

Ole Mathiesen
Departments of Gynecologic Oncology and Tumorbiology, The Norwegian Radium Hospital, Oslo, Norway

Alessandra Mazzoni
Experimental Immunology Branch, NCI, NIH, Bethesda, Maryland, USA

Martin McIntosh
Cancer Prevention Research Program, Fred Hutchinson Cancer Research Center, Seattle, Washington, USA, and Department of Biostatistics, University of Washington, Seattle, Washington, USA

Connette McMahon
Department of Obstetrics and Gynecology, Duke University Medical Center, Durham, NC 27710, USA

Usha Menon
St. Bartholomew's and the Royal London Medical and Dental School, London EC1M 6GR, UK

Delia Mezzanzanica
Unit of Molecular Therapies, Department of Experimental Oncology, Istituto Nazionale per lo Studio e la Cura dei Tumori, 20133, Milan, Italy

David Miles
ICRF Breast Cancer Biology Laboratory, Thomas Guy House, Guys Hospital, London SE1 9RT, UK

Gordon B. Mills
Department of Molecular Oncology, The University of Texas, M. D. Anderson Cancer Center, 1515 Holcombe Blvd, Box 317, Houston, Texas 77030, USA

Baruch Modan
Department of Clinical Epidemiology, Sheba Medical Center, Tel-Hashomer, Israel

Samuel C. Mok
Brigham and Women's Hospital, Harvard Medical School, Boston, MA 02115, USA

Robert Moore
ICRF Translational Oncology Laboratory, Barts and the London Queen Mary's Medical School, Charterhouse Square, London EC1M 6BQ, UK

Sarah J. Morland
Obstetrics and Gynaecology, University of Southampton, Princess Anne Hospital, Coxford Road, Southampton SO16 5YA, UK

M. Nardi
Regina Elena Cancer Institute, Roma, Italy

Faria Nasreen
St. Bartholomew's and the Royal London Schools of Medicine and Dentistry, Queen Mary Westfield University of London, London ECTA 7BE, UK

Donatella R. M. Negri
AM Experimental Immunology Branch, NCI, NIH, Bethesda, Maryland, USA; DRMN Laboratorio di Virologia, Istituto Superiore di Sanità, 00161, Rome, Italy

Phillippa J. Neville
Obstetrics and Gynaecology, University of Southampton, Princess Anne Hospital, Coxford Road, Southampton SO16 5YA, UK

Shu-wing Ng
Brigham and Women's Hospital, Harvard Medical School, Boston, MA 02115, USA

L. L. Nielsen
Department of Tumor Biology, Schering-Plough Research Institute

Koshiro Obata
Obstetrics and Gynaecology, University of Southampton, Princess Anne Hospital, Coxford Road, Southampton SO16 5YA, UK

David H. Oram
Gynecological Cancer Centre, St Bartholomew's Hospital, West Smithfield, London ECTA 7BE, UK

Robert F. Ozols
Division of Medical Science, Fox Chase Cancer Center, 7701 Burholme Avenue, Philadelphia, PA 19111, USA

Sergio Pecorelli
University of Brescia, Brescia, Italy

M.D. Pegram
Division of Hematology/Oncology, UCLA School of Medicine, Los Angeles, CA, USA

Hongqi Peng
Division of Medicine, University of Texas M.D. Anderson Cancer Center, Houston, TX 77030, USA

C.W. Perrett
Department of Obstetrics and Gynaecology, Royal Free Hospital School of Medicine, Rowland Hill, London NW3 2PF, UK

Ingemar Persson
Dept of Medical Epidemiology, Karolinska Institute, Box 281, 171 77 Stockholm, Sweden

James Petitte
Department of Poultry Science, College of Agriculture and Life Science, Box 7608, North Carolina State University, Raleigh, NC 27695, USA

Emmanuel Petricoin
Division of Cytokine Biology, Center for Biological Evaluation and Research, Food and Drug Administration, Bethesda, Maryland, USA

Paul D. Pharoah
University of Cambridge, Strangeways Research Laboratories, Wort's Causeway, Cambridge, UK

Dan Pinkel
University of California San Francisco, Cancer Research Center, San Francisco, California, USA

M. R. Pittelli
Ospedale San Gerardo, Monza, Italy

Daniel Plikoff
University of California San Francisco, Cancer Research Center, San Francisco, California, USA

Tim Plunkett
ICRF Breast Cancer Biology Laboratory, Thomas Guy House, Guys Hospital, London SE1 9RT, UK

R.H. Reznek
Department of Radiology, St Bartholomew's and Royal London School of Medicine and Dentistry, Queen Mary Westfield, University of London, London ECTA 7BE, UK

Gustavo C. Rodriguez
Division of Gynecologic Oncology, Department of Obstetrics and Gynecology, Duke University Medical Center, 3079, Durham, NC 27710, USA

I. Runnebaum
Division of Gynecologic Oncology, University of Ulm, Ulm, Germany

M.E. Rybak
Schering-Plough Research Institute, Kenilworth, NJ, USA

Thomas P. Salko
Schering-Plough Research Institute, Kenilworth, NJ, USA

Francisco Sapunar
Department of Medicine, Royal Marsden Hospital, Fulham Road, London SW3 6JJ, UK

Joellen S. Schildkraut
Department of Community and Family Medicine, Duke University Medical Center, Box 3079, Durham, NC 27710, USA

Kate Scott
ICRF Translational Oncology Laboratory, Barts and the London Queen Mary's Medical School, Charterhouse Square, London EC1M 6BQ, UK

Chris Scotton
ICRF Translational Oncology Laboratory, Barts and the London Queen Mary's Medical School, Charterhouse Square, London EC1M 6BQ, UK

Leonard W. Seymour
CRC Institute for Cancer Studies, University of Birmingham, Birmingham B15 2TA, UK

M. S. Shahin
University of Iowa Hospitals and Clinics, Iowa City, IA 52242-1009, USA

Jonathan Shamash
Department of Medical Oncology, St Bartholomew's Hospital, West Smithfield, London ECTA 7BE, UK

Laleh Shayestri
University of California San Francisco, Cancer Research Center, San Francisco, California, USA

Moira Shearer
ICRF Breast Cancer Biology Laboratory, Thomas Guy House, Guys Hospital, London SE1 9RT, UK

John H. Shepherd
Gynaecological Cancer Centre, St. Bartholomew's Hospital and the NHS Trust, West Smithfield, London EC1A 7BE, UK

Michael Siciliano
Department of Molecular Genetics, University of Texas M.D.
Anderson Cancer Center, Houston, TX 77030, USA

Kathy Siminovitch
University of Toronto, Toronto, Canada M5G 1X5

Naveena Singh
Department of Histopathology, St Bartholomew's and Royal
London School of Medicine and Dentistry, Queen Mary
Westfield, University of London, London ECTA 7BE, UK

Steven J. Skates
Biostatistics Center, Massachusetts General Hospital and Harvard
Medical School, Boston MA, USA

D.J. Slamon
Division of Hematology/Oncology, UCLA School of Medicine,
Los Angeles, CA, USA

Maurice Slevin
Department of Medical Oncology, St Bartholomew's Hospital,
West Smithfield, London ECTA 7BE, UK

Mark P. Smith
AstraZeneca Pharmaceuticals, Alderly House, Alderly Park,
Macclesfield, Cheshire, SE10 4TF, UK

Michael Smith
ICRF Breast Cancer Biology Laboratory, Thomas Guy House,
Guys Hospital, London SE1 9RT, UK

S. A. A. Sohaib
Department of Radiology, St Bartholomew's and Royal London
School of Medicine and Dentistry, Queen Mary Westfield,
University of London, London ECTA 7BE, UK

Michael R. Stratton
Section of Cancer Genetics, Institute of Cancer Research, Sutton,
Surrey SM2 5NG, UK

Jeffery P. Struewing
Laboratory of Population Genetics, NIH, 41 Library Dr., Building
41/D702, Bethesda, MD 20892–5055, USA

Christine E. Szarka
Department of Population Science, Fox Chase Cancer Center,
7701 Burholme Avenue, Philadelphia, PA 19111, USA

Kenneth J.W. Taylor
Department of Radiology, OBGYN and Surgery,
Yale University School of Medicine, New Haven, CT 06520, USA

Joyce Taylor-Papadimitriou
ICRF Breast Cancer Biology Laboratory, Thomas Guy House,
Guys Hospital, London SE1 9RT, UK

Ivana Teodorovic
EORTC Data Center, Brussels, Belgium

Nicola Thomas
Obstetrics and Gynaecology, University of Southampton,
Princess Anne Hospital, Coxford Road, Southampton SO16 5YA,
UK

Edward L. Trimble
Division of Cancer Treatment and Diagnosis, 6130 Executive
Boulevard, Suite 741, Bethesda, MD 20892-7436, USA

Claes Tropé
Department of Gynecologic Oncology and Tumorbiology, The
Norwegian Radium Hospital, Oslo, Norway

Nicole Urban
Cancer Prevention Research Program, Fred Hutchinson Cancer
Research Center, 1100 Fairview Avenue North, MP-804, Seattle,
WA 98109, USA, and Department of Health Services, University
of Washington, Seattle, Washington, USA

Maria E.L. van der Burg
University Hospital Rotterdam, Dijkzigt, Rotterdam,
The Netherlands

Ate G.J. van der Zee
Department of Gynaecological Oncology, University Hospital
Groningen, PO Box 30001, 9700 RB Groningen, The Netherlands
Bart Vanhaesebroeck
Imperial Cancer Research Fund, London, UK

Mat van Lent
The Rotterdam Cancer Institute, Daniel den Hoed Kliniek,
Rotterdam, The Netherlands

Ignace Vergote
Gynaecologic Oncology, University Hospitals Leuven,
Gasthuisberg, B-3000 Leuven, Belgium

Lise Walberg
Department of Tumorbiology, The Norwegian Radium Hospital,
Oslo, Norway

David Walmer
Department of Obstetrics and Gynecology, Division of
Reproductive Endocrinology, Duke University Medical Center,
Durham, NC 27710, USA

Christopher M. Ward
CRC Institute for Cancer Studies, University of Birmingham,
Birmingham B15 2TA, UK

William R. Welch
Brigham and Women's Hospital, Harvard Medical School,
Boston, MA 02115, USA

M. Wells
Division of Oncology and Cellular Pathology, University of Sheffield Medical School, Beech Hill Road, Sheffield S10 2RX, UK

Regina Whitaker
Division of Gynecologic Oncology, Duke University Medical Center, Durham NC 27710, USA

G. Bea A. Wisman
Department of Gynaecology, University Hospital Groningen, The Netherlands

Robert P. Woolas
Department of Gynaecological Oncology, St Marys Hospital, Portsmouth PO3 6AD, UK

Weiya Xia
Department of Cancer Biology, University of Texas M. D. Anderson Cancer Center, Houston, TX 77030, USA

Fengji Xu
Department of Urology, Peking Union Medical College, Bejing, Peoples' Republic of China

Gary K. Yiu
Brigham and Women's Hospital, Harvard Medical School, Boston, MA 02115, USA

Singxing Yu
Department of Molecular Oncology, The University of Texas, M. D. Anderson Cancer Center, Houston, Texas 77030, USA

Yinhua Yu
Division of Medicine, University of Texas, M. D. Anderson Cancer Center, Houston, TX 77030, USA

Shulei Zhao
Department of Cell Biology, Baylor College of Medicine, Houston, TX 77030, USA
Ronald P. Zweemer

Ronald P. Zweemer
Rustenbergerlaan 42, 2012 AP Haarlem, The Netherlands

Abbreviations

Ab	antibody	EORTC	European Organization for Research and Treatment of Cancer
AFP	α-fetoprotein	ERK	extracellular signal-regulated kinase
AI	apoptotic index	ER-α	oestrogen receptor-α
APC	adenomatous polyposis coli OR antigen-presenting cell	EST	expressed sequence tag
AR	androgen receptor	EVUS	endovaginal transducers utilizing high-frequency ultrasound
AUC	area under curve (dosing)	FACS	fluorescence-activated cell sorter
BCLC	Breast Cancer Linkage Consortium	FADD	Fas-associated death domain protein
bFGF	basic fibroblast growth factor	FAK	focal adhesion kinase
BOT	borderline ovarian tumour	FAP	familial adenomatous polyposis
BPO	bilateral prophylactic oophorectomy	FAP-1	Fas-associated phosphatase-1
BrdUrd	bromodeoxyuridine	FDA	Food and Drug Administration
BSA	bovine serum albumin	FDG	[^{18}F]deoxyglucose
BSO	bilateral salpingo-oophorectomy	FGF	fibroblast growth factor
CAP	cyclophosphamide, Adriamycin, platinum	FIGO	International Federation of Gynecology and Obstetrics
CBDCA	carboplatin		
CC	clomiphene citrate	FISH	fluorescence *in situ* hybridization
CDE	colour Doppler energy	FITC	fluoroscein isothiocyanate
CDI	colour Dopper imaging	FLICE	FADD-like ICE
cdk	cyclin-dependent kinase	αFR	α-folate receptor
CDR	complementary determinant region	FSH	follicle stimulating hormone
CEA	carcino-embryonic antigen	GAP	GTPase activating protein
CFTR	cystic fibrosis transport regulator	GCCG	Gynaecological Cancer Co-operative Group
CGAP	Cancer Genome Anatomy Project	GDP	guanosine diphosphate
CGH	comparative genomic hybridization	GFP	green fluorescent protein
CGN	Cancer Genetics Network	GM-CSF	granulocyte-macrophage colony stimulating factor
CHO	Chinese hamster ovary		
CHX	cycloheximide	GnRH	gonadotropin releasing hormone
CI	confidence interval	GTP	guanosine triphosphate
CMV	cytomegalovirus	HBC	hereditary breast cancer
CNS	clinical nurse specialist	HB-EGF	heparin-binding EGF
COC	combined oral contraceptive	HBOC	hereditary breast-ovarian cancer
CPYLS	incremental cost per YLS	hCG	human chorionic gonadotropin
CR	cumulative risk	HGPRT	hypoxanthine guanine phosphoribosyl transferase
CREB	cyclic AMP response element binding protein		
		5-HIAA	5-hydroxyindole acetic acid
CSF-1	colony-stimulating growth factor 1	HIF	hypoxia-inducible factor
CTL	cytotoxic T cell	HMFG	human milk fat globule
DDP	cisplatin	hMG	human menopausal gonadotropins
DLT	dose-limiting toxicity	HNPCC	hereditary non-polyposis colorectal cancer
DNA-PK	DNA-dependent protein kinase	HOC	hereditary ovarian cancer
2-D PAGE	two-dimensional polyacrylamide gel electrophoresis	HOSE	normal ovarian epithelial (cells)
		HPLC	high-performance liquid chromatography
E2	estradiol	HPM	histopathological marker
ECL	enhanced chemiluminescence	pHPMA	poly-*N*-(2-hydroxypropyl)methacrylamide
EGF	epidermal growth factor OR cisplatin, epirubicin, and infusional 5-fluorouracil	HRE	hypoxia response element
		hsr	homogeneously staining region
EGFR	epidermal growth factor receptor	hTR	human telomerase RNA (component)
ELISA	enzyme-linked immunosorbent assay	ICE	interleukin-1β converting enzyme
EMA	epithelial membrane antigen		

IEOC	invasive epithelial ovarian tumour	PCNA	proliferating cell nuclear antigen
IFN	interferon	PDGF	platelet-derived growth factor
IGF-I	insulin-like growth factor-I	PEB	parametric empirical Bayes (methods)
IL-1	interleukin-1	PEG	percutaneous endoscopic gastrostomy
ILK	integrin-linked kinase	PET	positron emission tomography
IM	intramuscularly	PH	pleckstrin homology (domain)
IP	intraperitoneally	pHPMA	poly-N-(2-hydroxypropyl)methacrylamide
ISH	*in situ* hybridization	PI	propidium iodine
i.v.	intravenously	PID	phosphotyrosine interacting domain
IVF	*in vitro* fertilization	PI3K	phosphatidylinositol 3-kinase
KGF	keratinocyte growth factor	PIK	phosphatidylinositol kinase
KITL	kit ligand	PJS	Peutz-Jeghers syndrome
KLH	keyhole limpet haemocyanin	PKB	protein kinase B
LASA	lipid-associated sialic acid	PLAP	placental-like alkaline phosphatase
LCM	laser capture microdissection	pLL/DNA	poly(l-lysine)/DNA
LDH	lactate dehydrogenase	PMN	polymorphonuclear leucocyte
LH	luteinizing hormone	PPV	positive predictive value
LI	labeling index	PR	progesterone receptor
LMP	low malignant potential	pRb	retinoblastoma gene product
LOD	log of the odds (score)	PSA	prostate-specific antigen
LOH	loss of heterozygosity	PSV	peak systolic velocity
LPA	lysophosphatidic acid	PtdIns	phosphatidylinositol
LPC	lysophosphatidyl choline	RB	retinoblastoma
LSA	lipid-associated sialic acid	RCT	randomized controlled trial
LT	leukotriene	RER	replication error
M1	mortalization stage 1	RI	resistive index
MAPK	mitogen-activated protein kinase	RIS	radio-immunoscintigraphy
MCP	monocyte chemoattractant protein	RIT	radio-immunotherapy
M-CSF	macrophage colony stimulating factor	RMI	risk of malignancy index
MEK	MAPK/ERK kinase	ROC	risk of ovarian cancer
MFI	mean fluorescence intensity		OR receiver operator characteristic
MI	morphology index score	ROCA	risk of ovarian cancer algorithm
MIBG	meta-iodobenzylguanidine	ROCC	risk of ovarian cancer calculation
MIBI	methoxyisobutyl isonitrile	RPA	RNase protection assay
MIP	macrophage inflammatory protein	RR	relative risk
MIS	Müllerian inhibitory substance	RT-PCR	reverse transcriptase polymerase chain reaction
MMP	matrix metalloprotease		
MMR	mismatch-repair	SAM	sheep-anti-mouse
MNC	mononuclear cell fraction	SDS-PAGE	sodium dodecyl sulfate polyacrylamide gel electrophoresis
4-MPR	N-(4-methoxyphenyl) retinamide		
MRI	magnetic resonance imaging	SELDI	surface-enhanced laser desorption and ionization
MTT	3-(4,5-dimethylthiazol-2-yl)-2,5-diphenyl tetrazolium bromide		
		SLL	second-look laparotomy
NF	neurofibromatosis	SPET	single photon emission tomography
NK	natural killer cells	SSC	serous surface carcinoma of the ovary
NOS	not otherwise specified	SSCP	single-strand conformation polymorphism
NPV	negative predictive value	STIR	short-tau inversion recovery
NSE	neuron-specific enolase	TAS	transabdominal ultrasound
OC	oral contraceptive	TATI	tumour-associated trypsin inhibitor
OCCR	ovarian cancer cluster-region	TCR	T-cell receptor
OCP	oral contraceptive pill	TGF-α	transforming growth factor-α
OSE	ovarian surface epithelial cells	TIL	tumour-infiltrating lymphocytes
PAMPS	pathogen-associated molecular patterns	TNF-α	tumor necrosis factor-α
PAS	periodic acid-Schiff	TPA	12-O-tetradecanoylphorbol-13 acetate ALSO tissue polypeptide antigen
PBMC	peripheral blood mononuclear cells		
PBS	phosphate-buffered saline	TRAP	telomeric repeat amplification protocol
PBST	PBS containing 0.1% Tween 20	TSG	tumour suppressor genes

TSP	thrombospondin	VHL	von Hippel-Lindau
TTP	time to progression	VNTR	variable number of tandem repeats
TVCD	transvaginal colour Doppler sonography	VPF	vascular permeability factor
TVU	transvaginal ultrasound	wt	wild type
UGF	urinary gonatropin fragment	YAC	yeast artificial chromosome
UPSC	uterine papillary serous carcinoma	YLS	years of life saved
VEGF	vascular endothelial growth factor		

Part I

Aetiology

1. Epidemiology of sporadic ovarian cancer

Daniel W. Cramer

Introduction

This chapter will be organized around a number of premises (Table 1.1) which I believe lead to the conclusion that genetic, environmental, and reproductive factors mediate risk for ovarian cancer largely through their effects on the ovarian/pituitary axis or through pelvic contamination with talc or menses, and that these risk factors may vary according to the histologic type of ovarian cancer.

Premise 1: Germ-line mutations play some role, even in 'sporadic' ovarian cancers

Germ-line mutations, including *BRCA1*, *BRCA2*, and the DNA mismatch repair genes, are clearly linked to 'hereditary' ovarian cancer, where more than one relative with breast or ovarian cancer is identified.[1] However, it is becoming apparent that such mutations are also involved in 'sporadic' ovarian cancer, where a family history of cancer is less evident. In a consecutive series of 116 women recently diagnosed with ovarian cancer, Rubin *et al.* found that 12 patients (10%) had germ-line mutations: nine in *BRCA1*, one with both *BRCA1* and *BRCA2*; and two with mutations in the DNA mismatch repair genes.[2] In a population-based study of 32 Ashkenazi Jewish women with invasive ovarian cancer, 14 (44%) had a *BRCA1/BRCA2* mutation: eight carried a 185delAG mutation of *BRCA1* and nine carried a 6174delT mutation of *BRCA2*.[3]

These are two of the three common mutations that occur with high frequency in Jewish women. Histologically, serous borderline tumors and mucinous tumors appear to be underrepresented among women with *BRCA1* or *BRCA2* mutations. A challenge for epidemiologists will be to determine how these germ-line mutations may interact with traditional risk factors for ovarian cancer. A recent important observation is that the protective effect of oral contraceptives (OCs) on ovarian cancer may pertain in women who carry a *BRCA1* or *BRCA2* mutation;[4] but the issue needs to be examined further, since another group claims that OCs may increase risk for breast cancer in carriers.[5]

Premise 2: Talc use in the genital area is a common environmental risk factor for ovarian cancer

The author has recently reviewed evidence regarding the association between the use of talc in genital hygiene and risk for ovarian cancer and presented some new data.[6] A 'meta-analysis' of 14 studies on this topic reveals a significantly elevated odds ratio for ovarian cancer associated with the use of talc: overall relative risk of 1.36, and 95% confidence interval of 1.24–1.49. In the author's study, risk was not apparent for women who used talc in nongenital areas and most apparent for women who used talc in multiple ways in the genital area; e.g. dusting after bathing and powdering underwear or sanitary napkin. Women who never personally used talc but whose husbands used it in their genital area

Table 1.1 Premises regarding the epidemiology of ovarian cancer

1. Germ-line mutations may play a role, even in 'sporadic' ovarian cancers
2. Talc use in the genital area is a common environmental risk factor for ovarian cancer
3. 'Pelvic contamination' with menstrual products may occur, leading to endometriosis, which may be a precursor to, and share risk factors with, ovarian cancer
4. Diet may affect ovarian cancer risk, but agreement on specific factors is lacking
5. Pregnancy may protect against ovarian cancer by one or more different mechanisms, understanding of which would help clarify pathogenesis
6. Exogenous hormones and drugs may influence ovarian cancer risk, most likely through effects on gonadotropins rather than ovulation
7. Despite differences in tumor histology, animal models may be relevant to human ovarian cancer and also suggest the importance of pituitary/gonadal disruption
8. Consideration of histologic type of ovarian cancer may further clarify its epidemiology

had an increased risk for ovarian cancer of borderline statistical significance. The association between talc and ovarian cancer was less apparent among women who had a tubal ligation. Among parous women, there was some evidence that risk for ovarian cancer associated with talc use was greater for women who had some exposure prior to their first pregnancy and not as apparent for women who began use of talc after a first pregnancy. A possible explanation for this is addressed in the discussion of premise 3. Finally, the talc relationship was most apparent for women with serous and undifferentiated tumors.

Patency of the female tract,[7] chemical relationship between talc and asbestos,[8] and evidence that asbestos exposure is associated with ovarian cancer[9] provide a biologic basis for the talc and ovarian cancer association. Confounding factors and lack of a clear dose response have been put forward as the main arguments against a causal relationship.[10] However, all of the major studies have adjusted for the key confounders, parity and oral contraceptive (OC) use. Furthermore, that no increased risk was associated with use of powders in non-genital areas and that use of cornstarch-based powders (even genitally) is not associated with elevated risk[11,12] are findings which suggest that characteristics of powder use rather than powder users are the important elements. Regarding the dose response, it is difficult to quantify the dose of an 'application of talc' that the pelvis might actually receive. Use during ovulatory cycles which might allow entrapment of talc deep into the stroma and other factors, such as patency of the female tract, may impact exposure. From a scientific standpoint, whether the talc/ovarian cancer association is causal warrants continued research and debate. From a public health standpoint, however, the risk/benefit analysis seems less complicated. Given what are solely aesthetic benefits for talc use and that 30–40% of women may use such products, I believe more formal public health warnings about avoiding talc in the genital area are warranted.

Premise 3: 'Pelvic contamination' with menstrual products may occur, leading to endometriosis, which may be a precursor to, and share risk factors with, ovarian cancer

A variety of other substances, besides talc, could contaminate the female pelvis, including menstrual fluid and chemicals in douches or spermicides. While no epidemiologic data suggest that the latter substances are linked to ovarian cancer, there is evidence that menstruation may play a role in this disease, possibly through its link to endometriosis. Pathologists report that ovarian cancer can arise in areas of endometriosis;[13] and a follow-up study of Swedish women hospitalized for endometriosis demonstrated an increased risk for subsequent ovarian cancer of about twofold overall, and about threefold if the ovaries were involved with endometriosis at the original diagnosis.[14]

A widely accepted theory for the origin of endometriosis is that it relates to menstrual regurgitation through the Fallopian tubes.[15] Menstrual factors such as heavy, frequent, and painful periods have been shown to be risk factors for endometriosis[16] and may also play a role in ovarian cancer. This author found moderate and severe menstrual pain to be a risk factor for ovarian cancer.[17] Green et al. reported that tubal ligation was especially protective for ovarian cancer among women who had heavy periods and suggested interruption of retrograde menstruation as the mechanism for the protective effect.[18] Thus, blockage of pelvic contaminants such as talc or menses from entering the pelvic cavity may be the best explanation for the protective effect of tubal ligation and hysterectomy (without oophorectomy).

Meigs argued that early pregnancy was an important preventive factor for endometriosis;[19] and this would be another example of a (protective) risk factor shared between endometriosis and ovarian cancer. One explanation for the protective effect of pregnancy on endometriosis may be that labor and delivery of a full-term infant permanently dilates the cervix, reducing the resistance to menstrual flow and the likelihood of retrograde menstruation. A second explanation might involve the 'decidual' reaction; i.e. differentiation of stromal cells that occurs primarily in the endometrium of the pregnant uterus but which also may be seen in the Fallopian tubes, pelvic peritoneum, and ovarian surface during pregnancy.[20] Whether this decidual reaction might induce a terminal differentiation of the pelvic peritoneum which reduces its susceptibility to carcinogenesis is a hypothesis worthy of further study. Finally, any link between risk factors for endometriosis and those for ovarian cancer may be strongest for the endometrioid and clear cell types of ovarian cancer, most likely to arise in the setting of endometriosis.[13]

Premise 4: Diet may affect ovarian cancer risk, but agreement on specific factors is lacking

The incidence of ovarian cancer varies about fivefold from the lowest rates, in the Orient and northern Africa, to the highest rates, in northern Europe and North America.[21] It is reasonable to propose that cultural differences, including diet, might play some role in this variation; but there is a lack of agreement on what the most important dietary factors might be. The geographic distribution of ovarian cancer correlates directly with per capita milk consumption and with frequency of the trait, lactase persistence, which allows digestion of milk sugar.[22] Observations that galactose (milk sugar) may be toxic to ovarian germ cells[23] and that ovarian toxicity can induce ovarian cancer experimentally (see premise 7) provide a biologic basis for a connection between milk products and ovarian cancer. Two studies have suggested increased risk with lactose consumption or milk products;[24,25] but this finding has not been confirmed in other studies[26,27]. Several studies have linked increased risk for ovarian cancer with animal fat or meat consumption[28–30] and egg or cholesterol consumption.[25] However, there may be the greatest consistency among studies that find a protective effect of vitamin A or carotene on ovarian cancer risk.[27, 31–33]

Except perhaps for vitamin A and carotene, inconsistency of dietary findings in relation to ovarian cancer risk may indicate that diet as a adult may be less relevant than diet earlier in life, or even dietary exposure as a fetus via maternal diet. Pregnant rodents fed a high-fat diet produced offspring who displayed more than a twofold increase in the occurrence mammary and ovarian tumors as they grew up, compared to control animals.[34] It is also relevant that mice fed high galactose during pregnancy produce female offspring with a significantly decreased endowment of germ cells.[23] Although the offspring were not followed to define subsequent occurrence of ovarian cancer, it is well known that risk for ovarian neoplasms is increased in animals born with a deficiency of germ cells.[35]

Premise 5: Pregnancy may protect against ovarian cancer by one or more different mechanisms, understanding of which would help clarify pathogenesis

A finding of virtually all studies of ovarian cancer is that childbirth exerts a protective effect; understanding how it does so would represent an importance advance. Table 1.2 lists possible explanations for the protective effect of pregnancy on ovarian cancer risk. In offering this list, I do not wish to imply that a single explanation is likely or that all possible mechanisms have been considered.

A 'trivial' explanation for the protective effect of pregnancy is that it is simply a marker for the 'healthy' ovary at lower risk for ovarian cancer than the ovary of an infertile woman. Perhaps consistent, there does appear to be a disproportionately greater decrease in risk in going from 0 to 1 pregnancy than in going from n to $n + 1$ pregnancies.[36] However, there is also a 'dose response' with protection offered by each subsequent pregnancy. Few studies have found reported infertility to be markedly higher for women with ovarian cancer compared to control subjects. These observations suggest that the protective effect of pregnancy goes beyond simply being a marker for a healthy ovary.

The most popular explanation for the protective effect of pregnancy is that it leads to a temporary cessation of ovulation.[37] This would reduce constant ovarian epithelial disruption and repair that may predispose to ovarian neoplasia, possibly through the accumulation of mutations in tumor suppressor genes such as

$p53$.[38] However, demographic features of ovarian cancer are not particularly compatible with this model. The incidence of ovarian cancer continues to increase throughout life—long after ovulation has stopped. The very low occurrence of ovarian cancer in Japan does not fit readily with incessant ovulation since this country has one of the lowest fertility rates in the world and virtually no use of oral contraceptives. Other risk factors, such as family history, seem hard to explain under an 'incessant ovulation' model. Finally, the disproportionate decrease in risk in going from 0 to 1 pregnancies is not easily explained by cessation of ovulation.

It is this author's opinion that the real importance of 'incessant ovulation' is that it causes stromal–epithelial admixture through inclusion cyst formation associated with ovulation. This permits epithelial cancers to be the predominant tumor type observed in humans as opposed to the stromal tumors in rodents, who ovulate less and lack stromal–epithelial admixture. It should also be appreciated that 'incessant ovulation' implies 'incessant menstruation' increasing the likelihood of pelvic contamination with menses and endometriosis.

The possibility that pregnancy induces a terminal differentiation of the ovarian surface epithelium and pelvic peritoneum (i.e. decidual reaction) has not been explored. Nor has the role of vaginal delivery in producing a simple mechanical effect in dilating the cervix and reducing the resistance to menstrual flow been considered. These mechanism were discussed under premise 3 and might be most relevant to risk factors that operate through pelvic contamination. These explanations would also fit with the marked effect of a single pregnancy, since decidual reaction and cervical dilation might be permanent changes occurring with the first pregnancy.

Finally, the possibility that pregnancy alters the pituitary gland to change the secretion of tropic hormones in later life should be explored. The size of the anterior pituitary increases dramatically during pregnancy;[39] and precipitous vascular changes following delivery may lead to pituitary failure in rare cases.[40] However, the degree of hypopituitarism is highly variable,[41] inviting the speculation that less dramatic functional changes in the pituitary occur in most women after delivery and lead to a reduction in the secretion of trophic hormones in later life. This theory is supported by a cross-sectional study of perimenopausal women which demonstrated a negative correlation between the number of prior pregnancies and luteinizing hormone levels,[42] an observation which might also help explain why there may be 'dose response' with number of pregnancies.

Table 1.2 Potential explanations for the protective effect of pregnancy

1. Pregnancy is a marker for a 'healthy' ovary, at inherently lower risk for ovarian cancer
2. Absence of pregnancy is associated with an increased number of ovulations—an event which increases risk for ovarian cancer
3. Pregnancy produces a decidual reaction that makes the ovarian and pelvic surface epithelium less susceptible to malignant transformation or endometriosis formation
4. Labor and vaginal delivery permanently dilates the cervix and reduces the resistance to menstrual flow and risk for endometriosis
5. Pregnancy permanently alters the pituitary gland to reduce the level of gonadotropins secreted in later life

Premise 6: Exogenous hormones and drugs may influence ovarian cancer risk, most likely through effects on gonadotropins rather than ovulation

In this section, the effect of several exogenous hormones and drugs on ovarian cancer risk will be discussed and the issue of whether associations are more likely to be mediated through ovulation or gonadotropins again considered. The drugs include: oral contraceptives, menopausal hormones, fertility drugs, and non-hormonal medications.

Next to parity, the most consistent epidemiologic finding for ovarian cancer is a protective effect of oral contraceptive (OC) use.[43] Compatible with the 'incessant ovulation' model, there is a fairly orderly dose response for greater protection with increasing years of use,[36] although some investigators have reported substantial decreases in risk with even short-term use.[43] Compatible with an effect mediated through gonadotropins, this author found evidence for a particular benefit of OC use in the late thirties when gonadotropin levels are known to be higher.[44] And, in a study of basal (menstrual phase) follicle stimulating hormone (FSH) levels, women who were not currently using OCs but had used them for more than 5 years had lower FSH compared to women who had never used OCs or used them only for a short time,[45] suggesting a residual downregulating effect of past OC use similar to that proposed for parity.

In sorting out the role of gonadotropin suppression versus cessation of ovulation, the relationship of menopausal hormones to ovarian cancer risk is important, because such agents may affect gonadotropins but not ovulation. A recent meta-analyses[46] reported that ever use of menopausal hormones was associated, if anything, with an increased risk for ovarian cancer: summary relative risk of 1.15 (1.05, 1.27). Although these data may appear contradictory to protection with gonadotropins suppression, it should be appreciated that almost all of the data reviewed related to use of unopposed estrogen regimens which may not lower gonadotropins to the same extent that opposed (estrogen plus progesterone) regimens do. The two studies with sufficient data to examine risk associated with opposed regimens have not found an elevated risk.[47,48] Based on the strong protection associated with OC use, use of continuous regimens (that combine estrogen and progesterone on a daily basis) are likely to have a protective effect.

Whether fertility drugs increase the risk for ovarian cancer has obvious relevance to the gonadotropin theory. If one finds that extracted human menopausal gonadotropins are associated with ovarian cancer, it is hard to escape the conclusion that endogenous gonadotropins may relate to ovarian cancer in the same age group of women from whom the gonadotropins are derived. However, the epidemiologic data linking past use of fertility drugs to subsequent risk of ovarian cancer is mixed. There have been several positive studies, at least two of which focused particular concern on tumors of borderline malignancy;[49–51] but an equal number of well-conducted negative studies.[52–54] Too numerous to cite here are dozens of case reports describing ovarian cancer

shortly following use of fertility drugs, which leads me to be more concerned about the effects of current use in women who may have an early ovarian neoplasm whose growth could be promoted by gonadotropins. Efforts should be made to rule out undiagnosed complex ovarian cysts before beginning fertility therapy.

Finally, in this section, I consider non-hormonal medications which might relate to ovarian cancer risk by effects on the ovarian/pituitary axis. Certain psychotropic medications, including the amphetamines, desipramine, and nortriptyline, have been reported to increase risk for ovarian cancer.[55] These are medications which are dopamine or norepinephrine re-uptake inhibitors and involve pathways which may influence gonadotropin secretion in various animal models.[56,57] Conversely, a non-hormonal medication which might reduce risk for ovarian cancer by lowering gonadotropins is acetaminophen (paracetamol). This author reported that regular use of acetaminophen on at least a weekly basis for 6 months or more was associated with a decreased risk for ovarian cancer, and the effect was more apparent for use on a daily basis.[17] Analgesic use *per se* did not appear to explain the effect, since no decreased risk was associated with aspirin or ibuprofen use. In another study, I found that women who used acetaminophen for menstrual pain had lower levels of gonadotropins and estradiol during the menstrual phase of their cycle[58] compared to women who did not use acetaminophen.

Premise 7: Despite differences in tumor histology, animal models are relevant to human ovarian cancer and also suggest the importance of pituitary/gonadal disruption

As reviewed by the author, classic animal models for ovarian cancer involved disruption of ovarian–pituitary feedback, either by prematurely destroying oocytes (using radiation or chemical toxins) or by transplanting the animal's ovary to its spleen, leading to enhanced metabolism of ovarian hormones before they could reach the hypothalamus or pituitary to exert feedback inhibition.[59] A role for gonadotopins was indicated by observations that ovarian tumors did not develop in rodents who were hypophysectomized before the experimental treatment, or who were given estrogen, which inhibited gonadotropin release.[59] More recently, it has been shown that gonadal stromal tumors invariably develop in mice with a targeted deletion of the α-inhibin gene, which produces the ovarian hormone inhibin, a downregulator of gonadotropins.[60] Again, a critical role for gonadotropins was demonstrated by cross-breeding experiments, showing the tumors did not develop in mice with the α-inhibin gene deletion who were also incapable of secreting gonadotropins due to gonadotropin releasing hormone (GnRH) deficiency.[61]

The relevance of stromal tumors in animals to the common epithelial types in women, may be based upon the difference in the degree of stromal–epithelial admixture in rodents compared to women (discussed earlier). The greater degree of stromal–epithelial admixture in women might permit epithelial tumors to be the manifestation of stromal stimulation in women, whereas stromal tumors would occur in rodents without abundant inclusion cyst formation. *In vitro* studies demonstrate that stroma may be involved in both epithelial differentiation and proliferation.[62] Thus not only are current models likely to be relevant, but the development of new models may bring fresh insights into the pathogenesis of ovarian cancer.

Premise 8: Consideration of the histologic subtype of epithelial ovarian cancer may further clarify its epidemiology

Variation in risk factors for ovarian cancer by epithelial subtype is suggested both by recent epidemiologic studies and by molecular genetic studies. We have already alluded to some of the epidemiologic differences: *BRCA1/2* associated with invasive non-mucinous tumors, talc associated with serous and undifferentiated tumors, and endometriosis associated with endometrioid and clear cell tumors. Reports are also increasing on how tumors may differ in the profile of somatic mutations. A full review of this topic is beyond the scope of this chapter. Examples include the tendency for K-*ras* mutations to be associated with mucinous tumors[63] and alterations in the DNA mismatch repair gene, *hMSH2*, to be more common in endometrioid tumors.[64]

In Table 1.3, we offer a suggested classification scheme for epidemiologic studies of ovarian cancer. Serous borderline should be distinguished from serous invasive tumors, based upon the infrequent occurrence of tumors displaying both elements.[65] However, this distinction is unnecessary for the mucinous tumors which frequently display borderline and invasive elements in the same specimen. We have suggested that the endometrioid and clear cell cancer should be distinguished based upon their possible link to endometriosis. This category would also include other cell types seen in the uterine cavity, such as the mixed Müllerian tumors and carcinosarcomas. Other and undifferentiated tumors remain as the final category. The ability to perform histology-specific epidemiologic analyses will require large and comprehensive ovarian cancer studies or collaborative studies to be conducted, which have uniform criteria for histologic classification.

Table 1.3 Suggested histologic subgroupings for epidemiologic studies of ovarian cancer

1. Serous borderline
2. Serous invasive
3. Mucinous (borderline and invasive combined)
4. Endometrioid and clear cell
5. Other and undifferentiated

Conclusion

Epidemiologic studies of ovarian cancer are valuable not only because they may identify modifiable risk factors for ovarian cancer, but also because they may help further understanding of the pathogenesis of the disease. My conclusion in reviewing such studies is that there are various genetic, environmental, and reproductive factors that mediate risk for ovarian cancer, largely through their effects on the ovarian/pituitary axis or through pelvic contamination with talc or menses, and that these risk factors may vary by the histologic type of ovarian cancer.

References

1. Claus, E.B. and Schwartz, P.E. (1995). Familial ovarian cancer. *Cancer,* 76, 1998–2003.
2. Rubin, S.C., Blackwood, A., Bandera, C. *et al.* (1998). BRCA1, BRCA2, and hereditary nonpolyposis colorectal cancer gene mutations in an unselected ovarian cancer population: relationship to family history and implications for genetic testing. *Am. J. Obstet. Gynecol.,* 178, 670–7.
3. Lu, K.H., Cramer, D.W., Muto, M.G. *et al.* (1999). A population-based study of BRCA1 and BRCA2 mutation in Jewish women with ovarian cancer. *Obstet. Gynecol.,* 93, 34–7.
4. Narod, S.A., Risch, H., Moslehi, R. *et al.* (1998). Oral contraceptives and the risk of hereditary ovarian cancer. *N. Engl. J. Med.,* 339, 424–8.
5. Ursin, G., Henderson, B.E., Haile, R.W. *et al.* (1997). Does oral contraceptive use increase the risk of breast cancer in women with BRCA1/BRCA2 mutations more than in other women? *Cancer Res.,* 57, 3678–81.
6. Cramer, D.W., Liberman, R.F., Titus-Ernstoff L. *et al.* (1999). Genital Talc Exposure And Risk For Ovarian Cancer. *Int. J. Cancer,* 81, 351–6.
7. Venter, P.F. and Iturralde, M. (1979). Migration of particulate radioactive tracer from the vagina to the peritoneal cavity and ovaries. *S. Afr. Med. J.,* 55, 917–19.
8. Rohl, A.N., Langer, A.M., Selikoff, I.J. *et al.* (1976). Consumer talcums and powders: mineral and chemical characterization. *J. Toxicol. Environ. Health.,* 2, 255–84.
9. Keal, E.E. (1960). Asbestosis and abdominal neoplasms. *Lancet,* 2, 1211–16.
10. Muscat, J.E. and Wynder, E.L. (1997). Perineal powder exposure and the risk of ovarian cancer (letter). *Am. J. Epidemiol.,* 146, 786.
11. Cook, L.S., Kamb, M.L., and Weiss, N.S. (1997). Perineal powder exposure and the risk of ovarian cancer. *Am. J. Epidemiol.,* 145, 459–65.
12. Chang, S. and Risch, H. (1997). Perineal talc exposure and risk of ovarian carcinoma. *Cancer,* 79, 2396–401.
13. Mostoufizadeh, M. and Scully, R.E. (1980). Malignant tumors arising in endometriosis. *Clin. Obstet. Gynecol.,* 23, 951–63.
14. Brinton, L.A., Gridley, G., Persson, I. *et al.* (1997). Cancer risk following a hospital discharge diagnosis of endometriosis. *Am. J. Obstet. Gynecol.,* 176, 572–9.
15. Sampson, J.A. (1940). The development of the implantation theory for the origin of endometriosis. *Am. J. Obstet. Gynecol.,* 40, 540–57.
16. Cramer, D.W., Wilson, E., Stillman, R.J. *et al.* (1986). The relation of endometriosis to menstrual characteristics, smoking, and exercise. *JAMA,* 255, 1904–8.
17. Cramer, D.W., Harlow, B.L., Titus-Ernstoff, L. *et al.* (1998). Over-the-counter analgesics and risk for ovarian cancer. *Lancet,* 351, 104–7.
18. Green, A., Purdie, D., Bain, C. *et al.* (1997). Tubal sterilization, hysterectomy and decreased risk of ovarian cancer. *Int. J. Cancer,* 71, 948–51.
19. Meigs, J.V. (1953). Endometriosis, Etiologic role of marriage, age and parity: conservative treatment. *Obstet. Gynecol.,* 2, 46.

20. Herr, J.C., Heidger, P.M., Scott, J.R. *et al.* (1978). Decidual cells in the human ovary at term I. Incidence, gross anatomy and ultrastructural features of merocrine secretion. *Am. J. Anat.*, **52**, 7–28.

21. Parkin, S.L. Whelan, J. Ferlay R., and Young, J. (1997). *Cancer incidence in five continents*, vol. VII. IARC Scientific Publications, No. 143.

22. Cramer, D.W. (1989). Lactase persistence and milk consumption as determinants of ovarian cancer risk. *Am. J. Epidemiol.*, **130**, 904–10.

23. Chen, Y.T., Mattison, D.R., Feigenbaum, L. *et al.* (1981). Reduction in oocyte number following prenatal exposure to a diet high in galactose. *Science*, **214**, 1145–7.

24. Cramer, D.W., Harlow, B.L., Willett, W.C. *et al.* (1989). Galactose consumption and metabolism in relation to the risk of ovarian cancer. *Lancet*, **2**, 66–71.

25. Kushi, L.H., Mink, P.J., Folsom, A.R. *et al.* (1999). Prospective study of diet and ovarian cancer. *Am. J. Epidemiol.*, **149**, 21–31.

26. Risch, H.A., Jain, M., Marrett, L.D., and Howe, G.R. (1994). Dietary lactose intake, lactose intolerance, and the risk of epithelial ovarian cancer in southern Ontario (Canada*). Cancer Causes and Control*, **5**, 540–8.

27. Engle, A., Muscat, J.E., and Harris, R.E. (1991). Nutritional risk factors and ovarian cancer. *Nutr. Cancer*, **15**, 239–47.

28. La Vecchia, C., Decarli, A., Negri, E. *et al.* (1987). Dietary factors and the risk of epithelial ovarian cancer. *J. Natl Cancer. Inst.*, **79**, 663–9.

29. Risch, H.A., Jain, M., Marrett, L.D., and Howe, G.R. (1994). Dictary fat intake and risk of epithelial ovarian cancer. *J. Natl. Cancer. Inst.*, **86**, 1409–15.

30. Shu, X.O., Gao, Y.T., Yuan, J.M. *et al.* (1989). Dietary factors and epithelial ovarian cancer. *Br. J. Cancer*, **59**, 92–6.

31. Byers, T., Marshall, J., Graham, S. *et al.* (1983). A case-control study of dietary and nondietary factors in ovarian cancer. *J. Natl Cancer Inst.*, **71**, 681–6.

32. Slattery, M.L., Schuman, K.L., West, D.W. *et al.* (1989). Nutrient intake and ovarian cancer. *Am. J. Epidemiol.*, **130**, 497–502.

33. Marshall, J., Freudenheim, J., Graham, S., and Brasure, J. (1993). Diet in the epidemiology of ovarian cancer in western New York. *FASEB J.*, **73**, A65.

34. Walker, B.E. and Kurth, L.A. (1995). Increased reproductive tract tumors in the female offspring of mice fed a high fat diet during the fetal stage of pregnancy. *Cancer Lett.*, **97**, 57–60.

35. Murphy, E.D. and Russell, E.S. (1963). Ovarian tumorigenesis following genic deletion of germ cells in hybrid mice. *Acta Un. Int. Cancer*, **19**, 779–82.

36. Whittemore, A.S., Harris, R., and Itnyre, J. (1992). Characteristics relating to ovarian cancer risk: collaborative analysis of 12 US case-control studies. *Am. J. Epidemiol.*, **136**, 1184–203.

37. Fathalla, M.F. (1971). Incessant ovulation – a factor in ovarian neoplasia. *Lancet*, **2**, 163.

38. Schildkraut, J.M., Bastos, E., and Berchuk, A. (1997). Relationship between lifetime ovulatory cycles and overexpression of mutant p53 in epithelial ovarian cancer. *J. Natl Cancer Inst.*, **89**, 932–8.

39. Goluboff, L.G. and Ezrin, C. (1969). Effect of pregnancy on the somatotroph and the prolactin cell of the human adenohypophysis. *J. Clin. Endocrinol. Metab.*, **29**, 1533–8.

40. Sheehan, H.L. (1939). Simmond's disease due to postpartum necrosis of the anterior pituitary. *Q. J. Med.*, **8**, 277.

41. Jackson, I.M.D., Whyte, W.G., and Garrey, M.M. (1969). Pituitary function following uncomplicated pregnancy in Sheehans's syndrome. *J. Clin. Endocrinol. Metab.*, **29**, 315–18.

42. Velasco, E., Malacarra, J.M., Cervantes, F. *et al.* (1990). Gonadotropin and prolactin serum levels during the perimenopausal period: correlation with diverse factors. *Fertil. Steril.*, **53**, 56–9.

43. Hankinson, S.E., Colditz, G.A., Hunter, D.J., and Rosner, B. (1992). A quantitative assessment of oral contraceptive use and risk of ovarian cancer. *Obstet. Gynecol.*, **80**, 708–41.

44. Harlow, B.L., Cramer, D.W., Geller, J.E. *et al.* (1991). The influence of lactose consumption on the association of oral contraceptive use and ovarian cancer risk. *Am. J. Epidemiol.*, **134**, 445–53.

45. Cramer, D.W., Barbieri, R.L., Xu, H., and Reichardt, J.K.V. (1994). Determinants of basal follicle stimulating hormone levels in premenopausal women. *J. Clin. Endocrinol. Metab.*, **79**, 1105–9.

46. Garg, P.P., Kerlikowske, K., Subak, L., and Grady, D. (1998). Hormone replacement therapy and the risk of ovarian carcinoma: a meta-analysis. *Obstet. Gynecol.*, **92**, 472–9.

47. Kaufman, D.W., Kelly, J.P., Welch, W.R. *et al.* (1989). Noncontraceptive estrogen use and epithelial ovarian cancer. *Am. J. Epidemiol.*, **130**, 1142–51.

48. Risch, H.A. (1996). Estrogen replacement therapy and risk of epithelial ovarian cancer. *Gynecol. Oncol.*, **63**, 254–7.

49. Rossing, M.A., Daling, J.R., Weiss, N.S. *et al.* (1994). Ovarian tumors in a cohort of infertile women. *N. Engl. J. Med.*, **331**, 771–6.

50. Shushan, A., Paltiel, O., Elchalal, U. *et al.* (1996). Human menopausal gonadotropin and the risks of epithelial ovarian cancer. *Fertil. Steril.*, **65**, 13–18.

51. Parazzini, F., Negri, E., La Vecchia, C. *et al.* (1998). Treatment for fertility an risk of ovarian tumors of borderline malignancy. *Gynecol. Oncol.*, **68**, 226–8.

52. Mosgaard, B.J., Lidegaard, O., Kjaer, S.K. *et al.* (1997). Infertility, fertility drugs, and invasive ovarian cancer: a case-control study. *Fertil. Steril.*, **67**, 1005–12.

53. Modan, B., Ron, E., Lerner-Geva, L. *et al.* (1998). Cancer incidence in a cohort of infertile women. *Am. J. Epidemiol.*, **147**, 1038–42.

54. Parazzini, F., Negri, E., LaVecchia, C. *et al.* (1997). Treatment for infertility and risks of invasive epithelial ovarian cancer. *Hum. Reprod.*, **123**, 2159–61.

55. Harlow, B.L., Cramer, D.W., Baron, J.A. *et al.* (1998). Psychotropic medication use and risks of epithelial ovarian cancer. *Cancer Epid. Biomarker. Prev.*, **7**, 697–702.

56. Donnelly, P.J. and Dailey, R.A. (1991). Effects of dopamine, norepinephrine and serotonin on secretion of luteinizing hormone, follicle-stimulating hormone, and prolactin in ovariectomized, pituitary stalk-transected ewew. *Domest. Anim. Endocrinol.*, **8**, 87–98.

57. Chang, J.P., Van Goor, F., and Acharya S. (1991). Influences of norepinephrine, adrenergic agonists and antagonists on gonadotropin secretion from dispersed pituitary cells of goldfish, *Carassius auratus. Neuroendocrinology*, **54**, 202–10.

58. Cramer, D.W., Liberman, R.F., Hornstein, M.D. *et al.* (1998). Basal hormone levels in women who use acetaminophen for menstrual pain. *Fertil. Steril.*, **70**, 731–3.

59. Cramer, D.W. and Welch, W.R. (1983). Determinants of ovarian cancer risk. II. Inferences regarding pathogenesis. *JNCI*, **71**, 717–21.

60. Matzuk, M.M., Finegold, M.J., Jyan-Gwo, J.S. *et al.* (1992). α-Inhibin is a tumor-suppressor gene with gonadal specificity in mice. *Nature*, **360**, 313–19.

61. Kumar, T.R., Wang, Y., and Matzuk, M.M. (1996). Gonadotropins are essential modifier factors for the gonadal tumor development in inhibin deficient mice. *Endocrinology*, **137**, 4210–16.

62. Cunha, G.R., Bigsby, R.M., Cooke, P.S., and Suginura, Y. (1985). Stromal–epithelial interactions in adult organs. *Cell Differ.*, **17**, 137–48.

63. Pieretti, M., Cavalieri, C., Conway, P.S. *et al.* (1995). Genetic alterations distinguish different types of ovarian tumors. *Int. J. Cancer*, **64**, 434–40.

64. Fujita, M., Enomoto, T., Yoshino, K. *et al.* (1995). Microsatellite instability and alterations in the *hMSH2* gene in human ovarian cancer. *Int. J. Cancer*, **64**, 361–6.

65. Young, R.H., Clement, P.B., and Scully, R.E. (1994). The ovary. In *Diagnostic surgical pathology,* (2nd edn), (ed. S.S. Sternberg), pp. 2213. Raven Press, New York.

2. Associations between infertility, its treatment and ovarian cancer risk

Ingemar Persson

Reasons for concern

The results, reported in 1992 by Whittemore,[1] from a pooled analysis of case-control studies from the USA on risk factors for ovarian cancer, caused substantial concern. The use of hormonal drugs to treat infertility problems in women was associated with a greatly increased risk of epithelial ovarian cancer, particularly in women who never became pregnant. Also because these 'fertility drugs' induce ovulations, increase gonadatropin levels (some regimens), and raise hormone levels in the ovary—changes believed to be key mechanisms in ovarian carcinogenesis—an adverse effect has been suspected. The use of fertility drugs has increased dramatically since the 1960s, and since the mid–1980s involved increasingly more potent stimulatory treatment regimens, as in *in vitro* fertilization (IVF) programs.[2] With this background of escalating use and trend towards more potent stimulatory regimens, and due to the fact that ovarian cancer is a highly lethal disease, any risk increase caused by hormonal infertility treatment would have an important public-health impact in women.

The purpose of this chapter is to review and evaluate the evidence of a possible link between fertility drugs and ovarian cancer risk. The available data reflect the effects in women treated up to the mid–1980s, i. e. not the effects of the recently introduced IVF programs.

Numerous reviews of the data on fertility drugs and ovarian cancer risk have been published elsewhere.[2–5]

Use of fertility drugs

The fertility drugs first introduced were follicle stimulatory agents (follicle stimulating hormone; FSH), marketed in the late 1950s. Clomiphene citrate (CC), for induction of ovulation through gonadotropin release, came into use during the 1960s. The fertility drugs addressed in this chapter include only CC, human menopausal gonadotropins (hMG)—containing both follicle stimulating hormones and luteinizing hormone (LH), and human chorionic gonadotropin (hCG). The indications for, and effects of, these treatment regimens are summarized in Table 2.1.

Clomiphene activates the intact hypothalamic–pituitary–ovarian system and induces ovulation, leading to an increase of the number of ovulations and an enhanced estradiol (E2) production. CC treatment is used mainly as a first-line treatment of unovulation, as part of a mild form of ovulatory infertility. Gonadotropin administrations (hMG and hCG) are given to treat a more pronounced unovulatory disturbance and in cases when the endocrine system fails to respond to estrogen (CC) treatment. The hMG/hCG treatment may, depending on dose, result in the stimulation of a large number of follicles ('super ovulations') and substantially elevated levels of ovarian hormones. In modern IVF programs, the treatment goal is to induce the maturation of a large number of follicles.

When assessing the affects of such fertility drug regimens on the ovarian epithelium, it seems important to take treatment

Table 2.1 Types, indications, and biological effects of infertility drug regimens

Type/name	Indications	Effects
Clomiphene citrate (CC)	Unovulation (WHO I) Artificial insemination Unexplained infertility IVF	↑ number of ovulations ↑ E2 levels
Human menopausal and chorionic gonadotropins (hMG, hCG)	Unovulatory infertility (WHO II) No effect of CC Oligo-ovulation Luteal phase deficiency IVF	↑ number of follicles 'Super ovulations' ↑↑ E2 levels

modality, dose, and duration of the treatment into account, because of possible differences in the magnitude of effects.

Risk factors and ovarian carcinogenesis

The knowledge on causes of ovarian cancer is far from complete. However, nulliparity, infertility, and family history are established risk factors of invasive epithelial cancer, whereas intake of combined oral contraceptives (COCs) and, tentatively, tubal ligation and hysterectomy are protective factors. For borderline ovarian tumors the roles of COCs and infertility are uncertain.[6–8] The relationships between age at menarche and menopause, age at first and last birth, and with hormone replacement therapy are uncertain as the research findings have been inconsistent.[2]

The findings from epidemiology, most importantly the effects of pregnancy and COCs, have led to the formulation of theories on the possible mechanisms for ovarian carcinogenesis. First, the incessant ovulation theory, introduced by Fathalla in 1972,[9] implies that the rupture of the follicle and scarring the ovarian epithelium, the subsequent repair process involving enhancement of cell proliferation, and entrapment of epithelial cells within the hormone-rich ovarian stroma, may lead to an increased probability for a malignant transformation. Secondly, the gonadotropin theory suggests that the ovarian epithelium is sensitive to, and stimulated by, high levels of gonadotropins, as for instance after menopause.[10] Finally, it has been hypothesized that high levels and continuous exposure to pregnancy and contraceptive hormones may affect the ovarian epithelium directly, e.g. progesterone/progestins by eliminating preformed malignant or premalignant epithelial cells through apoptosis.[11,12] Even though these theories lack empirical support in humans, they are relevant for the hypothesis for an adverse effect of fertility drugs on ovarian cancer risk, the basic idea being that these treatments augment ovarian epithelial cell proliferation and/or promote neoplastic growth.

The importance of infertility for ovarian cancer risk

Nulliparity has been linked consistently to an increased risk of ovarian cancer.[13] Whether this effect is explained by the absence of protection from a completed pregnancy, or partially or entirely by an underlying infertility state, is difficult to discern from data in epidemiological studies. One reason for this difficulty is the crude and unspecific ways of defining and measuring infertility (i.e. to distinguish voluntary from involuntary, and primary from secondary, types of infertility). Overall, studies have found that women reporting 'difficulties to conceive', 'unplanned childlessness', or 'many contraceptive-free years' were at a modestly increased risk of ovarian cancer, with relative risk (RR) estimates ranging from 1.5 to 2.[14,15] Specifically in *nulliparous* women, an attempted time to conceive exceeding 1 year was associated with about a twofold increased risk, as compared with a shorter time, RR 1.5–2.7.[1,16,17] Further, the underlying cause of infertility would likely be of importance. Thus, a few studies indicate that ovalutory dysfunction *per se* is linked to an increased risk with reported relative risk estimates of 2.1–3.7.[1,18]

In studies of the association between fertility drugs and ovarian cancer risk, infertility (depending on its type) may confound any association and is a major validity issue. One obvious difficulty has been to define the type of, and quantify the severity of, infertility. In the studies discussed below, only surrogate variables or no measures of infertility were available. A further fundamental problem is to disentangle the effects of the exposure from that of the treatment indication itself, i. e. an ovulatory type of infertility. In observational studies it may be impossible to address this problem of confounding by indication, since most evaluated infertile women with an ovulatory disturbance would receive hormonal fertility drugs.

Fertility drugs and ovarian cancer risk

Case reports

The first report of an ovarian cancer following CC and hMG treatments appeared in 1982.[19] Since then, altogether 16 reports have appeared on single patients who, at young ages, developed borderline epithelial or stroma cell tumors in most instances, or malignant epithelial cancers in a few instances.[2] Exposures listed in these reports included all types of hormonal infertility treatments, mostly CC and hMG. Even if some observations in these reports were remarkable, their weight of evidence for a causal adverse effect of fertility drugs is negligible. Detection bias might be one problem; the absence of a control group precludes an interpretation. Nevertheless, these case reports have helped to generate the hypotheses and have heightened the attention and interest concerning the long-term safety of hormonal fertility treatment.

Analytical studies

Included in this report are the results from four *cohort* studies (Table 2.2)[3,18,20,21] and four *case-control* studies (Table 2.3).[1,22–24]

Cohort studies
Ron et al.[20] reported from a cohort of about 2500 Israeli women, with a median age of about 29 years, who had been evaluated for primary and secondary infertility (about half of them exposed to CC or hMG). After about 12 years of follow-up, four ovarian cancer cases had occurred, without evidence of an excess risk for users of fertility drugs. Infertile women in the cohort had about a twofold (non-significant) risk increase as compared with women in the general population. Since the cohort women were still young at the time of follow-up, a limitation of the study was the very small number of cases of ovarian cancer.

Brinton et al.[21] studied some 2300 women seeking attention because of difficulties in conceiving. Hormonal treatment with

Table 2.2 Cohort studies of fertility drug treatments (FD) and ovarian cancer risk.

Study	Cohort	Exposure[a]	Results
Ron et al. (1987), Israel	2575; 28.7 yr	CC, hMG	12.3 yr: 4 cases Infertility, SIR = 2.1 (NS)[b] FD: cf. infertile women, no excess risk
Brinton et al. (1989), USA	2335; 28.6 yr	E or P	19.4 yr: 11 cases Infertility, SIR = 1.3 (NS) FD: cf. infertile women, SIR = 1.8 (NS)
Rossing et al. (1994), USA	3837; 29.7 yr	CC, hCG, hMG	12.3 yr: 11 cases (4 epit., 2 non-epit., 5 borderline)[c] Infertility (ovulatory), SIR = 3.7 (1.4–8.1) CC: cf. infertile women: 1–11 months, RR = 0.8; 12 months, RR = 11.1 (1.5–82)
Venn et al. (1995), Australia	10 358; 32 yr	IVF	5.2 yr: 6 cases (invasive epit.) IVF, cf. pop.: SIR = 1.7 (NS); no IVF: SIR = 1.8 (NS) IVF cf. infertile women: RR = 1.5 (NS)

Risk estimates given as standardized incidence ratio (SIR), when comparing to an external population, and as relative risk (RR), when comparing within the cohorts, together with 95% confidence intervals (95% CI).
[a]CC: clomiphene citrate; hMG: human menopausal gonadotropin; hCG: human chorionic gonadotropin; E: 'estrogens'; P: 'progestins'; IVF: *in vitro* fertilization.
[b]NS: non-significant
[c]Epit.: epithelial type of tumour

Table 2.3 Case-control studies of fertility drug treatments (FD) and ovarian cancer risk

Study	Cases/controls	Exposure	Results
Whittemore et al. (1992), USA	622/1101; pooled analyses, from 3/12 studies, including data on FD use	'Fertility drug use', unspecified	Infertility, RR = 1.0 FD use: 　no infertility, RR = 2.8 (1.3–6.1) 　infertility, RR = 2.9 (1.4–6.4) Never pregnant: 　infertility, RR = 2.1 (1.0–4.2) 　FD use: 　　no infertility, RR = 27.0 (2.3–315) 　　infertility, RR = 12.0 (2.0–71)
Franceschi et al. (1994), Italy	195/1339 epithelial	'Fertility drug use', unspecified	Infertility, RR = 0.8 FD use: 　no infertility, RR = 0.9 　infertility, RR = 1.3 (NS)
Shushan et al. (1996), Israel	164+36/408; epithel./ borderline	CC, hMG	Infertility, RR = 1.6 (1.0–2.6) FD use: 　no infertility, RR = 1.8 (1.0 3.3) 　　CC: RR = 1.0 　　hMG: RR = 3.2 (0.9–10.8) 　　mixed: RR = 1.6 (0.6–4.1)
Mosgaard et al. (1997), Denmark	684/1721; 87% epithel.	'Tablets, injections'; extrapolated type of fertility drug	Infertility, RR = 1.5 (1.2–2.0) FD use (CC, hMG): 　no infertility, RR = 1.2 (0.7–1.8) 　infertility, RR = 0.8 Never pregnant: 　infertility, RR = 2.9 (1.6–5.4) 　FD use: 　　no infertility, RR = 2.5 (NS) 　　infertility, RR = 0.8

Relative risk estimates (RR) and 95% confidence intervals (95% CI).

estrogens or progestins, given as the sole treatment, was not associated with an altered risk of ovarian cancer at 20 years of follow-up, based on 11 cases of ovarian cancer. Overall, women with ovulatory infertility had a non-significant 80% excess relative risk. Weaknesses of the study included the lack of detail on the treatment types and a 30% loss of the cohort women at follow-up.

Rossing et al.[18] reported on a cohort of over 3800 women accrued from several infertility clinics in the US. Over two-thirds of the cohort women had received CC treatment and some 4% hMG. After 12 years of follow-up, 11 ovarian tumors had been ascertained (four epithelial invasive, two non-epithelial, and five borderline). Use of hMG/FSH or CC was associated with about a threefold increased risk of ovarian tumors (non-significant risk estimates). Use of CC for less than 1 year conferred no risk increase, whereas such exposure exceeding 1 year was associated with an 11-fold increase (RR = 11.1; 95% CI 1.5–82). Interestingly, the risk for the cohort women compared with the population was only slightly increased (RR = 1.5) for invasive, and threefold (RR = 3.3; 1.1–7.8) for borderline tumors. Those with unovulatory ovarian dysfunction had an almost fourfold increase in the risk of tumors (RR = 3.7; 95% CI 1.4–8.1). One important feature of this study was the detailed information on exposure type and infertility background. The mixture of tumor types and small numbers of cases were, however, limitations of this study.

In the most recently published cohort study, by Venn et al.[3], the effects of different IVF modalities were evaluated in a cohort of over 10 000 Australian women—over half of them exposed to IVF—who were followed for about 5 years. Altogether, six cases of ovarian cancer were detected. In relation to the background population, the risk of IVF exposure was slightly (non-significantly) increased, as was the risk for the non-exposed cohort women. The risk among the infertile women in the cohort was not increased when comparing those with and without IVF exposure. Limitations of this study were the short follow-up, small number of cases, and the lack of detail regarding exposure.

Case-control studies

Whittemore et al.[1] analyzed the pooled data from 12 retrospective studies that included ovarian cancer cases diagnosed during the late 1950s through the mid–1980s. Three of these studies, with over 600 cases (aged 18–80 years) of invasive ovarian cancer, and about 1100 control subjects, yielded information on the effects of 'fertility drugs'(reported by 12% of the controls). Exposure, defined as ever-use of any kind of hormonal treatment in connection with infertility problems, was associated with about a threefold elevation in the risk for women either reporting or not reporting a problem of 'infertility'. However, when restricting the analysis to women who had never been pregnant, such fertility drug use was associated with a grossly increased risk, RR = 27 (95% CI 2.3–315), an estimate based on only 12 exposed cases and one control subject.

A separate analysis of about 90 cases of borderline tumors and 750 controls revealed a three- to fourfold higher risk for fertility drug use in women both with and without a history of infertility.[6] As mentioned, the suggestion of a very high excess risk in exposed never-pregnant women elicited concern in the early 1990s. The unspecific measurement of exposure and of type of infertility, the possibility for residual confounding due to other risk factors, and imprecision due to small numbers were serious limitations of this pooled study, rendering a cautious interpretation necessary.

The study by Franceschi et al.[22] included about 200 cases of epithelial ovarian cancer and over 1000 hospital-based controls in Italy, for an evaluation of the effects of 'fertility drug use', reported by only 2.5% of the controls. Such exposure was found unrelated to ovarian cancer risk, regardless of whether there was a history of infertility or not. A limitation of this study was the small numbers of exposed subjects.

In the Israeli study by Shushan et al.[23] some 160 cases of invasive epithelial and 40 borderline tumors were compared with over 400 control subjects, regarding exposure to CC and hMG treatments. Regardless of infertility background, neither ever-use of fertility drugs (RR = 1.8), nor of CC (RR = 1.0) or hMG (RR = 3.3; 95% CI 0.9–10.8) were associated with ovarian cancer risk. The estimate for hMG was based on only 11 exposed cases. Limitations of this study, apart from low statistical power, included the lack of data on cause of infertility, losses due to deaths, and likely bias in the control selection.

The largest and most recent case-control study by Mosgaard et al.[24] was performed in Denmark by making use of the National Cancer and Patient Registers. Some 680 ovarian cancer cases (of which about 90% were epithelial) and over 1700 population-based controls were included. Data on treatment indications (infertility defined as unsuccessful pregnancy attempt for 1 year or longer) and exposure type (extrapolated from the reported type of use, tablets or injections) were ascertained from questionnaires, responded by 81% of the survivors (63% of all cases) and 78% of the controls. Use of any type of fertility drugs (reported by 16% of the controls) was unrelated to ovarian cancer risk, with near base-line estimates in women with or without a history of infertility. Infertility, as defined above, was associated with a threefold increased risk in women who had never had a pregnancy before. This study has several strengths, but also weaknesses, e.g. a substantial loss of cases due to deaths (which might lead to selection bias), undefined causes of infertility, and an extrapolated classification of exposure type.

Interpretation of the epidemiological data

One key issue when interpreting the link between hormonal infertility treatment and ovarian cancer risk is the role of infertility itself. It would seem plausible that infertility, when caused by ovarian dysfunction, could also be associated with an excess risk of ovarian cancer. If so, there is the possibility that a relationship between treatment and cancer risk could be confounded by the treatment indication. Unfortunately, available epidemiological data are both inadequate with regard to infertility classification and numbers of subjects examined; further, these studies have produced inconsistent results. Therefore, the extent to which infertility has confounded the reported associations remains an unresolved problem.

The results of the eight epidemiologic studies are contradictory and rely on studies with varying methodological qualities. The very high risk estimates reported in the original pooled analysis[1] have not been replicated in subsequent studies. One study found a dose-dependent risk increase with clomiphene use,[18] whereas another large study failed to find any risk relationships with types of exposure, regardless of infertility or pregnancy status.[4]

The interpretation of the present data obviously needs to be cautious. The limitations of the reported studies are crucial. Importantly, the contradictory results could be explained by failures to define specific entities of ovarian tumors (epithelial invasive versus borderline or stroma cell tumors), to specify and quantify fertility drug exposure (type, dose, duration, recency, and latency of exposure), to consider the type of infertility (ovulatory or other), to achieve sufficient follow-up time, to accrue sufficiently large sample sizes, and to measure and adjust for relevant confounding factors (such as treatment indication and other risk factors). Further, results from these studies may not be relevant for exposure typical of new and modern hormonal infertility treatment modalities, like IVF.

Conclusions

Circumstantial evidence—based on the interpretation of ovarian cancer risk factors and those suggested carcinogenetic mechanisms that are compatible with epidemiological findings, along with numerous case reports—give reason to suspect a link between stimulatory fertility drugs and an adverse effect on ovarian cancer risk. However, empirical data from analytical epidemiological studies are contradictory and likely distorted by methodological deficiencies. Therefore, no firm conclusions can be drawn from the available data. However, the concern regarding the possible adverse effects of fertility drugs cannot be dismissed. The results of new and on-going research, using improved study designs, will be important.

References

1. Whittemore, A.S., Harris, R., and Itnyre, J. (1992). Characteristics relating to ovarian cancer risk: collaborative analysis of 12 US case-control studies. II. Invasive epithelial ovarian cancers in white women. *Am. J. Epidemiol.*, 136, 1184–203.
2. Glud, E., Krüger-Kjaer, S., Troisi, R. *et al.* (1998). Fertility drugs and ovarian cancer. *Epidemiol. Rev.*, 20 (2), 237–57.
3. Venn, A., Watson, L., Lumley, J. *et al.* (1995). Breast and ovarian cancer incidence after infertility and *in vitro* fertilisation. *Lancet*, 346, 995–1000.
4. Mosgaard, B.J., Lidegaard, O., and Andersen, A.N. (1997). The impact of parity, infertility and treatment with fertility drugs on the risk of ovarian cancer. *Acta Obstet. Gynecol. Scand.*, 76, 86–95.
5. Nugent D, Salha O, Bahlen A.H. *et al.* (1998). Ovarian neoplasia and subfertility treatments. *Br. J. Obstet. Gynaecol.*, 105, 584–91.
6. Harris, R., Whittemore, A.S., Itnyre, J. *et al.* (1992). Characteristics relating to ovarian cancer risk: collaborative analysis of 12 US case-control studies. III. Epithelial tumors of low malignant potential in white women. *Am. J. Epidemiol.*, 136, 1204–11.
7. Parazzini, F., Restelli, C., La Vecchia, C. *et al.* (1991). Risk factors for epithelial ovarian tumours of borderline malignancy. *Int. J. Epidemiol.*, 19–20, 287–307.
8. Harlow, B.L., Weiss, N.S., Roth, G.J. *et al.* (1988). Case-control study of borderline ovarian tumors: reproductive history and exposure to exogenous femal hormones. *Cancer Res.*, 48, 5849–52.
9. Fathalla, M.F. (1971). Incessant ovulation – a factor in ovarian neoplasia? *Lancet*, 2, 163.
10. Stadell, B.V. (1975). Letter: The etiology and prevention of ovarian cancer. *Am. J. Obstet. Gynecol.*, 123 (7), 772–4.
11. Adami, H.O., Hsieh, C.C., Lambe, M. *et al.* (1994). Parity, age and first childbirth, and risk of ovarian cancer. *Lancet*, 344, 1250–4.
12. Rodriguez, G.C., Walmer, D.K., Cline, M. *et al.* (1998). Effect of progestin on the ovarian epithelium of Macaques: cancer prevention through apoptosis? *J. Soc. Gynecol. Invest.*, 5, 271–6.
13. Negri, E., Franceschi, S., Tzonou, A. *et al.* (1991). Pooled analysis of 3 European case-control studies. I. Reproductive factors and risk of epithelial ovarian cancer. *Int. J. Cancer*, 49, 50–60.
14. Whittemore, A.S., Wu, M.L., Paffenbarger, P.S. Jr *et al.* (1989). Epithelial ovarian cancer and ability to conceive. *Cancer Res.*, 49, 4047–52.
15. Nasca, P.C., Greenwald, P., Chorost, S. *et al.* (1984). An epidemiologic case-control study of ovarian cancer and reproductive experience to cancer of the ovary. *Am. J. Epidemiol.*, 119, 705–13.
16. Risch, H.A., Hsieh, C.C., Howe, G.R. (1994). Parity, age at first childbirth and risk of ovarian cancer. *Lancet*, 344, 1250–4.
17. Mosgaard, B., Lidegaard, ø., Kjaer, S.K. *et al.* (1992). Infertility, fertility drugs and invasive ovarian cancer and reproductive factors. *Am. J. Epidemiol.*, 21, 23–9.
18. Rossing, M.A., Daling, J.R., Weiss, N.S. *et al.* (1994). Ovarian tumours in a cohort of infertile women. *N. Engl. J. Med.*, 331, 771–6.
19. Bamford, P.N. and Steele, S.J. (1982). Uterine and ovarian carcinoma in a patient receiving gonadotropin therapy: case report. *Br. J. Obstet. Gynaecol.*, 89, 962–4.
20. Ron, E., Lunenefeld, B., Menczer, J. *et al.* (1987). Cancer incidence in a cohort of infertile women. *Am. J. Epidemiol.*, 125, 780–90.
21. Brinton, L.A., Melton, L.J. III, Malkasian, G.D. Jr *et al.* (1989). Cancer risk after evaluation for infertility. *Am. J. Epidemiol.*, 129, 712–22.
22. Franceschi, S., La Vecchia, C., Negri, E. *et al.* (1994). Fertility drugs and risk of epithelial ovarian cancer in Italy. *Hum. Reprod.*, 9, 1673–5.
23. Shushan, A., Paltiel, O., Iscovich, J. *et al.* (1988). Human menopausal gonadotropin and the risk of epithelial ovarian cancer. *Fertil. Steril.*, 49, 551–3.
24. Mosgaard, B., Lidegaard, ø., Kjaer, S.K. *et al.* (1997). Infertility, fertility drugs and invasive ovarian cancer: a case-control study. *Fertil. Steril.*, 67, 1005–12.

3. The molecular basis of sporadic ovarian cancer

Angeles Alvarez and Andrew Berchuck

Introduction

Malignant transformation of a normal ovarian epithelial cell is caused by genetic alterations that disrupt regulation of proliferation, programmed cell death, and senescence (Table 3.1). About 10% of epithelial ovarian cancers arise in women who have inherited mutations in cancer susceptibility genes such as *BRCA1* or *BRCA2*. The genetics of hereditary ovarian cancers are discussed in Chapters 4–8. The vast majority of ovarian cancers arise due to the accumulation of genetic damage over the course of a lifetime, and are referred to as sporadic cancers. Over the past 15 years, several of the alterations involved in the development of sporadic ovarian cancers have been identified, but much remains unknown regarding their molecular pathogenesis. It is anticipated that all of the genes in the human genome will be identified in the near future, which will provide the framework for studies aimed at completing our understanding of this complex disease. This should facilitate the development of new approaches to early diagnosis, treatment, and prevention that will decrease ovarian cancer mortality.

Most ovarian cancers are characterized by a high degree of genetic damage that is manifest at both the chromosomal and molecular levels. Gains and losses of large portions of chromosomes, as well as complex translocations, were described initially, using classic karyotype analysis. In one study of 23 ovarian cancers, the average number of chromosomal alterations was seven (range 2–14).[1] More recently, studies using a technique called comparative genomic hybridization (CGH) have confirmed that most ovarian cancers have gains or losses of large segments of chromosomes. In one study of 44 ovarian cancers, there were 13 areas of chromosomal gain and five areas of chromosomal loss that were seen in at least 20% of cases.[2] The most common areas

of chromosomal loss were 16q and 17pter–q21, whereas the most frequent areas of chromosomal gain were 3q25–26 and 8q24. In another study which included 20 sporadic ovarian cancers, the average number of alterations in each cancer was 7.5, and gains were more than twice as common as losses.[3] In agreement with the studies noted above,[2] losses on 17p and gains on 8q23–24 and 3q26 were confirmed in two other studies to be among the most frequent events in ovarian cancers.[3,4]

It has been suggested that differences exist in the pattern of genetic alterations in serous, mucinous, and endometrioid ovarian cancers.[5] In one CGH study, gains at 1q were observed frequently in endometrioid and serous tumours. Increased copy number at 10q was seen in endometrioid tumours only, whereas gains at 11q occurred mostly in serous tumours. In mucinous tumours, the most common copy number change was a gain at 17q. The findings of this small study, which included only 24 well or moderately differentiated cancers, can not be considered definitive, but they add weight to the theory that there are differences in the molecular pathogenesis of various histologic types of ovarian cancers.

Although chromosomal gains are detected more often than losses using CGH, deletion of one allele of many genetic loci has been noted using loss of heterozygosity (LOH) analysis (Fig. 3.1). LOH has been demonstrated to occur at a high frequency on many chromosomal arms; including 5q,[6,7] 6q,[8–11] 7p,[6,12] 11p,[13] 11q,[14–17] 13q,[6,18] 14q,[19] 17p,[20] 17q,[21] 22q,[22] and others.[6,18,23] It is unclear whether the extent of these genetic alterations reflects the need to inactivate multiple tumor suppressor genes, or is the result of generalized genomic instability. Currently, with the identification and characterization of thousands of genes through the efforts of the human genome project, it is now possible to assess simultaneously expression of a large array of genes. This promises to speed the pace of genetic discoveries in ovarian cancer in the next decade.

One consistent finding of various studies has been that poorly differentiated, advanced-stage cancers have more genetic alterations than early stage, well-differentiated, or borderline cases.[2,18] For example, in one CGH study, the average number of alterations was 5.4 in low-grade ovarian cancers compared to 11.2 in high-grade cases.[2] This finding could be interpreted as reflective of accumulation of genetic changes with evolution of a cancer. On the other hand, it is equally plausible that advanced stage, poorly

Table 3.1 Cellular processes that inhibit malignant transformation

1. Tumor suppressor genes restrain inappropriate proliferation
2. DNA repair genes that fix mutations
3. Apoptosis of genetically damaged cells
4. Finite replicative capacity of most adult cells, due to lack of telomerase, leads to senescence

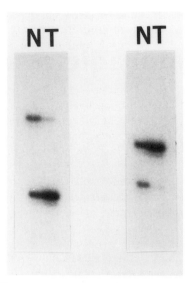

Fig. 3.1 Loss of heterozygosity analysis for the *p53* gene in ovarian cancer. Tumor: normal pairs in which the upper allele has been lost in the patient on the left and the lower allele has been lost in the patient on the right.

differentiated cancers are intrinsically more virulent, even early in their development, by virtue of their specific mutations or increased genomic instability. If this latter theory is correct, this could have significant implications for early diagnosis of ovarian cancer. Cancers that are inherently more virulent might metastasize fairly rapidly and be less amenable to early detection.

Etiology of genetic alterations

In addition to identifying the specific genetic changes involved in ovarian carcinogenesis, an understanding of the etiology of this damage is essential—particularly if we hope to develop effective prevention strategies. Like other sporadic cancers, most epithelial ovarian carcinomas are thought to develop due to accumulation of a series of genetic alterations over a lifetime. The causes of the genetic damage that underlies the development of these cancers are not completely understood (Table 3.2), but epidemiologic and molecular studies have begun to shed some light on the etiology of ovarian cancer. There is evidence to suggest that sporadic ovarian cancer generally is a monoclonal disease that originates in the ovarian surface epithelium or underlying inclusion cysts.[24] About 10% of ovarian cancers arise in women who carry mutations in cancer susceptibility genes (*BRCA1, BRCA2*, DNA repair genes) and there is evidence that some cancers that arise in the peritoneum of these patients may be polyclonal.[25] The etiology of

Table 3.2 Theories regarding the etiology of genetic damage in ovarian cancer

1. Spontaneous mutations due to epithelial proliferation after ovulation
2. Stimulation of epithelial proliferation by steroids and/or gonadotropins
3. Talc or other carcinogens that migrate up the genital tract
4. Lack of progestin-induced apoptosis of genetically damaged cells

acquired genetic damage in the ovarian epithelium remains uncertain, but exogenous carcinogens, other than perhaps talc,[26] have not been strongly implicated.

It has been suggested that ovulation may be the main cause of mutations in the ovarian epithelium. Several lines of evidence link ovulation and epithelial ovarian cancer. First, most animals, such as rats and mice, ovulate reflexively when stimulated appropriately and have a low incidence of epithelial ovarian cancer. In contrast, chickens and women ovulate repetitively and have the highest incidence of epithelial ovarian cancer. Conversely, women with Turner's syndrome, who are anovulatory, rarely develop epithelial ovarian cancer. The observation that pregnancy and oral contraceptive pill use, which decrease lifetime ovulatory cycles, are protective against ovarian cancer[27] is also consistent with the theory that ovulation is the main driving force underlying the accumulation of genetic damage in the ovarian epithelium.

It is not known with certainty why repetitive ovulation facilitates the development of ovarian cancer, and several factors, including stimulation by gonadotropins, may play a role. One appealing theory is that mutations in the epithelium may result from errors in DNA synthesis that occur during proliferation required to repair ovulatory defects. There is evidence to suggest that spontaneous mutations are more likely to occur in cells that are proliferating relative to those at rest.[28] Although the process of DNA synthesis occurs with a high degree of fidelity, it is estimated that spontaneous errors may occur about once every million bases. Several families of DNA repair genes exist, but some types of mutations more readily elude surveillance and repair and become fixed in the genome. In addition, the efficiency of these DNA repair systems may vary between individuals due to inherited differences in activity of various alleles of DNA repair genes.

A decreased rate of mutations in the ovarian epithelium probably is not solely responsible for the protective effect of pregnancy and oral contraceptive pills against ovarian cancer. This effect is greater in magnitude than would be predicted based on the extent that ovulation is interrupted. Five years of oral contraceptive use decreases risk by approximately 50%, while decreasing lifetime ovulatory cycles by only about 10–20%.[27] Recently, however, it has been shown that administration of the progestin levonorgestrel, either alone or in combination with estrogen, stimulates apoptosis of ovarian epithelial cells in macaques.[29] This suggests that the progestagenic milieu of pregnancy and the pill might protect against ovarian cancer by increasing apoptosis of ovarian epithelial cells, thereby cleansing the ovary of cells that have acquired genetic damage.

Mechanisms of malignant transformation

The mutations that lead to the development of ovarian and other cancers primarily target genes involved in regulating proliferation, programmed cell death (apoptosis) and senescence—processes that determine the number of cells in a population (Table 3.1). Development of a cancer results from disruption of these complex regulatory pathways, with the net effect being an increased number of cells. Mutations that inactivate DNA repair genes also occur in some types of cancers and may accelerate the accumulation of cancer-causing mutations, but this has not yet been demonstrated to be a prominent feature of sporadic ovarian cancers.

In addition to growth of a primary tumor, cancers are characterized by acquisition of a metastatic phenotype. Ovarian cancers have the ability to invade the surrounding stroma, due to production of proteases that degrade connective tissue and produce angiogenic factors that stimulate the development of new blood vessels to support their growth and spread. Although these molecular pathways are integral to the process of cancer progression, there is little evidence to date to suggest that evolution of the metastatic phenotype is directly attributable to mutations in genes that encode proteases or other molecules involved in invasion and metastasis.

Proliferation

The rate of proliferation is a major determinant of the number of cells in a population. To prevent excessive proliferation, DNA synthesis and cell division ordinarily are restrained. When proliferation is appropriate, these inhibitory mechanisms are turned off and growth stimulatory signals are generated. Malignant tumors are characterized by alterations in genes that control proliferation. There is increased activity of genes that stimulate proliferation (oncogenes) and loss of growth inhibitory (tumor suppressor) genes (Table 3.3). In the past, it was thought that cancer might arise entirely because of more rapid proliferation or a higher fraction of cells proliferating. It is now clear that this was an overly simplistic view. Although increased proliferation is a characteristic of many cancers, the fraction of cancer cells actively dividing and the transition time of the cell cycle are not strikingly different than that seen in some normal cells. Increased proliferation is only one of several factors that contributes to cancerous growth.

The fraction of ovarian cancer cells that are actively proliferating can be measured using various techniques. One approach is to assess the DNA content of cells in a sample. This can be accomplished with flow cytometry using disaggregated nuclei, or in frozen sections using image analysis. The fraction of cells with a DNA content consistent with S phase can be distinguished from those in the G_1 or G_2/M phases to calculate a proliferation index. In one study, about 25% of ovarian cancers had an S-phase fraction below 5% and this correlated with early stage and favorable survival.[30] Proliferation can also be assessed using immunohistochemical techniques to identify cells that express Ki67 or PCNA, antigens that are expressed only in actively proliferating cells. In

Table 3.3 Classes of genes involved in growth regulatory pathways and malignant transformation

Growth stimulatory (oncogenes)	
Peptide growth factors	**Corresponding receptors**
Epidermal growth factor (EGF) and transforming growth factor (TGF-α)	EGF receptor
heregulin	erbB2 (HER-2/neu)
	erbB3, erbB4
Insulin-like growth factors (IGF-I and IGF-II)	IGF-I and -II receptors
Platelet-derived growth factor (PDGF)	PDGF receptor
Fibroblast growth factors (FGFs)	FGF receptors
Macrophage-colony stimulating factor (M-CSF)	M-CSF receptor (fms)
Cytoplasmic factors	**Examples**
Non-receptor tyrosine kinases	abl, src, PIK3CA
G proteins	K-ras, H-ras
Serine/threonine kinases	AKT2
Nuclear factors	**Examples**
Transcription factors	myc, jun, fos
Cell cycle progression factors	Cyclins, E2F
Growth inhibitory (tumor suppressor genes)	
Extranuclear factors	**Examples**
Cell membrane factors	Transforming growth factor-βs 1–3 and their type I and II receptors
Cell adhesion factors	Cadherins, APC
Phosphatases	PTEN
Nuclear factors	**Examples**
Cell cycle inhibitors	Rb, p53, p16, p27
Unknown function	BRCA1, BRCA2

most such studies, there has been a correlation between higher proliferation indicies (>5–15%) and more advanced stage, worse grade, and poor survival.[31–33]

Apoptosis

Cells are capable of activating a suicide pathway of programmed cell death referred to as apoptosis. Apoptosis is an active energy-dependent process that involves cleavage of the DNA by endonucleases and proteins by proteases. Morphologically, apoptosis is characterized by condensation of chromatin and cellular shrinkage. This is in contrast to the process of necrosis, which is characterized by loss of osmoregulation and cellular fragmentation.

Since the size of a population of cells is normally static, due to a balance between the birth rate and the death rate, growth of a neoplasm theoretically could result due to either increased proliferation or decreased apoptosis. In addition to restraining the number of cells in a population, apoptosis may serve an important role in preventing malignant transformation by specifically eliminating cells that have undergone mutations. Following exposure of cells to mutagenic stimuli, including radiation and carcinogenic drugs, the cell cycle is arrested so that DNA damage may be repaired. If DNA repair is not sufficient, apoptosis occurs, so cells that have undergone significant damage do not survive. This serves as an anti-cancer surveillance mechanism by which mutated cells are eliminated before they become fully transformed. The *p53* tumor suppressor gene is a critical regulator of cell cycle arrest and apoptosis in response to DNA damage, but apoptosis may also be triggered via other pathways under different circumstances.

The molecular events that affect cell death in response to various stimuli have only been partially elucidated thus far, but it appears that a family of genes encoding proteins that reside in the mitochondrial membrane are directly involved.[34] The *bcl–2* gene was first of these genes to be identified, and was found at a translocation breakpoint in B-cell lymphomas. Expression of *bcl–2* acts to inhibit apoptosis[35] and, paradoxically, persistence of *bcl–2* expression in ovarian cancers has been associated with favorable prognosis.[36,37] The *bcl-XL* gene, a structural and functional homologue of *bcl–2*, also inhibits apoptosis and has been shown to play a role in preventing apoptosis of ovarian cancer cells in response to chemotherapy.[38] Conversely, other related genes such as *bax*, and *bcl-XS* have pro-apoptotic activity. High *bax* expression has been reported in 60% of newly diagnosed ovarian cancers and was associated with a favorable response to therapy.[39]

It remains unclear exactly how Bcl–2 and these other mitochondrial proteins act to regulate apoptosis, but those that increase membrane permeability stimulate apoptosis while those that decrease permeability prevent apoptosis. Activation of a family of cytosolic proteolytic enzymes called caspases also occurs during apoptosis, leading to breakdown of cellular proteins.

Senescence

Normal cells are only capable of undergoing division a finite number of times before becoming senescent. Recently, it has been shown that cellular senescence is due to shortening of repetitive DNA sequences (TTAGGG), called telomeres, that cap the ends of each chromosome. Telomeres are thought to be involved in chromosome stabilization and in preventing recombination during mitosis. At birth chromosomes have long telomeric sequences that become progressively shorter each time a cell divides. Malignant cells appear to avoid senescence by turning on expression of telomerase activity that acts to lengthen the telomeres.[40,41] Telomerase is a ribonucleoprotein complex and both the protein and RNA subunits have been identified. The RNA component serves as a template for telomere extension and the protein subunit acts to catalyze the synthesis of new telomeric repeats.

Because telomerase expression in most normal tissues is restricted to development, it has been suggested that telomerase might be useful diagnostic marker in patients with cancer. Not surprisingly, several groups have shown that telomerase activity is detectable in most ovarian cancers.[42–44] It has been suggested that persistence of telomerase activity in peritoneal washings after primary therapy for advanced ovarian cancer may predict the presence of microscopic residual disease in some cases, despite negative cytologic washings and biopsies.[43] Demonstration of the utility of this approach awaits the completion of more definitive studies.

Growth stimulatory pathways:

Oncogenes

Oncogenes encode proteins normally involved in stimulating proliferation, but when these gene products are overactive they contribute to the process of malignant transformation. Oncogenes can be activated via several mechanisms. In some cancers, amplification of oncogenes with resultant overexpression of the corresponding protein has been noted. Some oncogenes may become overactive when affected by point mutations. Finally, oncogenes may be translocated from one chromosomal location to another and then come under the influence of promoter sequences that cause overexpression of the gene. This latter mechanism frequently occurs in leukemias and lymphomas, but has not been demonstrated in gynecologic cancers or other solid tumors.

In cell culture systems in the laboratory, many genes that are involved in normal growth stimulatory pathways can elicit transformation when altered to overactive forms. On this basis, a large number of genes have been classified as oncogenes (Fig. 3.2, Table 3.4). Studies in human cancers have suggested that the actual spectrum of genes altered in the development of human cancers may be more limited. A number of genes that elicit transformation when activated *in vitro* have not been documented to undergo alterations in human cancers. In this section, the various classes of oncogenes involved in ovarian cancer will be discussed.

Peptide growth factors

Peptide growth factors in the extracellular space can stimulate a cascade of molecular events that leads to proliferation by binding to cell membrane receptors. Unlike endocrine hormones, which are secreted into the bloodstream to act in distant target organs, peptide growth factors usually act in the local environment where

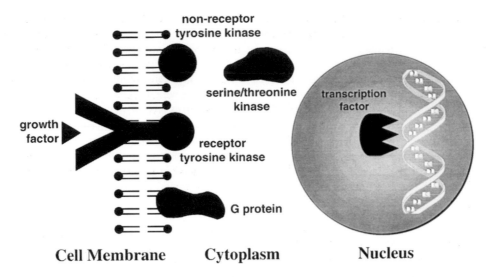

Fig. 3.2 Classes of oncogenes.

they have been secreted. The concept that autocrine growth stimulation might be a key strategy by which cancer cell proliferation becomes autonomous is intellectually appealing and has received considerable attention. In this model, it is postulated that cancers secrete stimulatory growth factors which then interact with receptors on the same cell. Although increased production of stimulatory growth factors may play a role in enhancing proliferation associated with malignant transformation, they also are involved in development, stromal–epithelial communication, tissue regeneration, and wound healing.

It has been shown that ovarian cancers produce or are capable of responding to various peptide growth factors. For example, epidermal growth factor (EGF)[45] and transforming growth factor-α (TGF-α)[46] are produced by some ovarian cancers that also express the receptor that binds these peptides (EGF receptor).[47,48] Some cancers produce insulin-like growth factor-I (IGF-I), IGF-I binding protein, and express type 1 IGF receptor.[49] Platelet-derived growth factor (PDGF) also is expressed by many types of epithelial cells, including human ovarian cancer cell lines, but

these cells are not usually responsive to PDGF.[50–52] In addition, ovarian cancers produce basic fibroblast growth factor (FGF) and its receptor, and basic FGF acts as a mitogen in some ovarian cancers.[53] Ovarian cancers produce macrophage-colony stimulating factor (M-CSF)[54] and serum levels of M-CSF are elevated in some patients.[55] Since the M-CSF receptor (*fms*) is expressed by many ovarian cancers,[56] this could comprise an autocrine growth stimulatory pathway in some cancers. In addition, M-CSF could act in a paracrine fashion to stimulate recruitment and activation of macrophages. Since macrophage products such as interleukin–1 (IL–1), IL–6, and tumor necrosis factor-α have been shown to stimulate proliferation of some ovarian cancer cell lines,[57–59] the potential for paracrine stimulation of the cancer by macrophages also exists. In addition to expression of peptide growth factors and their receptors, ascites of patients with ovarian cancer contains phospholipid factors that stimulate proliferation of ovarian cancer cells.[60,61]

Several groups also have demonstrated that normal ovarian epithelial cells produce, and are responsive to, many of the same

Table 3.4 Molecular alterations in sporadic ovarian cancers

	Function	Alteration	Approximate frequency
Oncogenes			
HER-2/*neu*	Tyrosine kinase	Overexpression	20%
K-*ras*	G protein	Mutation	5%
AKT2	Serine/threonine kinase	Amplification	10%
PIK3CA	Serine/threonine kinase	Amplification	?40%
c-myc	Transcription	Overexpression factor	20–30%
Tumor suppressor genes			
BRCA1	?DNA repair	Mutation/deletion	5%
p53	Transcription factor	Mutation/deletion	60%
p16	Cdk inhibitor	Homozygous deletion/methylation	?15%
p27	Cdk inhibitor	Decreased expression	?40%

peptide growth factors as malignant ovarian epithelial cells.[48,62–64] Thus, despite circumstantial evidence demonstrating the potential for autocrine and paracrine growth regulation of ovarian cancer cells by peptide growth factors, it remains unclear whether alterations in expression of growth factors are critical in the development of ovarian cancer. Peptide growth factors may function as necessary cofactors rather than as the driving force behind malignant transformation.

Growth factor receptors, including the epidermal growth factor receptor family (EGF receptor, HER–2/neu)

Cell membrane receptors that bind peptide growth factors are composed of an extracellular ligand-binding domain, a membrane-spanning region, and a cytoplasmic tyrosine kinase domain. Binding of a growth factor to the extracellular domain results in aggregation and conformational shifts in the receptor and activation of the inner tyrosine kinase.[65,66] This kinase phosphorylates tyrosine residues on both the growth factor receptor (autophosphorylation) and targets in the cell interior, leading to activation of secondary signals. For example, phosphorylation of phospholipase C leads to breakdown of cell membrane phospholipids and generation of diacylglycerol and inositol trisphosphate, both of which play a role in propagation of the mitogenic signal.

The role of the epidermal growth factor (EGF) receptor family of transmembrane receptors and their ligands in growth regulation and transformation has been a prominent focus in cancer research.[67] EGF is a peptide growth factor of 53 amino acids that maintains its secondary structure by virtue of disulfide bonds between cysteine residues. At least five other peptide growth factors, including transforming growth factor-α (TGF-α) also interact with and activate the EGF receptor. EGF, TGF-α and other EGF receptor ligands are produced as pro-forms that are inserted into the cell membrane. The membrane-anchored growth factor can interact with receptors on adjacent cells, a phenomenon known as juxtacrine growth regulation. Alternatively, the active peptide then can be cleaved and released into the extracellular space. The free peptide may interact with receptors on the same (autocrine) or nearby (paracrine) cells to stimulate growth.

The EGF receptor is expressed ubiquitously in both epithelial and stromal cells, and plays a role in growth stimulation of most cell types. The EGF receptor has been shown to be amplified in some squamous cancers, and the EGF receptor can be targeted therapeutically with monoclonal antibodies.[68] EGF receptor is expressed in normal ovarian epithelium and, although the level of expression varies between cancers, this is not a strong predictor of clinical behavior.[69]

The EGF receptor family of receptors is also often referred to as the erbB family because the first member identified was the v-erbB oncogene. The second member of the family (erbB2) was initially called neu because it was found to be the transforming gene responsible for the generation of neuroblastomas in rats treated with a chemical carcinogen. This human EGF receptor-like molecule was named both HER–2/neu and erbB2 by investigators working in the field. The transforming activity of neu in the animal model was due to the presence of a mutation in the transmembrane portion of the molecule that results in constitutive activation of the inner tyrosine kinase domain. Biochemical studies of HER–2/neu have shown that activation of this receptor is not driven by ligand binding, but rather is dependent on activation of other members of the erbB family (erbB3, erbB4) that heterodimerize with erbB2 and activate its tyrosine kinase domain.[70]

In contrast to EGF receptor, which is normally expressed in both stromal and epithelial cells, HER–2/neu is expressed primarily in epithelial cells. The level of HER–2/neu is increased in some human breast, ovarian, and other cancers due to amplification,[71,72] and the SKOV3 ovarian cancer cell line and the SKBR3 breast cancer cell line both have amplification of this gene. In human cancers, HER–2/neu may also be overexpressed due to alterations in regulation of transcription in the absence of gene amplification. Regardless of the underlying mechanism, it has been shown that overexpression occurs in about 20% of ovarian cancers and 30% of breast cancers, and correlates with aggressive features. The level of overexpression in breast cancers is generally higher than in ovarian cancers, however, and some studies have not found overexpression of HER–2/neu to adversely affect prognosis in ovarian cancer.[73,74] It has been shown that transfection of HER–2/neu into normal ovarian epithelial cells can induce a malignant phenotype in vitro, including the ability of cells to grow in an anchorage-independent fashion and to form tumors in nude mice.

As noted above, activation of the erbB3 and 4 transmembrane receptors is requisite for HER–2/neu kinase activity. At least four families of ligands, collectively called neuregulins (e.g. heregulin, neu differentiating factor), bind to erbB3 and 4.[70] Interestingly, there is considerable promiscuity between erbB ligands and receptors. For example, amphiregulin can activate both the EGF receptor (erbB1) and erbB3. And one of the more recently described ligands (epiregulin) can activate heterodimers of any of the erbB family members; and these heterodimers are more potent growth stimulators than homodimers of any individual erbB receptor. Although their molecular signaling mechanisms have not yet been fully elucidated, the erbB family of receptors has also been exploited as therapeutic targets. Monoclonal antibodies that interact with HER–2/neu can decrease growth of breast and ovarian cancer cell lines that overexpress this receptor.[75,76] In addition, these antibodies may enhance the sensitivity of cancers to cytotoxic chemotherapy by interfering with repair of DNA adducts.[77] Recently an anti-HER–2/neu antibody that induces breast cancer regression has been approved for clinical use by the Food and Drug Administration (FDA).[78] It is possible that this approach might also benefit some women whose ovarian cancers overexpress HER–2/neu.

Other kinases

Following interaction of peptide growth factors and their receptors, secondary molecular signals are generated to transmit the mitogenic stimulus towards the nucleus. This function is served by a multitude of complex and overlapping signal transduction pathways that occur in the inner cell membrane and cytoplasm. Many of these signals involve phosphorylation of proteins by enzymes known as kinases.[79] Cellular processes other than growth also are regulated by kinases, but one family of kinases appears to have evolved specifically for the purpose of transmitting growth stimulatory signals. These tyrosine kinases transfer a phosphate group from ATP to tyrosine residues of target proteins. Some kinases that phosphorylate proteins on serine and/or threonine residues also are involved in stimulating proliferation. Although several families of intracellular kinases have been identified that can elicit transformation when activated *in vitro*, it remains uncertain whether structural alterations in most of these molecules play a role in the development of human cancers. The activity of kinases is regulated by phosphatases, which act in opposition to the kinases by removing phosphates from the target proteins.[80] It has been shown that a number of phosphatases are expressed by ovarian cancers and that some of these oppose the kinase activity of HER–2/*neu*.[81]

AKT2 is a gene on chromosome 19q that encodes a serine–threonine protein kinase. *AKT2* has been shown to be amplified and overexpressed in two of eight ovarian cancer cell lines and two of 15 primary epithelial ovarian cancers.[82] This study was confirmed by a larger series of 132 primary ovarian cancers in which 14% had *AKT2* amplification or overexpression. *AKT2* amplification/overexpression was found have a statistically significant association with higher grade and worse survival.[83] Further studies are needed to confirm the functional significance of *AKT2* overexpression in ovarian cancers.

The region of chromosome 3p26 that includes the regulatory subunit of phosphatidylinositol 3 kinase (PIK3CA) has been shown to be amplified in some ovarian cancer cell lines and 40% of primary ovarian cancers, using comparative genomic hybridization.[84] Interestingly, the *AKT2* gene is one of the downstream targets of PIK3CA. Thus, theoretically, amplification of either of these two genes leads to excessive activation of this mitogenic pathway.

G proteins

G proteins represent another class of molecules involved in transmission of growth stimulatory signals in towards the nucleus.[85,86] They are located on the inner aspect of the cell membrane and have intrinsic GTPase activity that catalyzes the exchange of GTP (guanosine triphosphate) for GDP (guanosine diphosphate). In their active GTP-bound form, G proteins interact with kinases that are involved in relaying the mitogenic signal. Conversely, hydrolysis of GTP to GDP, which is stimulated by GTPase activating proteins (GAPs), leads to inactivation of G proteins. The genes for the Ras family of G proteins are among the most frequently mutated oncogenes in human cancers (e.g. gastrointestinal and endometrial cancers). Activation of *ras* genes usually involves point mutations in codons 12, 13, or 61 that result in constitutively activated molecules.

Mutations in the *ras* genes do not appear to be a common feature of invasive serous epithelial ovarian cancers.[87–89] K-*ras* mutations have been noted more frequently in mucinous ovarian cancers, but these tumors comprise only a small fraction of epithelial ovarian cancers. In contrast, K-*ras* mutations are common in borderline epithelial ovarian tumors, occurring in 20–50% of cases.[90,91] Thus, studies of the K-*ras* oncogene suggest that the molecular pathology of borderline tumors differs from that of invasive epithelial ovarian cancers.

Nuclear factors

If proliferation is to occur in response to signals generated in the cytoplasm, these events must lead to activation of nuclear factors responsible for DNA replication and cell division. Expression of several genes that encode nuclear proteins increases dramatically within minutes of treatment of normal cells with peptide growth factors. Once induced, the products of these genes bind to specific DNA regulatory elements and induce transcription of genes involved in DNA synthesis and cell division. When inappropriately overexpressed, however, these transcription factors can act as oncogenes. Among the nuclear transcription factors involved in stimulating proliferation, amplification and/or overexpression of members of the *myc* family has most often been implicated in the development of human cancers.[92,93] Myc proteins are key regulators of mammalian cell proliferation, and treatment of cells with *myc* antisense oligonucleotides inhibits proliferation. It has been shown that Myc acts as part of a heterodimeric complex with the protein Max to initiate transcription of other genes involved in cell cycle progression.[92]

Amplification of the c-*myc* oncogene occurs in some epithelial ovarian cancers. In five small studies, c-*myc* was reported to be amplified in a total of 24 of 77 cases (31%).[94–98] In a more recent study in which 51 epithelial ovarian cancers were analyzed, a similar incidence of c-*myc* overexpression was observed (37%).[99] c-*myc* overexpression was more frequently observed in advanced-stage serous adenocarcinomas, suggesting a role for tumor progression.

Growth inhibitory pathways: tumor suppressor genes

Tumor suppressor genes encode proteins normally involved in inhibiting proliferation, and inactivation of these genes plays a role in the development of most cancers. Knudson's 'two-hit' model established the paradigm that both alleles must be inactivated in order to exert a phenotypic effect on tumorigenesis.[100] The location and the type of the inactivating mutations in tumor suppressor genes may vary from one cancer to the next. Frequently, mutations in tumor suppressor genes alter the base sequence, such that the encoded protein product is truncated due to generation of a premature stop codon. Truncated protein products may result from several types of mutational events, including nonsense mutations, in which a single base substitution changes that sequence from a specific amino acid to a stop codon (AAG to TAG). In addition, microdeletions or insertions of one or several nucleotides that disrupt the reading frame of the DNA (frameshifts) also lead to the generation of stop codons downstream in the gene. In some cases, missense mutations occur which change only a single amino acid in the encoded protein. A mutation in one allele, whether germline or somatic, is then revealed following somatic inactivation of the homologous wild-type allele. In theory, the same spectrum of mutational events could contribute to inactivation of the second allele, but what is typically observed in tumors is homozygosity or hemizygosity for the first mutation, indicating 'loss' of the wild-type allele. The loss of heterozygosity (LOH) has become recognized as the hallmark of tumor suppressor gene inactivation.

There is also evidence that some tumor suppressor genes may be inactivated due to methylation of the promoter region of the gene.[101] The promoter is an area proximal to the coding sequence that regulates whether or not the gene is transcribed from DNA into RNA. When the promoter is methylated it is resistant to activation and the gene is essentially silenced, despite remaining structurally intact. Like oncogenes, tumor suppressor gene products are found throughout the cell (Table 3.4). In this section the various classes of tumor suppressor genes involved in sporadic epithelial ovarian cancers will be reviewed.

Extranuclear tumor suppressor genes

Although most tumor suppressor gene products are nuclear proteins, some extranuclear tumor suppressors have been identified. Theoretically, any protein that normally is involved in inhibition of proliferation could conceivably act as a tumor suppressor. In this regard, phosphatases, which normally oppose the action of the tyrosine kinases by dephosphorylating tyrosine residues, are appealing candidates.[80] Analysis of deletions on chromosome 10q23 in human cancers led to the discovery of the *PTEN* gene[102] In addition to its phosphatase activity, PTEN is homologous to the cytoskeleton proteins tensin and actin and it has been postulated that PTEN might act to inhibit invasion and metastasis through modulation of the cytoskeleton.[103] Interestingly, it has been shown that PIK3CA and AKT2 kinase activity can be specifically opposed by the PTEN phosphatase. *PTEN* mutations are rare in serous ovarian cancers, perhaps because amplification of *PIK3CA* or *AKT2* abrogates the need for loss of *PTEN* tumor suppressor function. In contrast, *PTEN* mutations occur in about 20% of endometrioid ovarian cancers.[104]

Transforming growth factor-β

The transforming growth factor-β (TGF-β) family of growth factors inhibits proliferation of normal epithelial cells.[105] It is thought that TGF-β causes cell-cycle arrest in G_1 by triggering pathways that result in inhibition of cyclin-dependent kinases. Three closely related forms of TGF-β have been discovered which are encoded by separate genes (TGF-β1, TGF-β2, TGF-β3). All three forms of TGF-β are 25 kDa homodimers with subunits bound together by disulfide bonds. TGF-β is secreted from cells in an inactive form bound to a portion of its precursor molecule from which it must be cleaved to release biologically active TGF-β. Active TGF-β interacts with type I and type II cell surface TGF-β receptors and initiates serine/threonine kinase activity.[106] Prominent intracellular targets include a class of molecules, called Smads, that translocate to the nucleus and act as transcriptional regulators.[107] Although mutations in the TGF-β receptors and Smads have been reported in some cancers, this does not appear to be a feature of ovarian cancers.

Normal ovarian epithelial cells produce, activate, and are growth inhibited by TGF-β;[108] however, most immortalized ovarian cancer cell lines have lost the ability to either produce, activate, or respond to TGF-β.[51,108–112] This suggested that TGF-β might normally act as an autocrine growth inhibitory factor in normal ovarian epithelium, and that loss of this pathway might play a role in the development of some ovarian cancers. Although convenient to work with, immortalized cell lines frequently have undergone profound genetic alterations in tissue culture. Examination of primary ovarian cancers obtained directly from patients revealed that in almost all cases cancers were sensitive to the growth inhibitory effect of TGF-β.[113] Thus, it remains unclear whether alterations in the TGF-β pathway play a role in the development of ovarian cancers.

p53 tumor suppressor gene

Mutation of the *p53* tumor suppressor gene is the most frequent genetic event described thus far in human cancers (Fig. 3.3).[114–116] The *p53* gene encodes a 393 amino-acid protein that appears to play a central role in the regulation of both proliferation and apoptosis.[117–119] In normal cells, p53 protein resides in the nucleus and exerts its tumor suppressor activity by binding to transcriptional regulatory elements of genes, such as the cyclin-dependent kinase (cdk) inhibitor *p21*, that act to arrest cells in G_1. Beyond simply inhibiting proliferation, normal p53 is thought to play a role in preventing cancer by stimulating apoptosis of cells that have undergone excessive genetic damage.[120] In this regard, p53 has been described as the 'guardian of the genome' since it delays entry into S phase until the genome has been cleansed of mutations. If DNA repair is inadequate, p53 may initiate apoptosis, thereby eliminating cells with genetic damage.

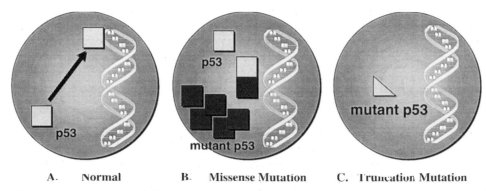

A.   Normal   B.   Missense Mutation   C.   Truncation Mutation

Fig. 3.3 Inactivation of the *p53* tumor suppressor gene by 'dominant negative' missense mutation or by truncation mutation and deletion.

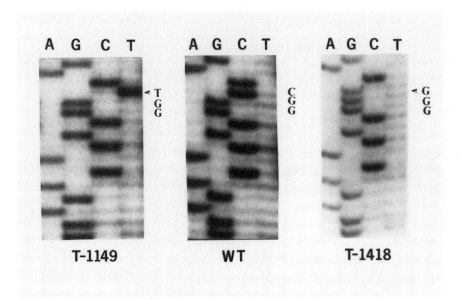

Fig. 3.4 Transition and transversion mutations of codon 282 of the *p53* gene in ovarian cancers. WT, wild-type codon 282 sequence (CGG); T-1149, ovarian cancer with transition mutation (C → T) at codon 282; T-1418, ovarian cancer with transversion mutation (C → G) at codon 282.

Many cancers have missense mutations in one copy of the *p53* gene that result in substitution of a single amino acid in exons 5 through 8, which encode the DNA-binding domains (Figs 3.4 and 3.5). Although these mutant *p53* genes encode full-length proteins, they are unable to bind to DNA and regulate transcription of other genes. Mutation of one copy of the *p53* gene is often accompanied by deletion of the other copy, leaving the cancer cell with only mutant p53 protein. If the cancer cell does retain one normal copy of the *p53* gene, the mutant p53 protein can form a complex with wild-type p53 protein and prevent it from interacting with DNA. Because inactivation of both *p53* alleles is not required for loss of p53 function, mutant *p53* is said to act in a 'dominant negative' fashion. While normal cells have low levels of p53 protein because it is rapidly degraded, missense mutations encode protein products that are resistant to degradation and overaccumulate in the nucleus; and overexpression of mutant p53 protein can be detected immunohistochemically. A smaller fraction of cancers have mutations in the *p53* gene that encode truncated protein products.[121] Whereas missense mutations in the *p53* gene cluster in exons 5–8, truncation mutations are more evenly dispersed throughout the gene, presumably because they inactivate the p53 protein regardless of their location (Fig. 3.5). In cases of *p53* truncation mutations, deletion of the other allele occurs as the second event, as is seen with other tumor suppressor genes (Fig. 3.1).

Alteration of the *p53* tumor suppressor gene is the most frequent genetic event described thus far in ovarian cancers.[121–128] The frequency of overexpression of mutant *p53* is significantly higher in advanced stage III/IV disease (40–60%) relative to stage I cases (10–20%). In addition, *p53* inactivation is uncommon in borderline tumors.[129] The higher frequency of *p53* overexpression in advanced stage cases may indicate that this is a 'late event' in ovarian carcinogenesis. Alternatively, the loss of *p53* may confer a more aggressive metastatic phenotype. In advanced-stage ovarian cancer, there is a suggestion that overexpression of *p53* may be associated with somewhat poorer chances of survival.[122,124–128] The literature is not entirely consistent and most studies have not been large enough or optimally designed to yield reliable prognostic information. Finally, although there is a high concordance between *p53* missense mutations and protein overexpression, about 20% of advanced ovarian cancers contain mutations that result in truncated protein products that generally are not overexpressed.[121] Overall, about 70% of advanced ovarian cancers have either missense or truncation mutations in the *p53* gene.

The finding that overexpression of mutant *p53* tumor suppressor genes is associated with high lifetime ovulatory cycles is consistent with the hypothesis that ovulation-associated proliferation may be the cause of these mutations in the ovarian epithelium.[130] In addition, most of the *p53* point mutations are transitions rather than transversions,[20,131] which also suggests that these mutations occur spontaneously, rather than due to exogenous carcinogens.

It has been suggested that loss of *p53* might confer a chemoresistant phenotype, because p53 plays a role in chemotherapy-induced apoptosis. In this regard, several studies have examined the correlation between chemosensitivity and *p53* mutation in ovarian cancers *in vitro*.[36,132–135] Some have suggested a relationship between *p53* mutation and loss of chemosensitivity, but in other equally valid studies such a relationship has not been observed.[136] The status of the *p53* gene is probably one of a number of factors that determines sensitivity to chemotherapy.

BRCA1

Inherited mutations of the *BRCA1* gene on chromosome 17q are the most frequent cause of hereditary ovarian cancers. Prior to the identification of *BRCA1*, it had been anticipated that somatic

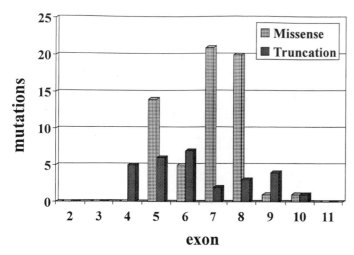

Fig. 3.5 Spectrum of *p53* mutations in advanced ovarian cancers (*n* = 58).

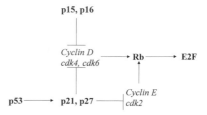

Fig. 3.6 Regulation of G_1 progression by p53 cyclins, cdks, cdk inhibitors, and Rb.

mutations in *BRCA1* would be common in ovarian cancers, since more than half of these cancers exhibit loss of heterozygosity on chromosome 17q.[21,137,138] Initially, two small studies reported somatic mutations in *BRCA1* in about 10% of 54 ovarian cancers,[139,140] but somatic mutations were not seen in two larger studies.[138,141] In these initial studies, mutational screening was performed using single-stranded conformation analysis.

More recently, a large study in which complete sequencing of the *BRCA1* gene was performed in 103 ovarian cancers, somatic mutations were found in at least seven cases.[142] In contrast to women with germline *BRCA1* mutations whose median age at ovarian cancer diagnosis is typically in the mid-forties, the median age of women with somatic mutations was about 60. Similar to ovarian cancers with germline *BRCA1* mutations, all of the ovarian cancers with somatic *BRCA1* mutations were serous. In addition, loss of the wild-type *BRCA1* allele invariably accompanied somatic *BRCA1* mutations. These data are supportive of the hypothesis that loss of *BRCA1* function occurs by way of the classic tumor suppressor paradigm, with mutation of one copy and deletion of the other. The *BRCA2* gene, which is responsible for some hereditary ovarian cancer cases, also has been examined for somatic mutations, but none have been identified.[143]

Retinoblastoma tumor suppressor gene

Initiation of the cell cycle with resultant cell division is dependent on progression through the G_1 phase of the cycle into the DNA-synthetic S phase. The retinoblastoma gene (*Rb*), which was the first tumor suppressor gene discovered, plays a central role in actively regulating this process.[144,145] In the early G_1 phase of the cell cycle Rb protein binds to the E2F transcription factor and prevents it from activating transcription of other genes involved in cell-cycle progression. When Rb is phosphorylated, E2F is released and stimulates entry into the DNA synthesis phase of the cell cycle (Fig. 3.6). Mutations in the *Rb* gene have been noted primarily in retinoblastomas and sarcomas, but rarely in other types of cancers. Loss of heterozygosity at the *Rb* locus occurs in about

30% of ovarian cancers, but mutations in the gene have not been detected[146] and functional Rb protein is present despite loss of one copy of the gene.[147]

Cyclins, cyclin-dependent kinases, and cdk inhibitors

Phosphorylation of Rb serves as a final common pathway with respect to initiation of proliferation; and this process is tightly controlled because of its critical importance (Fig. 3.6). Rb is phosphorylated by a family of cyclin-dependent kinases (cdk2, 4, 6) and associated cyclins (cyclin D and E), which act as regulatory subunits. Conversely, a family of cdk inhibitors (p15, p16, p21, p27) has been described that prevents phosphorylation of Rb by cyclin–cdk complexes. Although many of the intricacies of regulation of G_1 progression remain poorly understood, it is clear that inappropriately high activity of cyclins and cdks, or loss of cdk inhibitors, facilitates malignant transformation. Several alterations in these classes of genes have been described in human cancers, including overexpression of cyclin D and loss of p16.

The p16 cdk inhibitor is the most frequently altered of the genes involved in regulating Rb phosphorylation.[101] The *p16* gene on chromosome 9p21 encodes a protein that inhibits cdk4 or cdk6/cyclin D complexes from phosphorylating Rb. Initially it was noted that both copies of the *p16* gene are deleted in a high fraction of immortalized cancer cell lines, including the SKOV3 ovarian cancer cell line.[148] The hypothesis that *p16* loss plays a significant role in malignant transformation was strengthened by the finding that it is inactivated in some familial melanoma kindreds. Although the *p16* gene also is inactivated by mutations or deletion of both alleles in some sporadic cancers, this occurs much less frequently than in immortalized cell lines. More commonly, however, the *p16* gene appears to be silenced due to methylation of its promoter, which prevents transcription.

The *p16* gene has been studied extensively in ovarian cancers, but the results of various studies are conflicting. Some studies have reported that the *p16* gene is homozygously deleted or the promoter methylated in a fraction of cases,[149–151] whereas other studies have not found *p16* deletions, mutations, or methylation.[152–154] The inconsistency of these various reports likely reflects the technical difficulty of assaying promoter methylation and homozygous deletions in primary tumor samples. In addition, some groups have reported that some ovarian cancers have very high levels of p16 protein,[155] but the underlying mechanism and significance of this observation has not yet been elucidated.

Finally, the p14arf protein arises from an alternative reading frame of the *p16* gene and has been shown to increase p53 expression by decreasing its degradation.[156] Deletions of the *p16* locus would also lead to loss of p14arf expression, which also could have significant consequences for regulation of G_1 progression.

There is some evidence to suggest that decreased activity of other cdk inhibitors may also play a role in the development of some cancers. In this regard, reduced expression of p27, which is encoded by a gene on chromosome 12p, has been noted in some cancers due to increased p27 degradation. About one-third of ovarian cancers have been noted to have decreased p27 expression and this correlated with poor outcome.[157,158] In addition, over-expression of cyclin D and/or cyclin E has been noted in some cancers. The cyclin D gene on chromosome 11q13 is translocated or amplified in some human cancers. Although the levels of cyclin D appear to be high in some ovarian cancers, overexpression has not been shown to be due to amplification or translocation.[158,159] Likewise, cyclin E levels are high in some ovarian cancers, particularly clear cell tumors.[160]

Other cyclins, cdks, and regulatory molecules such as the chk family are involved in regulating progression from G_2 to M. Alterations in these pathways clearly play a role in the development of some cancers, but the intricacies of G_2/M transition are less well understood than those of G_1/S. Studies of G_2/M in ovarian cancers to date are preliminary and have not yielded evidence of significant alterations.

References

1. Gallion, H.H., Powell, D.E., Smith, L.W. *et al.* (1990). Chromosome abnormalities in human epithelial ovarian malignancies. *Gynecol. Oncol.*, 38, 473–7.

2. Iwabuchi, H., Sakamoto, M., Sakunaga, H. *et al.* (1995). Genetic analysis of benign, low-grade, and high-grade ovarian tumors. *Cancer Res.*, 55, 6172–80.

3. Elledge, R.M. and Allred, D.C. (1994). The p53 tumor suppressor gene in breast cancer. *Breast Cancer Res. Treat* 32, 39–47.

4. Sonoda, G., Palazzo, J., du Manoir, S. *et al.* (1997). Comparative genomic hybridization detects frequent overrepresentation of chromosomal material from 3q26, 8q24, and 20q13 in human ovarian carcinomas. *Genes Chromos. Cancer*, 20, 320–8.

5. Tapper, J., Butzow, R., Wahlstrom, T. *et al.* (1997). Evidence for divergence of DNA copy number changes in serous, mucinous and endometrioid ovarian carcinomas. *Br. J. Cancer*, 75, 1782–7.

6. Cliby, W., Ritland, S., Dodson, M. *et al.* (1993). Human epithelial ovarian cancer allelotype. *Cancer Res.*, 53, 2393–8.

7. Tavassoli, M., Steingrimsdottir, H., Pierce, E. *et al.* (1996). Loss of heterozygosity on chromosome 5q in ovarian cancer is frequently accompanied by TP53 mutation and identifies a tumour suppressor gene locus at 5q13.1–21. *Br. J. Cancer*, 74, 115–19.

8. Saito, S., Sirahama, S., Matsushima, M. *et al.* (1996). Definition of a commonly deleted region in ovarian cancers to a 300-kb segment of chromosome 6q27. *Cancer Res.*, 56, 5586–9.

9. Tibiletti, M.G., Bernasconi, B., Furlan, D. *et al.* (1996). Early involvement of 6q in surface epithelial ovarian tumors. *Cancer Res.*, 56, 4493–8.

10. Colitti, C.V., Rodabaugh, K.J., Welch, W.R. *et al.* (1998). A novel 4 cM minimal deletion unit on chromosome 6q25.1–q25.2 associated with high grade invasive epithelial ovarian carcinomas. *Oncogene*, 16, 555–9.

11. Shridhar, V., Staub, J., Huntley, B. *et al.* (1999). A novel region of deletion on chromosome 6q23.3 spanning less than 500 Kb in high grade invasive epithelial ovarian cancer. *Oncogene*, 18, 3913–18.

12. Watson, R.H., Neville, P.J., Roy, W.J.J. *et al.* (1998). Loss of heterozygosity on chromosomes 7p, 7q, 9p and 11q is an early event in ovarian tumorigenesis. *Oncogene*, 17, 207–12.

13. Lu, K.H., Weitzel, J.N., Kodali, S. *et al.* (1997). A novel 4-cM minimally deleted region on chromosome 11p15.1 associated with high grade non-mucinous epithelial ovarian carcinomas. *Cancer Res.*, 57, 387–90.

14. Gabra, H., Langdon, S.P., Watson, J.E. *et al.* (1995). Loss of heterozygosity at 11q22 correlates with low progesterone receptor content in epithelial ovarian cancer. *Clin. Cancer Res.*, 1, 945–53.

15. Launonen, V., Stenback, F., Puistola, U. *et al.* (1998). Chromosome 11q22.3–q25 LOH in ovarian cancer: association with a more aggressive disease course and involved subregions. *Gynecol. Oncol.*, 71, 299–304.

16. Davis, M., Hitchcock, A., Foulkes, W.D. and Campbell, I.G. (1996). Refinement of two chromosome 11q regions of loss of heterozygosity in ovarian cancer. *Cancer Res.*, 56, 741–4.

17. Gabra, H., Watson, J.E., Taylor, K.J. *et al.* (1996). Definition and refinement of a region of loss of heterozygosity at 11q23.3–q24.3 in epithelial ovarian cancer associated with poor prognosis. *Cancer Res.*, 56, 950–4.

18. Dodson, M.K., Hartmann, L.C., Cliby, W.A. *et al.* (1993). Comparison of loss of heterozygosity patterns in invasive low-grade and high-grade epithelial ovarian carcinomas. *Cancer Res.*, 53, 4456–60.

19. Bandera, C.A., Takahashi, H., Behbakht, K. *et al.* (1997). Deletion mapping of two potential chromosome 14 tumor suppressor gene loci in ovarian carcinoma. *Cancer Res.*, 57, 513–15.

20. Kohler, M.F., Marks, J.R., Wiseman, R.W. *et al.* (1993). Spectrum of mutation and frequency of allelic deletion of the p53 gene in ovarian cancer. *J. Natl Cancer Inst.*, 85, 1513–19.

21. Jacobs, I.J., Smith, S.A., Wiseman, R.W. *et al.* (1993). A deletion unit on chromosome 17q in epithelial ovarian tumors distal to the familial breast/ovarian cancer locus. *Cancer Res.*, 53, 1218–21.

22. Bryan, E.J., Watson, R.H., Davis, M. *et al.* (1996). Localization of an ovarian cancer tumor suppressor gene to a 0.5-cM region between D22S284 and CYP2D, on chromosome 22q. *Cancer Res.*, 56, 719–21.

23. Gallion, H.H., Powell, D.E., Morrow, J.K. *et al.* (1992). Molecular genetic changes in human epithelial ovarian malignancies. *Gynecol. Oncol.*, 47, 137–42.

24. Jacobs, I.J., Kohler, M.F., Wiseman, R.W. *et al.* (1992). Clonal origin of epithelial ovarian carcinoma: analysis by loss of heterozygosity, p53 mutation, and X-chromosome inactivation. *J. Natl Cancer Inst.*, 84, 1793–8.

25. Schorge, J.O., Muto, M.G., Welch, W.R. *et al.* (1998). Molecular evidence for multifocal papillary serous carcinoma of the peritoneum in patients with germline BRCA1 mutations. *J. Natl Cancer Inst.*, 90, 841–5.

26. Harlow, B.L., Cramer, D.W., Bell, D.A. and Welch, W.R. (1992). Perineal exposure to talc and ovarian cancer risk. *Obstet. Gynecol.*, 80, 19–26.

27. Whittemore, A.S., Harris, R. and Itnyre, J. (1992). Characteristics relating to ovarian cancer risk. Collaborative analysis of twelve US case-control studies: IV. The pathogenesis of epithelial ovarian cancer. *Am. J. Epidemiol.*, 136, 1212–20.

28. Ames, B.N. and Gold, L.S. (1990). Too many rodent carcinogens: Mitogenesis increases mutagenesis. *Science*, 249, 970–1.

29. Rodriguez, G.C., Walmer, D.K., Cline, M. *et al.* (1998). Effect of progestin on the ovarian epithelium of macaques: Cancer prevention through apoptosis? *J. Soc. Gynecol. Invest.*, 5, 271–6.

30. Reles, A.E., Gee, C., Schellschmidt, I. *et al.* (1998). Prognostic significance of DNA content and S-phase fraction in epithelial ovarian carcinomas analyzed by image cytometry. *Gynecol. Oncol.*, 71, 3–13.

31. Layfield, L.J., Saria, E.A., Berchuck, A. *et al.* (1997). Prognostic value of MIB–1 in advanced ovarian carcinoma as determined using automated immunohistochemistry and quantitative image analysis. *J. Surg. Oncol.*, 66, 230–6.

32. Hartmann, L.C., Sebo, T.J., Kamel, N.A. *et al.* (1992). Proliferating cell nuclear antigen in epithelial ovarian cancer: relation to results at second-look laparotomy and survival. *Gynecol. Oncol.*, **47**, 191–5.

33. Garzetti, G.G., Ciavattini, A., Goteri, G. *et al.* (1995). Ki67 antigen immunostaining (MIB 1 monoclonal antibody) in serous ovarian tumors: index of proliferative activity with prognostic significance. *Gynecol. Oncol.*, **56**, 169–74.

34. Green, D.R. and Reed, J.C. (1998). Mitochondria and apoptosis. *Science*, **281**, 1309–12.

35. Korsmeyer, S.J. (1999). BCL–2 gene family and the regulation of programmed cell death. *Cancer Res.*, **59**, 1693s–1700s.

36. Herod, J.J., Eliopoulos, A.G., Warwick, J. *et al.* (1996). The prognostic significance of Bcl–2 and p53 expression in ovarian carcinoma. *Cancer Res.*, **56**, 2178–84.

37. Henriksen, R., Wilander, E. and Oberg, K. (1995). Expression and prognostic significance of Bcl–2 in ovarian tumours. *Br. J. Cancer*, **72**, 1324–9.

38. Liu, J.R., Fletcher, B., Page, C. *et al.* (1998). Bcl-xL is expressed in ovarian carcinoma and modulates chemotherapy-induced apoptosis. *Gynecol. Oncol.*, **70**, 398–403.

39. Tai, Y.T., Lee, S., Niloff, E. *et al.* (1998). BAX protein expression and clinical outcome in epithelial ovarian cancer. *J. Clin. Oncol.*, **16**, 2583–90.

40. Holt, S.E., Shay, J.W. and Wright, W.E. (1996). Refining the telomere–telomerase hypothesis of aging and cancer. *Nat. Biotech.*, **14**, 836–9.

41. Shay, J.W. (1998). Telomerase in cancer: diagnostic, prognostic, and therapeutic implications. *Cancer J. from Sci. Am.*, **4** (Suppl. 1), S26–34.

42. Kyo, S., Takakura, M., Tanaka, M. *et al.* (1998). Quantitative differences in telomerase activity among malignant, premalignant, and benign ovarian lesions. *Clin. Cancer Res.*, **4**, 399–405.

43. Duggan, B.D., Wan, M., Yu, M.C. *et al.* (1998). Detection of ovarian cancer cells: comparison of a telomerase assay and cytologic examination. *J. Natl Cancer Inst.*, **90**, 238–42.

44. Wan, M., Li, W.Z., Duggan, B.D., *et al.* (1997). Telomerase activity in benign and malignant epithelial ovarian tumors. *J. Natl Cancer Inst.*, **89**, 437–41.

45. Bauknecht, T., Kiechle, M., Bauer, G. and Siebers, J.W. (1986). Characterization of growth factors in human ovarian carcinomas. *Cancer Res.*, **46**, 2614–18.

46. Kommoss, F., Wintzer, H.O., Von Kleist, S. *et al.* (1990). In situ distribution of transforming growth factor-α in normal human tissues and in malignant tumours of the ovary. *J. Pathol.*, **162**, 223–30.

47. Morishige, K., Kurachi, H., Amemiya, K. *et al.* (1991). Evidence for the involvement of transforming growth factor-α and epidermal growth factor receptor autocrine growth mechanism in primary human ovarian cancers *in vitro*. *Cancer Res.*, **51**, 5322–8.

48. Rodriguez, G.C., Berchuck, A., Whitaker, R.S. *et al.* (1991). Epidermal growth factor receptor expression in normal ovarian epithelium and ovarian cancer. II. Relationship between receptor expression and response to epidermal growth factor. *Am. J. Obstet. Gynecol.*, **164**, 745–50.

49. Yee, D., Morales, F.R., Hamilton, T.C. and Von Hoff, D.D. (1991). Expression of insulin-like growth factor I, its binding proteins, and its receptor in ovarian cancer. *Cancer Res.*, **51**, 5107–12.

50. Sariban, E., Sitaras, N.M., Antoniades, H.N. *et al.* (1988). Expression of platelelt-derived growth factor (PDGF)-related transcripts and synthesis of biologically active PDGF-like proteins by human malignant epithelial cell lines. *J. Clin. Invest.*, **82**, 1157–64.

51. Berchuck, A., Olt, G.J., Everitt, L. *et al.* (1990). The role of peptide growth factors in epithelial ovarian cancer. *Obstet. Gynecol.*, **75**, 255–62.

52. Henrikson, R., Funa, K., Wilander, E. *et al.* (1993). Expression and prognostic significance of platelet-derived growth factor and its receptors in epithelial ovarian neoplasms. *Cancer Res.*, **53**, 4550–4.

53. Di Blasio, A.M., Cremononesi, L., Vigano, P. *et al.* (1993). Basic fibroblast growth factor and its receptor messenger ribonucleic acids are expressed in human ovarian epithelial neoplasms. *Am. J. Obstet. Gynecol.*, **169**, 1517–23.

54. Ramakrishnan, S., Xu, F.J., Brandt, S.J., *et al.* (1989). Constitutive production of macrophage colony-stimulating factor by human ovarian and breast cancer cell lines. *J. Clin. Invest.*, **83**, 921–6.

55. Kacinski, B.M., Stanley, E.R., Carter, D. *et al.* (1989). Circulating levels of CSF–1 (M-CSF) a lymphohematopoietic cytokine may be a useful marker of disease status in patients with malignant ovarian neoplasms. *Int. J. Radiat. Oncol. Biol. Phys.*, **17**, 159–64.

56. Kacinski, B.M., Carter, D., Mittal, K. *et al.* (1990). Ovarian adenocarcinomas express *fms*-complementary transcripts and *fms* antigen, often with coexpression of CSF–1. *Am. J. Pathol.*, **137** (1), 135–47.

57. Wu, S., Rodabaugh, K., Martinez-Maza, O. *et al.* (1992). Stimulation of ovarian tumor cell proliferation with monocyte products including interleukin–1, interleukin–6 and tumor necrosis factor-α. *Am. J. Obstet. Gynecol.*, **166**, 997–1007.

58. Wu, S., Boyer, C.M., Whitaker, R.S. *et al.* (1993). Tumor necrosis factor-α as an autocrine and paracrine growth factor for ovarian cancer: Monokine induction of tumor cell proliferation and tumor necrosis factor-α expression. *Cancer Res.*, **53**, 1939–44.

59. Naylor, S.M., Stamp, G.W.H., Foulkes, W.D. *et al.* (1993). Tumor necrosis factor and its receptors in human ovarian cancer *J. Clin. Invest.*, **91**, 2194–206.

60. Fang, X., Gibson, S., Flowers, M. *et al.* (1997). Lysophosphatidylcholine stimulates activator protein 1 and the c- Jun N-terminal kinase activity. *J. Biol. Chem.*, **272**, 13683–9.

61. Mills, G.B., May, C., Hill, M. *et al.* (1990). Ascitic fluid from human ovarian cancer patients contains growth factors necessary for intraperitoneal growth of human ovarian adenocarcinoma cells. *J. Clin. Invest.*, **86**, 851–5.

62. Siemans, C.H. and Auersperg, N. (1991). Serial propagation of human ovarian surface epithelium in culture. *J. Cell Physiol.*, **134**, 347–56.

63. Lidor, Y.J., Xu, F.J., Martinez-Maza, O. *et al.* (1993). Constitutive production of macrophage colony stimulating factor and interleukin–6 by human ovarian surface epithelial cells. *Exp. Cell Res.*, **207**, 332–9.

64. Ziltener, H.J., Maines-Bandiera, S., Schrader, J.W. and Auersperg, N. (1993). Secretion of bioactive interleukin–1, interleukin–6 and colony-stimulating factors by human ovarian surface epithelium. *Biol. Reprod.*, **49**, 635–41.

65. Pinkas-Kramarski, R., Shelly, M., Guarino, B.C. *et al.* (1998). ErbB tyrosine kinases and the two neuregulin families constitute a ligand-receptor network. *Mol. Cell Biol.*, **18**, 6090–101.

66. Weiss, A. and Schlessinger, J. (1998). Switching signals on or off by receptor dimerization. *Cell*, **94**, 277–80.

67. Gullick, W.J. (1998). Type I growth factor receptors: current status and future work. *Biochem. Soc. Symp.*, **63**, 193–8.

68. Fan, Z. and Mendelsohn, J. (1998). Therapeutic application of antigrowth factor receptor antibodies. *Curr. Opin. Oncol.*, **10**, 67–73.

69. Berchuck, A., Rodriguez, G.C., Kamel, A. *et al.* (1991). Epidermal growth factor receptor expression in normal ovarian epithelium and ovarian cancer: I. Correlation of receptor expression with prognostic factors in patients with ovarian cancer. *Am. J. Obstet. Gynecol.*, **164**, 669–74.

70. Alroy, I. and Yarden, Y. (1997). The ErbB signaling network in embryogenesis and oncogenesis: signal diversification through combinatorial ligand-receptor interactions. *FEBS Lett.*, **410**, 83–6.

71. Slamon, D.J., Godolphin, W., Jones, L.A. *et al.* (1989). Studies of HER–2/*neu* proto-oncogene in human breast and ovarian cancer. *Science*, **244**, 707–12.

72. Berchuck, A., Kamel, A., Whitaker, R. *et al.* (1990). Overexpression of HER–2/*neu* is associated with poor survival in advanced epithelial ovarian cancer. *Cancer Res.*, **50**, 4087–91.

73. Rubin, S.C., Finstad, C.L., Wong, G.Y. *et al.* (1993). Prognostic significance of HER–2/*neu* expression in advanced ovarian cancer. *Am. J. Obstet. Gynecol.*, **168**, 162–9.

74. Kacinski, B.M., Mayer, A.G., King, B.L. *et al.* (1992). *Neu* protein overexpression in benign, borderline, and malignant ovarian neoplasms. *Gynecol. Oncol.*, **44**, 245–53.

75. Rodriguez, G.C., Boente, M.P., Berchuck, A. *et al.* (1993). The effect of antibodies and immunotoxins reactive with HER- 2/*neu* on growth of

ovarian and breast cancer cell lines. *Am. J. Obstet. Gynecol.*, **168**, 228–32.

76. Pietras, R.J., Pegram, M.D., Finn, R.S. *et al.* (1998). Remission of human breast cancer xenografts on therapy with humanized monoclonal antibody to HER–2 receptor and DNA-reactive drugs. *Oncogene*, **17**, 2235–49.

77. Pegram, M.D., Finn, R.S., Arzoo, K. *et al.* (1997). The effect of HER–2/*neu* overexpression on chemotherapeutic drug sensitivity in human breast and ovarian cancer cells. *Oncogene,* **15**, 537–47.

78. Pegram, M.D., Lipton, A., Hayes, D.F. *et al.* (1998). Phase II study of receptor-enhanced chemosensitivity using recombinant humanized anti-p185HER2/neu monoclonal antibody plus cisplatin in patients with HER2/neu-overexpressing metastatic breast cancer refractory to chemotherapy treatment. *J. Clin. Oncol.*, **16**, 2659–71.

79. Schwartzberg, P.L. (1998). The many faces of Src: multiple functions of a prototypical tyrosine kinase. *Oncogene*, **17**, 1463–8.

80. Parsons, R. (1998). Phosphatases and tumorigenesis. *Curr. Opin. Oncol.*, **10**, 88–91.

81. Wiener, J.R., Kassim, S.K., Yu, Y. *et al.* (1996). Transfection of human ovarian cancer cells with the HER–2/neu receptor tyrosine kinase induces a selective increase in PTP-H1, PTP–1B, PTP-alpha expression. *Gynecol. Oncol.*, **61**, 233–40.

82. Cheng, J.Q., Godwin, A.K., Bellacosa, A. *et al.* (1992). AKT2, a putative oncogene encoding a member of a subfamily of protein-serine/threonine kinases, is amplified in human ovarian carcinomas. *Proc. Natl Acad. Sci. USA*, **89**, 9267–71.

83. Bellacosa, A., de Feo, D., Godwin, A.K. *et al.* (1995). Molecular alterations of the AKT2 oncogene in ovarian and breast carcinomas. *Int. J. Cancer*, **64**, 280–5.

84. Shayesteh, L., Lu, Y., Kuo, W.L. *et al.* (1999). PIK3CA is implicated as an oncogene in ovarian cancer. *Nature Genet.*, **21**, 99–102.

85. Campbell, S.L., Khosravi-Far, R., Rossman, K.L. *et al.* (1998). Increasing complexity of Ras signaling. *Oncogene*, **17**, 1395–1413.

86. Gutkind, J.S. (1998). Cell growth control by G protein-coupled receptors: from signal transduction to signal integration. *Oncogene*, **17**, 1331–42.

87. Enomoto, T., Inoue, M., Perantoni, A.O. *et al.* (1990). K-*ras* activation in neoplasms of the human female reproductive tract. *Cancer Res.*, **50**, 6139–45.

88. Feig, L.A., Bast, R.C. Jr, Knapp, R.C. and Cooper, G.M. (1984). Somatic activation of *ras*K gene in a human ovarian carcinoma. *Science*, **223**, 698–701.

89. Haas, M., Isakov, J. and Howell, S.B. Evidence against *ras* activation in human ovarian carcinomas. *Mol. Biol. Med.*, **4**, 265–75.

90. Teneriello, M.G., Ebina, M., Linnoila, R.I. *et al.* (1993). p53 and ki-*ras* gene mutations in epithelial ovarian neoplasms. *Cancer Res.*, **53**, 3103–8.

91. Mok, S.C.H., Bell, D.A., Knapp, R.C. *et al.* (1993). Mutation of K-*ras* protooncogene in human ovarian epithelial tumors of borderline malignancy. *Cancer Res.*, **53**, 1489–92.

92. Facchini, L.M. and Penn, L.Z. (1998). The molecular role of Myc in growth and transformation: recent discoveries lead to new insights. *FASEB J.*, **12**, 633–51.

93. Bouchard, C., Staller, P. and Eilers, M. (1998). Control of cell proliferation by Myc. *Trends Cell Biol.*, **8**, 202–6.

94. Baker, V.V., Borst, M.P., Dixon, D., *et al.* (1990). c-*myc* amplification in ovarian cancer. *Gynecol. Oncol.*, **38**, 340–2.

95. Zhou, D.J., Gonzalez-Cadavid, N., Ahuja, H. *et al.* (1988). A unique pattern of proto-oncogene abnormalities in ovarian adenocarcinomas. *Cancer*, **62**, 1573–6.

96. Serova, D.M. (1987). Amplification of c-*myc* proto-oncogene in primary tumors, metastases and blood leukocytes of patients with ovarian cancer. *Eksp. Onkol.*, **9**, 25–7.

97. Sasano, H., Garrett, C., Wilkinson, D. *et al.* (1990). Protoocogene amplification and tumor ploidy in human ovarian neoplasms. *Hum. Pathol.*, **21** (4), 382–91.

98. Berns, E.M.J.J., Klijn, J.G.M., Henzen-Logmans, S.C. *et al.* (1992). Receptors for hormones and growth factors (onco)-gene amplification in human ovarian cancer. *Int. J. Cancer*, **52**, 218–24.

99. Tashiro, H., Niyazaki, K., Okamura, H. *et al.* (1992). c-*myc* overexpression in human primary ovarian tumors: Its relevance to tumor progression. *Int. J. Cancer*, **50**, 828–33.

100. Knudson, A.G. (1997). Hereditary predisposition to cancer. *Ann. NY Acad. Sci.*, **833**, 58–67.

101. Liggett, W.H.J. and Sidransky, D. (1998). Role of the p16 tumor suppressor gene in cancer. *J. Clin. Oncol.*, **16**, 1197–206.

102. Steck, P.A., Pershouse, M.A., Jasser, S.A. *et al.* (1997). Identification of a candidate tumour suppressor gene, MMAC1, at chromosome 10q23.3 that is mutated in multiple advanced cancers. *Nature Genet.*, **15**, 356–62.

103. Li, J., Yen, C., Liaw, D. *et al.* (1997). PTEN, a putative protein tyrosine phosphatase gene mutated in human brain, breast, and prostate cancer. *Science*, **275**, 1943–7.

104. Obata, K., Morland, S.J., Watson, R.H. *et al.* (1998). Frequent PTEN/MMAC mutations in endometrioid but not serous or mucinous epithelial ovarian tumors. *Cancer Res.*, **58**, 2095–7.

105. Serra, R. and Moses, H.L. (1996). Tumor suppressor genes in the TGF-beta signaling pathway? *Nature Med.*, **2**, 390–1.

106. Shi, Y., Wang, Y.F., Jayaraman, L. *et al.* (1998). Crystal structure of a Smad MH1 domain bound to DNA: insights on DNA binding in TGF-beta signaling. *Cell*, **94**, 585–94.

107. Kretzschmar, M. and Massague, J. (1998). SMADs: mediators and regulators of TGF-beta signaling. *Curr. Opin. Genet. Devel.*, **8**, 103–11.

108. Berchuck, A., Rodriguez, G.C., Olt, G.J. *et al.* (1992). Regulation of growth of normal ovarian epithelial cells and ovarian cancer cell lines by transforming growth factor-β. *Am. J. Obstet. Gynecol.*, **166**, 676–84.

109. Marth, C., Lang, T., Koza, A. *et al.* (1990). Transforming growth factor-beta and ovarian carcinoma cells: regulation of proliferation and surface antigen expression. *Cancer Lett.*, **51**, 221–5.

110. Bartlett, J.M.S., Rabiasz, G.J., Scott, W.N. *et al.* (1992). Transforming growth factor-β mRNA expression in growth control of human ovarian carcinoma cells. *Br. J. Cancer*, **65**, 655–60.

111. Jozan, S., Guerrin, M., Mazars, P. *et al.* (1992). Transforming growth factor-β–1 (TGF-β–1) inhibits growth of a human a human ovarian cancer cell line (OVCCR–1) and is expressed in human ovarian tumors. *Int. J. Cancer*, **52**, 766–70.

112. Zhou, L.I. and Leung, B.S. (1992). Growth regulation of ovarian cancer cells by epidermal growth factor and transforming growth factors-α and β–1. *Biochem. Biophys. Acta*, **1080**, 130–6.

113. Hurteau, J., Rodriguez, G.C., Whitaker, R.S. *et al.* (1994). Effect of transforming growth factor-β on on proliferation of human ovarian cancer cells obtained from ascites. *Cancer*, **74**, 93–9.

114. Berchuck, A., Kohler, M.F., Marks, J.R. *et al.* (1994). The p53 tumor suppressor gene frequently is altered in gynecologic cancers. *Am. J. Obstet. Gynecol.*, **170**, 246–52.

115. Wang, X.W. and Harris, C.C. (1997). p53 tumor-suppressor gene: clues to molecular carcinogenesis. *J. Cell Physiol.*, **173**, 247–55.

116. Hainaut, P., Hernandez, T., Robinson, A. *et al.* (1998). IARC Database of p53 gene mutations in human tumors and cell lines: updated compilation, revised formats and new visualisation tools. *Nucleic Acids Res.*, **26**, 205–13.

117. Lamb, P. and Crawford, L. (1986). Characterization of the human p53 gene. *Mol. Cell. Biol.*, **6**, 1379–85.

118. Braithwaite, A.W., Sturzbecher, H.W., Addison, C. *et al.* (1987). Mouse p53 inhibits SV40 origin-dependent DNA replication. *Nature*, **329**, 458–60.

119. Rotter, V., Abutbul, H. and Ben Zeev, A. (1983). P53 transformation-related protein accumulates in the nucleus of transformed fibroblasts in association with the chromatin and is found in the cytoplasm of non-transformed fibroblasts. *EMBO J.*, **2**, 1041–7.

120. Kuerbitz, S.J., Plunkett, B.S., Walsh, W.V. and Kastan, M.B. (1992). Wild-type p53 is a cell cycle checkpoint determinant following irradiation. *Proc Natl Acad Sci USA*, **89**, 7491–5.

121. Casey, G., Lopez, M.E., Ramos, J.C. *et al.* (1996). DNA sequence analysis of exons 2 through 11 and immunohistochemical staining are required to detect all known p53 alterations in human malignancies. *Oncogene*, **13**, 1971–81.

122. Marks, J.R., Davidoff, A.M., Kerns, B. *et al.* (1991). Overexpression and mutation of p53 in epithelial ovarian cancer. *Cancer Res.*, **51**, 2979–84.

123. Kohler, M.F., Kerns, B.J., Humphrey, P.A. *et al.* (1993). Mutation and overexpression of p53 in early-stage epithelial ovarian cancer. *Obstet. Gynecol.*, **81**, 643–50.

124. Hartmann, L., Podratz, K., Keeney, G. *et al.* (1994). Prognostic significance of p53 immunostaining in epithelial ovarian cancer. *J. Clin. Oncol.*, **12**, 64–9.

125. Eltabbakh, G.H., Belinson, J.L., Kennedy, A.W. *et al.* (1997). p53 overexpression is not an independent prognostic factor for patients with primary ovarian epithelial cancer. *Cancer*, **80**, 892–8.

126. Henriksen, R., Strang, P., Backstrom, T. *et al.* (1994). Ki–67 immunostaining and DNA flow cytometry as prognostic factors in epithelial ovarian cancers. *Anticancer Res.*, **14**, 603–8.

127. Berns, E.M., Klijn, J.G., van Putten, W.L. *et al.* (1998). p53 protein accumulation predicts poor response to tamoxifen therapy of patients with recurrent breast cancer. *J. Clin. Oncol.*, **16**, 121–7.

128. van der Zee, A.G., Hollema, H., Suurmeijer, A.J. *et al.* (1995). Value of P-glycoprotein, glutathione S-transferase pi, c-erbB–2, and p53 as prognostic factors in ovarian carcinomas. *J. Clin. Oncol.*, **13**, 70–8.

129. Berchuck, A., Kohler, M.F., Hopkins, M.P., *et al.* (1994). Overexpression of the p53 tumor suppressor gene is not a feature of benign and early stage borderline epithelial ovarian tumors. *Gynecol. Oncol.*, **52**, 232–6.

130. Schildkraut, J.M., Bastos, E. and Berchuck, A. (1997). Relationship between lifetime ovulatory cycles and overexpression of mutant p53 in epithelial ovarian cancer. *J. Natl Cancer Inst.*, **89**, 932–8.

131. Kupryjanczyk, J., Thor, A.D., Beauchamp, R. *et al.* (1993). p53 mutations and protein accumulation in human ovarian cancer. *Proc Natl Acad Sci USA*, **90**, 4961–5.

132. Brown, R., Clugston, C., Burns, P. *et al.* (1993). Increased accumulation of p53 protein in cisplatin-resistant ovarian cell lines. *Int. J. Cancer*, **55**, 678–84.

133. Eliopoulos, A.G., Kerr, D.J., Herod, J. *et al.* (1995). The control of apoptosis and drug resistance in ovarian cancer: influence of p53 and Bcl–2. *Oncogen*, **11**, 1217–28.

134. Righetti, S.C., Della, T.G., Pilotti, S. *et al.* (1995). A comparative study of p53 gene mutations, protein accumulation, and response to cisplatin-based chemotherapy in advanced ovarian carcinoma. *Cancer Res.*, **56**, 689–93.

135. Perego, P., Giarola, M., Righetti, S.C. *et al.* (1996). Association between cisplatin resistance and mutation of p53 gene and reduced bax expression in ovarian carcinoma cell systems. *Cancer Res.*, **56**, 556–62.

136. Havrilesky, L.J., Elbendary, A., Hurteau, J.A. *et al.* (1995). Chemotherapy-induced apoptosis in epithelial ovarian cancers. *Obstet. Gynecol.*, **85**, 1007–10.

137. Schildkraut, J.M., Collins, N.K., Dent, G.A. *et al.* (1995). Loss of heterozygosity on chromosome 17q11–21 in cancers of women who have both breast and ovarian cancer. *Am. J. Obstet. Gynecol.*, **172**, 908–13.

138. Takahashi, H., Behbakht, K., McGovern, P.E. *et al.* (1995). Mutation analysis of the BRCA1 gene in ovarian cancers. *Cancer Res.*, **55**, 2998–3002.

139. Merajver, S.D., Pham, T.M., Caduff, R.F. *et al.* (1995). Somatic mutations in the BRCA1 gene in sporadic ovarian tumours. *Nature Genet.*, **9**, 439–43.

140. Hosking, L., Trowsdale, J., Nicolai, H. *et al.* (1995). A somatic BRCA1 mutation in an ovarian tumour. *Nature Genet.*, **9**, 343–4.

141. Futreal, P.A., Liu, Q., Shattuck-Eidens, D. *et al.* (1994). BRCA1 mutations in primary breast and ovarian carcinomas. *Science*, **266**, 120–2.

142. Berchuck, A., Heron, K., Carney, M.E. *et al.* (1998). Frequency of germline and somatic BRCA1 mutations in ovarian cancer. *Clin. Cancer Res.*, **4**, 2433–7.

143. Lancaster, J.M., Wooster, R., Mangion, J. *et al.* (1996). BRCA2 mutations in primary breast and ovarian cancers. *Nature Genet.*, **13**, 1–5.

144. Ewen, M.E. (1998). Regulation of the cell cycle by the Rb tumor suppressor family. *Result Probl. Cell Different.*, **22**, 149–79.

145. Bartek, J., Bartkova, J. and Lukas, J. (1997). The retinoblastoma protein pathway in cell cycle control and cancer. *Exp. Cell Res.*, **237**, 1–6.

146. Sasano, H., Comerford, J., Silverberg, S.G. and Garrett, C.T. An analysis of anormalities of the Retinoblastoma gene in human ovarian and endometrial carcinoma. *Cancer*, **66**, 2150–4.

147. Dodson, M.K., Cliby, W.A., Xu, H.J. *et al.* (1994). Evidence of functional RB protein in epithelial ovarian carcinomas despite loss of heterozygosity at the RB locus. *Cancer Res.*, **54**, 610–13.

148. Kamb, A. (1998). Cyclin-dependent kinase inhibitors and human cancer. *Curr. Top. Microbiol. Immunol.*, **227**, 139–48.

149. Kanuma, T., Nishida, J., Gima, T. *et al.* (1997). Alterations of the p16INK4A gene in human ovarian cancers. *Mol. Carcinog.*, 18, 134–41.

150. Niederacher, D., Yan, H.Y., An, H.X., *et al.* (1999). CDKN2A gene inactivation in epithelial sporadic ovarian cancer. *Br. J. Cancer*, **80**, 1920–6.

151. Schultz, D.C., Vanderveer, L., Buetow, K.H. *et al.* (1995). Characterization of chromosome 9 in human ovarian neoplasia identifies frequent genetic imbalance on 9q and rare alterations involving 9p, including CDKN2. *Cancer Res.*, **55**, 2150–7.

152. Schuyer, M., van Staveren, I.L., Klijn, J.G. *et al.* (1996). Sporadic CDKN2 (MTS1/p16ink4) gene alterations in human ovarian tumours. *Br. J. Cancer*, **74**, 1069–73.

153. Shih, Y.C., Kerr, J., Liu, J. *et al.* (1997). Rare mutations and no hypermethylation at the CDKN2A locus in epithelial ovarian tumours. *Int. J. Cancer*, **70**, 508–11.

154. Ryan, A., Al-Jehani, R.M., Mulligan, K.T., Jacobs, I.J. (1998). No evidence exists for methylation inactivation of the p16 tumor suppressor gene in ovarian carcinogenesis. *Gynecol. Oncol.*, **68**, 14–17.

155. Shigemasa, K., Hu, C., West, C.M. *et al.* (1997). p16 overexpression: a potential early indicator of transformation in ovarian carcinoma. *J. Soc. Gynecol. Investig.*, **4**, 95–102.

156. Kamijo, T., Weber, J.D., Zambetti, G. *et al.* (1998). Functional and physical interactions of the ARF tumor suppressor with p53 and Mdm2. *Proc Natl Acad Sci USA*, **95**, 8292–7.

157. Masciullo, V., Sgambato, A., Pacilio, C. *et al.* (1999). Frequent loss of expression of the cyclin-dependent kinase inhibitor p27 in epithelial ovarian cancer. *Cancer Res.*, **59**, 3790–4.

158. Sui, L., Tokuda, M., Ohno, M. *et al.* (1999). The concurrent expression of p27(kip1) and cyclin D1 in epithelial ovarian tumors. *Gynecol. Oncol.*, **73**, 202–9.

159. Worsley, S.D., Ponder, B.A., Davies, B.R. (1997). Overexpression of cyclin D1 in epithelial ovarian cancers. *Gynecol. Oncol.*, **64**, 189–95.

160. Session, D.R., Lee, G.S., Choi, J. and Wolgemuth, D.J. (1999). Expression of cyclin E in gynecologic malignancies. *Gynecol. Oncol.*, **72**, 32–7.

4. Overview of the aetiology of familial ovarian cancer

Ronald P. Zweemer

Introduction

Ovarian cancer represents the fourth or fifth most significant cause of cancer-related deaths and is the most frequent cause of death from gynaecological malignancy in the western world. In the UK approximately 5000 new cases are diagnosed each year.[1] The first report on ovarian cancer suggesting a possible inherited predisposition for the disease, by Kimbrough in 1929, describes a case of 'coincident carcinoma of the ovary in twins'.[2] In the 1980s Lynch *et al.* described several families with a high genetic risk for ovarian cancer, based on family studies.[3] At the same time, the first familial ovarian cancer registry was set up. The Gilda Radner Familial Ovarian Cancer Registry has provided a valuable database for further studies.

Approximately 1% of women are affected by ovarian cancer; some families will therefore have a history of ovarian cancer in two or more relatives, just by chance. Some 15% of all ovarian cancer patients thus report a positive family history for the disease. These familial cases of ovarian cancer could be explained by chance, common lifestyle or exposure to carcinogenic factors, or shared genetic susceptibility. An estimated 10% of all ovarian cancers are currently thought to be the result of a highly penetrant autosomal dominant susceptibility factor. The two major genetic targets of hereditary ovarian cancer have now been identified as the tumour suppressor genes *BRCA1* and *BRCA2*. It is estimated that some 95% of all hereditary ovarian cancers are linked to either of these two genes; however, little is still known about the genetic events occurring in the initiation and progression of BRCA-related ovarian cancer. This chapter aims to provide an overview on the aetiology of hereditary ovarian cancer.

Characteristics of hereditary ovarian cancer families

Evidence for a hereditary component in ovarian cancer was derived from three observations. First, a family history of ovarian cancer has long been recognized as the greatest risk factor for developing the disease[4,5] besides age. This effect is especially strong in families with more than one relative affected. Where the population risk of ovarian cancer is approximately 1 : 80, the risk increases to 1 : 30 when one first-degree relative is affected (mother or sister) and may be as high as 1 : 4 when two first-degree relatives are affected.[6] Secondly, population-based epidemiological studies have shown that there is a significant excess risk of several types of cancer among the relatives of ovarian cancer patients; these include breast cancer, colorectal, and stomach cancer.[7] Finally, several case reports have described families in which the occurrence of ovarian cancer, sometimes in combination with other types of cancer, appears to follow a pattern of autosomal dominant inheritance.[3] When such families are evaluated, three distinct clinical patterns of familial ovarian cancer can be recognized:

(1) hereditary breast–ovarian cancer (HBOC)—families with a pattern of autosomal dominant inheritance of ovarian and (usually early onset) breast cancer;
(2) hereditary ovarian cancer (HOC)—families with clear autosomal dominant inheritance of ovarian cancer, but without apparent excess of breast cancer; and
(3) hereditary non-polyposis colorectal cancer (HNPCC)—families with an autosomal dominant pattern of early onset colorectal cancer, often in combination with endometrial cancer and sometimes ovarian cancer.

Since it has become clear that mutations in the *BRCA1* and *BRCA2* genes are responsible for the majority of both HBOC and HOC families, the clinical distinction between these two syndromes may have become obsolete

The hereditary (breast–) ovarian cancer syndrome

Proof that a genetic predisposition is responsible for familial clustering of ovarian cancer can only be established by demonstration of an underlying gene defect. Genetic studies into the cause of hereditary breast–ovarian cancer started with linkage analysis of several families by the Breast Cancer Linkage Consortium. Linkage analysis demonstrates the co-segregation of a specific genetic marker and the disease. In 1990, Hall *et al.* identified a susceptibility locus on chromosome 17q21 in a study of 23 families with autosomal dominant breast cancer.[8] The same locus was confirmed to show linkage to the ovarian and breast cancer cases in five large HBOC families.[9] The second step in proving the hereditary nature of ovarian cancer in these families was provided by the identification of a putative tumour suppressor gene, named BReast CAncer 1 (*BRCA1*).[10] Finally, if the gene which predisposes to (breast and) ovarian cancer is a tumour suppressor gene, based on Knudsen's hypothesis, it would be expected that a tumour from a mutation carrier would show loss of heterozygosity (LOH) of the wild-type (normal) *BRCA*-allele. In a study of four breast ovarian cancer families Smith *et al.*[11] indeed found that all nine tumours in these families showed allelic loss of the wild-type *BRCA1* allele.

BRCA1

The *BRCA1* gene consists of 22 coding exons distributed over 100 kb of genomic DNA. It has 5592 bp of coding sequence and encodes a protein of 1863 amino acids. To date more than 300 distinct mutations have been described, scattered throughout the gene. Although there are some well-defined founder mutations,[12,13] there are no specific hot spots in the gene and only a minority of mutations are recurrent. Approximately 80% of all mutations are nonsense or frameshift mutations, causing a truncation of the protein. It has been suggested that the position of the mutation may influence penetrance as well as tissue specificity. Gayther *et al.*[14] found a significant correlation between the localization of the mutation in the gene and the ratio of breast and ovarian cancers within a family. Mutations in the 3' third of the gene were associated with a lower risk of ovarian cancer. The findings have not been confirmed by subsequent studies. In the Ashkenazi Jewish population, two *BRCA1* founder mutations are common: 185delAG and 5382insC. From a study of 5318 subjects, the estimated risk of breast and ovarian cancer was found to be 56% and 16% for breast and ovarian cancer by the age of 70 years, respectively. A second study[15] found even lower penetrance for breast cancer: 36% for these mutations. These results differ markedly from previous estimates based on high-risk cancer families, where the risk of ovarian cancer for *BRCA1* mutation carriers was estimated at 40–60%.[16,17] It is important to realize, however, that the studies in the Ashkenazi Jewish population were performed without selection on the basis of a strong family history. It is very well possible that environmental circumstances and/or modifier genes may influence the penetrance of a specific type of cancer between and within families. Phelan *et al.*[18] suggested that the risk of ovarian cancer in women with a *BRCA1* mutation might be increased for those who carry one of two rare variants of the *HRAS* variable number of tandem repeats (VNTR) compared to women with the common allele. The same rare *HRAS* allele may also predispose to ovarian cancer in the general population.[19] An 'environmental' influence on the penetrance of *BRCA* mutations was shown by Narod *et al.*,[20] who studied 207 patients with *BRCA1* or *BRCA2* mutations and ovarian cancer, and compared oral contraceptive use with sisters who served as controls. Their findings suggested that the use of oral contraceptives protects against ovarian cancer in carriers of *BRCA* mutations.

Localization and cloning of the second BReast CAncer gene, *BRCA2*, soon followed the identification of *BRCA1*.

BRCA2

In 1994, Wooster *et al.* localized the second breast–ovarian cancer gene at chromosome 13q12–13 in a study of 15 high-risk breast cancer families that were unlinked to *BRCA1*.[21] Only months later, the same group identified the gene by showing segregation of inactivating mutations of mostly breast cancer in families linked with the 13q locus.[22] The *BRCA2* gene consists of 26 coding exons distributed over approximately 70 kb of genomic DNA. It has 10 254 bp of coding sequence and encodes a protein of 3418 amino acids, which has little homology to previously identified proteins.[23] To date, some 100 distinct mutations have been described and, as is the case for *BRCA1*, these are scattered throughout the coding sequence and, apart from several distinct founder mutations,[24,25] there are no specific hot spots. The most frequent type of *BRCA2* mutations are frameshifts, most commonly deletions. It appears that missense mutations are rarer than in *BRCA1*. The contribution of *BRCA2* to hereditary breast cancer (HBC) appears to be similar to the contribution of *BRCA1*, whereas only a minority of cases of HBOC and HOC are caused by *BRCA2* germline mutations. Although the overall penetrance for ovarian cancer in *BRCA2* germline mutation carriers is estimated at approximately 25%,[17] Gayther *et al.*[26] found evidence for an 'ovarian cancer cluster-region' (OCCR) in exon 11. Mutations in this OCCR were suggested to confer a higher risk of ovarian cancer.

The *BRCA2* gene appears to be subject to frequent sequence variation, thus complicating the distinction between disease-associated mutations and sequence variants that are not associated with disease. Wagner *et al.*[27] found 82 sequence variants, of which 79 were not obviously associated with disease whereas eight sequence variants of unknown significance were specific to breast–ovarian cancer families and were not detected in controls.

Ford *et al.*[17] evaluated the contribution of both *BRCA1* and *BRCA2* to the total hereditary breast–ovarian cancer burden and found that the majority (81%) of hereditary breast–ovarian cancer families were due to *BRCA1*. An additional 14% was estimated to be due to *BRCA2*. Of hereditary breast cancer cases, 16% could not be explained by either *BRCA1* or *BRCA2*, suggesting a role for a third breast cancer susceptibility gene. For hereditary ovarian cancer, however, only 5% remain unexplained.

The function of BRCA1 and BRCA2

Studies of the function of *BRCA1* and *BRCA2* are still in their infancy. The report of a normal woman who inherited two mutant copies of the *BRCA1* gene indicates that *BRCA1* is probably not required for normal growth and development.[28] The genes function as tumour suppressor genes, since the wild-type copy is invariably deleted in the tumour of BRCA-related breast and ovarian cancer patients.[11] The 7.8kb *BRCA1* mRNA transcript is expressed most abundantly in the testis and thymus and, at lower levels in the breast and ovary. The *BRCA2* mRNA transcript shows a similar tissue-specific expression.[23,29] Chen *et al.*[30] found a 220kDa nuclear phosphoprotein to be the *BRCA1* gene product. They localized the protein mainly in the cytoplasm. Others have localized the *BRCA1* protein in the perinuclear compartment of the endoplasmic reticulum–Golgi complex and inside cytoplasmic tubes invaginating the nucleus,[31] thus suggesting a role in the cell cycle. Although *BRCA1* and *BRCA2* are unrelated at the sequence level, there are some intriguing similarities. Both have a large exon 11, which contains more than half of the coding sequence. In both genes, translation starts at codon 2 and both are relatively A–T rich. Defining the biochemical and biological functions that are responsible for tumorigenesis in large genes such as *BRCA1* and *BRCA2* has proven to be difficult. Both genes probably have several functional domains. The presence of a 'zinc-finger' motif suggests a role as a transcription factor for the *BRCA1* protein. *BRCA2* also has homology with known transcription factors.[32] Association of *BRCA1* and *BRCA2* with the DNA repair gene *RAD51* indicates that the genes may be cofactors in the Rad51-dependent DNA repair of double-strand breaks. Recent studies have shown a physical association between *BRCA1* and p53 and suggested that they may be cooperatively involved in the apoptosis of cancer cells.[33] Finally. it has been suggested that the BRCA proteins possess the properties of a 'granin' and are secreted in secretory vesicles;[34] granins have thus far only been identified in (neuro) endocrine processes and are unknown in other tumour suppressor genes.

In summary, both *BRCA1* and *BRCA2* are probably involved in specific pathways of DNA repair. Both are likely to be involved in specific carcinogenic pathways in conjunction with other genes. *BRCA1* and *BRCA2* were, for example, found to bind and complex with Rad51, a protein involved in the repair of double-strand DNA breaks.[35,36] The inactivation of *BRCA1* or *BRCA2* may therefore lead to an increased frequency of DNA breaks, leading to alteration of other genes involved in growth regulation and transformation.[37]

An alternative insight into the function of *BRCA1* and *BRCA2* has been provided by Kinzler and Vogelstein.[38] In contrast with the distinction between oncogenes and tumour suppressor genes, they made a distinction between gatekeeper genes and caretaker genes in the determination of cancer. Gatekeepers are genes that regulate the growth of tumours directly, by inhibiting cell growth or promoting cell death. Each cell type has only one (or a few) gatekeepers, and inactivation of the given gatekeeper leads to a very specific tissue distribution of cancer; for example, inherited mutations of the retinoblastoma (RB1), von Hippel–Lindau (VHL), neurofibromatosis type I (NF1), and adenomatous polyposis coli (APC) genes lead to tumours of the retina, kidney, Schwann cells, and colon, respectively. Both the maternal and the paternal copies of the gene must be altered for tumour development. It is in connection with these gatekeeper, or tumour suppressor, genes that the Knudson two-hit hypothesis was advanced. In contrast, inactivation of a caretaker gene does not promote tumour initiation directly. Rather, neoplasia occurs indirectly; inactivation leads to genetic instability that results in increased mutation of all genes, including gatekeepers. Once a tumour is initiated by inactivation of a gatekeeper gene, it may progress rapidly due to an accelerated rate of mutation in other genes that directly control cell birth or death. Known caretaker genes include the nucleotide-excision-repair genes that are responsible for xeroderma pigmentosum and mismatch-repair genes that cause HNPCC. Kinzler and Vogelstein proposed that *BRCA1* and *BRCA2* should be added to the list of caretaker genes. Consistent with this hypothesis, mutations in *BRCA1* and *BRCA2* are rarely found in sporadic cancers, and the risk of cancer arising in people with *BRCA* mutations is relatively low. The distinction between gatekeepers and caretakers has important practical, as well as theoretical, ramifications. Tumours that have defective caretaker genes present an additional therapeutic target. Such tumours would be expected to respond favourably to therapeutic agents that reduce the type of genomic damage that is normally detected or repaired by the particular caretaker gene involved.

HNPCC-associated hereditary ovarian cancer

Hereditary non-polyposis colorectal cancer (HNPCC) is characterized by the autosomal dominant inheritance of early onset colorectal cancer, without the multiple adenomas that constitute familial adenomatous polyposis (FAP). Endometrial cancer is relatively common in HNPCC families and should be considered part of the syndrome. Other cancers, including epithelial ovarian cancer, are encountered in HNPCC families, but are infrequent. Germline mutations in one of five mismatch repair genes are responsible for the syndrome. *hMSH2* (chromosome 2p), *hMLH1* (chromosome 3p), *hPMS1* (chromosome 2q), *hPMS2* (chromosome 7p), and *hMSH6* (chromosome 2p) are all part of a family of genes involved in the repair of DNA-replication errors. Froggatt *et al.*[39] calculated age-related risks of colorectal, endometrial, and ovarian cancers in 76 carriers of a common *MSH2* mutation. The penetrance at age 60 years for all cancers was 86%. For colorectal cancer, penetrance was estimated at 57%. There was a high risk of endometrial cancer (50% at age 60 years) and premenopausal ovarian cancer (20% at 50 years). Tumours arising in patients with germline mutations in one of the mismatch repair genes are, in the vast majority of cases, genetically unstable and have an RER (replication error) phenotype which can easily be detected by studying somatic length alterations in simple nucleotide repeat sequences. In contrast with ovarian cancers in the hereditary breast ovarian cancer syndrome, tumours of HNPCC patients therefore have a specific genetic characteristic, which suggests the underlying cause of the disease. Although mutations in all five genes have been detected in HNPCC-related colorectal cancers, 90% of mutations occur in either the *hMSH2* or *hMLH1* gene. Mutation detection of these genes is particularly arduous since they are large—2.2–2.8 kb of coding sequence—and, as for *BRCA1* and *BRCA2* mutations, are not confined to specific hot spots. The contribution of germline mutations in one of these five mismatch-repair (MMR) genes to the total burden of hereditary ovarian cancer is limited, and probably accounts for less than 2% of hereditary ovarian cancer cases.

Characteristics of hereditary ovarian cancer patients

The initial studies on hereditary breast–ovarian cancer were performed on highly selected, large families with many affected and unaffected relatives. Linkage analysis is usually not suitable for clinical practice because most families are small and, especially in the case of ovarian cancer, family members have often died. The cloning of BRCA1 and BRCA2 allows direct mutation analysis in individual patients. It has therefore become possible to investigate the role of these genes in a much larger group of families with possible hereditary ovarian cancer. Since the cloning of BRCA1 and BRCA2, it has proved to be difficult to predict the presence of a BRCA1 or BRCA2 mutation in a specific family. This is due partly to the sensitivity of the presently available tests. More importantly, however, the familial pattern of ovarian (and/or breast) cancer is often inconclusive. It has been shown that BRCA1 and BRCA2 together are responsible for 95% of families with an autosomal dominant pattern of inheritance,[17] usually defined as families with three or more first-degree relatives affected in two successive generations. However, BRCA1 and BRCA2 mutations have also been detected in seemingly sporadic cases of ovarian cancer, and are relatively common in families with some familial clustering of the disease. In these situations the question arises whether individual characteristics of ovarian cancer patients may indicate hereditary disease.

Studies to characterize the clinical characteristics of hereditary ovarian cancer are few, especially when compared to hereditary breast cancer. Such studies are complicated to perform. First, ovarian cancer is relatively uncommon. The risk of developing breast cancer in a patient with a BRCA1 or BRCA2 mutation is at least two times the ovarian cancer risk. In addition, the studies that are performed are often difficult to compare. Some studies have defined hereditary ovarian cancer clinically, based on the number of affected relatives in a given family. Other studies have only included BRCA1 or BRCA2 mutation carriers, disregarding family history. The first are likely to have included so-called phenocopies in their analyses. A phenocopy is a coincidental case within a family with a hereditary predisposition. The second type of study may include cases with mutations of unknown penetrance. Finally, selection bias is difficult to avoid in any study of hereditary cancer, as families with specific characteristics, such as unusually young age of onset or unfavourable survival, are more likely to come forward for genetic evaluation.

Age at diagnosis

Cancer resulting from a hereditary predisposition is often manifested at a relatively young age. It is thought that patients who have already inherited a genetic defect require fewer additional (somatic) genetic events for the development of a malignancy. Several studies have found that this does not apply for ovarian cancer.[40–42] Other studies have found differences in age of onset of ovarian cancer.[43–45] In the latter studies an earlier age of onset of approximately 8 years was found for hereditary cases.

Survival

Several studies have investigated survival of patients with hereditary ovarian cancer, and the results have been conflicting. A study by Rubin et al.[44] found a median survival of 77 months in 43 BRCA1 mutation carriers with ovarian cancers, compared to 29 months for age- and stage-matched controls. No other study has found such highly statistically significant differences. The study has been much criticized because of the possibility of surveillance bias and the likelihood of differences in treatment strategies for both groups. A recent study by Pharoah et al.[46] has found the opposite. Hereditary cases, with and without proven mutations, had a statistically significant worse survival rate. A third study, by Johannsson et al.,[47] of 38 BRCA1 mutation carriers found a similar (when matched for age and stage) or better (when not matched) survival in hereditary cases for the first 2.5 years, after which survival for hereditary cases was worse.

Histopathological characteristics

Most ovarian tumours (80–90%) are epithelial in origin and arise from the coelomic epithelium. The remainder arise from germ cell or sex cord/stromal cells. A hereditary component in the latter group is rare and includes granulosa-cell tumours in patients with the Peutz–Jeghers syndrome.[48] BRCA1 and BRCA2, as well as HNPCC-related, ovarian cancer cases have consistently been found to be epithelial in origin. Piver et al., in 1993, were the first to suggest that mucinous carcinomas of the ovary are underrepresented in hereditary ovarian cancer cases.[49] Other studies have since confirmed this finding and have shown that hereditary ovarian cancers are more often of the serous type.[41,43,44,50,51] Some authors also describe an overrepresentation of endometrioid carcinoma.[41] Hereditary breast cancers have been found to be characterized by a lower mean aneuploidy index, higher proliferation rates, and high S-phase fractions.[52] For ovarian cancer such quantitative pathological differences have not been described. A relatively high frequency of poorly differentiated ovarian tumours has been described in hereditary disease.[47] Grading ovarian carcinoma is notoriously difficult, and different grading systems are in use. Therefore it is difficult to compare data on grade in hereditary ovarian cancer with controls, often derived from cancer registries.

A study of our own group revealed a more advanced stage of disease at the time of diagnosis (30 families), a finding recently confirmed by Pharoah et al.[46]

Somatic genetic events in the carcinogenesis of hereditary ovarian cancer

Cancer is caused by abnormalities in the genetic mechanisms that control cellular growth and proliferation. Usually such genetic abnormalities are acquired, but in patients with a genetic predisposition to cancer, a genetic alteration is inherited. There is strong evidence that carcinogenesis is a multistep process with an estimated 4–6 steps required for a detectable tumour to develop. Molecular genetic analyses of malignant tumours consistently reveal a multitude of genetic abnormalities. Especially in colonic cancer, it has been shown that the critical factor for the development of a malignancy is the accumulation of specific mutations in oncogenes and tumour suppressor genes.

With the observation that hereditary ovarian cancer is usually due to an inherited mutation in either the BRCA1 or BRCA2 tumour suppressor gene, it was anticipated that somatic (non-hereditary) BRCA1 and BRCA2 mutations would be as important in the development of sporadic ovarian cancer. However, fewer somatic mutations in BRCA1 or BRCA2 have been identified than was anticipated, suggesting a fundamental molecular difference between hereditary and sporadic ovarian cancer. Both BRCA1 and BRCA2 function as tumour suppressor genes, and the development of a cancer is thought to require an accumulation of somatic genetic events in addition to the inherited germline predisposition. Loss of the wild-type allele is likely to be an early, initiating event, but little is still known about the nature or frequency of subsequent events in initiation and progression of ovarian cancers associated with BRCA germline mutations. It is possible that the somatic genetic events that occur in sporadic ovarian cancer are similar to those in BRCA-associated cancers. Alternatively, a germline BRCA mutation may represent a separate pathway of molecular carcinogenesis associated with distinct somatic genetic events.

To unravel the pathway of carcinogenesis in hereditary ovarian cancer, studies have been performed to compare the somatic genetic events occurring in hereditary and sporadic ovarian cancer. Studies of BRCA-related breast cancer compared to sporadic breast cancer may occasionally be of interest in this repeat.

The p53 gene

The p53 tumour suppressor gene has recently been under investigation for a possible relation with BRCA1 and/or BRCA2 in hereditary cancer. These studies initiated from the observation that a mutation in p53 is the most frequent somatic molecular event in sporadic ovarian cancer. A number of studies have reported a high frequency of p53 overexpression and/or mutations in ovarian cancer, varying from 15% in early stages up to 81% in advanced stages.[53,54] Missense mutations are the most common mutations of the p53 gene[54] and a strong correlation between such mutations and immunohistochemical staining has been found. Immunohistochemically detected p53 overexpression has been studied by Auranen et al.[55] in a cohort of ovarian cancer patients with a positive family history and sporadic controls. No differences were detected in p53 overexpression between familial and sporadic cases. Unfortunately, mutation analysis for BRCA1 and BRCA2 was not performed in this study, and since most familial cases in the study had only one other relative with ovarian cancer, the study group is likely to be diluted with patients who do not have such mutations.

In contrast with this study, an analysis of p53 in BRCA-related breast cancers revealed a very high prevalence of somatic p53 mutations. Crook et al.[56] studied seven breast cancers and one ovarian cancer in four families with a known BRCA1 mutation and found somatic p53 mutations in all. It was postulated that a somatic p53 mutation might be a prerequisite for tumour development in BRCA1 germline mutation carriers. There is additional evidence for this notion from recent experimental data.[57] However, a similar clinical study by Schlichtholz et al.[58] could not confirm these findings as p53 mutations were detected in only 3 out of 14 BRCA1-related breast cancers.

Little research has been performed into the relation between somatic p53 mutations and germline BRCA mutations in ovarian cancer. Our group has recently studied p53 overexpression by immunohistochemistry in 30 ovarian cancer patients with BRCA1 and nine with BRCA2 germline mutations. Immunostaining was compared with sporadic ovarian cancer cases, which were tested and found negative for BRCA1 and BRCA2 germline mutations. A similar rate of p53 overexpression was detected in BRCA1- and BRCA2-related ovarian cancers, compared to BRCA1- and BRCA2-negative controls.[59] Not all p53 mutations result in protein overexpression that can be detected immunohistochemically. Insertion, deletion, nonsense, splice site, and missense mutations outside exons 5 through 9 may result in weak or negative immunohistochemical staining.[60,61] Therefore possible differences in the distribution of this type of mutations may have been missed by studying immunohistochemical staining alone. Only one study has included p53 mutation analysis in addition to immunohistochemistry.[62] p53 mutations were detected in 80% of BRCA-related ovarian cancers, which is higher than the expected rate of approximately 55% in sporadic ovarian cancer. The spectrum of p53 mutations detected was unremarkable compared with those seen in sporadic ovarian cancer, single nucleotide substitutions were most common, with more transitions than transversions. Interestingly, there was a statistically significant greater fraction of nucleotide insertions and deletions in BRCA2-related ovarian cancers (5/8) compared with BRCA1-related cases (3/24). It is uncertain, however, whether data from this study are representative of all BRCA1 mutations, since 20 of the 29 BRCA1-related ovarian cancer cases harboured the same 185delAG founder mutation and all 11 BRCA2 mutations were of the 6174delT type. From the limited data available, it seems likely that p53 is a common, but probably not critical, somatic genetic event in hereditary BRCA-related ovarian carcinogenesis.

The role of other genes commonly involved in (sporadic) ovarian cancer

Little is known about the role of specific oncogenes such as HER–2/neu and K-ras in hereditary ovarian cancer. From the available data it is likely that mutations and/or overexpression are rare in BRCA-related tumours. Rhei et al.[62] found no mutations in codon 12 or 13 of the K-ras oncogene after sequencing 40 BRCA1- and BRCA2-related ovarian cancers. The prevalence of such mutations in unselected ovarian cancer cases is generally considered to be around 5–10%. It is noteworthy, however, that K-ras mutations are more common in mucinous and borderline ovarian tumours than in invasive serous tumours. Since almost all *BRCA*-related ovarian cancers are of the serous type, a low prevalence of K-*ras* mutations can be expected and a histologically matched case-control study would be required to compare the true prevalence of K-*ras* mutations in hereditary and sporadic ovarian cancer.

HER2/*neu* overexpression was observed by Auranen et al.[55] in 70% of familial cases, which is significantly higher than that reported for unselected ovarian cancer. Although overexpression as detected by immunohistochemistry may be the result of gene amplification, immunostaining also has been demonstrated in the absence of gene amplification. Rhei et al.[62] used a semiquantitative differential PCR to assess HER2/*neu* expression and found no evidence of amplification among 40 *BRCA*-related ovarian cancers. There was no amplification of, c-*myc* or *AKT2* either.

These data suggest that hereditary *BRCA*-related ovarian cancer may differ from sporadic ovarian cancer with respect to the involvement of specific tumour suppressor and oncogenes. It is likely that they share a specific, but limited spectrum of somatic genetic alterations in several genes, including *p53*, but not including other genes such as K-*ras* and HER2/*neu*.

Genome-wide comparison of hereditary and sporadic ovarian cancer

The relatively new technique of comparative genomic hybridization (CGH) enables a genome-wide search for chromosomal regions that have either an increased in copy number (amplification or gain) or are lost in a given tumour. Regions showing gain may harbour oncogenes involved in the carcinogenesis of the tumour, whereas regions with losses may contain a tumour suppressor gene(s). The technique is based on the competitive hybridization of tumour and control DNA on normal metaphase chromosomes.[63] Although CGH enables genome-wide screening for chromosomal gains and losses, the minimal size of detection is approximately 10 Mb. Smaller chromosomal losses or gains will therefore be missed. Recently Tapper et al.[64] performed a CGH-analysis on 16 *BRCA1*- and four *BRCA2*-related ovarian cancers and compared these results with a stage- and grade-matched sporadic control group. Their results revealed a striking similarity between sporadic and *BRCA*-related cases, with the exception of a region on chromosome 2q where the *BRCA1*-related tumours showed more gains. It is difficult to speculate about which gene might be responsible for this finding. Chromosome 2q harbours a large number of genes that could potentially be involved in cancer initiation and progression.

References

1. Office of Population Censuses, and Surveys (1994). *Cancer Statistics Registrations 1989.* Her Majesty's Stationery Office, London.
2. Kimbrough, R.A. (1929). Coincidental carcinoma of the ovary in twins. *J. Obstset. Gynecol.*, 18, 148–9.
3. Lynch, H.T., Albano, W.A., Lynch, J.F. *et al.* (1982). Surveillance and management of patients of high genetic risk for ovarian carcinoma. *Obstet. Gynecol.*, 59, 589–96.
4. Lurain, J.R. and Piver, M.S. (1979). Familial ovarian cancer. *Gynecol. Oncol.*, 8, 185–92.
5. Boyd, J. and Rubin, S.C. (1997). Hereditary ovarian cancer: molecular genetics and clinical implications. *Gynecol. Oncol.*, 64, 196–206.
6. Schildkraut, J.M. and Thompson, W.D. (1988). Familial ovarian cancer: a population-based control study. *Am. J. Epidemiol.*, 128, 456–66.
7. Ponder, B.A.J. (1996). Familial ovarian cancer. In *Genetic predisposition to cancer*, (ed. R.A. Eeles, B.A.J. Ponder, D.F. Easton and A. Horwich), pp. 290–6. Chapman & Hall, London.
8. Hall, J.M. Lee, M.K. Newman, B. *et al.* (1990). Linkage of early-onset familial breast cancer to chromosome 17q21. *Science*, 250, 1684–9.
9. Narod, S.A. Feunteun, J., Lynch, H.T. *et al.* (1991). Familial breast–ovarian cancer locus on chromosome 17q12–q23. *Lancet*, 338, 82–3.
10. Miki, Y., Swensen, J., Shattuck-Eidens, D. *et al.* (1994). A strong candidate for the breast and ovarian cancer susceptibility gene BRCA1. *Science*, 266, 66–71.
11. Smith, S.A. Easton, D.F. Evans, D.G. and Ponder, B.A. (1992). Allele losses in the region 17q12–21 in familial breast and ovarian cancer involve the wild-type chromosome. *Nature Genet.*, 2, 128–31.
12. Struewing, J.P., Abeliovich, D., Peretz, T. *et al.* (1995). The carrier frequency of the BRCA1 185delAG mutation is approximately 1 percent in Ashkenazi Jewish individuals. *Nature Genet.*, 11, 198–200.
13. Peelen, T., van Vliet, V.M., Petrij-Bosch, A. *et al.* (1997). High proportion of novel mutations in BRCA1 with strong founder effects among Dutch and Belgian hereditary breast and ovarian cancer families. *Am. J. Hum. Genet.*, 60, 1041–9.
14. Gayther, S.A., Warren, W., Mazoyer, S. *et al.* (1995). Germline mutations of the BRCA1 gene in breast and ovarian cancer families provide evidence for a genotype-phenotype correlation. *Nature Genet.*, 11, 428–33.
15. Fodor, F.H., Weston, A., Bleiweiss, I.J. *et al.* (1998). Frequency and carrier risk associated with common BRCA1 and BRCA2 mutations in Ashkenazi Jewish breast cancer patients. *Am. J. Hum. Genet.*, 63, 45–51.
16. Ford, D., Easton, D.F., Bishop, D.T. *et al.* (1994). Risks of cancer in BRCA1-mutation carriers. Breast Cancer Linkage Consortium. *Lancet*, 343, 692–5.
17. Ford, D., Easton, D.F., Stratton, M. *et al.* (1998). Genetic heterogeneity and penetrance analysis of the BRCA1 and BRCA2 genes in breast cancer families. The Breast Cancer Linkage Consortium. *Am. J. Hum. Genet.*, 62, 676–89.
18. Phelan, C.M., Rebbeck, T.R., Weber, B.L. *et al.* (1996). Ovarian cancer risk in BRCA1 carriers is modified by the HRAS1 variable number of tandem repeat (VNTR) locus. *Nature Genet.*, 12, 309–11.
19. Weitzel, J.N. Ding, S., Larson, G.P. *et al.* (2000). The HRAS1 minisatelite locus and risk of ovarian cancer. *Cancer Res.*, 60, 259–61.
20. Narod, S.A., Risch, H., Moslehi, R. *et al.* (1998). Hereditary Ovarian Cancer Clinical Study Group. Oral contraceptives and the risk of hereditary ovarian cancer. *N. Engl. J. Med.*, 339, 424–8.
21. Wooster, R., Neuhausen, S.L., Mangion, J. *et al.* (1994). Localization of a breast cancer susceptibility gene, BRCA2, to chromosome 13q12–13. *Science*, 265, 2088–90.
22. Wooster, R., Bignell, G., Lancaster, J. *et al.* (1995). Identification of the breast cancer susceptibility gene BRCA2. *Nature*, 378, 789–92.
23. Tavtigian, S.V., Simard, J., Rommens, J. *et al.* (1996). The complete BRCA2 gene and mutations in chromosome 13q-linked kindreds. *Nature Genet.*, 12, 333–7.
24. Levy-Lahad, E., Catane, R., Eisenberg, S. *et al.* (1997). Founder BRCA1 and BRCA2 mutations in Ashkenazi Jews in Israel: frequency and differential penetrance in ovarian cancer and in breast–ovarian cancer families. *Am. J. Hum. Genet.*, 60, 1059–67.
25. Thorlacius, S., Sigurdsson, S., Bjarnadottir, H. *et al.* (1997). Study of a single BRCA2 mutation with high carrier frequency in a small population. *Am. J. Hum. Genet.*, 60, 1079–84.
26. Gayther, S.A., Mangion, J., Russell, P. *et al.* (1997). Variation of risks of breast and ovarian cancer associated with different germline mutations of the BRCA2 gene. *Nature Genet.*, 15, 103–5.
27. Wagner, T.M.U., Hirtenlehner, K., Shen, P. *et al.* (1999). Global sequence diversity of BRCA2: analysis of 71 breast cancer families and 95 control individuals of worldwide populations. *Hum. Molec. Genet.*, 8, 413–23.

28. Boyd, M., Harris, F., McFarlane, R. *et al.* (1995). A human BRCA1 gene knockout. *Nature*, **375**, 541–2.

29. Sharan, S.K. and Bradley, A. (1997a). Murine Brca2: sequence, map position, and expression pattern. *Genomics*, **40**, 234–41.

30. Chen, Y., Chen, C.-F., Riley, D.J. *et al.* (1995). Aberrant subcellular localization of BRCA1 in breast cancer. *Science*, **270**, 789–91.

31. Coene, E., Van Oostveldt, P., Willems, K. *et al.* (1997). BRCA1 is localized in cytoplasmic tube-like invaginations in the nucleus. [Letter]*Nature Genet.*, **116**, 122–4.

32. Milner, J., Ponder, B., Hughes-Davies, L. *et al.* (1997). Transcriptional activation functions in BRCA2. *Nature*, **386**, 772–3.

33. Zhang, H., Somasundaram, K., Peng, Y. *et al.* (1998). Brca1 physically associates with p53 and stimulates its transcriptional activity. *Oncogene*, **16**, 1713–21.

34. Jensen, R.A. Thompson, M.E. Jetton, T.L. *et al.* (1996). BRCA1 is secreted and exhibits properties of a granin. *Nature Genet.*, **12**, 303–8.

35. Scully, R., Chen, J., Plug, A. *et al.* (1997). Association of BRCA1 with Rad51 in mitotic and meiotic cells. *Cell*, **88**, 265–75.

36. Sharan, S.K., Morimatsu, M., Albrecht, U. *et al.* (1997). Embryonic lethality and radiation hypersensitivity mediated by Rad51 in mice lacking Brca2. *Nature*, **386**, 804–10.

37. Berchuck, A., Schildkraut, J.M., Marks, J.R. and Futreal, P.A. (1999). Managing hereditary ovarian cancer risk. *Cancer (supplement)*, **86**, 1697–704.

38. Kinzler, K.W. and Vogelstein, B. (1997). Gatekeepers and caretakers. *Nature*, **386**, 761–3.

39. Froggatt, N.J., Green, J., Brassett, C. *et al.* (1999). A common MSH2 mutation in English and North American HNPCC families: origin, phenotypic expression, and sex specific differences in colorectal cancer. *J. Med. Genet.*, **36**, 97–102.

40. Greggi, S., Genuardi, M., Benedetti-Panici, P. *et al.* (1990). Analysis of 138 consecutive ovarian cancer patients: incidence and characteristics of familial cases. *Gynecol. Oncol.*, **39**, 300–4.

41. Chang, J., Fryatt, I., Ponder, B. *et al.* (1995). A matched control study of familial epithelial ovarian cancer: patient characteristics, response to chemotherapy and outcome. *Ann. Oncol.*, **6**, 80–2.

42. Narod, S.A., Madlenski, L., Bradley, L. *et al.* (1994). Hereditary and familial ovarian cancer in Southern Ontario. *Cancer*, **74**, 2341–6.

43. Bewtra, C., Watson, P., Conway, T. *et al.* (1992). Hereditary ovarian cancer: A clinicopathological study. *Int. J. Gynecol. Pathol.*, **11**, 180–7.

44. Rubin, S.C., Benjamin, I., Behbakht, K. *et al.* (1996). Clinical and pathological features of ovarian cancer in women with germ-line mutations of BRCA1. *N. Engl. J. Med.*, **335**, 1413–16.

45. Zweemer, R.P., Verheijen, R.H.M., Gille, J.J.P. *et al.* (1998). Clinical and genetic evaluation of 30 ovarian cancer families. *Am. J. Obstet. Gynecol.*, **178**, 85–90.

46. Pharoah, P.D.P., Easton, D.F., Stockton, D.L. *et al.* (1999). Survival in familial, *brca1*-associated, and *brca2*-associated epithelial ovarian cancer. *Cancer Res.*, **59**, 868–71.

47. Johannsson, O.T., Ranstam, J., Borg, A. and Olsson, H. (1998). Survival of BRCA1 breast and ovarian cancer patients: a population-based study from southern Sweden. *J. Clin. Oncol.*, **16**, 397–404.

48. Ferry, J.A., Young, R.H., Engel, G. and Scully, R.E. (1994). Oxyphilic Sertoli cell tumor of the ovary: a report of three cases, two in patients with the Peutz–Jeghers syndrome. *Int. J. Gynecol. Pathol.*, **13**, 259–66.

49. Piver, M.S., Baker, T.R., Jishi, M.F. *et al.* (1993). Familial ovarian cancer: a report of 658 families from the Gilda Radner Familial Ovarian Cancer Registry 1981–1991. *Cancer*, **71**, 582–8.

50. Katagiri, T., Emi, M., Ito, I. *et al.* (1996). Mutations in the BRCA1 gene in Japanese breast cancer patients. *Hum. Mut.*, **7**, 334–9.

51. Johannsson, O.T., IdVall, I., Anderson, C. *et al.* (1997). Tumour biological features of BRCA1-induced breast and ovarian cancer. *Eur. J. Cancer*, **33**, 362–71.

52. Breast Cancer Linkage Consortium (1997). Pathology of familial breast cancer: differences between breast cancers in carriers of BRCA1 or BRCA2 mutations and sporadic cases. *Lancet*, **349**, 1505–10.

53. Berchuck, A., Kohler, M.F., Marks, J.R. *et al.* (1994). The p53 tumour suppressor gene frequently is altered in gynecologic cancers. *Am. J. Obstet. Gynecol.*, **170**, 246–52.

54. Kupryjanczyk, J., Thor, A.D., Beauchamp, R. *et al.* (1993). p53 gene mutations and protein accumulation in human ovarian cancer. *Proc. Natl Acad. Sci. USA*, **90**, 4961–5.

55. Auranen, A., Grenman, S. and Klemi, P.-J. (1997). Immunohistochemically detectd p53 and HER–2/*neu* expression and nuclear DNA content in familial epithelial ovarian carcinomas *Cancer*, **79**, 2147–53.

56. Crook, T., Crossland, S., Crompton, M.R. *et al.* (1997). p53 mutations in BRCA1-associated familial breast cancer. [Letter]*Lancet*, **350**, 638–9.

57. Brugarolas, J. and Jacks, T. (1997). Double indemnity: p53, BRCA and cancer. p53 mutation partially rescues developmental arrest in Brca1 and Brca2 null mice, suggesting a role for familial breast cancer genes in DNA damage repair. *Nature Med.*, **3**, 721–2.

58. Schlichtholtz, B., Bouchind'homme, B., Pages, P. *et al.* (1998). p53 mutations associated familial breast cancer. *Lancet*, **352**, 622.

59. Zweemer, R.P., Shaw, P.A., Verheijen, R.H.M. *et al.* (1999). p53 overexpression is frequent in ovarian cancers associated with BRCA1 and BRCA2 germline mutations. *J. Clin. Pathol.*, **52**, 372–5.

60. Casey, G., Lopez, M.E., Ramos, J.C. *et al.* (1996). DNA sequence analysis of exons 2 through 11 and immunohistochemical staining are required to detect all known p53 alterations in human malignancies. *Oncogene*, **13**, 1971–81.

61. Skilling, J.S., Sood, A., Niemann, T. *et al.* (1996). An abundance of p53 null mutations in ovarian carcinoma. *Oncogene*, **13**, 117–23.

62. Rhei, E., Bogomolniy, F., Federici, M.G. *et al.* (1998). Molecular genetic characterisation of BRCA1 and BRCA2-linked hereditary ovarian cancers. *Cancer Res.*, **58**, 3193–6.

63. Kallioniemi, O.P., Kallioniemi, A., Sudar, D. *et al.* (1993). Comparative genomic hybridization: a rapid new method for detecting and mapping DNA amplification in tumours. *Semin. Cancer Biol.*, **4**, 41–6.

64. Tapper, J., Sarantaus, L., Vahteristo, P. *et al.* (1998). Genetic changes in inherited and sporadic ovarian carcinomas by comparative genomic hybridization: Extensive similarity exept for a difference at chromosome 2q24–q32. *Cancer Res.*, **58**, 2715–19.

5. The prevalence of mutations in *BRCA1* and *BRCA2*

Michael R. Stratton

Introduction

Following the localization[1,2] and isolation[3,4] of the breast/ovarian cancer susceptibility genes *BRCA1* and *BRCA2*, the spectrum of disease-associated mutations in various populations has been investigated in detail (Breast Information Core at http://www.nhgri.nih.gov/Intramural_research/Lab_transfer/Bic/. The breast and ovarian cancer risks associated with mutations in the genes have been estimated[5] and other cancer types to which mutation carriers are predisposed have been identified.[6] Variations in cancer risks between different mutations in the genes have been described[7,8] and the pathological features of breast and ovarian cancers arising in mutation carriers have been characterized.[9]

The prevalence of *BRCA1* and *BRCA2* mutations has been less exhaustively investigated. This has been attributable predominantly to the complexity of analysis (due to the large sizes of the two genes and diversity of mutations) and the substantial numbers of samples required to obtain reliable estimates. However, the information is important. Together with estimates of the risks of cancer associated with mutations in the genes, it determines the cost-benefit implications for individuals, health services, and insurance companies of genetic testing on a population scale.

The prevalence of *BRCA1* and *BRCA2* mutations depends upon the method of ascertainment of the cases evaluated and the ethnic groups from which they are drawn. Ideally, one would wish to know the prevalence of mutations in families with multiple cases of breast and/or ovarian cancer, in population-based series of cases of breast and ovarian cancer unselected for family history (at all ages), and in the general population (unselected for disease status). Currently, many prevalence estimates have been provided for multiple-case families, fewer for unselected series of breast–ovarian cancer cases and rarely for the general population.

Gene prevalence data

The prevalence of BRCA1 and BRCA2 mutations in multiple-case breast–ovarian cancer families

Because genetic linkage analysis of multiple-case families using markers on chromosomes 13q and 17q can be used to evaluate the presence of a mutation in *BRCA1* and *BRCA2*, and because the likelihood of finding mutations is high, even in small series, many estimates of the proportion of such families that are due to *BRCA1* and *BRCA2* have been published. Unfortunately, most of these family sets do not faithfully reflect the characteristics of breast–ovarian cancer families in the population, and many of these estimates are therefore influenced by biases in the methods of family ascertainment. Thus, selection for very large numbers of breast cancer cases, for the presence of ovarian cancer cases, or for very early onset disease influences the prevalence of mutations in *BRCA1* and *BRCA2*.

The Breast Cancer Linkage Consortium (BCLC) has analysed the largest series of breast–ovarian cancer families for the contribution of *BRCA1* and *BRCA2* mutations.[5] In its most recent analysis of 211 families with at least four cases of breast cancer under age 60 or any ovarian cancer, 54% were attributed to *BRCA1*, 27% to *BRCA2*, and 19% to other genes. However, of families with both breast and ovarian cancer, 74% were attributed to *BRCA1*, 16% to *BRCA2*, and 10% to other genes. Indeed, when families with at least two cases of ovarian cancer were considered, 80% were attributed to *BRCA1*, 18% to *BRCA2*, and only 2% to other genes. Therefore *BRCA1* and *BRCA2* appear to account for most families with both breast and ovarian cancer, with *BRCA1* accounting for the large majority.

Amongst families with female breast cancer only, the picture is different. Overall, 35% of such families are estimated as being due to *BRCA1*, 36% to *BRCA2*, and 29% to other genes.[5] When these data are broken down by number of cases per family, interesting differences are observed. In families with six or more breast cancers, 29% are due to *BRCA1*, 66% to *BRCA2*, and only 5% to other genes, showing that large familial clusters are predominantly attributable to *BRCA1* and *BRCA2*. Conversely, the contribution of *BRCA1* and *BRCA2* to families with four or five breast cancer cases is more limited, with 50% attributable to *BRCA1* and *BRCA2* combined, and 50% to other genes. In its analyses, the BCLC has not included breast cancer clusters with fewer than four cases; however, other studies indicate that less than 20% of families with three cases of early onset breast cancer have a *BRCA1* or *BRCA2* mutation (ref. 10 and Stratton, unpublished data). Since these small familial clusters are much more common than larger multiple-case families, the data suggest that a considerable proportion of the predisposition to breast cancer is yet to be elucidated and that the remaining genes are of lower penetrance than *BRCA1* and *BRCA2*.

The prevalence of BRCA1 and BRCA2 mutations in breast cancer cases unselected for family history

There is much less information on the prevalence of mutations in series of breast cancer cases unselected for family history than there is for multiple-case families. Therefore, the contribution of mutations in *BRCA1* and *BRCA2* to the population incidence of breast cancer has not been estimated accurately. As indicated above, this is largely due to the substantial numbers of cases required to obtain robust estimates, the large sizes of the two genes and hence the laborious nature of the task.

In certain populations or ethnic groups, however, there exists a very restricted set of *BRCA1* and *BRCA2* founding mutations, rendering analysis of large numbers of samples relatively straightforward. Until recently, it was only in such populations that estimates of the prevalence of mutations amongst breast cancer cases had been obtained. For example, in Ashkenazi Jews most mutations in *BRCA1* and *BRCA2* are *BRCA1* 185delAG, *BRCA1* 5382insC, and *BRCA2* 6174delT. *BRCA1* 185delAG is found in 20% of Ashkenazi Jewish breast cancer cases diagnosed under the age of 42, whereas *BRCA2* 6174delT accounts for 8% of cases.[11–13] Therefore amongst Ashkenazi Jews, *BRCA1* mutations appear to make a greater contribution to early onset breast cancer than *BRCA2* mutations. However, in cases diagnosed over age 50, *BRCA1* and *BRCA2* mutations are each found in 4–5% cases.[13] Conversely, in Iceland, a single *BRCA2* mutation, 999del5, accounts for 24% of breast cancer cases diagnosed under the age of 40, whereas *BRCA1* makes a very small contribution.[14,15] The discrepancy between these observations is primarily a consequence of the histories of the Ashkenazi and Icelandic populations, which have resulted in the current populations originating from a relatively small number of individuals. In addition, different *BRCA1* and *BRCA2* mutations may be associated with slightly different risks of breast and ovarian cancer, and these variations may also influence the contribution of each gene to the disease. Whatever the underlying reasons, these distortions mean that the results of these studies are not directly applicable to large, outbred populations.

To clarify the contribution of mutations in *BRCA1* and *BRCA2* to breast cancer incidence in outbred populations, we recently examined a population-based series of 617 early onset breast cancer cases from the UK for mutations in both *BRCA1* and *BRCA2*.[16] The estimates provided by this study should be more generally applicable than those from the Ashkenazi or Icelandic studies, although ultimately each population may require its own estimates. The diverse origins of the British population and the lack of the founder effect that is seen in the Ashkenazi and Icelandic populations is reflected in this study by the number of distinct mutations detected: 25 distinct *BRCA1/2* mutations being detected in 30 individuals.[16]

This study showed that 5.9% of British women diagnosed with breast cancer under the age of 36 years carried *BRCA1* mutations, whereas 3.5% carried *BRCA2* mutations. In women diagnosed between the ages of 36 and 45, 1.9% carried *BRCA1* mutations and 2.2% carried *BRCA2* mutations. Therefore, *BRCA1* mutations predominate slightly in very early onset cases, probably as a result of a higher penetrance than *BRCA2* at an early age. At later ages,

however, *BRCA2* mutations appear to contribute equally. These observed prevalences are likely to be underestimates, as the sensitivity of the mutation detection technique used is not complete. Large genomic deletions, mutations in introns or promoter regions, and a small minority of base substitutions are not detected. Moreover, some of the rare missense amino-acid changes which were classified as of unknown significance may be disease causing. By comparing the number of mutations found in families clearly linked to either gene, the sensitivity of CSGE (conformation sensitive gel electrophoresis) and other similar techniques has been estimated at 63%.[5] Adjusting for incomplete sensitivity, our estimate of the proportion of breast cancers that are due to these genes is 9.4% below age 36 and 6.6% between ages 36 and 45.

Although cases diagnosed at ages over 45 were not examined in this study, predictions made on the basis of these results and *BRCA1/2* penetrance estimates indicate that *BRCA2* may make a greater contribution than *BRCA1* mutations to later onset breast cancer (*BRCA2* mutations accounting for 0.84% of cases aged 50–69, with *BRCA1* accounting for 0.49%), and that for all breast cancer diagnosed up to age 69, 1.5% cases are due to *BRCA2* and 1.3% to *BRCA1*.

The prevalence of mutations obtained in this study is generally in agreement with the limited amount of other data available. The prevalence of *BRCA1* mutations among breast cancer patients in the UK has previously been estimated at 7.5% for those diagnosed below age 30, 5.1% at age 30–39 and 2.2% at age 40–49.[17] These estimates were obtained using the penetrance estimates for breast and ovarian cancer in *BRCA1* mutation carriers derived from the multiple-case BCLC linkage families, and assuming that the excesses of ovarian cancer in relatives of breast cancer patients, and of breast cancer in relatives of ovarian cancer, are due to *BRCA1*. The observed frequencies of 3.5% (9/254) cases diagnosed under age 36, and 1.9% (7/363) cases diagnosed between 36 and 45, for *BRCA1* are comparable to these predictions, particularly after adjustment for the sensitivity of mutation detection. The results obtained in this study are also not significantly lower than recently published results for *BRCA1* in a US population-based study of an outbred population, in which 6.2% (12/193) cases diagnosed before age 35 carried *BRCA1* mutations.[18]

Despite the previous lack of information, the prevailing view amongst clinicians and geneticists seems to be that *BRCA1* makes a greater contribution to breast cancer incidence than *BRCA2*. An important conclusion from the study[16] is therefore that, in the UK (and hence probably in many other outbred populations), mutations in *BRCA2* (14/617, 2.3%) make a contribution similar to that of *BRCA1* (16/617, 2.6%) to early onset breast cancer, and may account for more cases up to age 70. Currently, there is no published information on the prevalence of *BRCA2* in other outbred population-based series of cancer cases. In a hospital-based series of 73 cases diagnosed under age 32, *BRCA2* mutations were detected in 2.7% cases, compared to 12.3% cases with mutations in *BRCA1*.[19,20] However, this study was conducted in the Boston (Massachusetts) area, which has a substantial Ashkenazi Jewish population, and four of the mutations detected were *BRCA1* 185delAG, which has a high prevalence amongst Ashkenazi Jews. Therefore its wider relevance is questionable.

The prevalence of BRCA1 and BRCA2 mutations in ovarian cancer cases unselected for a family history

In Ashkenazi Jews, 20–60% of ovarian cancer cases carry mutations in *BRCA1* and *BRCA2*.[13, 21,22] In Iceland, only 8% of ovarian cancer cases carry *BRCA2* 999del5, reflecting the relatively low ovarian cancer risk associated with *BRCA2* mutations.[14] A study of 374 British ovarian cancer cases unselected for family history found *BRCA1* mutations in 3.5%.[23] This is consistent with an indirect estimate for the British population, which predicted that 2.8% of ovarian cancer is due to *BRCA1* mutations.[17]

The prevalence of BRCA1 and BRCA2 mutations in the general population

There are few reliable direct estimates of the prevalence of mutations in the general population, because the numbers to be screened need to be so large. The Ashkenazi and Icelandic populations are again exceptions because of their restricted number of mutations. Amongst Ashkenazi Jews, approximately 1.1% carry *BRCA1* 185delAG, 0.1% carry *BRCA1* 5382insC, and 1.5% carry *BRCA2* 6174delT.[24] Therefore, approximately 2.5% of Ashkenazi Jews carry a mutation in one or other gene. This is remarkably high compared to what has been expected and, to some extent, demonstrated for other populations. It therefore has substantial significance for the Ashkenazi population but little relevance for other groups. In Iceland, approximately 1 in 200 individuals carries *BRCA2* 999del5[14,15] and there appears to be a very small contribution from *BRCA1* or other *BRCA2* mutations.

There are currently no direct estimates of *BRCA1* and *BRCA2* mutation prevalence for large outbred populations. However, we have recently provided indirect estimates, based upon assumptions concerning the penetrances of *BRCA1* and *BRCA2* and the results from the analyses of British early onset breast cancer cases, reported above. These indicate that *BRCA1* mutation carriers account for 0.11% of the British population and *BRCA2* mutation carriers for 0.12%.[16] The estimate for *BRCA1* is similar to the value (0.12%) previously derived from the familial association of breast and ovarian cancers.[17]

Conclusions

Accurate estimates of the prevalence of *BRCA1* and *BRCA2* mutations are important for rational implementation of presymptomatic testing for breast cancer susceptibility. Ideally, these estimates should be provided for breast and ovarian cancer cases ascertained in several different ways and for different ethnic groups. Mutations in *BRCA1* and *BRCA2* account for most families with multiple cases of both breast and ovarian cancer, or with many (six or more) early onset breast cancers. However, in smaller familial clusters (for example, three breast cancer cases under age 60) *BRCA1* and *BRCA2* mutations appear much less common (approximately 20%). The prevalence of *BRCA1* and *BRCA2* mutations in breast cancer cases unselected for a family history has been less extensively studied. Estimates have been derived for

the Ashkenazi Jewish and Icelandic populations, but these are of limited relevance to larger outbred populations. In Britain, *BRCA1* and *BRCA2* mutations are detectable in 5.9% cases diagnosed before age 36, and in 4.1% cases diagnosed between ages 36 and 45. In the general population (unselected for disease status), direct estimates of mutation prevalence have only been provided for the Ashkenazi Jewish and Icelandic populations. However, on the basis of recent penetrance estimates and the results from the analysis of British early onset breast cancer cases, indirect estimates of 0.11% for *BRCA1* and 0.12% for *BRCA2* mutation carriers in the general population have been obtained.

These results have implications for the cost-effectiveness of wider implementation of *BRCA1* and *BRCA2* mutation analysis. In most populations only a small proportion of early onset breast cancer cases carry a mutation in one or other gene. Moreover, it appears that only a small proportion of the familial risk of breast cancer is attributable to these genes. In these populations, it would seem reasonable to consider offering presymptomatic diagnostic testing to individuals with a strong family history of early onset breast cancer or ovarian cancer. These considerations should be different amongst Ashkenazi Jews, because the general population prevalence of mutations in the *BRCA1* and *BRCA2* is five- to tenfold higher.

Acknowledgements

We would like to thank the women who agreed to take part in this study and members of the UK Case Control Study Group who facilitated this work. The original study was partly funded by the ICRF. We would like to thank the Cancer Research Campaign and Breakthrough Breast Cancer for their support.

References

1. Hall, J.M., Lee M.K. and Newman, B. *et al.* (1990). Linkage of early-onset familial breast cancer to chromosome 17q21. *Science*, **250**, 1684–9.
2. Wooster, R., Neuhausen, S.L., Mangion, J. *et al.* (1994). Localization of a breast cancer susceptibility gene, BRCA2, to chromosome 13q12–13. *Science*, **265**, 2088–90.
3. Miki, Y., Swensen, J., Shattuck-Eidens, D. *et al.* (1994). A strong candidate for the breast and ovarian cancer susceptibility gene BRCA1. *Science*, **266**, 66–71.
4. Wooster, R., Bignell, G., Lancaster, J. *et al.* (1995). Identification of the breast cancer susceptibility gene BRCA2. *Nature*, **378**, 789–92.
5. Ford, D., Easton, D.F., Stratton, M. *et al.* (1998). Genetic heterogeneity and penetrance analysis of the BRCA1 and BRCA2 genes in breast cancer families. The Breast Cancer Linkage Consortium. *Am. J. Hum. Genet.*, **62**, 676–89.
6. Ford, D., Easton, D.F., Bishop, D.T. *et al.* (1994). Risks of cancer in BRCA1-mutation carriers. Breast Cancer Linkage Consortium. *Lancet*, **343**, 692–5.
7. Gayther, S.A., Mangion, J., Russell, P. *et al.* (1997). Variation of risks of breast and ovarian cancer associated with different germline mutations of the BRCA2 gene. *Nature Genet.*, **15**, 103–5.
8. Gayther, S.A., Warren, W., Mazoyer, S. *et al.* (1995). Germline mutations of the BRCA1 gene in breast and ovarian cancer families provide evidence for a genotype-phenotype correlation. *Nature Genet.*, **11**, 428–33.

9. Breast Cancer Linkage Consortium (1997). Pathology of familial breast cancer: differences between breast cancers in carriers of BRCA1 or BRCA2 mutations and sporadic cases. *Lancet*, **349**, 1505–10.

10. Ligtenberg, M.J., Hogervorst, F.B., Willems, H.W. *et al.* (1999). Characteristics of small breast and/or ovarian cancer families with germline mutations in BRCA1 and BRCA2. *Br. J. Cancer*, **79**, 1475–8.

11. Neuhausen, S., Gilewski, T., Norton, L. *et al.* (1996). Recurrent BRCA2 6174delT mutations in Ashkenazi Jewish women affected by breast cancer. *Naure Genet.*, **13**, 126–8.

12. Offit, K., Gilewski, T., McGuire, P. *et al.* (1996). Germline BRCA1 185delAG mutations in Jewish women with breast cancer. *Lancet*, **347**, 1643–5.

13. Abeliovich, D., Kaduri, L., Lerer, I. *et al.* (1997). The founder mutations 185delAG and 5382insC in BRCA1 and 6174delT in BRCA2 appear in 60% of ovarian cancer and 30% of early-onset breast cancer patients among Ashkenazi women. *Am. J. Hum Genet.*, **60**, 505–14.

14. Johannesdottir, G., Gudmundsson, J., Bergthorsson, J.T. *et al.* (1996). High prevalence of the 999del5 mutation in Icelandic breast and ovarian cancer patients. *Cancer Res.*, **56**, 3663–5.

15. Thorlacius, S., Sigurdsson, S., Bjarnadottir, H. *et al.* (1997). Study of a single BRCA2 mutation with high carrier frequency in a small population. *Am. J. Hum. Genet.*, **60**, 1079–84.

16. Peto, J., Collins, N., Barfoot, R. *et al.* (1999). Prevalence of BRCA1 and BRCA2 gene mutations in patients with early-onset breast cancer. *J. Natl. Cancer Inst.*, **91**, 943–9.

17. Ford, D., Easton, D. F. and Peto, J. (1995). Estimates of the gene frequency of BRCA1 and its contribution to breast and ovarian cancer incidence. *Am. J. Hum. Genet.*, **57**, 1457–62.

18. Newman, B., Mu, H., Butler, L. M. *et al.* (1998). Frequency of breast cancer attributable to BRCA1 in a population-based series of American women. *J. Am. Med. Assoc.*, **279**, 915–21.

19. Krainer, M., Silva-Arrieta, S., FitzGerald, M.G. *et al.* (1997). Differential contributions of BRCA1 and BRCA2 to early-onset breast cancer. *N. Engl. J. Med.*, **336**, 1416–21.

20. FitzGerald, M.G., MacDonald, D.J., Krainer, M. *et al.* (1996). Germ-line BRCA1 mutations in Jewish and non-Jewish women with early-onset breast cancer. *N. Engl. J. Med.*, **334**, 143–9.

21. Beller, U., Halle, D., Catane, R. *et al.* (1997). High frequency of BRCA1 and BRCA2 germline mutations in Ashkenazi Jewish ovarian cancer patients, regardless of family history. *Gynecol. Oncol.*, **67**, 123–6.

22. Modan, B., Gak, E., Sade-Bruchim, R.B. *et al.* (1996). High frequency of BRCA1 185delAG mutation in ovarian cancer in Israel. National Israel Study of Ovarian Cancer. *J. Am. Med. Assoc.*, **276**, 1823–5.

23. J.F., Gayther, S.A., Russell, P. *et al.* (1997). Contribution of BRCA1 mutations to ovarian cancer. *N. Engl. J. Med.*, **336**, 1125–30.

24. Roa, B.B., Boyd, A.A., Volcik, K. *et al.* (1996). Ashkenazi Jewish population frequencies for common mutations in BRCA1 and BRCA2. *Nature Genet.*, **14** 185–7.

6. The penetrance of *BRCA1/2* mutations

Jeffery P. Struewing

Introduction

Second to breast cancer, ovarian cancer is the next most common malignancy occurring in women who carry germline mutations in the *BRCA1* and *BRCA2* genes. It is one of the strongest indicators that a *BRCA1* mutation, and to a lesser extent *BRCA2* mutation, is present within a family: breast cancer families with at least one case of ovarian cancer are much more likely to be segregating a mutation than families without. Estimates of the absolute risk of ovarian cancer among mutation carriers (penetrance) are about twice as high for *BRCA1* compared to *BRCA2*. Most penetrance estimates have been derived from the Breast Cancer Linkage Consortium (BCLC) families and have averaged about 50% for *BRCA1* and about 25% for *BRCA2* by age 70. A subset of *BRCA1* mutation-positive families appear to have a very high risk of ovarian cancer (over 80%), although this has not been linked thus far to any specific mutation(s). A community-based study of three founder mutations in the Ashkenazi Jewish population estimated a 16% risk of ovarian cancer by age 70. The prospective incidence of ovarian cancer among *BRCA1* mutation carriers, ascertained from breast/ovarian cancer families, appears to be over 70% by age 70. An individual mutation carrier's risk of ovarian cancer is difficult to predict, but the apparent heterogeneity in risk between individuals/families suggests that important modifiers may exist. Identification of these modifiers may allow more precise risk estimates and provide targets for intervention.

BRCA1/2 and the association with ovarian cancer

Ovarian cancer is approximately one-tenth as frequent as breast cancer and its inherited forms have been studied largely in the context of inherited breast cancer families. Soon after the initial localization of the *BRCA1* locus among families with multiple cases of breast cancer,[1] it was confirmed by another genetic linkage study in families with both breast and ovarian cancer.[2] Subsequent studies have shown consistently that when a breast cancer family has at least one case of ovarian cancer, the likelihood of the family having a *BRCA1* mutation is much greater.[3–5] Although the association is not as strong, a case of ovarian cancer also increases the likelihood of a breast cancer family having a *BRCA2* mutation. Thus, while ovarian cancer is relatively rare, and most *BRCA1/2* positive families identified to date have only cases of breast cancer, ovarian cancer is one of the strongest indicators that a *BRCA1/2* mutation might be present.

The risk of ovarian cancer among *BRCA1/2* mutation carriers

Breast Cancer Linkage Consortium

Most studies on the risk of cancer among *BRCA1/2* mutation carriers have been conducted on a large data set of families with multiple, early onset cases of breast cancer, known as the Breast Cancer Linkage Consortium (BCLC).[3] Eligibility criteria have varied somewhat, but generally include families with at least five cases of breast cancer diagnosed before age 50. The focus initially was on families with living cases of breast cancer in order to analyze samples for genetic linkage studies. Early analyses based on 33 families showing genetic linkage to the *BRCA1* locus estimated the cumulative risk of ovarian cancer among mutation carriers to be approximately 22% by age 50 and 44% by age 70, using a LOD score maximization method, and 29% by age 50 and 62% by age 70 using the incidence of ovarian cancer after breast cancer (second cancers) method (Fig. 6.1).[6,7] These analyses assumed no

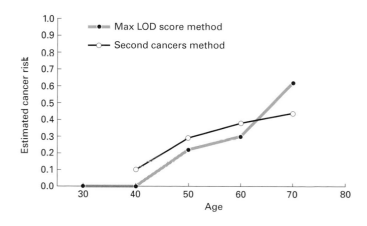

Fig. 6.1 Estimated cumulative ovarian cancer risk for *BRCA1* mutation carriers in Breast Cancer Linkage Consortium linked families under allelic homogeneity.

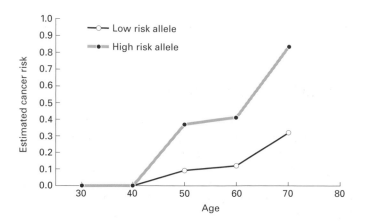

Fig. 6.2 Estimated cumulative Ovarian Cancer Risk for *BRCA1* mutation carriers in Breast Cancer Linkage Consortium linked families under allelic heterogeneity.

heterogeneity, meaning that the estimated cancer was the same for all carriers as a whole. Again, based on genetic linkage information, but allowing for heterogeneity, analyses suggested two risk categories for *BRCA1* families, a low-risk form resulting in a 32% cumulative incidence by age 70 and a high-risk form associated with an 84% risk by age 70 (Fig. 6.2).[8]

Ovarian cancer risk estimates for carriers of *BRCA2* mutations have generally been lower and with a later age at onset than for *BRCA1*, with estimates of negligible risk to age 50 and a cumulative risk of 27% by age 70 using the LOD score maximization method.[5,9] Estimates of ovarian cancer risk have also been calculated for *BRCA2* mutation-positive families, grouped by the location of the mutation, either 5′ of the ovarian cancer cluster-region (OCRR), within the OCRR, a region of 3000 bp in the middle of the gene, or 3′ to the OCRR.[10] Risk estimates for carriers of mutations 5′ of the OCRR were similar to the overall estimates using

the LOD score method, while they were high for mutations within the OCRR (75% by age 70), and low for mutations 3′ of the OCRR (5% by age 70) (Fig. 6.3).

Washington Ashkenazi Survey

Within the Jewish population, most being Ashkenazi Jews in the United States, there are three relatively common founder mutations in *BRCA1/2*. The combined frequency of the 185delAG and 5382insC mutations in *BRCA1* and 6174delT in *BRCA2* is approximately 2.3%. The relative ease with which these three single mutations may be assayed, compared to testing for all possible mutations in the over 15 kb of coding sequence in these two genes in most populations, makes more population-based studies possible. The Washington Ashkenazi Survey was a cross-sectional study conducted in the Washington DC area, in which 5318 Jews volunteered by giving a small blood sample and completing a questionnaire on personal and family history of cancer.[11] Approximately 75% of participants did not have a close relative with breast or ovarian cancer. By comparing the incidence of cancer in the mothers, sisters, and daughters of the 120 volunteers who tested positive for one of the three founder mutations to the incidence in the female relatives of the non-carriers, estimates of the cumulative risk of cancer for mutation carriers were obtained.

There were 12 reported cases of ovarian cancer among the 306 female relatives of mutation carriers compared to 121 cases among 13 018 relatives of non-carriers. Using the kin-cohort method, the estimated cumulative risk of ovarian cancer for mutation carriers was 16% (95% confidence limits = 6–28%) by age 70 (Fig. 6.4). The large confidence interval highlights the fact that even in this large study, only 12 'observations' occurred in the relatives of carriers, larger studies will be required to further refine these estimates. There were no statistically significant differences in the risk estimates for carriers of the three individual mutations, but the risk of ovarian cancer among the 6174delT mutation in *BRCA2* did not increase until after age 60.

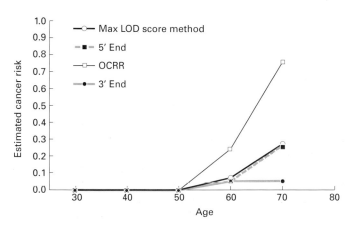

Fig. 6.3 Estimated cumulative ovarian cancer risk for *BRCA2* mutation carriers in Breast Cancer Linkage Consortium linked families. LOD score method assumes homogeneity; other methods assume heterogeneity, according to Gayther *et al.* 1997.[10]

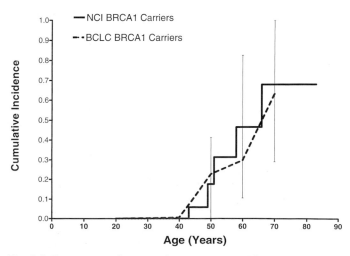

Fig. 6.4 Comparison of estimated ovarian cancer risk estimates between the Washington Ashkenazi Study (95% confidence limits) and Breast Cancer Linkage Consortium.

Other studies

Few other studies have estimated the risk of ovarian cancer among *BRCA1/2* mutation carriers. Even in studies that are family based, there are usually not enough mutation carriers identified nor enough individuals with ovarian cancer to make reliable estimates.[12] A segregation analysis based on several ovarian cancer case-control studies estimated ovarian cancer risks of 9% by age 50 and 22% by age 70.[13] Given that the families studied were ascertained from ovarian cancer probands, most of the familial clustering would be expected to be due to *BRCA1* mutations.

One population-based study in the UK analyzed the entire *BRCA1* gene in 374 women with epithelial ovarian cancer.[14] They identified 13 probable mutations and estimated that approximately 5% of the cases might carry *BRCA1* mutations. A small, population based case-control study in the US identified one of three founder mutations in 14 (44%) of 32 Jewish women with ovarian cancer and in none of 33 controls.[15] While absolute risks of cancer cannot be obtained from such case-control comparisons, relative risks can be estimated. In these two studies, however, controls were either untested or were of insufficient number to determine the control frequency of mutations. However, given that the likely carrier frequency for *BRCA1/2* mutations among 'controls' in the UK is likely to be much less than 1%,[16] and is approximately 2% among Jewish 'controls', these observed carrier frequencies among cases would be consistent with very high relative risks of ovarian cancer among mutation carriers.

Prospective cancer incidence

An historical cohort approach is being used to obtain prospective cancer incidence among *BRCA1* mutation carriers from high-risk families from the US National Cancer Institute's (NCI) Familial Cancer Registry of the Genetic Epidemiology Branch, some of which are part of the BCLC set of families. Families with at least two cases of epithelial ovarian cancer were eligible, and there were 16 families with identified *BRCA1* mutations.[17] There were an average of 2.8 cases of ovarian cancer and 2.9 cases of breast cancer per family. Preliminary analyses have been completed on 53 female mutation carriers who were free of breast and ovarian cancer at the time of their family's ascertainment. Their average age at ascertainment was 31 years and they were followed for an average of 18 years (>1000 person-years of observation). All cancers and years of observation that occurred up to the time of family ascertainment were excluded from analysis. Years of observation for life-table analyses of breast and ovarian cancer occurrence began at the date of family ascertainment or at age 20, whichever occurred later. Observation continued until the development of breast (or ovarian) cancer or, for unaffected individuals, until the date of bilateral removal of the breasts (or ovaries), death, or 31 December 1996, whichever occurred first. With regard to the two outcomes of breast cancer and ovarian cancer, women who developed one type of cancer or had bilateral surgery to remove the organs were not censored for the occurrence of the other cancer.

There were 16 incident breast cancers and five incident ovarian cancers among *BRCA1* mutation carriers since ascertainment. The cumulative incidence of ovarian cancer among carriers was 17% by age 50 and 70% by age 70.

Genetic heterogeneity

The spectrum of cancers that are associated with inherited mutations in the *BRCA1* and *BRCA2* genes is quite limited, involving primarily breast and ovarian cancer. But these two cancers do not always occur together in individuals or families. In fact, some mutation-positive families present with only breast cancer, some with only ovarian cancer, and some with both cancers. It is possible, but very unlikely, that this is due solely to allelic heterogeneity, that is, that certain specific mutations (or alleles) of these genes predispose to one cancer, and other alleles to the other cancer. While there is some evidence for a stronger predisposition to ovarian cancer with mutations in various regions of these genes,[10,18] this association is weak and some families with the same mutation have primarily breast cancer and others have primarily ovarian cancer. Another explanation for the observed heterogeneity is that non-*BRCA1/2* factors modify the expression of mutations. These may be other genetic loci or environmental factors.[19,20]

The prospective cancer incidence in the NCI families suggests that other factors may modify the expression of mutations in these genes in individuals and families. The NCI families were ascertained largely through ovarian cancer cases. If this relative preponderance for ovarian cancer was a chance phenomenon, then the cancer occurrence after ascertainment would shift back toward more breast cancers, and the future risk of ovarian cancer would revert back toward the 'mean'. The observed ovarian cancer incidence, however, continues to be very high, suggesting that there is some factor that modifies the expression of *BRCA1* toward ovarian cancer in these families. The identification of such factors will be both important and challenging.

Summary and implications

Estimates of the absolute risk of ovarian cancer among *BRCA1/2* mutation carriers (penetrance) are difficult to make. Based on analyses in high-risk families, it appears that the risk of ovarian cancer is about twice as high for *BRCA1* compared to *BRCA2*, being about 50% for *BRCA1* and 25% for *BRCA2* by age 70. A subset of *BRCA1* mutation-positive families appear to have a very high risk of ovarian cancer (over 80%), although this has not been linked so far to any specific mutation(s). A population-based study suggested that the risk of ovarian cancer may be considerably lower, around 20% by age 70. Expanded studies will be necessary to better characterize the true risk of ovarian cancer.

An individual mutation carrier's risk of ovarian cancer is difficult to predict. If the mutation carrier is from a family with multiple cases of breast and ovarian cancer, similar to the BCLC families, it appears that their prospective risk of both ovarian and breast cancer are very high. If such a family history is not present, precise risk estimates are not possible—the risk may indeed still be very high (or very low), but there would be little on which to base an estimate. The apparent heterogeneity in risk between individuals/families suggests that important modifiers may exist. Identification of these modifiers may allow more precise risk estimates and provide targets for intervention.

Acknowledgments

Most of the work summarized here is due to the efforts of many others, and I thank all my co-authors, especially Margaret Tucker, Patricia Hartge, Sholom Wacholder, and Larry Brody, and to colleagues who conducted the preliminary analyses of the NCI family historical cohort, particularly Dave Kaufman.

References

1. Hall, J.M., Lee, M.K., Newman, B. *et al.* (1990). Linkage of early-onset familial breast cancer to chromosome 17q21. *Science*, **250**, 1684–9.
2. Narod, S.A., Feunteun, J., Lynch, H.T. *et al.* (1991). Familial breast-ovarian cancer locus on chromosome 17q12-q23. *Lancet*, **338**, 82–3.
3. Breast Cancer Linkage Consortium (1993). Genetic linkage analysis in familial breast and ovarian cancer: results from 214 families. *Am. J. Hum. Genet.*, **52**, 678–701.
4. Narod, S.A., Ford, D., Devilee, P. *et al.* (1995). An evaluation of genetic heterogeneity in 145 breast-ovarian cancer families. Breast Cancer Linkage Consortium. *Am. J. Hum. Genet.*, **56**, 254–64.
5. Ford, D., Easton, D.F., Stratton, M. *et al.* (1998). Genetic heterogeneity and penetrance analysis of the *BRCA*1 and *BRCA*2 genes in breast cancer families. The Breast Cancer Linkage Consortium. *Am. J. Hum. Genet.*, **62**, 676–89.
6. Ford, D., Easton, D.F., Bishop, D.T. *et al.* (1993). The risks of cancer in *BRCA*1 mutation carriers. *Am. J. Hum. Genet.*, **53**, Abstract 298.
7. Ford, D., Easton, D.F., Bishop, D.T. *et al.* (1994). Risks of cancer in *BRCA*1-mutation carriers. Breast Cancer Linkage Consortium. *Lancet*, **343**, 692–5.
8. Easton, D.F., Ford, D. and Bishop, D.T. (1995). Breast and ovarian cancer incidence in *BRCA*1-mutation carriers. Breast Cancer Linkage Consortium. *Am. J. Hum. Genet.*, **56**, 265–71.
9. Easton, D.F., Steele, L., Fields, P. *et al.* (1997). Cancer risks in two large breast cancer families linked to *BRCA*2 on chromosome 13q12–13. *Am. J. Hum. Genet.*, **61**, 120–8.
10. Gayther, S.A., Mangion, J., Russell, P. *et al.* (1997). Variation of risks of breast and ovarian cancer associated with different germline mutations of the *BRCA*2 gene. *Nature Genet.*, **15**, 103–5.
11. Struewing, J.P., Hartge, P., Wacholder, S. *et al.* (1997). The risk of cancer associated with specific mutations of *BRCA*1 and *BRCA*2 among Ashkenazi Jews. *N. Engl. J. Med.*, **336**, 1401–8.
12. Thorlacius, S., Struewing, J.P., Hartge, P. *et al.* (1998). Population-based study of risk of breast cancer in carriers of *BRCA*2 mutation. *Lancet*, **352**, 1337–9.
13. Whittemore, A.S., Gong, G. and Itnyre, J. (1997). Prevalence and contribution of *BRCA*1 mutations in breast cancer and ovarian cancer: results from three U.S. population-based case-control studies of ovarian cancer. *Am. J. Hum. Genet.*, **60**, 496–504.
14. Stratton, J.F., Gayther, S.A., Russell, P. *et al.* (1997). Contribution of *BRCA*1 mutations to ovarian cancer. *N. Engl. J. Med.*, **336**, 1125–30.
15. Lu, K.H., Cramer, D.W., Muto, M.G. *et al.* (1999). A population-based study of *BRCA*1 and *BRCA*2 mutations in Jewish women with epithelial ovarian cancer. *Obstet. Gynecol.*, **93**, 34–7.
16. Ford, D., Easton, D.F. and Peto, J. (1995). Estimates of the gene frequency of *BRCA*1 and its contribution to breast and ovarian cancer incidence. *Am. J. Hum. Genet.*, **57**, 1457–62.
17. Struewing, J.P., Brody, L.C., Erdos, M.R. *et al.* (1995). Detection of eight *BRCA*1 mutations in 10 breast/ovarian cancer families, including 1 family with male breast cancer. *Am. J. Hum. Genet.*, **57**, 1–7.
18. Gayther, S.A., Waren, W., Mazoyer, S. *et al.* (1995). Germline mutations of the *BRCA*1 gene in breast and ovarian cancer families provide evidence for a genotype-phenotype correlation. *Nature Genet.*, **11**, 428–33.
19. Narod, S.A., Goldgar, D., Cannon-Albright, L. *et al.* (1995). Risk modifiers in carriers of *BRCA*1 mutations. *Int. J. Cancer*, **64**, 394–8.
20. Narod, S.A., Risch, H., Moslehi, R. *et al.* (1998). Oral contraceptives and the risk of hereditary ovarian cancer. *N. Engl. J. Med.*, **339**, 424–8.

7. Founder mutations of *BRCA1/2*

Uziel Beller, Baruch Modan, Ofer Lavie, Bella Kaufman, Galit Hirsh-Yechzkel, Orit Gotfeld, Angela Chetrit, Raphael Catane, and Ephrat Levy-Lahad

Definition of the population

The Israeli population, and specifically Ashkenazi Jews (of European ancestry), present as a high risk group for the development of hereditary ovarian cancer. Three high-frequency founder mutations are known in this ethnic group, i.e. *BRCA1* 185delAG (1.0%), *BRCA1* 5382insC (0.1%), and *BRCA2* 6174delT (1.4%). These are all frameshift mutations leading to premature truncation of the associated proteins. The combined frequency of these mutations in the Ashkenazi population is 2.5%.[1] This frequency is higher than the total *BRCA1* mutation found in the general Caucasian population (0.12%). Therefore, in Israel, where about half the population is of Ashkenazi origin, over 35 000 women are estimated to be carriers. The Israeli high-risk population may therefore benefit from effective screening and prevention measures, and can serve as a test population for the evaluation of these strategies.

Interestingly, even among non-Ashkenazi Jewish patients of Iraqi and other origins, an identical founder mutation (*BRCA1* 185delAG) was identified, with frequencies ranging from 0.47% to 1.1%.[2,3] This mutation is found on an identical haplotype in the different Jewish subgroups, suggesting that it may have occurred prior to the dispersion of the Jewish people in the Diaspora, around the sixth century BC. Despite these frequencies, the morbidity from ovarian cancer differs between the Ashkenazi and the non-Ashkenazi population, suggesting that other genetic or environmental factors may account for ethnic diversity in cancer rates.

A recent analysis of the three common mutations was performed on 387 epithelial ovarian cancer patients in the National Israeli Study of Ovarian Cancer (NISOC; personal communication), which has registered close to 1500 ovarian cancer patients since it was initiated 5 years ago. Among these patients of all ethnic origins, 18.9% were carriers of *BRCA1* mutations and 6.2% of *BRCA2*; a total carrier rate of 25.1%. Separating these patients into two major ethnic-origin groups, revealed a carrier rate of 29.6% (22.7% *BRCA1* and 6.9% *BRCA2*) among Ashkenazi Jews and 12.3% (6.7% *BRCA1* and 5.6% *BRCA2*) among non-Ashkenazi patients, for the same three founder mutations. This contrasts sharply with the observed mutation rate in other popu-lations, where inherited mutations account for only 5–10% of ovarian cancer.

Our experience with these high-frequency mutations includes an anecdotal case of a 50-year-old woman who requested genetic counselling following her mother's death due to ovarian cancer.[4] Interestingly, this woman underwent premature menopause at age 31 and never used hormone replacement therapy (HRT). DNA analysis revealed her to be a carrier of two mutations—*BRCA1* 185delAG and *BRCA2* 6174delT. She elected to undergo prophylactic bilateral salpingo-oophorectomy (BSO). Her 25-year-old daughter also inherited both of these mutations. As we discuss later in this manuscript, it may be that the reduction in ovulation cycles and lack of HRT use contributed to the protection of this woman from developing ovarian cancer.

The intriguing question is why, despite this high frequency rate, the incidence of ovarian cancer for Jewish women in Israel is similar to that observed in other Western countries (15.5/100 000). It appears that the penetrance of these mutations is lower than previously estimated. We have shown in the past that the most common mutation, *BRCA2* 6174delT (1.4% in the general population), is associated with significantly lower risk than the *BRCA1* mutations.[5] Indeed, in the Ashkenazi patients of the NISOC group, the frequency of *BRCA2* 6174delT mutation was a quarter that of the *BRCA1* mutations, despite the fact that in the general Ashkenazi population *BRCA2* is more frequent than *BRCA1*. A search for other epidemiological factors and genetic somatic events are in progress to try to delineate this issue.

Prognostic significance of *BRCA1/2* mutation

Previous studies on the prognosis and survival in *BRCA1/2*-associated cancer have yielded conflicting results, suggesting that *BRCA1* carriers had either better, worse, or similar prognosis, compared with non-carriers.[6–8] A presentation from the NISOC at the Society of Gynecologic Oncology meeting in 1998 showed no survival benefit for carriers of the *BRCA1* 185delAG mutation. However, recently the group from the Memorial

Sloan Kettering Cancer Center analysed their data and demon-strated once again an advantage for mutation carriers.[9] The only published study comparing BRCA1 and BRCA2 directly found decreased survival of patients with ovarian cancer associ-ated with BRCA2 but not BRCA1 mutations.[8]

To better understand the role of BRCA1/2 mutations in ovarian cancer patients, as well as the effect of different risk factors, includ-ing hormonal, environmental, and different clinical parameters among these patients, we evaluated our single institution group of Ashkenazi ovarian cancer patients. Forty-eight Ashkenazi ovarian cancer patients were ascertained sequentially at Shaare Zedek Medical Center (SZMC) from January 1994 to March 1998. Twenty-eight were consecutive patients diagnosed on or after 1 January 1994, and 20 were women diagnosed earlier and referred to either the Gynecologic Oncology service or the Cancer Genetics clinic.

Risk factors and disease characteristics were compared between three groups: (1) non-carriers; (2) BRCA1 mutation carriers; and (3) BRCA2 mutation carriers. Family pedigrees were drawn as far back and laterally as possible in all subjects. Data analysed included: age at onset, stage, histology, grade, course of disease, time to progression (TTP), and cumulative survival. Other details noted were reproductive hormonal body mass index (BMI), number of pregnancies, number of abortions, breast feeding duration, age at menarche, age of menopause, oral contraceptive use, ovulation induction, and HRT) and environmental factors (smoking, past surgery, and perineal talc exposure). These data were obtained from patient interviews and patients' medical charts. All participants received genetic counselling and gave informed consent, and the study was approved by the ethical review board. Mutation analysis was performed as previously published. We tested for the three common mutations: BRCA1 185delAG and 5382insC, and BRCA2 6174delT.

Of these patients, 26 (54%) were non-carriers and 22 (46%) carriers. Of the carriers, 14 (29%) were BRCA1 carriers (11 were 185delAG and 3 were 5382insC) and 8 (17%) were BRCA2 carri-ers (6174delT).

Reproductive factors which differed among the three groups included mean number of pregnancies (regardless of outcome), which was smaller in BRCA1 carriers (3.7) compared to non-car-riers (5.2, $P = 0.06$) and BRCA2 carriers (5.1, $P = 0.08$). Mean number of abortions differed only for BRCA2 carriers (2.8) versus BRCA1 carriers (1.4, $P = 0.18$). History of oral contraceptive use was 23% in BRCA1 carriers, 27% in non-carriers, and 0% among BRCA2 carriers. Rates of previous HRT were 63% in BRCA1 carri-ers, 27% in non-carriers, and 14% in BRCA2 carriers. Any history of hormone use (oral contraceptive and/or HRT) was more fre-quent in BRCA1 versus BRCA2 carriers ($P = 0.06$). There was no statistical difference in breast feeding duration or age at menarche between the three groups.

No significant difference between the three groups was found for other factors, including height, weight, smoking, and previous operations, as well as talc use (perineal talc use is practically non-existent in Israel). As to a family history of breast–ovarian cancer, non-carriers had significantly fewer affected first-degree relatives (0.29) compared to BRCA1 (1.03, $P = 0.006$) and BRCA2 (1.22, $P = 0.07$) carriers. Family history was not significantly different in BRCA1 versus BRCA2 carriers.

Mean age at diagnosis was significantly younger in BRCA1 car-riers (50.7) compared to both non-carriers (58.9) and BRCA2 car-riers (65.3). Age of onset in BRCA2 carriers was not significantly different from that of non-carriers. Stage at diagnosis was similar in all three groups. Most patients were diagnosed in stage IIIc. Tumour histology was not significantly different among the three groups: in 39/43 (79%) women for whom information was avail-able, the carcinoma was serous. As to the disease course, there were significant differences between the three groups. Time to progression (TTP) was significantly longer in BRCA2 carriers compared to BRCA1 carriers, with a hazard ratio of 8.6 ($P = 0.01$): in BRCA2 carriers, median TTP was not reached, compared to a median TTP of 24 months in BRCA1 carriers. Non-carriers had a median TTP of 22 months, which is not significantly different from BRCA1 carriers and is not significantly shorter (hazard ratio 4.0; $P = 0.08$) than that of BRCA2 carriers.

Cumulative survival was also significantly longer in BRCA2 car-riers compared to BRCA1 carriers (hazard ratio 11.4; $P = 0.04$) and non-carriers (hazard ratio 13.2; $P = 0.02$). There was no significant difference between BRCA1 carriers and non-carriers. Cumulative survival was longer than usual in the group as a whole, because a survival bias was introduced by the 20 referral cases diagnosed before 1/1994 who were long survivors. However, similar trends approaching statistical significance were observed in the 28 con-secutive cases in our series, in whom there is no survival bias.

We have shown in the past a lower cancer risk and lower pene-trance for BRCA2 ovarian cancer patients (older age at diagnosis). This is the first demonstration of improved prognosis in BRCA2-associated ovarian cancer, both in terms of time to progression and of cumulative survival. Altogether, this implies that BRCA2-associated ovarian cancer has a less virulent course. These results are different than those observed by Frank et al.,[8] and may reflect ascertainment bias or a specific allelic effect of the BRCA2 6174delT mutation. In the study by Frank et al. only one of 38 ovarian cancer patients was a 6174delT carrier, and she was diagnosed at age 61. Differential onset and survival in BRCA2 versus BRCA1 and non-carriers raises the possibility that the biology of ovarian cancer may also be related to mutation status. Hormonal and reproductive factors may therefore have differing effects in these three sub-groups. Indeed, we found that among affected women, hormonal use was most common in BRCA1 carriers, intermediate in non-carriers, and lowest in BRCA2 carriers. This suggests that hormonal exposure may increase cancer risk in BRCA1 carriers and/or that it may be protective in BRCA2 carriers. Obviously this should be tested by comparing affected to unaffected carriers. An interesting analogy would be to compare BRCA2 carriers to estrogen and progesterone receptor positive breast cancer, where there is older age at diagnosis selective estrogen receptor modulators, (SERMs) are protective, and prognosis is better.

Our results may have implications for both treatment of affected carriers and for preventive strategies in non-affected car-riers. The current recommendation for ovarian cancer prevention in carriers is prophylactic oophorectomy at age 35–40. In BRCA2 carriers this procedure could perhaps be delayed by 5–10 years. It will be important to clarify the disparate roles of hormonal manipulation in BRCA1/BRCA2 carriers, taking into account not only their risk for ovarian cancer, but also for breast cancer.

Uterine papillary serous carcinoma

Women found to be carriers of one of the three common founder mutations are usually referred for prophylactic oophorectomy when childbearing is no longer desired. This procedure is usually performed by the laparoscopic technique, with early ambulation and fast recovery.

Over the past 3 years we have encountered two patients who underwent prophylactic BSO due to strong personal and family histories of breast and ovarian cancer. Unfortunately, these patients later developed advanced, primary uterine papillary serous carcinoma (UPSC), a tumour with known histological and clinical behaviour similar to that of ovarian cancer. As a result we have attempted to evaluate a possible association between *BRCA1/2* carrier status and this aggressive endometrial tumour.

Five of seven patients had a personal or family history of breast–ovarian cancer. Preliminary analysis of DNA and blood samples from seven Ashkenazi patients with UPSC revealed two (28.5%) patients who were carriers of a *BRCA1* germ-line mutation. Both women had a family history of ovarian cancer and one also had breast cancer. This carrier rate is similar to that seen in our larger series of ovarian cancer patients. Endometrial tissue samples from these two patients were analysed for loss of heterozygosity (LOH). In one case, the tumour was extremely invasive and it was impossible to isolate tumour from normal tissue. In this case, the wild-type allele was not completely absent in DNA extracted from the tumour sample, but it was significantly reduced compared to the 185delAG allele. In the second case, where a purer tumour sample was available, there was loss of heterozygosity (LOH) for *BRCA1* and only the 5382insC allele was observed in the tumour tissue, indicating loss of the wild-type allele. These results indicate that the endometrial tumour observed in these two carriers was causally related to the *BRCA1* mutation carrier state and was not a chance association.

This important observation requires further verification in a larger group of patients with UPSC and, if substantiated, may have implications for decision-making prior to prophylactic measures. At the moment, many women choose to have a hysterectomy at the time of BSO, for non-oncological reasons. If indeed carriers are at increased risk of developing UPSC, one could strengthen the indication for hysterectomy and add this procedure to the prophylactic strategy.

Summary

The Israeli population is defined as a high-risk group because of the frequency of carriers in the general population. However, the issues involved in the clinical implementation of current data regarding hereditary ovarian cancer have not yet been resolved. The prognostic significance of mutation carriers among patients, the role of screening in this high-risk population, and the prophylactic strategies recommended to healthy carriers, need to be evaluated and analysed further.

It is therefore extremely important to be cautious and to keep our high-risk population, and the physicians involved in counselling them, up to date with the current information, since the relevant decision-making may change frequently.

Acknowledgements

The *BRCA1/BRCA2* analysis at the Shaare Zedek Medical Center was supported in part by a grant from the ICRF (Israel Cancer Research Fund) to ELL and RC, and by a gift from the Basker family, in loving memory of Eileen Basker. We thank Ms Gaya Klein for excellent technical assistance.

References

1. Roa, B.B., Boyd, A.A., Volcik, K. and Richards, C.S. (1996). Ashkenazi Jewish population frequencies for common mutations in BRCA1 and BRCA2. *Nature Genet.*, **14**, 185–7.
2. Bruchim Bar Sade, R., Theodor, I., Gak E. *et al.* (1997). Could the 185delAG BRCA1 mutation be an ancient Jewish mutation? *Eur. J. Hum. Genet.*, **5**, 413–16.
3. Bruchim Bar-Sade, R., Kruglikova, A., Modan, B. *et al.* (1998). The 185delAG BRCA1 mutation originated before the dispersion of Jews in the Diaspora and is not limited to Ashkenazim. *Hum. Mol. Genet.*, **7** (5), 801–5.
4. Friedman, E., Bruchim Bar-Sade, R., Kruglikova, A. *et al.* (1998). Double heterrozygotes for the Ashkenazi founder mutation in BRCA1 and BRCA2 genes. *Am. J. Hum. Genet.*, **63** (4), 1224–7.
5. Levy-Lahad, E., Catane, R., Eisenberg, S. *et al.* (1997). Founder BRCA1 and BRCA2 mutations in Ashknazi Jews in Israel: frequency and differential penetrance in ovarian cancer in breast/ ovarian cancer families. *Am. J. Hum. Genet.*, **60**, 1059–67.
6. Rubin, S.C., Benjamin, I., Behbakht, K. *et al.* (1996). Clinical and pathological features of ovarian cancer in women with germline mutations in BRCA1. *N. Engl. J. Med.*, **336** (19), 1413–16.
7. Johansson, O..T., Idvall, I., Anderson, C. *et al.* (1997). Tumor biological features of BRCA1 induced breast and ovarian cancer. *Eur. J. Cancer*, **33**, 362–71.
8. Frank, T.S., Monley, S.A., Olutunmilay, I. *et al.* (1998) Sequence analysis of BRCA1 abd BRCA2: correlation of mutations with family history and ovarian cancer risk. *J. Clin. Oncol.*, **16** (7), 2417–25.
9. Boyd, J., Sonoda, Y., Federici, M.G. *et al.* (1999). Clinical and pathological features of hereditary ovarian cancer associated with germline mutations in BRCA1 or BRCA2. Society of Gynecologic Oncology Meeting, San Francisco, March.

8.   Clinical implications of genetic testing

Andrew Berchuck, P. Andrew Futreal, and Joellen S. Schildkraut

Introduction

Since the discovery of the *BRCA1* and *BRCA2* cancer susceptibility genes about 5 years ago, it has become clear that germ-line mutations in these genes account for the vast majority of hereditary ovarian cancers, as well as a significant fraction of hereditary breast cancers. Genetic testing is now widely available and should serve as the primary basis for management of most familial breast–ovarian cancer. The aim of this chapter is to discuss the clinical implications of genetic testing. Although a consensus has begun to emerge regarding some issues, genetic testing is a relatively new development and many areas of controversy remain. For example, the most effective strategy for prevention and early diagnosis of cancer in mutation carriers has not yet been determined. In addition, many of the social, ethical, and legal issues that accompany cancer susceptibility testing remain unresolved.

Genetic testing

About 10% of epithelial ovarian cancers are thought to arise in women who carry mutations in high-penetrance cancer suscepti-

bility genes. Germ-line mutations in *BRCA1* are seen in 4–6% of ovarian cancers[1,2] and mutations in *BRCA2* in about 2–4% of cases.[3,4] Although mutational analysis of *BRCA1* and *BRCA2* remains labor intensive, genetic testing is now widely available. Mutations have been observed throughout these large genes and approximately 80–90% of the mutations predict truncated protein products (Fig. 8.1).[5,6] Missense mutations that encode full-length protein products in which a single amino acid is altered occur in about 10–15% of hereditary cases.[7] In some families it may be difficult to distinguish disease-causing mutations from rare polymorphisms. If a missense alteration has previously been associated with familial breast–ovarian cancer in the literature, this suggests that the sequence variant represents a deleterious mutation. Likewise, if other family members are available and willing to be tested, segregation of a missense alteration with cancer in a family suggests, but does not prove, its significance. As the function of *BRCA1* and *BRCA2* is elucidated in normal cells, this may facilitate the development of assays that can be used to determine whether individual missense alterations actually disrupt the function of these proteins.

Presently, the significance of many missense mutations that alter a single amino acid are uncertain, and the results of genetic

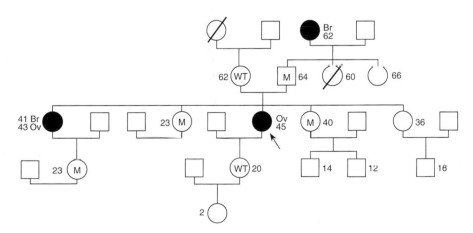

Fig. 8.1 Hereditary ovarian cancer pedigree with *BRCA1* mutation. The age of family members and type of cancers are noted. Individuals denoted 'M' have a G to T mutation in the exon 5 splice site of *BRCA1* that results in a truncated 75 amino-acid protein product, whereas those denoted 'WT' have normal *BRCA1*. The 40-year-old sister of the proband underwent prophylactic oophorectomy and mastectomy after learning that she was a *BRCA1* mutation carrier.

testing must be considered indeterminate in these cases. An indeterminate result presents a difficult clinical dilemma. In these instances, and those in which no sequence variation is seen in *BRCA1* or *BRCA2* despite a strong family history of breast–ovarian cancer, clinical decisions must still be based on the family history, as was the practice prior to the identification of *BRCA1* and *BRCA2*. It is possible that some of these families may harbor mutations in other, as yet undiscovered, cancer susceptibility genes. Alternatively, clustering of breast and/or ovarian cancer in some families may simply represent chance rather than the result of a genetic predisposition. In either event, an indeterminate or negative test result in the context of a strong family history remains problematic.

Because cancer genetic susceptibility testing is relatively new, a consensus has not been reached regarding guidelines for testing in clinical practice. Although mutations in *BRCA1* and *BRCA2* have been noted in some women in the absence of a family history of breast or ovarian cancer, the incidence is low and cost considerations currently prohibit mutational screening in the general population. Those who believe that it is reasonable to test 'high-risk' individuals generally advocate testing when the family history suggests at least a 10–20% probability of finding a mutation. In practical terms, this means a history of two individuals in a family who have had either ovarian cancer at any age or breast cancer prior to age 50 and are either first- or second-degree relatives. Although this is a reasonable guideline, it will exclude from testing some families that harbor mutations. To better quantify the probability of finding a mutation in a given individual in a family, Berry and others have constructed complex mathematical models that account for factors such as the age of cancer diagnosis in affected individuals, the current age of unaffected individuals, the number of unaffected individuals, and the exact relationships of all family members.[8,9] Such models may have significant clinical utility in the future, particularly if genetic testing for cancer susceptibility is ordered directly by primary-care physicians.

We have analyzed our initial experience with genetic testing in the Duke University Hereditary Cancer Clinic. This multidisciplinary clinic includes oncologists (medical, surgical, gynecological), epidemiologists, genetic counselors, and an ethicist. Over 400 pedigrees have been entered into a familial cancer database. From this database, 201 affected probands (184 breast cancer, 17 ovarian cancer) agreed to have blood drawn for genetic testing. All those invited to undergo testing had a predicted probability of carrying either a *BRCA1* or *BRCA2* mutation of at least 10–20%. The entire *BRCA1* and *BRCA2* genes were screened for mutations using single-stranded conformation analysis and heteroduplex analysis, and variant bands were sequenced. Mutations were identified in 41/201 (21%) affected probands (28 *BRCA1*, 13 *BRCA2*). Relatives of probands with mutations have been invited to undergo testing as well. More recently, we have been working with several other institutions that were selected to participate in the Cancer Genetics Network (CGN), which has been funded by the National Cancer Institute. The purpose of the CGN is to set up a common infrastructure for accruing cancer-prone families and performing genetic testing. After this initial work is completed, the CGN will initiate studies that address various clinical issues.

Since the benefits of genetic testing remain hypothetical, it is important that women receive educational material and counseling explaining the postulated risks and benefits prior to deciding to undergo testing. In the Duke Hereditary Cancer Clinic, a rigorous process of education and informed consent takes place prior to genetic testing. We are conducting a formal study that examines the effect of various pre-test educational approaches on acceptance of testing. Some patients receive standard educational materials, while others receive tailored materials based on their age, race, socio-economic status, and other factors. In addition, post-test counseling and follow-up are crucial to help women work through various issues, including decisions regarding prophylactic surgery. The involvement of genetic counselors is invaluable as they are well trained in the nuances of helping individuals through the entire genetic testing process. Depression and anxiety are frequent, regardless of whether one receives a positive or negative test result.[10] Finally, confidentiality remains a critical issue in cancer susceptibility testing. Misuse of genetic information could have potentially devastating consequences, including difficulty in securing employment and life, health, or disability insurance. Fortunately, the potential for such discrimination has rarely been realized to date.

Pathologic and clinical features of hereditary ovarian cancers

Large clinical studies of *BRCA1*- and *BRCA2*-associated ovarian cancer have been difficult to perform because few institutions have identified large numbers of cases. Thus far, it appears that the strongest clinical correlate of *BRCA1* mutation is papillary serous histology. In summarizing five hospital-based studies,[1,2,11–13] 94% (59/63) of *BRCA1*-associated ovarian cancers have been serous. Although this is the most commonly observed histologic type of epithelial ovarian cancer, it generally accounts for only about half to two-thirds of cases. In view of the consistency of these reports, it now seems reasonably certain that serous histology is a hallmark of ovarian cancers with *BRCA1* mutations. Most women with *BRCA1*-associated ovarian cancer present with advanced-stage invasive disease, but some early stage and borderline cancers have been noted.

It has been suggested that survival of *BRCA1* mutation carriers with ovarian cancer may be relatively favorable compared to that of controls. Rubin *et al.* performed a collaborative study that included several institutions in the United States.[14] They reviewed the clinical and pathologic characteristics of ovarian cancers that developed in 53 *BRCA1* carriers. The average age at diagnosis was 48 years (range 28–78). Most of the cancers were poorly differentiated (70%) and there were only two borderline tumors. Survival of 43 *BRCA1* carriers with advanced-stage ovarian cancer was compared to that of controls matched for stage, age, grade, and histologic type. Actuarial median 5-year survival was 77 months in *BRCA1* carriers and 29 months in non-carriers, and this difference was highly significant. Likewise, recently it was reported at the 1999 meeting of the Society of Gynecologic Oncologists that women with ovarian cancer at Memorial Sloan Kettering Cancer

Center who carry the Ashkenazi mutations in *BRCA1*, but not *BRCA2*, had more favorable survival relative to controls.

Studies from other groups have not confirmed the favorable survival of *BRCA1* carriers, however. A population-based study examined survival in 38 Swedish women with *BRCA1*-associated ovarian cancers from 21 families, relative to a large population of Swedish women with ovarian cancer in whom *BRCA1* status was unknown.[15] Stage I/II cases accounted for 31% of the study group and 69% had stage III/IV disease. Although an initial survival advantage was noted for the first 2–3 years in *BRCA1*-associated cases, this difference did not persist over time. In addition, the familial ovarian cancer study group in the United Kingdom examined survival in 151 patients from 57 *BRCA1* and *BRCA2* families compared to that seen in 119 patients from 62 families in which a *BRCA1/2* mutation was not identified. Overall survival at 5 years was 21% in cases from *BRCA1* mutation families, 25% in *BRCA2* mutation families, and 19% in families with no identified mutation.[16]

Prevention and early detection of ovarian cancer

With the discovery of genes responsible for hereditary ovarian cancer, there is reason to believe that we can move beyond the old paradigm of simply recommending prophylactic oophorectomy on the basis of a strong family history. In families in which a deleterious mutation in *BRCA1* or *BRCA2* is demonstrated, women who are found not to be carriers can be reassured that their risk of ovarian cancer is not elevated. Conversely, carriers should be considered candidates for various early detection and/or prevention strategies.

Screening has been advocated as a possible approach to decreasing ovarian cancer mortality in women who carry germ-line *BRCA1* or *BRCA2* mutations, but significant obstacles exist. First, a histologically definable preinvasive lesion has not yet been identified conclusively in the ovary. As a result, efforts have focused on early detection of invasive cancers that still are confined to the ovaries, but this is difficult due to the small size and inaccessibility of the ovaries. Most serous and endometrioid ovarian cancers produce CA125, and serum levels of this marker often are elevated in women with ovarian cancer. However, so far CA125 has not been proven cost-effective for ovarian cancer screening, for several reasons, including the low incidence of ovarian cancer in the population, the relatively low sensitivity of CA125 for detection of early stage disease, and low specificity (because CA125 is often elevated in women with benign diseases).[17] Strategies to improve the utility of serum markers, include repeating the CA125 in individuals with low-level elevations rather than immediately initiating further evaluation, and the use of other serum markers (such as OVX1 or LPA) that may complement CA125. Transvaginal ultrasound also has been proposed as a method of screening for ovarian cancer.[18] Most ovarian enlargement seen by ultrasound does not represent ovarian cancer, but the presence of complex architecture, mural nodules, and neovascularization (as detected by Doppler) increases the likelihood of malignancy. Similar to serum markers, ultrasound suffers from low cost-effectiveness due to its relatively low positive predictive value in a screening setting, because most ovarian masses are not malignant.

Although CA125 and ultrasound are not currently recommended for screening in the general population, screening with these modalities might be more practical in *BRCA1* and *BRCA2* carriers, in whom the incidence of ovarian cancer is much higher. Even if the lifetime risk of invasive ovarian cancer is assumed to be only 15% in carriers, this represents about a tenfold increased relative risk compared to the general population. Early detection strategies that employ CA125 or ultrasound are worthy of formal study in mutation carriers. In the interim, these tests seem reasonable to recommend for women during the reproductive years when oophorectomy would involve loss of fertility and premature menopause, and in peri- and postmenopausal women who have not undergone oophorectomy.

Another strategy that has been suggested to decrease the risk of ovarian cancer in women with germ-line *BRCA1* or *BRCA2* mutations is the use of oral contraceptives. Long-term use of the oral contraceptive pill decreases the risk of ovarian cancer in the general population by as much as 60–80%. Other factors, such as high parity and breastfeeding, which, like the pill, inhibit total lifetime ovulations, also decrease ovarian cancer risk. A recent study of *BRCA1* and *BRCA2* carriers with ovarian cancer and their unaffected sisters suggested that birth control pill use also is protective against ovarian cancer in these families.[19] The magnitude of protection afforded by the pill (>50% in those who used the pill for more than 3 years) was similar to that seen in studies in the general population. The finding that oral contraceptive users in the Gilda Radner familial ovarian cancer registry had a lower incidence of ovarian cancer than non-users is also encouraging.[20] Oral contraceptives might be a particularly attractive alternative for young women who have not yet completed childbearing, but there is concern that oral contraceptive use might increase the risk of breast cancer. Although the above-noted study of the pill in *BRCA1/2* mutation carriers was not designed to detect an increased risk of breast cancer, it is reassuring that no such risk was observed.

Prophylactic oophorectomy

Although surgical prophylaxis is associated with significant cost, oophorectomy appears to be a reasonable option in mutation carriers, for several reasons (Table 8.1). First, this procedure can be performed laparoscopically in an outpatient setting; and although surgical morbidity and mortality can occur, the incidence of serious complications is low. In addition, most women do not view removal of the ovaries as cosmetically mutilating, and oophorectomy causes only modest changes in body image and self-esteem. Finally, estrogen replacement can be administered either orally or transdermally, thereby avoiding the deleterious side-effects of premature menopause, including vasomotor symptoms, urogenital atrophy, osteoporosis, and heart disease. Although there is some concern that estrogen replacement might

Table 8.1 Pros and cons of prophylactic oophorectomy

Pros
  decreases ovarian cancer incidence and mortality
  can be delayed to allow completion of childbearing
  laparoscopic approach
  little effect on body image or self-esteem
  estrogen replacement can prevent surgical menopause
Cons
  cost of prophylactic surgery may not be covered by insurance
  potential morbidity and mortality
  potential for primary peritoneal carcinoma
  estrogen replacement may increase breast cancer risk

increase the risk of breast cancer in these women, this risk already is exceedingly high. In addition, systemic estrogen levels are lower in premenopausal women after hormone replacement than if the ovaries had been left in place. Because the incidence of ovarian cancer in BRCA1 and BRCA2 carriers does not begin to rise dramatically until about age 40,[21] prophylactic oophorectomy can be delayed until after childbearing is completed. Lynch *et al.* reported that 76% of high-risk women undergoing genetic testing would strongly consider oophorectomy.[10]

Histologic examination has suggested that ovaries removed prophylactically from women with a strong family history of ovarian cancer have a higher frequency of epithelial architectural abnormalities and cytologic atypia. This phenomenon, often referred to as ovarian dysplasia or ovarian intraepithelial neoplasia, was observed initially in women undergoing prophylactic oophorectomy because their identical twin sisters had developed ovarian cancer.[22] The spectrum of epithelial abnormalities subsequently described includes surface epithelial pseudostratification, atypia, and papillomatosis; deep cortical invaginations of the surface epithelium, frequently with multiple papillary projections within small cystic spaces; and epithelial inclusion cysts, frequently with epithelial hyperplasia and papillary formations.[23] Similar alterations have also been reported in normal ovarian epithelium adjacent to early ovarian cancers and in the contralateral normal ovary in Stage I ovarian cancers.[24,25] These studies provide evidence to suggest that prophylactic removal of the ovaries in high-risk women serves to remove premalignant lesions before they progress to fully invasive cancers. On the other hand, studies of prophylactically removed ovaries in BRCA1 or BRCA2 carriers from Harvard and the Memorial Sloan Kettering Cancer Center were reported not to have an increased frequency of 'premalignant' histologic abnormalities (1999 meeting of the Society of Gynecologic Oncologists).

However, the benefit of oophorectomy in mutation carriers has not been demonstrated conclusively, and there are reasons to believe that the protective effect of oophorectomy may be less than intuitively expected. First, although the lifetime risk of ovarian cancer in BRCA1 carriers was reported to be as high as 60% in some initial series, more recent studies have suggested that this risk is significantly lower (15–30%).[26,27] The lifetime risk of ovarian cancer in BRCA2 carriers is probably about 10%. Thus, even in known mutation carriers, somewhere in the range of 3–10 prophylactic oophorectomies must be performed for each case of ovarian cancer prevented. A significant fraction of families with

BRCA1 or BRCA2 mutations do not include any ovarian cancer cases, and women in these families may be less highly motivated to pursue prophylactic oophorectomy. Likewise, in the absence of an understanding of the variable penetrance of ovarian cancer genes in mutation carriers, the bias of many physicians is to recommend prophylactic oophorectomy more strongly to mutation carriers in families in which ovarian cancer has already been diagnosed in other women.

The occurrence of peritoneal papillary serous carcinoma, indistinguishable histologically or macroscopically from ovarian cancer, represents another potential drawback to prophylactic oophorectomy. Initially, Tobacman *et al.* reported primary peritoneal carcinoma in 3 of 28 women who had undergone oophorectomy in the National Cancer Institute's registry of cancer-prone families.[28] Cancers were diagnosed 1, 5, and 11 years later. In the Gilda Radner Familial Ovarian Cancer Registry, carcinomatosis developed in only 6 out of 324 women (2%) who had undergone prophylactic oophorectomy from 1 to 27 years previously.[29] Only 102 of these women had at least two first-degree relatives with ovarian cancer, but five of the six cases in which primary peritoneal carcinoma developed were from this group, and the other case had three second-degree relatives with ovarian cancer. This report preceded the identification of BRCA1 and BRCA2, and it is unclear what fraction of women in the registry were actually mutation carriers.

More recently, Struewing *et al.* examined the effect of oophorectomy on the risk of serous carcinoma of the ovary or peritoneum in women with a first-degree relative with ovarian cancer in the National Cancer Institute registry of cancer-prone families.[30] In 44 women who had oophorectomy, two peritoneal cancers arose in 460 person-years. In contrast, in 346 who did not undergo oophorectomy, eight ovarian cancers arose in about 1600 person-years. When these data were compared to the Connecticut Tumor Registry, there was approximately a 24-fold excess of cancer among non-oophorectomized women and a 13-fold excess risk among oophorectomized women. Although the methodology utilized in this study was not optimal, it suggested that oophorectomy reduced the risk of subsequent serous carcinoma of the ovary or peritoneum by about half.

In addition to these registry reports, other cases reports have been published substantiating the occurrence of peritoneal carcinoma after oophorectomy.[31,32] The origin of these 'primary peritoneal' cancers is somewhat unclear. In some cases that were thought to arise in the peritoneal cavity after oophorectomy, careful retrospective examination of the ovaries revealed the presence of microscopic foci of cancer that were not appreciated at the time of the initial pathologic examination.[32] This may occur due to sampling error if only a single section is examined in a normal-appearing ovary. In addition, cases have been reported in which early ovarian cancer was already noted to be present at the time of prophylactic oophorectomy.[33] It was suggested that the entire peritoneal cavity should be inspected carefully, and perhaps biopsies and cytologic washings should be obtained when this procedure is performed. In addition, the pathologist should be alerted as to the indication for surgery, and multiple sections should be examined from each ovary to exclude the presence of occult carcinoma or other abnormal histologic changes.

The occurrence of primary peritoneal papillary serous carcinoma after oophorectomy is thought to reflect the common origin of the ovarian epithelium and peritoneum from embryonic mesoderm. It also is conceivable that some cases of peritoneal carcinomatosis may arise from ectopic ovarian tissue or endometriosis. Whereas most sporadic ovarian cancers have been found to be monoclonal, with peritoneal implants representing metastases from an ovarian primary,[34] evidence has emerged to suggest that some peritoneal carcinomas may arise multifocally. Clonality analysis revealed that 5/22 cases of primary peritoneal carcinoma appeared to have a polyclonal origin, including all three cases in which *BRCA1* mutations had been identified.[35] In 14 cases in which mutations in *BRCA1* had not been found, only two had a polyclonal origin. If multifocal tumorigenesis in the peritoneal cavity is a frequent occurrence in carriers, this certainly could limit the efficacy of prophylactic oophorectomy.

Breast cancer screening and prevention

Although ovarian cancer is the focus of the Helene Harris Memorial Trust, it is important to acknowledge that breast cancer is the most common cancer in women who carry *BRCA1* or *BRCA2* mutations. Breast examination and mammography are well-accepted screening tests, which have been demonstrated to facilitate early detection of breast cancer and to decrease breast cancer deaths.[36] As a result, breast cancer survival is about 70%, compared to only 30% for ovarian cancer. All women who carry *BRCA1* or *BRCA2* mutations should avail themselves of breast cancer screening.

In addition, there are also convincing data suggesting that chemoprevention of breast cancer is an attainable goal. Initially, in a National Surgical Adjuvant Breast and Bowel Project (NSABP) study, a decreased risk of contralateral breast cancer was noted in women with breast cancer who took the anti-estrogen, tamoxifen, compared to women with breast cancer who did not take tamoxifen.[37] This unanticipated observation led to a formal trial by the NSABP of tamoxifen as a breast cancer preventive agent in women with a strong family history of breast cancer. About a 50% reduction in breast cancer incidence was noted in the tamoxifen arm of the study, relative to untreated controls.[38] The relative risk of endometrial cancer in tamoxifen users was increased about 2.5-fold, but the more selective anti-estrogen raloxifene, which does not have an agonist effect on the endometrium, has also been noted to decrease the incidence of breast cancer. One disadvantage of an anti-estrogen preventive strategy in young women would be the potential for symptoms of estrogen deficiency, such as anovulation and hot flushes. Although tamoxifen therapy may not be the most attractive alternative for young women who carry *BRCA1* or *BRCA2* mutations, it might be a very reasonable strategy in older women.

Finally, there is strong evidence that prophylactic mastectomy probably decreases the incidence of breast cancer by about 90% in mutation carriers.[39] The major drawback to this approach is that mastectomy, even with breast reconstruction, leads to marked alterations in self-esteem and body image. Although some women will continue to choose mastectomy, screening and/or chemoprevention with anti-estrogens may prove to have higher patient acceptance and to be equally effective in reducing breast cancer mortality.

Acknowledgements

Supported by the Department of Defense Ovarian Cancer Research Program and the Duke Breast Cancer Specialized Program of Research Excellence.

References

1. Stratton, J.F., Gayther, S.A., Russell, P. *et al.* (1997). Contribution of BRCA1 mutations to ovarian cancer. *N. Engl. J. Med.*, **336**, 1125–30.
2. Berchuck, A., Heron, K., Carney, M.E. *et al.* (1998). Frequency of germline and somatic BRCA1 mutations in ovarian cancer. *Clin. Cancer Res.*, **4**, 2433–7.
3. Foster, K.A., Harrington, P., Kerr, J. *et al.* (1996). Somatic and germline mutations of the BRCA2 gene in sporadic ovarian cancer. *Cancer Res.*, **56**, 3622–5.
4. Rubin, S.C., Blackwood, M.A., Bandera, C. *et al.* (1998). BRCA1, BRCA2, and hereditary nonpolyposis colorectal cancer gene mutations in an unselected ovarian cancer population: relationship to family history and implications for genetic testing. *Am. J. Obstet. Gynecol.*, **178**, 670–7.
5. Couch, F.J. and Weber, B.L.(1996). Mutations and polymorphisms in the familial early-onset breast cancer (BRCA1) gene. *Hum. Mutat.*, **8**, 8–18.
6. Shattuck-Eidens, D., Oliphant, A., McClure, M. *et al.* (1997). BRCA1 sequence analysis in women at high risk for susceptibility mutations. Risk factor analysis and implications for genetic testing. *J. Am. Med. Assoc.*, **278**, 1242–50.
7. Frank, T.S., Manley, S.A., Olopade, O.I. *et al.* (1998). Sequence analysis of BRCA1 and BRCA2: Correlation of mutations with family history and ovarian cancer risk. *J. Clin. Oncol.*, **17**, 2417–25.
8. Parmigiani, G., Berry, D., and Aguilar, O. (1998). Determining carrier probabilities for breast cancer-susceptibility genes BRCA1 and BRCA2. *Am. J. Hum. Genet.*, **62**, 145–58.
9. Berry, D.A., Parmigiani, G., Sanchez, J., Schildkraut, J., and Winer, E. (1997). Probability of carrying a mutation of breast–ovarian cancer gene BRCA1 based on family history. *J. Natl Cancer Inst.*, **89**, 227–38.
10. Lynch, H.T., Lemon, S.J., Durham, C. *et al.* (1997). A descriptive study of BRCA1 testing and reactions to disclosure of test results. *Cancer*, **79**, 2219–28.
11. Takahashi, H., Behbakht, K., McGovern, P.E. *et al.* (1995). Mutation analysis of the BRCA1 gene in ovarian cancers. *Cancer Res.*, **55**, 2998–3002.
12. Matsushima, M., Kobayashi, K., Emi, M. *et al.* (1995). Mutation analysis of the BRCA1 gene in 76 Japanese ovarian cancer patients: four germline mutations, but no evidence of somatic mutation. *Hum. Mol. Genet.*, **4**, 1953–6.
13. Takano, M., Aida, H., Tsuneki, I. *et al.* (1997). Mutational analysis of BRCA1 gene in ovarian and breast–ovarian cancer families in Japan. *Jpn J. Cancer Res.*, **88**, 407–13.
14. Rubin, S.C., Benjamin, I., Behbakht, K. *et al.* (1996). Clinical and pathological features of ovarian cancer in women with germ-line mutations of BRCA1. *N. Engl. J. Med.*, **335**, 1413–16.
15. Johannsson, O.T., Ranstam, J., Borg, A., and Olsson, H. (1998). Survival of BRCA1 breast and ovarian cancer patients: a population-based study from southern Sweden. *J. Clin. Oncol.*, **16**, 397–404.
16. Pharoah, P.D., Easton, D.F., Stockton, D.L., Gayther, S., and Ponder, B.A. (1999). Survival in familial, BRCA1-associated, and BRCA2-associated epithelial ovarian cancer. United Kingdom Coordinating Committee for

Cancer Research (UKCCCR) Familial Ovarian Cancer Study Group. *Cancer Res.*, **59**, 868–71.

17. Rosenthal, A.N. (1998). Screening for gynecologic cancers. *Curr. Opin. Oncol.*, **10**, 447–51.

18. Collins, W.P., Bourne, T.H., and Campbell, S. (1998). Screening strategies for ovarian cancer. *Curr. Opin. Obstet. Gynecol.*, **10**, 33–9.

19. Narod, S.A., Risch, H., Moslehi, R. *et al.* (1998). Oral contraceptives and the risk of hereditary ovarian cancer. Hereditary Ovarian Cancer Clinical Study Group. *N. Engl. J. Med.*, **339**, 424–8.

20. Piver, M.S., Baker, T.R., Jishi, M.F. *et al.* (1993). Familial ovarian cancer. A report of 658 families from the Gilda Radner Familial Ovarian Cancer Registry 1981–1991. *Cancer*, **71**, 582–8.

21. Ford, D., Easton, D.F., Bishop, D.T., Narod, S.A., and Goldgar, D. E. (1994). Risks of cancer in BRCA1-mutation carriers. Breast Cancer Linkage Consortium. *Lancet*, **343**, 692–5.

22. Gusberg, S.B. and Deligdisch, L. (1984). Ovarian dysplasia. A study of identical twins. *Cancer*, **54**, 1–4.

23. Salazar, H., Godwin, A.K., Daly, M.B. *et al.* (1996). Microscopic benign and invasive malignant neoplasms and a cancer-prone phenotype in prophylactic oophorectomies. *J. Natl Cancer Inst.*, **88**, 1810–20.

24. Plaxe, S.C., Deligdisch, L., Dottino, P.R., and Cohen, C.J. (1990). Ovarian intraepithelial neoplasia demonstrated in patients with stage I ovarian carcinoma. *Gynecol. Oncol.*, **38**, 367–72.

25. Resta, L., Russo, S., Colucci, G.A. and Prat, J. (1993). Morphologic precursors of ovarian epithelial tumors. *Obstet. Gynecol.*, **82**, 181–6.

26. Whittemore, A.S., Gong, G., and Itnyre, J. (1997). Prevalence and contribution of BRCA1 mutations in breast cancer and ovarian cancer: results from three U.S. population-based case-control studies of ovarian cancer. *Am. J. Hum. Genet.*, **60**, 496–504.

27. Struewing, J.P., Hartge, P., Wacholder, S. *et al.* (1997). The risk of cancer associated with specific mutations of BRCA1 and BRCA2 among Ashkenazi Jews. *N. Engl. J. Med.*, **336**, 1401–8.

28. Tobacman, J.K., Greene, M.H., Tucker, M.A., Costa, J., Kase, R., Fraumeni, J.F. Jr (1982). Intra-abdominal carcinomatosis after prophylactic oophorectomy in ovarian-cancer-prone families. *Lancet*, **2**, 795–7.

29. Piver, M.S., Jishi, M.F., Tsukada, Y., and Nava, G. (1993). Primary peritoneal carcinoma after prophylactic oophorectomy in women with a family history of ovarian cancer. A report of the Gilda Radner Familial Ovarian Cancer Registry. *Cancer*, **71**, 2751–5.

30. Struewing, J.P., Watson, P., Easton, D.F., Ponder, B.A., Lynch, H.T., and Tucker, M.A. (1995). Prophylactic oophorectomy in inherited breast/ovarian cancer families. *Monogr. Natl Cancer Inst.*, 33–35.

31. Weber, A.M., Hewett, W.J., Gajewski, W.H., and Curry, S.L. (1992). Serous carcinoma of the peritoneum after oophorectomy. *Obstet. Gynecol.*, **80**, 558–60.

32. Chen, K.T., Schooley, J.L., and Flam, M.S. (1985). Peritoneal carcinomatosis after prophylactic oophorectomy in familial ovarian cancer syndrome. *Obstet. Gynecol.*, **66**, 93S–94S.

33. Menczer, J. and Ben-Baruch, G. (1991). Familial ovarian cancer in Israeli Jewish women. *Obstet. Gynecol.*, **77**, 276–7.

34. Jacobs, I.J., Kohler, M., Wiseman, R. *et al.* (1992). Clonal origin of epithelial ovarian cancer: Analysis by loss of heterozygosity, p53 mutation and X-chromosome inactivation. *J. Natl Cancer Inst.*, **84**, 1793–8.

35. Schorge, J.O., Muto, M.G., Welch, W.R. *et al.* (1998). Molecular evidence for multifocal papillary serous carcinoma of the peritoneum in patients with germline BRCA1 mutations. *J. Natl Cancer Inst.*, **90**, 841–5.

36. Hoskins, K.F., Stopfer, J.E., Calzone, K.A. *et al.* (1995). Assessment and counseling for women with a family history of breast cancer. A guide for clinicians. *J. Am. Med. Assoc.*, **273**, 577–85.

37. Fisher, B., Costantino, J., Redmond, C. *et al.* (1989). A randomized clinical trial evaluating tamoxifen in the treatment of patients with node-negative breast cancer who have estrogen-receptor-positive tumors. *N. Engl. J. Med.*, **320**, 479–84.

38. Fisher, B., Costantino, J.P., Wickerham, D.L. *et al.* (1998). Tamoxifen for prevention of breast cancer: report of the National Surgical Adjuvant Breast and Bowel Project P–1 Study. *J. Natl Cancer Inst.*, **90**, 1371–88.

39. Hartmann, L.C., Schaid, D.J., Woods, J.E. *et al.* (1999). Efficacy of bilateral prophylactic mastectomy in women with a family history of breast cancer. *N. Engl. J. Med.*, **340**, 77–84.

Part 2
Natural history and pathology

9. Pathology of epithelial ovarian cancer

Harold Fox and Naveena Singh

Introduction

The malignant epithelial tumours of the ovary are adenocarcinomas, accounting for 90% of all malignant disease of the ovary. There are five main forms of ovarian adenocarcinoma:

(1) serous adenocarcinomas;
(2) mucinous carcinomas;
(3) endometrioid carcinomas;
(4) transitional cell carcinomas (malignant Brenner tumours); and
(5) clear cell adenocarcinomas.

Some malignant epithelial neoplasms are so poorly differentiated that no diagnosis more specific than 'undifferentiated carcinoma' can be made, whereas a significant proportion of epithelial tumours contain more than one type of epithelium, it being not uncommon, for instance, to encounter a mixture of serous carcinoma and mucinous carcinoma within a given neoplasm. These latter tumours are classified in terms of the predominant type of epithelium and are only diagnosed as 'mixed' if the second epithelial component is a prominent feature of the tumour.

Histogenesis

There is considerable evidence that most epithelial neoplasms arise, either directly or indirectly, from the surface epithelium, or serosa, of the ovary.[1,2] The ovarian serosa is the direct descendant, and exact postnatal equivalent, of the coelomic epithelium which, during embryogenesis, overlies the parent structure of the ovary, the nephrogenital ridge. As the embryo develops, the coelomic epithelium of the nephrogenital ridge gives rise, by a process of evagination, to the Müllerian ducts from which the endocervical epithelium, the endometrium, and the epithelium of the Fallopian tube develop. The Wolffian ducts, from which parts of the urinary system develop, also arise from the coelomic epithelium of the nephrogenital ridge. It is a basic histogenetic concept in ovarian neoplasia that tumours are derived from undifferentiated cells which have the same potentiality for differentiation as do the embryonic cells from which the adult tissue was derived. Hence, undifferentiated cells in the ovarian serosa can undergo a neoplas-

tic change while retaining their embryonic potentiality to differentiate along various Müllerian pathways. Thus differentiation of neoplastic cells along a tubal pathway produces the serous group of neoplasms; differentiation along an endocervical route results in mucinous neoplasms; and differentiation along endometrial lines yields the endometrioid tumours. The transitional cell carcinomas (and their benign counterparts, the Brenner tumours) are formed of urinary tract-type epithelium and appear to arise from the surface epithelium by a process of Wolffian, rather than Müllerian, differentiation. It is not surprising that there is a residual capacity for Wolffian differentiation in undifferentiated ovarian serosal cells, in view of the origin of the Wolffian ducts from the coelomic epithelium of the nephrogenital ridge. The clear cell carcinomas are of Müllerian nature and are best considered as a variant of an endometrioid tumour.

This concept of the epithelial tumours of the ovary having a common origin from the surface epithelium but showing different patterns of differentiation is almost certainly true, but is too all-embracing, for some epithelial tumours are of different histogenesis. Thus some endometrioid and clear cell carcinomas arise in, and from, foci of ovarian endometriosis, their direct origin from, and their common lineage with, the endometriotic focus having been confirmed by showing that the endometriosis and the tumour share the same genetic alterations.[3] It is difficult to assess the proportion of ovarian adenocarcinomas that develop in this fashion, for a neoplasm may, as it grows, obliterate any residual evidence of a preceding precursor lesion, but circumstantial evidence suggests that about 30% of endometrioid carcinomas and 50% of clear cell carcinomas arise from pre-existing endometriosis.[4]

It is also possible that not all mucinous carcinomas develop from the ovarian serosa, for some, indeed many, are formed not of endocervical-type epithelium but of gastrointestinal-type epithelium. Neoplasms of this type may arise from the ovarian serosa via a process of gastrointestinal metaplasia, a change now known to occur with some frequency in Müllerian tissues, but there is a possibility that some are monodermal teratomas.

Actual origin directly from the ovarian serosa is very difficult to prove in most ovarian adenocarcinomas, for these have usually attained a large size at initial diagnosis and no site of origin can be determined. However, a small number of very early ovarian adenocarcinomas have been described which did appear to involve the surface epithelium,[5] whereas changes such as nuclear pleomorphism, irregularity of nuclear chromatin, stratification, and loss of nuclear polarity, thought to represent ovarian 'dysplasia' or 'intraepithelial neoplasia', have been described in the surface epithelium adjacent to ovarian adenocarcinomas.[6,7] Expression of the p53 protein, indicative of a mutation in the tumour suppressor gene *p53*, is also frequently detectable in the serosa adjacent to an adenocarcinoma,[8] but nevertheless, the status of 'ovarian intraepithelial neoplasia' or 'ovarian dysplasia' as a precursor lesion remains uncertain. Abnormalities of this type have not been detected in the serosa of the ovaries of women who are at high risk of developing ovarian carcinoma,[9–11] while doubt has recently been cast upon the validity of a number of the original observations of 'ovarian dysplasia'.[12]

It is, in fact, probable that some ovarian adenocarcinomas do not arise directly from the serosa but from inclusion cysts which result from invagination of the serosa. Credence has been lent to this view by reports that the contralateral ovaries from women with unilateral ovarian adenocarcinoma contain an increased number of inclusion cysts,[13] that inclusion cysts associated with ovarian adenocarcinoma have a high incidence of cytological atypia, and that the epithelium in these cysts may show overexpression of the oncogene c-*erbB–2* and p53 protein expression.[8] It must be noted, however, that an increased incidence of inclusion cysts in association with adenocarcinoma has not been confirmed in all studies.[14] An increased incidence of inclusion cysts has been noted in some studies of ovaries from women at high risk for ovarian cancer,[10,15] but not in all.[9]

The question as to whether or not ovarian adenocarcinomas arise with any frequency from pre-existing cystadenomas or tumours of borderline malignancy is still not fully decided. There are usually no morphological features in serous adenocarcinomas to suggest an origin from a benign or borderline neoplasm, whereas molecular and genetic analyses of serous tumours have shown different, rather than similar, patterns of genetic alterations in benign, borderline, and malignant tumours.[16] By contrast, a high proportion of mucinous adenocarcinomas contain apparently benign epithelium,[17] whereas identical genetic changes have been noted in benign, borderline, and malignant mucinous neoplasms.[18,19] These findings may indicate that mucinous adenocarcinomas not uncommonly develop from pre-existing benign neoplasms, but it is possible that the apparently benign epithelium actually represents a more differentiated subpopulation of malignant cells rather than the remnants of a precursor lesion.

Although, as remarked, it is generally believed that most ovarian adenocarcinomas arise, either directly or indirectly, from the ovarian serosa, there is a quite strongly argued minority view that ovarian adenocarcinomas arise from structures that can, perhaps in a rather loose fashion, be regarded as the secondary Müllerian system, these including paraovarian and paratubal cysts, the rete ovarii, and endometriosis.[20] While there is little doubt that ovarian carcinomas can originate in foci of endometriosis (see above), the evidence that they are derived from paraovarian cysts or the rete ovarii is not compelling.

Aetiology

It has emerged from epidemiological studies, with considerable clarity, that population groups with a high incidence of ovarian cancer are those which, on average, have small families, and that within any given population nulliparity is an important risk factor.[21,22] It could be, and indeed has been, argued that it is not nulliparity which is the real risk factor, the apparent relationship between the nulliparous state and ovarian cancer simply reflecting a tendency for infertile women with ovarian malfunction to develop this form of neoplasia. Ovarian cancer is, however, unduly common in nuns, and nulliparous women who have never been married have the same risk as do married nulliparous women. These facts not only suggest that infertility *per se* is not an independent risk factor, but also that the elevated risk in nulliparous women is attributable to deprivation of a direct protective effect conferred by pregnancy. That this is the case is shown by the fact that the more pregnancies a woman has, the less is her chance of developing ovarian adenocarcinoma. It is of note, however, that the first pregnancy has a greater protective effect than later pregnancies, and that the pregnancy need not be completed, for failed gestations (e.g. ectopic pregnancies and abortions) also reduce the risk of ovarian cancer, although the magnitude of protection is less than that obtained from a full-term pregnancy.[21–23] In some studies, the age at which the first pregnancy occurred did not appear to be of any significance, although in one population-based case-control study the older the woman at the time of her first gestation, the greater the degree of protection.[24] The protective effect of pregnancy appears to last for only about 10 years, with a progressively increasing risk of ovarian cancer after that period.[25]

Breast feeding also decreases the risk of ovarian cancer, and the measure of protection increases with the length of the breast feeding period.[26] Studies of the effects of age of menarche and of menopause on the risk of ovarian cancer have not yielded any consistent pattern, but there has been general agreement, in a very large number of studies, that the use of combined oral contraceptives diminishes considerably the risk of ovarian carcinoma, the magnitude of the risk reduction increasing with lengthening duration of usage.[22,27] The effect of oral contraceptives on ovarian cancer risk persists for at least 10–15 years after use has ceased,[28] but it is of note that the protective effect of oral contraception usage is most marked in older women, a possible indication that the early high-potency contraceptives were more protective than those in current use.

As discussed already, fertility *per se* does not appear to be a significant risk factor for ovarian cancer,[29] but it has been suggested that there is a subset of infertile women, those who have received drug therapy, who are at increased risk of developing ovarian adenocarcinoma.[22] In one later study it was found that only the use of clomiphene citrate was associated with an increased risk of ovarian cancer,[30] whereas in another no association at all was found between the use of fertility drugs and ovarian cancer.[31]

Both hysterectomy and tubal ligation reduce the risk for ovarian adenocarcinoma,[32–35] and there is some evidence that hysterectomy before the age of 40 confers greater protection than does a similar operation after this age.[22]

Other factors

Genetic factors are clearly important in the aetiology of a relatively small percentage of ovarian carcinomas; these are discussed elsewhere in this volume.

The protective effect of hysterectomy and of tubal ligation has led some to suggest that an ascending carcinogen is involved in ovarian neoplasia, and the finger of guilt has been pointed at talc,[36,37] but overall the evidence in favour of a causal connection between talc and ovarian cancer has not been proven.[38,39] The protective effect of tubal ligation and hysterectomy appears to result mainly from a reduction in the incidence of endometrioid and clear cell carcinomas[40] and hence may simply result from a decreased incidence of endometriosis.

There have been repetitive claims that dietary factors play a role in ovarian carcinogenesis, dietary fat intake being particularly implicated in this respect. The evidence for this is, however, far from convincing.[41] It has also been maintained that milk consumption and lactose intake are related to the risk for ovarian cancer, but this could not be confirmed in two later studies.[42,43]

Pathogenesis

Consideration of all the factors known either to increase or decrease the risk of ovarian adenocarcinoma allows for the formulation of two aetiological hypotheses. The first of these is the 'incessant ovulation' hypothesis, which argues that any factor that reduces the number of ovulations during a woman's reproductive life will decrease the risk of ovarian epithelial neoplasia.[44] The possible mechanisms by which repetitive ovulation could influence the development of ovarian adenocarcinoma include an increased formation of inclusion cysts, repeated bathing of the surface epithelium by oestrogen-rich follicular fluid, excess production of growth factors or cytokines, or an aberration of the repeated repair process which follows the trauma to the surface epithelium consequent upon ovulation. Most of the data with regard to reproductive factors are in accord with the incessant ovulation hypothesis, in particular the protective effects of pregnancy, oral contraception, and breast feeding, all of which inhibit ovulation. The protective effects of hysterectomy and tubal ligation can also be, at least partially, explained in these terms, for there is a tendency for anovulatory cycles to occur after both procedures. Further support for the excessive ovulation hypothesis comes from the observation that there is a correlation between the frequency of *p53* mutations in ovarian carcinomas and the number of prior ovulatory cycles,[45] although, it must be admitted, a subsequent study failed to confirm this finding.[46] Arguments against the excessive ovulation hypothesis include the weak, if any, influences of age of menarche and menopause, the greater risk reduction offered by pregnancy than a similar period of oral contraception, and the differential protective effect of first and subsequent pregnancies.

The alternative hypothesis is that raised gonadotrophin levels play an aetiological role in the development of ovarian adenocarcinoma, and that any factor reducing the levels of these hormones would protect against ovarian cancer.[47] However, the hypergonadotrophic hypothesis does not accord with the protective effects of breast feeding, hysterectomy, or tubal ligation, or with the lack of any reduction in risk with oestrogen replacement therapy[22] which, if anything, tends to be associated with a slightly increased incidence of ovarian cancer.[48,49]

It is clear that neither of the two aetiological theories would explain all the known epidemiological data, and it is perhaps unduly simplistic to believe that any single factor can be held responsible for this disease.

Pathology of malignant epithelial tumours

Amongst malignant epithelial ovarian tumours serous adenocarcinomas are the most common form, accounting for between 40 and 50% of cases. Endometrioid and mucinous adenocarcinomas form about 20% and 10% of the total, respectively, whereas clear cell carcinomas account for between 5 and 10% of adenocarcinomas. Malignant Brenner tumours are uncommon, although their infrequency has, in the past, been markedly overestimated.

Gross appearances

Little point is served in attempting to describe the gross appearance of each individual type of ovarian adenocarcinoma, for specific features are generally absent. The tumours are usually bulky, typically measuring between 15 and 30 cm in diameter, and may have a smooth or bosselated outer surface, which can be studded with papillae. On section the neoplasm may be cystic, partially cystic, or solid throughout. Cystic areas may be unilocular or, more commonly, multiloculated, and can contain either serous or mucinous fluid, which may be turbid, bloodstained, or frankly haemorrhagic. Fleshy or firm mural nodules often protrude into cystic spaces, while, particularly but not specifically in serous adenocarcinomas, the cyst cavities may be partly or wholly filled with soft, friable villi. Solid areas may be crumbly, soft, fleshy, firm, or rubbery, and are commonly white, whitish-yellow, or grey. Foci of haemorrhage and necrosis, often extensive, are a characteristic feature.

Histological appearances

Well-differentiated serous adenocarcinomas have a predominantly papillary pattern (Fig. 9.1a). The papillae tend to be fine, often branching, and not infrequently fused at their tips. They have a delicate connective tissue support and a covering, but invading, epithelium, in which the constituent cells bear an anarchic resemblance to those normally found in the tubal epithelium. However, a purely papillary pattern is relatively uncommon and there are often a few areas showing an irregular acinar pattern, the acini tending to have slit-like lumens. Poorly differentiated serous adenocarcinomas have a predominantly solid histological appearance, with sheets of small, relatively uniform cells, sometimes showing a syncytial-like pattern, admixed with poorly formed glandular acini or abortive papillae. Serous tumours of moderate differentiation occupy an intermediate position, often containing a melange of papillary, acinar, and solid areas. Psammoma bodies, which are small, laminated calcospherites (Fig. 9.1 b), are a characteristic, but not specific, feature of serous adenocarcinomas and are seen most commonly, and most conspicuously, in well-differentiated neoplasms.

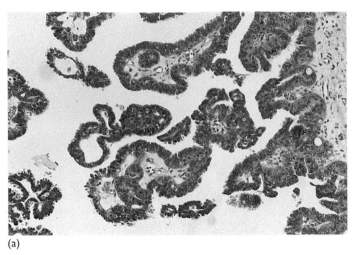

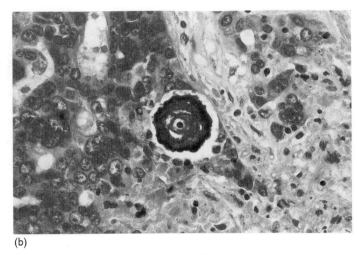

(a)   (b)

Fig. 9.1 (a) Papillary pattern in invasive serous adenocarcinoma (haematoxylin and eosin ×100). (b) Laminated calcospherite or psammoma body in serous adenocarcinoma (haematoxylin and eosin ×400).

Well-differentiated mucinous adenocarcinomas (Fig. 9.2) tend to show a locular and acinar pattern, the lining epithelium being recognizably formed of columnar mucus-secreting cells which show varying degrees of multilayering, mitotic activity, and atypia; goblet cells are commonly seen. Stromal invasion is evident, but it is not uncommon for well-differentiated tumours, if extensively sampled, to also contain areas having the appearance of a benign mucinous cystadenoma, or areas showing the appearance of a tumour of borderline malignancy. Poorly differentiated mucinous adenocarcinomas may be formed largely of solid sheets of anaplastic cells which are interspersed with poorly formed glandular acini. There may be clusters or single infiltrating cells, while signet-ring cells may be a noticeable feature. In all grades of mucinous carcinoma there may be extrusion of mucus into the stroma; this is sometimes extensive, with the formation of large pools of mucus in which tumour cells appear to be floating (pseudomyxoma ovarii).

Endometrioid adenocarcinomas have a histological appearance which is very similar to, indeed virtually identical with, that of an endometrioid adenocarcinoma of the endometrium (Fig. 9.3). Most endometrioid adenocarcinomas are well differentiated and have a well-formed acinar pattern, with the cells lining the acini often showing multilayering and irregular budding. The cells resemble those of the glandular epithelium of a proliferative-phase endometrium, but show a greater degree of pleomorphism and atypia. The stroma of the tumour resembles that of the ovary rather than that of the endometrium, and stromal invasion is usually readily apparent. A papillary pattern may be present in some areas and may even predominate. The papillae are, however, blunter and broader than those in a serous adenocarcinoma. Squamous metaplasia is a common occurrence, whereas a clear cell pattern is often focally present. Moderately differentiated adenocarcinomas show a more complex microglandular pattern with a greater degree of pleomorphism, whereas poorly differentiated

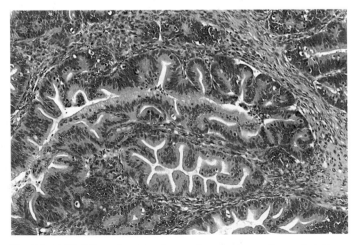

Fig. 9.2 Well-differentiated mucinous adenocarcinoma (haematoxylin and eosin ×100).

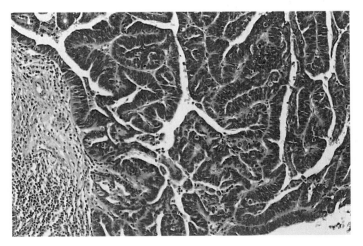

Fig. 9.3 Well-differentiated endometrioid adenocarcinoma with a papillary pattern (haematoxylin and eosin ×100).

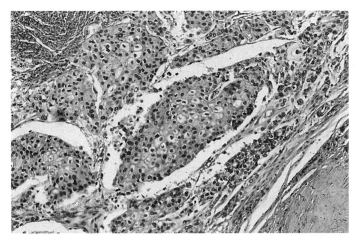

Fig. 9.4 Invasive transitional cell carcinoma of ovary (malignant Brenner tumour). (Haematoxylin and eosin ×100).

endometrioid tumours have a predominantly solid growth pattern with residual microglandular areas. Some endometrioid tumours adopt a pattern resembling a Sertoli cell neoplasm,[50] but in such cases there is usually a transition, in at least some areas, to a more conventional endometrioid appearance. It should be noted that the term 'malignant endometrioid tumour of the ovary' encompasses all the various neoplasms which may also occur in the endometrium, such as carcinosarcomas, adenosarcomas, adenosquamous carcinomas, and endometrioid stromal sarcomas.

Malignant Brenner tumours have generally been regarded as rare neoplasms but it is probable that their apparent infrequency has been overemphasized by an insistence upon unnecessarily rigid and restrictive diagnostic criteria. In essence, a malignant Brenner tumour is a transitional cell carcinoma which resembles neoplasms of similar type found in the bladder (Fig. 9.4). The tumour may grow in a solid fashion but papillary areas may also be present; areas of squamous differentiation are common, while

foci of adenocarcinomatous differentiation are sometimes apparent. It has traditionally been insisted upon that a malignant Brenner tumour can only be diagnosed if there is an observable transition from benign Brenner elements, but this implies that a malignant Brenner tumour invariably originates from a previously present benign neoplasm, a view not held for any other form of ovarian carcinoma. However, a distinction has been drawn between malignant Brenner tumours, which are associated with benign Brenner elements, and pure transitional cell carcinomas.[51]

Clear cell adenocarcinomas show a variety of architectural patterns, which may occur singly or in any combination within an individual neoplasm. In the diffuse pattern there are sheets of polyhedral cells with distinct boundaries, abundant clear cytoplasm, and eccentric, angular nuclei. The tubulocystic pattern (Fig. 9.5a) is characterized by tubules and cysts, which may be lined by flattened, cuboidal, or columnar clear cells, or by hobnail cells (Fig. 9.5b), the latter having prominent nuclei which occupy the bulbous tips of the cells and protrude into the lumen. In the papillary pattern, the papillae may be simple or complex and have delicate mesenchymal cores which often show hyalinization. The papillae are covered by clear, hobnail, or nondescript cuboidal cells. Oxyphilic cells, with abundant eosinophilic cytoplasm, are often present in clear cell adenocarcinomas and sometimes predominate.

Spread of ovarian carcinoma

Bilateral involvement of the ovaries by adenocarcinoma is common and it is often far from clear whether this is due to metastatic spread or to multicentric origin. It appears highly probable, however, that spread to the contralateral ovary contributes substantially to the incidence of bilaterality, for the frequency of bilateral involvement increases progressively with advancing clinical stage. Possible routes of spread to the opposite ovary include transperitoneal seeding, cell migration through the tubes and

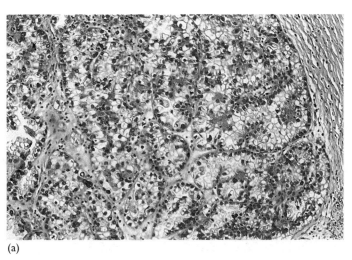

(a)

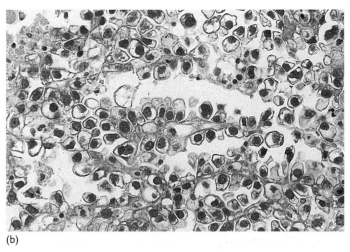

(b)

Fig. 9.5 (a) Clear cell adenocarcinoma with tubulocystic architecture (haematoxylin and eosin ×100). (b) Hobnail cells with clear cytoplasm in clear cell adenocarcinoma (haematoxylin and eosin ×400).

endometrial cavity, and lymphatic spread via anastomoses between ovarian and uterine lymphatic vessels. The uterus is frequently involved by tumour, either because of direct extension or because of retrograde lymphatic spread, while extension to the endometrium may be either via the lymphatics or by lumenal migration of tumour cells through the tube.

Transperitoneal spread is very common and is not limited to those neoplasms with external excrescences, occurring with almost equal frequency in tumours with an apparently intact capsule. Direct seeding leads to implants on the pelvic peritoneum, in the pouch of Douglas, and in the omentum. Deposits in the pouch of Douglas may grow through to the vagina, but those in the pelvic peritoneum tend to spread over the surface, leading to widespread adhesions. Tumour cells also seed directly into the small amount of normally present peritoneal fluid, and are carried by this to be deposited in the paracolic gutters and on the undersurface of the right leaf of the diaphragm, spread to the left diaphragm not occurring because the phrenico-colic ligament blocks the upward movement of the fluid on this side.[52]. Tumour cells are also seeded out to involve the gastrointestinal tract, often to form multiple, small, superficial nodules on the peritoneum of the small bowel. Involvement of large areas of the wall of the sigmoid colon or rectum is common, while less frequently there is diffuse infiltration of the mesentery.[53]

Lymphatic spread is a common feature of ovarian carcinoma. Six to eight lymphatic channels accompany the ovarian blood vessels to the para-aortic nodes, but lymphatic vessels also run via the broad ligament to the obturator nodes. As there are numerous anastomoses between the obturator nodes and the iliac and para-aortic nodes, the retroperitoneal nodes which drain the ovary are interconnected to the level of the aortic bifurcation.[54] In autopsy studies of ovarian carcinoma patients, metastases in the pelvic lymph nodes have been found in between 48 and 80% of cases, and metastases in the para-aortic nodes in between 58 and 78%.[55] Nodal metastasis is, however, not a late event, for even in women with apparent stage I disease nodal metastases are found in between 14 and 24%.[56] The incidence of nodal metastasis doubles in patients with apparent stage II disease and exceeds 70% in stage III.[57] The topographic distribution of nodes involved by ovarian carcinoma is unpredictable, but metastases confined to the pelvic nodes are somewhat more common than are metastases confined to the paraortic nodes, while in 44% of patients both sets of nodes are involved.[56]

Haematogenous spread of ovarian carcinoma is uncommon, but occurs, usually late in the course of the disease, to sites such as the liver, spleen, lungs, brain, and bone.

Prognostic pathological factors

The overall 5-year survival rate for women with ovarian carcinoma is in the region of 30% and the most important prognostic factor is the surgicopathologic stage at the time of initial diagnosis. However, staging is not of absolute prognostic value to the individual patient, for some women with stage I or II disease die quite quickly, while others with stage III or IV disease survive for surprisingly long periods.

The histological type of ovarian carcinoma has been thought by many to be of prognostic importance, it often being claimed that endometrioid and mucinous adenocarcinomas have a relatively good prognosis, that serous carcinomas have an unusually poor prognosis, and that the outlook for women with clear cell adenocarcinomas lies somewhere between these two extremes.[58] Evidence for the prognostic value of histological type has, however, been based upon univariate analysis, and multivariate analysis has generally shown that, stage for stage and grade for grade, the histological type of an ovarian adenocarcinoma is of little or no prognostic significance.[59–61] This conclusion applies, however, largely to serous and endometrioid adenocarcinomas, and there is still some dispute about the prognostic significance of mucinous, clear cell, and transitional cell patterns. Although early stage mucinous carcinomas have as good a prognosis as endometrioid and serous tumours at the same stage, they appear to have a significantly worse prognosis than their serous and endometrioid counterparts in stage III and IV ovarian cancer, possibly because of their resistance to platinum therapy.[62] Clear cell carcinomas are widely thought to have an unusually poor prognosis,[63–65] but some have thought that this applies only to early stage disease[66] while others have considered that this gloomy outlook also applies to patients with advanced tumours[62,65,67] partly, if not entirely, because of a particular resistance of this type of ovarian carcinoma to platinum-based chemotherapy. In some studies, however, the prognosis for clear cell adenocarcinomas did not appear to differ significantly from that of other forms of ovarian adenocarcinoma.[68–70] It certainly seems the case that an unusually high proportion of clear cell adenocarcinomas present as bulky stage I disease, and that a high proportion of such early cases recur,[64,69,71] but nevertheless the 5-year survival rate for women with stage I clear cell carcinoma appears to be similar to that of patients with other forms of stage I adenocarcinoma. It remains a moot point as to whether the histological pattern within a clear cell carcinoma is of prognostic significance or not.[65,72] The transitional cell carcinomas were originally thought to have a poor prognosis[51] but later reports claimed that these neoplasms are associated with a relatively good outlook, even when at an advanced stage, and respond unusually well to chemotherapy.[73,74] A subsequent study showed, however, that transitional cell carcinomas did not appear to be associated with a particularly favourable prognosis or a better response rate to chemotherapy.[75]

The prognostic value of histological grading of ovarian carcinoma has been widely accepted[59,60,76] but it is, in fact, far from clear how these neoplasms should be graded. The Broders' system, in which the percentage of undifferentiated cells is assessed, has been found useful by some but is highly subjective and difficult to apply in a consistent pattern. More commonly, ovarian carcinomas have been variously graded in architectural terms, by the degree of nuclear atypia or by a combination of nuclear and architectural features.[60,77–81] No particular agreed grading system has been universally adopted and all are subjective in nature; furthermore, in many studies the grading system has not been clearly defined. It is therefore not surprising that there are very high inter- and intraobserver differences in the assessment of ovarian carcinoma grades.[82,83] A further point is that it has not been agreed whether any particular grading system is applicable to all histological types of ovarian carcinoma, many feeling that clear cell carcinomas cannot be graded. In an attempt to overcome these difficulties a new grading system, thought to be applicable to all types of ovarian carcinoma, has been proposed, which combines carefully defined architectural features and nuclear grade with an equally carefully defined mitotic count.[84] However, doubts have been expressed about the reproducibility of even a carefully defined grading system such as this, and it has been argued that all attempts to define a universally applicable grading system for ovarian carcinoma are misguided in so far as this disease is not a single entity.[85]

In the past few decades the introduction of quantitative techniques have allowed for a more objective and consistent approach to the grading of ovarian carcinomas. Tumour aneuploidy, demonstrated by DNA flow cytometry, has been shown, in most studies, to be an important independent adverse prognostic factor in both early and late stage ovarian epithelial cancer,[86–93] although, admittedly, there have been a significant number of dissenters from this view.[94–97] In general terms, tumour aneuploidy tends to correlate with serous or clear cell histology, advanced stage, large tumour bulk, presence of residual tumour, and retroperitoneal lymph node metastases.

Quantitative morphometric and stereologic analysis of tumours using automated image analysis systems provides information that is both objective and reproducible.[98] Measurements that can be made in such systems include mean nuclear area, volume, longest axis, and shortest axis, while such parameters as the volume percentage epithelium (i.e. the percentage of the volume of a tumour that is formed of epithelium) and the mitotic activity index can also be assessed quantitatively. Techniques such as these have been applied to ovarian adenocarcinomas and it has been shown that estimation of the mitotic activity index and the volume percentage epithelium allows for stratification of tumours into 'high-risk' and 'low-risk' groups,[99,100] while the addition of the mean nuclear area to these variables adds a further element of prognostic precision, this latter measurement probably being the single best indicator of clinical outcome in early ovarian cancer.[101–103]

Oestrogen and progesterone receptors are present in a high proportion of ovarian adenocarcinomas and there have been both claims and denials that expression of these receptors is associated with a relatively good prognosis,[104,105] no clear agreement having been attained.[106]

Within the past few years the search for prognostic factors in ovarian carcinomas has widened to include studies of cell proliferation markers, expression of proto-oncogenes and their products, and mutations within tumour suppressor genes. Two cell proliferation markers have been studied, PCNA and Ki–67.[107] Staining for the cell proliferation marker PCNA (proliferating cell nuclear antigen) has yielded conflicting results about the prognostic value of this marker in ovarian adenocarcinoma,[108,109] and while the range of Ki–67-positive cells in ovarian carcinomas is variable, high values have correlated with poor patient survival in some studies[110] but not in others.[111]

Mutation of the tumour suppressor gene *p53* with positive immunostaining for p53 protein is common in ovarian carcinomas and has been related to poor tumour differentiation and an adverse clinical outcome in patients with stage I ovarian carcinomas.[112] Some have found that, overall, detectable p53 in ovarian

carcinomas is associated with poor tumour differentiation and with decreased survival,[113,114] but others have been unable to show any correlation between p53 expression and either tumour-related features or an adverse clinical outcome.[115,116] It is a reasonable conclusion that the prognostic significance of mutation and overexpression of p53 in ovarian cancer remains somewhat uncertain.[117]

It has been suggested that c-*myc* overexpression in ovarian carcinomas is associated with unusually aggressive tumour behaviour,[118] but expression of the *ras* oncogene product p21 has not been shown to have any correlation with tumour characteristics or clinical outcome.[119] Overexpression of the c-*erbB–2* oncogene is common in ovarian adenocarcinomas but there has been considerable disagreement about the prognostic significance of this finding, some noting that c-*erbB–2* expression is associated with a poor prognosis[120,121] and others finding it has no prognostic significance.[122,123]

References

1. Langley, F.A. and Fox, H. (1995). Ovarian tumours: classification, histogenesis and aetiology. In *Haines and Taylor: textbook of obstetrical and gynaecological pathology*, (4th edn), (ed. H. Fox), pp. 727–42. Churchill Livingstone, New York.

2. Auersperg, N., Edelson, M.I., Mok, S.C., Johnson, S.W. and Hamilton, T.C. (1998). The biology of ovarian cancer. *Sem. Oncol.*, **25**, 281–304.

3. Jiang, X., Morland, S.J., Hitchcock, A., Thomas, E.J. and Campbell, I.G. (1998). Allelotyping of endometriosis with adjacent ovarian carcinoma reveals evidence of a commmon lineage. *Cancer Res.*, **58**, 1707–12.

4. Toki, T., Fujii, S. and Silverberg, S.G. (1996). A clinicopathologic study on the association of endometriosis and carcinoma of the ovary using a scoring system. *Int. J. Gynecol. Cancer*, **6**, 68–75.

5. Bell, D.A. and Scully, R.E. (1994). Early *de novo* ovarian carcinoma: a study of fourteen cases. *Cancer,* **73**, 1859–64.

6. Plaxe, S.C., Deligdisch, L., Dottino, P.R. and Cohen, C.J. (1990). Ovarian intraepithelial neoplasia demonstrated in patients with stage I ovarian carcinoma. *Gynecol. Oncol.*, **38**, 367–72.

7. Deligdisch, L. (1997). Ovarian dysplasia: a review. *Int. J. Gynecol. Cancer*, **7**, 94–8.

8. Hutson, R., Ramsdale, J. and Wells, M. (1995). p53 protein expression in putative precursor lesions of epithelial ovarian cancer. *Histopathology*, **27**, 367–71.

9. Sherman, M.E., Lee, J.S., Burks, R.T. Struewing, J.P., Kurman, R.J. and Hartge, P. (1999). Histopathologic features of ovaries at increased risk for carcinoma: a case control analysis. *Int. J. Gynecol. Pathol.*, **18**, 151–7.

10. Werness, B.A., Afify, A.M., Bielat, K.L., Eltabbakh, G.H., Piver, M.S. and Paterson, J.M. (1999). Altered surface and cyst epithelium of ovaries removed prophylactically from women with a family history of ovarian cancer. *Hum. Pathol.*, **30**, 151–7.

11. Stratton, J.F., Buckley, C.H., Lowe, D. *et al.* (1999). Comparison of prophlactic oophorectomy specimens from carriers and noncarriers of a BRAC1 or BRCA2 gene mutation. *J Natl Cancer Inst.*, **91**, 626–8.

12. Werness, B.A. and Eltabbakh, G.H. (2000). Ovarian dysplasia identified by cul-de-sac aspiration: a re-examination of previously reported cases. *Int. J. Gynecol. Pathol.*, **19**, 190–1.

13. Mittal, K.R., Zeleniuch-Jacquotte, A., Cooper, R. and Demopoulos, R.I. (1993). Contralateral ovary in unilateral ovarian carcinoma: a search for preneoplastic lesions. *Int. J. Gynecol. Pathol.*, **12**, 59–63.

14. Westhoff, C., Murphy, C., Heller, D. and Halim, A. (1993). Is ovarian cancer associated with an increased frequency of germinal inclusion cysts? *Am. J. Epidemiol.*, **138**, 90–3.

15. Salazar, H., Godwin, A.K., Daly, M.B. *et al.* (1996). Microscopic benign and invasive malignant neoplasms and a cancer-prone phenotype in prophylactic oophorectomies. *J. Natl Cancer Inst.*, **88**, 1810–20.

16. McCluskey, L.L. and Dubeau, L. (1997). Biology of ovarian cancer. *Curr. Opin. Oncol.*, **9**, 465–70.

17. Puls, L.E., Powell, D.E., Gallion, H.H., Hunter, J.E., Kryscio, R.J. and Vannagell, J.R. (1992). Transition from benign to malignant epithelium in mucinous and serous cystadenocarcinoma. *Gynecol. Oncol.*, **47**, 53–7.

18. Werness, B.A., DiCioccio, R.A. and Piver, M.S. (1997). Identical, unique p53 mutations in a primary ovarian mucinous adenocarcinoma and a synchronous contralateral ovarian mucinous tumor of low malignant potential suggest a common clonal origin. *Hum. Pathol.*, **28**, 626–30.

19. Mandai, M., Konishi, I., Kuroda, H. *et al.* (1998). Heterogenous distribution of K-ras-mutated epithelia in mucinous ovarian tumors with special reference to histopathology. *Hum. Pathol.*, **29**, 34–40.

20. Dubeau, L. (1999). The cell of origin of ovarian epithelial tumors and the ovarian surface epithelium dogma: does the emperor have no clothes? *Gynecol. Oncol.*, **72**, 437–42.

21. Parazzini, F., Franceschi, S., La Vecchia, C. and Fasoli, M. (1991). The epidemiology of ovarian cancer. *Gynecol. Oncol.*, **42**, 9–23.

22. Whittemore, A.S., Harris, R. and Imyre, J. (1992). Characteristics relating to ovarian cancer risk: collaborative analysis of 12 US case control studies. *Am. J. Epidemiol.*, **136**, 1184–203.

23. Negri. E., Franceschi, S., Tzonou, A. *et al.* (1991). Pooled analysis of 3 European case-control studies. I. Reproductive factors and risk of epithelial ovarian cancer. *Int. J. Cancer*, **49**, 50–6.

24. Adami, H.-O., Hsieh, C.C., Lambe, M. *et al.* (1994). Parity, age at first childbirth, and risk of ovarian cancer. *Lancet*, **344**, 1250–4.

25. Cooper, G.S., Schildkraut, J.M., Whittemore, A.S. and Marchbanks, P.A. (1999). Pregnancy frequency and risk of ovarian cancer. *Cancer Causes Control*, **10**, 397–402.

26. Rosenblatt, K.A. and Thomas, D.B. (1993). Lactation and the risk of epithelial ovarian cancer. *Int. J. Epidemiol.*, **22**, 192–7.

27. Franseschi, S., Parazzini, F., Negri, E. *et al.* (1991). Pooled analysis of 3 European case-control studies of epithelial ovarian cancer. III. Oral contraceptive use. *Int. J. Cancer*, **49**, 61–5.

28. La Vecchia, C. and Franceschi, S. (1999). Oral contraceptives and ovarian cancer. *Europ. J. Cancer Prevent.*, **8**, 761–3.

29. Modan, B., Ron, E., Lerna-Geva, L., *et al.* (1998). Cancer incidence in a cohort of infertile women. *Am. J. Epidemiol.*, **147**, 1038–42.

30. Rossing, M.A., Daling, J.R., Weiss, N.S., Moore, D.E. and Self, S.G. (1994). Ovarian tumors in a cohort of infertile women. *N. Engl. J. Med.*, **331**, 771–6.

31. Franceschi, S., La Vecchia, C., Negri, E. *et al.* (1994). Fertility drugs and risk of epithelial ovarian cancer in Italy. *Hum. Reprod.*, **9**, 1673–5.

32. Parazinni, F., Negri, E. and La Vecchia C. (1993). Hysterectomy, oophorectomy, and subequent ovarian cancer risk. *Obstet. Gynecol.*, **81**, 363–6.

33. Green, A., Purdie, D., Bain, C. *et al.* (1997). Tubal sterilisation, hysterectomy and decreased risk of ovarian cancer: Survey of Women's Health Study Group. *Int. J. Cancer*, **71**, 948–51.

34. Miracle-McMahill, H.L., Calle, E.E., Kosinski, A.S. *et al.* (1997). Tubal ligation and fatal ovarian cancer in a large prospective cohort study. *Am. J. Epidemiol.*, **145**, 349–57.

35. Cornelison, T.L., Natarajan, N., Piver, M.S. and Mettlin, C.J. (1997). Tubal ligation and the risk of ovarian carcinoma. *Cancer Detect. Prevent.*, **21**, 1–6.

36. Harlow, B.L., Cramer, D.W., Bell, D.A. and Welch, W.R. (1992). Perineal exposure to talc and ovarian cancer risk. *Obstet. Gynecol.*, **80**, 19–23.

37. Cramer, D.W., Liberman, R.F., Titus-Ernsoff, L. *et al.* (1997). Genital talc exposure and risk of ovarian cancer. *Int. J. Cancer*, **81**, 351–6.

38. Wong, C., Hempling, R.E., Piver, M.S., Natarajan, N. and Mettlin, C.J. (1999). Perineal talc exposure and subsequent epithelial ovarian cancer: a case control study. *Obstet. Gynecol.*, **93**, 372–6.

39. Gertig, D.M., Hunter, D.J., Cramer, D.W. *et al.* (2000). Prospective study of talc use and ovarian cancer. *J. Natl Cancer Inst.*, **92**, 249–52.

40. Rosenblatt, K.A. and Thomas, D. (1996). Reduced risk of ovarian cancer in women with a tubal ligation or hysterectomy. *Cancer Epidemiol. Biomark. Prevent.*, **5**, 933–5.

41. Doyle, P. and dos Santos Silva, I. (1996). Pathogenesis and epidemiology of ovarian cancer. In *Gynecologic oncology: current diagnosis and treatment*, (ed. H.M. Shingleton, W.C. Fowler Jr, J.A. Jordan, and W.D. Lawrence), pp. 165–73. Saunders, London.

42. Risch, H.A., Jain, M., Marrett., L.D. and Howe, G.R. (1994). Dietary lactose intake, lactose intolerance and the risk of epithelial ovarian cancer in southern Ontario (Canada). *Cancer Causes Control*, **5**, 540–8.

43. Herrington, L.J., Weiss, N.S., Beresford, S.A. *et al.* (1995). Lactose and galactose intake and metabolism in relation to the risk of epithelial ovarian cancer. *Am. J. Epidemiol.*, **141**, 407–16.

44. Fathalla, M.F. (1971). Incessant ovulation—a factor in ovarian neoplasia? *Lancet*, **ii**, 163.

45. Schildkraut, J.M., Bastos, E. and Berchuck, A. (1997). Relationship between lifetime ovulatory cycles and overexpression of mutant p53 in epithelial ovarian cancer. *J. Natl Cancer Inst.*, **89**, 932–8.

46. Webb, P.M., Green, A., Cummings, M.C., Purdie, D.M., Walsh, M.D. and Chevenix-Trench, G. (1998). Relationship between number of ovulatory cycles and accumulation of mutant p53 in epithelial ovarian cancer. *J Natl Cancer Inst.*, **90**, 1729–34.

47. Stadel, B.V. (1975). The etiology and prevention of ovarian cancer. *Am. J. Obstet. Gynecol.*, **123**, 772–4.

48. Garg, P.P., Kerlikowske, K., Subak, L. and Grady, D. (1998). Hormone replacement therapy and the risk of epithelial ovarian carcinoma: a meta-analysis. *Obstet. Gynecol.*, **92**, 472–9.

49. Negri, E., Tzonou, A., Beral, V. *et al.* (1999). Hormonal therapy for menopause and ovarian cancer in a colaborative re-analysis of European studies. *Int. J. Cancer*, **15**, 848–51.

50. Young, R.H., Prat, J. and Scully, R.E. (1982). Ovarian endometrioid carcinomas resembling sex cord-stromal tumors: a clinicopathologic analysis of 13 cases. *Am. J. Surg. Pathol.*, **5**, 513–22.

51. Austin, R.M. and Norris, H.J. (1987). Malignant Brenner tumors and transitional cell carcinoma of the ovary. *Int. J. Gynecol. Pathol.*, **6**, 29–39.

52. Fuks, Z. (1980). Patterns of spread of ovarian carcinoma: relation to therapeutic strategies. In *Ovarian cancer*, (ed. C.E. Newman, C.H.J. Ford and J.E. Jordan), pp. 39–51. Pergamon, Oxford.

53. Wu, P.-C., Lang, J.-H., Huang, R.-L., Liu, J., Tang, M.-Y. and Lian, L.-J. (1989). Intestinal metastasis and operation in ovarian cancer: a report on 62 cases. *Ballière's Clin. Obstet. Gynaecol.*, **3**, 95–108.

54. Pickel, H., Lahousen, M., Stetner, H. and Girardi, F. (1989). The spread of ovarian cancer. *Ballière's Clin. Obstet. Gynaecol.*, **3**, 3–12.

55. Rose, P.G., Piver, M.S., Tsukada, Y. and Lau, T. (1989). Metastatic patterns in histologic variants of ovarian cancer: a autopsy study. *Cancer*, **64**, 1508–13.

56. Burghardt, E., Girardi, F., Lahousen, M., Tamussino, K. and Stettner, H. (1991). Patterns of pelvic and paraaortic lymph node involvement in ovarian cancer. *Gynecol. Oncol.*, **40**, 103–6.

57. Burghardt, E., Lahousen, M. and Stettner, H. (1990). Die operative Behandlung des Ovarialkarzinoms. *Geburtsh. Frauenheilk.*, **50**, 670–7.

58. Kolstad, P. (1986). *Clinical gynecologic oncology: the Norwegian experience.* Norwegian University Press, Oslo.

59. Sorbe, B., Frankendal, B.O. and Veress, B. (1982). Importance of histologic grading in the prognosis of epithelial ovarian carcinoma. *Obstet. Gynecol.*, **59**, 576–82.

60. Swenerton, K.D., Hislop, T.G., Spinelli, J., LeRiche, J.C, Yang, N. and Boyes, D.A. (1985). Ovarian carcinoma: a multivariate analysis of prognostic factors. *Obstet. Gynecol.*, **5**, 264–70.

61. Zwart, J., Geisler, J.P. and Geisler, H.P. (1998). Five year survival in patients with endometrioid carcinoma of the ovary versus those with serous carcinoma. *Europ. J. Gynecol. Oncol.*, **19**, 225–8.

62. Omura, G.A., Brady, M.F., Homesley, H.D. *et al.* (1991). Long term follow up and prognostic factor analysis in advanced ovarian cancer: the Gynecologic Oncology Group experience. *J. Clin. Oncol.*, **9**, 1138–50.

63. Jenison, E.L., Montag, A.G., Griffiths, C.H. *et al.* (1989). Clear cell adeno-carcinoma of the ovary: a clinical analysis and comparison with serous carcinoma. *Gynecol. Oncol.*, **32**, 762–72.

64. Crozier, M.A., Copeland, C.J., Silva, E.G. *et al.* (1989). Clear cell carcinoma of the ovary: a study of 59 cases. *Gynecol. Oncol.*, **35**, 199–203.

65. Imachi, M., Tsukamoto, N., Shimamoto, T., *et al.* (1991). Clear cell carcinoma of the ovary: a clinicopathologic analysis of 34 cases. *Int. J. Gynecol. Cancer*, **1**, 113–20.

66. O'Brien, M.E.R., Schofield, J.B., Tan, S. *et al.* (1993). Clear cell epithelial ovarian cancer (mesonephroid): bad prognosis only in early stages. *Gynecol. Oncol.*, **49**, 250–4.

67. Goff, B.A., Sainz de la Cuesta, R., Muntz, H.G. *et al.* (1996). Clear cell carcinoma of the ovary: a distinct histologic type with poor prognosis and resistance to platinum-based chemotherapy in Stage III disease. *Gynecol. Oncol.*, **60**, 412–17.

68. Shevchuk, M.M., Winkler-Monsanto, B., Fenoglio, C.M. *et al.* (1981). Clear cell carcinoma of the ovary: a clinicopathologic study with review of the literature. *Cancer*, **47**, 1344–51.

69. Kennedy, A.W., Biscotti, C.V., Hart, W.R. *et al.* (1989). Ovarian clear cell carcinoma. *Gynecol. Oncol.*, **32**, 342–9.

70. Brescia, R.J., Dubin, N. and Demopoulos, R. (1989). Endometrioid and clear cell carcinoma of the ovary: factors affecting survival. *Int. J. Gynecol. Pathol.*, **8**, 132–8.

71. Behbakht, K., Randall, T.C., Benjamin, I. *et al.* (1998). Clinical characteristics of clear cell carcinoma of the ovary. *Gynecol. Oncol.*, **70**, 255–8.

72. Montag, A.G., Jenison, E.L., Griffiths, C.T. *et al.* (1989). Ovarian clear cell carcinoma: a clinicopathologic analysis of 44 cases. *Int. J. Gynecol. Pathol.*, **8**, 85–96.

73. Silva, E.G., Robey-Cafferty, S.S., Gershenson, D.M. *et al.* (1990). Ovarian carcinoma with transitional cell carcinoma pattern. *Am. J. Clin. Pathol.*, **63**, 839–47.

74. Gershenson, D.M., Silva, E.G., Mitchell, M.F. *et al.* (1993). Transitional cell carcinoma of the ovary: a matched controlled study of advanced-stage patients treated with cisplatin-based chemotherapy. *Am. J. Obstet. Gynecol.*, **168**, 1178–87.

75. Hollingsworth, H.C., Steinberg, S.M., Silverberg, S.G. *et al.* (1996). Advanced stage transitional cell carcinoma of the ovary. *Hum. Pathol.*, **27**, 1267–72.

76. Hogberg, T., Carstensen, J. and Simonsen, E. (1993). Treatment results and prognostic factors in a population-based study of epithelial ovarian cancer. *Gynecol. Oncol.*, **48**, 38–49.

77. Jacobs, A.J., Deligdisch, L., Deppe, G. *et al.* (1982). Histologic correlates of virulence in ovarian adenocarcinoma. *Am. J. Obstet. Gynecol.*, **143**, 574–80.

78. Sigurdsson, K., Alm, P. and Gusberg, B. (1983). Prognostic factors in malignant epithelial ovarian tumors. *Gynecol. Oncol.*, **15**, 370–80.

79. Silverberg, S.G. (1989). Prognostic significance of pathologic features of ovarian carcinoma. *Curr. Top. Pathol.*, **78**, 85–109.

80. Dembo, A.J., Davy, M., Stenwig, A.E. *et al.* (1990). Prognostic factors in patients with stage I epithelial ovarian cancer. *Obstet. Gynecol.*, **75**, 263–73.

81. Eisner, R.E., Teng, F., Oliviera, M. *et al.* (1994). The influence of tumor grade, distribution and extent of carcinomatosis in minimal residual stage III ovarian cancer after optimal cytoreductive surgery. *Gynecol. Oncol.*, **55**, 108–11.

82. Baak, J.P.A., Langley, F.A., Talerman, A. and Delemarre, J.F.M. (1987). The prognostic variability of ovarian tumor grading by different pathologists. *Gynecol. Oncol.*, **27**, 166–72.

83. Bertelsen, K., Holund, B. and Andersen, E. (1993). Reproducibility and prognostic value of histologic type and grade in early epithelial ovarian cancer. *Intern. J. Gynecol. Cancer*, **3**, 72–9.

84. Shimizu, Y., Kamoi, S., Amada, S. *et al.* (1998). Toward the development of a universal grading system for ovarian epithelial carcinoma: I. Prognostic significance of histopathologic features—problems involved in the architectural grading system. *Gynecol. Oncol.*, **70**, 2–12.

85. Silva, E.G. and Gershenson, D.M. (1998). Editorial. Standardized histologic grading of epithelial ovarian cancer: elusive after all these years. *Gynecol. Oncol.*, **70**, 1.

86. Vergote, I.B., Kaern, J., Abeler, V.M. *et al.* (1993). Analysis of prognostic factors in stage I epithelial ovarian carcinoma: importance of degree of differentiation and DNA ploidy in predicting relapse. *Am. J. Obstet. Gynecol.*, **169**, 40–52.

87. Gajewski, W.H., Fuller, A.F., Pastel-Ley, C. *et al.* (1994). Prognostic significance of DNA content in epithelial ovarian cancer. *Gynecol. Oncol.*, **53**, 5–12.

88. Kaern, J., Trope, C.G., Kristensen, C.B. *et al.* (1994). Evaluation of DNA ploidy and S-phase fraction as prognostic parameters in advanced epithelial ovarian carcinoma. *Am. J. Obstet. Gynecol.*, **170**, 479–87.

89. Zanetta, G., Keeney, G.L., Cha, S.S., Wieand, H.S., Katzmann, J.A. and Podratz, K.C. (1996). DNA index by flow cytometry analysis: an additional prognostic factor in advanced ovarian carcinoma without residual disease after initial operation. *Gynecol. Oncol.*, **62**, 208–12.

90. Schueler, J.A., Trimbos, J.B., Burg, M., Cornelisse, C.J., Hermans, J. and Fleuren, G.J. (1996). DNA index reflects the biological behaviour of ovarian carcinoma stage I-IIa. *Gynecol. Oncol.*, **62**, 59–66.

91. Kimball, R.E., Schlaerth, J.B., Kute, T. *et al.* (1997). Flow cytometric analysis of lymph node metastases in advanced ovarian carcinoma: clinical and biologic significance. *Am. J. Obstet. Gynecol.*, **176**, 1326–7.

92. Silvestrini, R., Daidone, M.G., Veneroni, S. *et al.* (1998). The clinical predictivity of biomarkers of stage III–IV epithelial ovarian cancer in a prospective randomized treatment protocol. *Cancer*, **82**, 159–67.

93. Trope, C. and Kaern, J. (1999). DNA ploidy in epithelial ovarian cancer: a new independent prognostic factor. *CME J. Gynecol. Oncol.*, **4**, 154–60.

94. Rice, L.W., Mark, S.D., Berkowitz, R.S., Goff, B.A. and Lage, J.M. (1995). Clinicopathologic variables, operative characteristics, and DNA ploidy in predicting outcome in ovarian epithelial carcinoma. *Obstet. Gynecol.*, **86**, 379–85.

95. Resnik, E., Trujillo, Y.P. and Taxy, J.B. (1997). Long term survival and DNA ploidy in advanced epithelial ovarian cancer. *J. Surg. Oncol.*, **64**, 299–303.

96. Curling, M., Stenning, S., Hudson, C.N. and Watson, J.V. (1998). Multivariate analyses of DNA index, p53, myc and clinicopathological status of patients with ovarian cancer. *J. Clin. Pathol.*, **51**, 455–61.

97. Reles, A.E., Gee, C., Schellschmidt, I. *et al.* (1998). Prognostic significance of DNA content and S-phase fraction in epithelial ovarian carcinomas analyzed by image cytometry. *Gynecol. Oncol.*, **71**, 3–13.

98. Burton, J. and Wells, M. (1999). Quantitative pathological prognostic factors in epithelial ovarian cancer. *CME J. Gynecol. Oncol.*, **4**, 151–3.

99. Baak, J.P.A., Langley, F.A., Talerman, A. and Delemarre, J.F.M. (1986). Morphometric data in the prognosis of ovarian tumours in addition to FIGO stage, histologic type and grade. *J. Clin. Pathol.*, **39**, 1340–6.

100. Baak, J.P.A., Wisse-Brekelmans, E.C.M., Uyterlinde, A.M. and Schipper, N.W. (1987). Evaluation of the prognostic value of morphometric features and cellular DNA content in FIGO 1 ovarian cancer patients. *Anal. Quant. Cytol. Histol.*, **9**, 287–90.

101. Diest, P.J. van, Baak, J.P.A., Brugghe, J. *et al.* (1994). Quantitative prognostic features as predictors of long-term survival in patients with advanced ovarian cancer treated with cisplatin. *Int. J. Gynecol. Cancer*, **3**, 174–80.

102. Brinkhuis, M., Lund, B., Meijer, G.A. and Baak, J.P.A. (1996). Quantitative pathologic variables as prognostic factors for overall survial in Danish patients with FIGO stage III ovarian cancer. *Int. J. Gynecol. Cancer*, **6**, 168–74.

103. Brugghe, J., Baak, J.P.A., Wiltshaw, E., Brinkhuis, M., Meijer, G.A. and Fisher, C. (1998). Quantitative prognostic features in FIGO stage I ovarian cancer patients without postoperative treatment. *Gynecol. Oncol.*, **68**, 47–56.

104. Slotman, B.J., Narta, J.J.P. and Rao, B.R. (1990). Survival of patients with ovarian cancer: apart from stage and grade, tumor progesterone receptor content is a prognostic indicator. *Cancer*, **66**, 740–4.

105. Scambia, G., Benedetti-Panici, P., Ferrandina. G. *et al.* (1995). Epidermal growth factor, oestrogen and progesterone receptor expression in primary ovarian cancer: correlation with clinical outcome and response to chemotherapy. *Br. J. Cancer*, **72**, 361.

106. Bonte, J. (1999). Steroid hormone receptors as possible prognostic factors in epithelial ovarian carcinoma. *CME J. Gynecol. Oncol.*, **4**, 178–9.

107. Geisler, J.P., Geisler, H.E., Tammela, J., Miller, G.A., Wiemann, M.C. and Zhou, Z. (1999). Molecular biologic markers in ovarian carcinoma. *CME J. Gynecol. Oncol.*, **4**, 210–14.

108. Guo, L.-N., Wilkinson, N., Buckley, C.H., Fox, H., Hale, R.J. and Chawner, L. (1992). Proliferating cell nuclear antigen (PCNA) immunoreactivity in ovarian serous and mucinous neoplasms: diagnostic and prognostic value. *Int. J. Gynecol. Cancer*, **3**, 391–4.

109. Nakopoulou, L., Janinis, J., Panagos, G., Comin, G. and Davaris, P. (1993). The immunohistochemical expression of proliferating cell nuclear antigen (PCNA/Cyclin) in malignant and benign epithelial ovarian neoplasms and correlation with prognosis. *Europ. J. Cancer*, **29A**, 1599–601.

110. Kerns, B.M., Jordan, P.A., Faerman, L.L., Berchuck, A. and Bast, R.C. (1994). Determination of proliferation index with MIB–1 in advanced ovarian cancer using quantitative image analysis. *Am. J. Clin. Pathol.*, **101**, 192–7.

111. de Nictolis, M., Garbisa, S., Lucarini, G. *et al.* (1996). 72 kilo-dalton type IV collagenase, type IV collagen, and Ki67 in serous tumors of the ovary: a clinicopathologic, immunohistochemical, and serological study. *Int. J. Gynecol. Pathol.*, **15**, 102–9.

112. Levesque, M.A., Katsaros, D., Yu, H. *et al.* (1995). Mutant p53 protein overexpression is associated with poor outcome in patients with well or moderately differentiated ovarian carcinoma. *Cancer*, **75**, 1327–38.

113. Hartmann, L.C., Podratz, K.C., Keeney, G.L. *et al.* (1994). Prognostic significance of p53 immunostaining in epithelial ovarian cancer. *J. Clin. Oncol.*, **12**, 64–9.

114. Wen, W.-H., Reles, A., Runnebaum, I.B. *et al.* (1999). p53 mutations and expression in ovarian cancers: correlation with overall survival. *Int. J. Gynecol. Pathol.*, **18**, 29–41.

115. Niwa, K., Itoh, M., Murase, T. *et al.* (1994). Alteration of p53 gene in ovarian carcinoma: clinicopathological correlation and prognostic significance. *Br. J. Cancer*, **70**, 1191–7.

116. Allan, L.A., Campbell, M.K., Eccles, R.C.F. *et al.* (1996). The significance of p53 mutation and over-expression in ovarian cancer prognosis. *Int. J. Gynecol. Cancer*, **6**, 483–90.

117. Berchuck, A., Lambers, A. and Schildkraut, J.M. (1999). Relationship between alterations in the p53 tumor suppressive gene and prognosis of ovarian cancer. *CME J. Gynecol. Oncol.*, **4**, 215–18.

118. Bauknecht, T., Bermelin, G. and Kommoss, F. (1990). Clinical significance of oncogenes and growth factors in ovarian carcinoma. *J. Steroid Biochem. Med. Biol.*, **37**, 855–62.

119. Scambia, G., Catozzi, L., Panici, P.B. *et al.* (1993). Expression of ras p21 protein in normal and neoplastic ovarian tissues: correlation with histopathologic features and receptors for estrogen, progesterone, and epidermal growth factor. *Am. J. Obstet. Gynecol.*, **168**, 71–8.

120. Felip, E., Del Campo, J.M., Rubio, D., Vidal, M.T., Colomer, R. and Bermejo, B. (1995). Overexpression of c-erbB–2 in epithelial ovarian cancer. *Cancer*, **75**, 2147–52.

121. Meden, H., Marx, D., Rab, T., Kron, M., Schauer, A. and Kuhn, W. (1995). EGF-R and overexpression of the oncogene c-erbB–2 in ovarian cancer: immunohistochemical findings and prognostic value. *J. Obstet. Gynaecol.*, **21**, 167–78.

122. Leeson, S.C., Morphopoulos, G., Buckley, C.H. and Hale, R.J. (1995). c-erbB2 oncogene expression in stage 1 epithelial ovarian cancer. *Br. J. Obstet. Gynaecol.*, **102**, 65–7.

123. Fajac, A., Bernard, J., Lhomme, C. *et al.* (1995). c-erbB–2 gene amplification and protein expression in ovarian epithelial tumors: evaluation of their respective prognostic significance by multivariate analysis. *Int. J. Cancer*, **64**, 146–51.

10. Pathology of borderline ovarian malignancy

Harold Fox

Introduction

Ovarian tumours of borderline malignancy are a well-delineated and clearly defined group, the diagnosis of which is a positive one, based upon specific histological findings. Many are unhappy with the term 'ovarian tumours of borderline malignancy' and have attempted to introduce terms such as 'tumours of low malignant potential', 'atypically proliferating tumours', 'proliferative tumours', and 'tumours of low-grade malignancy'. There are cogent conceptual and semantic arguments against the use of all these terms, and it should be noted that all tumours, whatever their degree of malignancy, are proliferating and that the expression 'atypical proliferation', if it means anything at all, can be applied with equal justification to both tumours of borderline malignancy and to frank adenocarcinomas. It is true that the word 'borderline' hints at uncertainty and hesitation but, nevertheless, it conveys accurately the somewhat equivocal nature of these neoplasms and is still the terminology of choice.[1]

Only mucinous and serous tumours of borderline malignancy have been clearly defined in clinicopathological terms. Endometrioid, clear cell, and Brenner tumours of borderline malignancy have been described, but the status of these neoplasms remains uncertain and their clinical course is ill defined.

Many reports of the behaviour and management of ovarian tumours of borderline malignancy consider the serous and mucinous types together as if they were a single homogeneous group in respect to pathology, clinical course, and management. This approach is increasingly seen to be invalid and, apart from considerations of nomenclature and definition, the mucinous and serous tumours require separate consideration.

Definition

The World Health Organization definition of a tumour of borderline malignancy[2] is imprecise, and that of the Ovarian Tumour Panel of the Royal College of Obstetricians and Gynaecologists[3] is much to be preferred. The Panel defined a borderline tumour as one in which the epithelial component shows some, or all, of the characteristics of malignancy but in which there is no stromal invasion. It will be recognized that this definition takes no account of the degree of epithelial abnormality and employs lack of stromal invasion as the cardinal defining feature of these neoplasms. It should also be noted that the presence or absence of apparent extraovarian spread plays no role in the definition of a neoplasm of borderline malignancy, and that even if extensive extraovarian lesions are present, the ovarian tumour will still be placed in the borderline category if it fulfils the histological criteria for that diagnosis. The definition employed in the recently published Armed Forces Institute of Pathology fascicle on ovarian tumours[4] is broadly in agreement with that of the Ovarian Tumour Panel, but differs in recognizing those with very severe atypia ('intraepithelial carcinoma') as a specific subgroup of borderline neoplasms.

Insistence on the prime diagnostic importance of a lack of stromal invasion, although undoubtedly the correct approach, has nevertheless led to some conceptual and practical problems. Thus, because difficulties may be encountered in deciding whether stromal invasion is present or not, there has been an increasing tendency to insist on a lack of 'destructive' invasion;[5] unfortunately, 'destructive' has not been defined in this context and hence its recognition may be highly subjective. Identification of stromal invasion may be particularly difficult in those mucinous tumours of borderline malignancy, which have a complex glandular pattern with many epithelial outpouchings. This has led to the proposal that in such neoplasms those showing a marked overgrowth of atypical epithelial cells with cellular stratification of four or more cell layers in thickness should be classed as mucinous carcinomas, even in the absence of overt stromal invasion.[6–8] This concept has won some support,[5,9,10,11] but others have not found it to confer any added prognostic precision and have argued against its use.[12–17]

Some have been tempted to equate borderline ovarian tumours with non-invasive neoplasia in other sites, such as the cervix.[18] Enthusiasm for this comparison should, however, be tempered by the fact that the stroma underlying the abnormal epithelium in a borderline tumour is, unlike that of the cervix, a component of the neoplasm rather than normal tissue stroma. Further, the term 'ovarian intraepithelial neoplasia' has also been applied to a quite different lesion, namely, the presence of atypical cells in the surface epithelium of the ovary.[19]

Although evidence of stromal invasion negates a diagnosis of borderline malignancy, there have, nevertheless, been several reports of 'microinvasion' of the stroma of both serous and mucinous tumours which otherwise showed the typical features of a neoplasm of borderline malignancy;[17,20–22] such neoplasms followed the same clinical course and had the same prognosis as did borderline tumours without microinvasion. Conceptually, neoplasms with microinvasion are not of borderline malignancy but clinically they are not adenocarcinomas.

Serous tumours of borderline malignancy

These are usually cystic and differ macroscopicaly from a benign papillary serous cystadenoma only by an unusually luxuriant proliferation of fine papillae on their inner surface and by the presence of exophytic papillary excrescences on their outer surface. A proportion resemble a benign serous surface papillary tumour but tend to have a rather more complex and dense papillary pattern. Histologically, these neoplasms are formed of rather fine, branching papillae (Fig. 10.1). In those with only minimal apithelial atypia, the cellular mantle of the papillae can be clearly recognized as being tubal in type, but in tumours with marked epithelial abnormalities this resemblance tends to be lost and the cells become predominantly round or cuboidal. The epithelial component of the tumour shows fa variable degree of multilayering and has a marked tendency to form cellular buds or tufts; these buds may break off to float freely within the cyst, whereas fusion of the tips of adjacent epithelial buds may result in a honeycomb pattern. Nuclear crowding, atypia, and hyperchromatism are of variable degree but mitotic figures are uncommon; psammoma bodies are frequently present. In most of these neoplasms there is a very sharp interface between epithelium and stroma, and the possibility of stromal invasion can be excluded with relative ease (Fig. 10.2); furthermore, the borderline pattern tends to be consistent throughout, it being rather unusual to encounter an intermingling with areas showing a benign appearance or with areas showing a focal evolution into a frank adenocarcinoma.

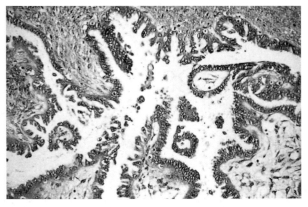

Fig. 10.1 Typical pattern of ovarian papillary serous tumour of borderline malignancy (haematoxylin and eosin). (Republished by kind permission of the editor and publishers of *Current Diagnostic Pathology*.)

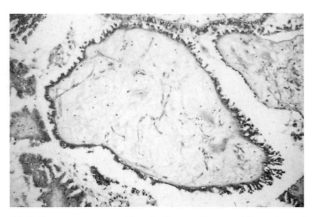

Fig. 10.2 Serous tumour of borderline malignancy. There is a sharp interface between epithelium and strome and this allows for easy recognition of the presence or absence of stromal invasion. (Haematoxylin and eosin.) (Republished by kind permission of the editor and publishers of *Current Diagnostic Pathology*.)

There is a very high incidence of bilaterality in serous tumours of borderline malignancy, the reported frequency ranging in different series from 26 to 66%.[12,23–33] The variation in the reported incidence of bilaterality probably reflects the fact that involvement of the contralateral ovary to that containing an obvious neoplasm may not be apparent to the naked eye, not infrequently being recognized only on histological examination. It is virtually certain that the presence of bilateral tumours represents the synchronous development of two primary neoplasms rather than spread of one tumour to the contralateral side.

A further, and often disconcerting, feature of serous borderline tumours is that in a significant proportion of cases, variously reported as being between 16% and 48%, but averaging at about 35%, there is, at initial diagnosis, apparent extraovarian spread in the form of tumour implants in the pelvic peritoneum and infracolic omentum.[12,23–25,27–38] Histologically the extraovarian lesions may be plastered onto the surface of the peritoneum or lie in the subperitoneal connective tissue and show a variety of patterns.[39–41] Some have a fully benign appearance and consist of simple tubules lined by tubal-type epithelium or indifferent cuboidal cells; psammoma bodies may be present. Others consist of papillae lying within mesothelial-lined spaces. There is some degree of epithelial atypia and multilayering but no invasion, and the appearances resemble closely those seen in a serous tumour of borderline malignancy (Fig. 10.3). In a small minority of cases the subserosal 'implants' are invasive, with infiltrating epithelial cells which have the appearances of an adenocarcinoma (Fig. 10.4). In any given patient there may be an admixture of different patterns, with some lesions having a benign appearance, others resembling a borderline tumour, and, rarely, yet others resembling an adenocarcinoma.[40]

There has been, over the years, much argument as to whether the extraovarian lesions represent true implantation metatases or whether they are independent of the ovarian neoplasm and develop *in situ* within the secondary Müllerian system, i.e. the submesothelial connective tissues.[42,43] It is, in fact, quite probable that the superficial lesions are true seeding deposits from serous

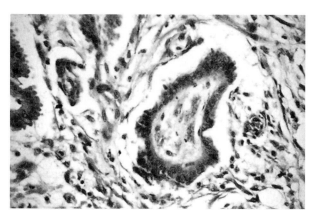

Fig. 10.3 A non-invasive peritoneal lesion associated with an ovarian serous tumour of borderline malignancy (haematoxylin and eosin). (Republished by kind permission of the editor and publishers of *Current Diagnostic Pathology*.)

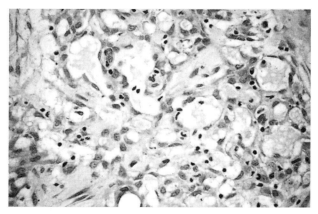

Fig. 10.4 An invasive peritoneal lesion associated with an ovarian serous tumour of borderline malignancy (haematoxylin and eosin). (Republished by kind permission of the editor and publishers of *Current Diagnostic Pathology*.)

tumours of borderline malignancy which show an exophytic growth pattern,[44] but there is strong evidence that the subserosal lesions are independent of the ovarian tumour and develop *in situ*. Thus, those with a fully benign appearance clearly correspond to the well-recognized condition of endosalpingosis,[45,46] which can occur in the absence of an ovarian neoplasm and can also be found in association with a benign ovarian tumour.[47] Those showing some degree of atypia but no evidence of invasion are sometimes categorized as 'atypical endosalpingosis'[48] and can also occur in the absence of any ovarian tumour, often being classed under such circumstances as primary serous borderline tumours of the peritoneum;[49,50] the frequently found admixture of atypical and typical endosalpingosis indicates a common derivation. Further, the invasive lesions can similarly occur independently of an ovarian tumour as primary peritoneal adenocarcinomas[47] which are also thought to be derived from foci of endosalpingosis.[51] Finally, a clonality study which utilized X-chromosome inactivation analysis of the androgen receptor locus has provided clear evidence for the multifocal and diverse origin of ovarian and peritoneal lesions.[52]

In recent studies, in which a full staging procedure had been performed, the long-term survival rate (excluding deaths from other causes) for patients with stage I serous tumours of borderline malignancy neoplasms has been virtually 100%.[30,31,53–63] This excellent prognosis was confirmed by Kurman and Trimble (1993)[64] who surveyed 22 reported series of serous ovarian tumours of borderline malignancy and came to the conclusion that, if deaths due to complications of treatment were excluded, the long-term survival rate for patients with stage I disease was 99%. Patients with stage I disease do, however, appear to be at risk for the eventual development of serous adenocarcinoma. Kurman and Trimble[64] estimated that the risk of such a complication was only 0.7%, but in a recent series 10 out of 160 patients developed a serous adenocarcinoma after time intervals ranging from 8 to 39 years.[65] It could be argued that this was due to small areas of adenocarcinoma being overlooked in the initial pathological assessment of the neoplasm, but adenocarcinomas arising in a serous tumour of borderline malignancy tend to be aggressive and usually lead to death within 4 years.[66]

The long-term survival rate for women with extraovarian disease has been reported as between 75 and 79%.[58,59] It is widely thought that the prognosis in such cases depends upon the nature of the peritoneal lesions, those patients in whom the peritoneal lesions have a non-invasive pattern having an excellent prognosis, and those with invasive implants tending to develop progressive peritoneal disease which takes the form of a low-grade peritoneal serous adenocarcinoma,[39,41,59,67,68] although it has not been everyone's experience that invasive lesions are necessarily associated with a poor prognosis or that only invasive lesions progress.[33,37,40,58,69] Indeed, in two recent studies the progression rate in patients with serous borderline tumours and invasive peritoneal lesions was 31%, whereas that for women with similar tumours and non-invasive peritoneal lesions was 30%.[70,71] It has been suggested that all invasive lesions are in fact true metastases from a subgroup of non-invasive ovarian tumours characterized by a complex papillary architecture with fibrous stalks covered by proliferating, rounded cells showing a filigree pattern (Fig. 10.5),

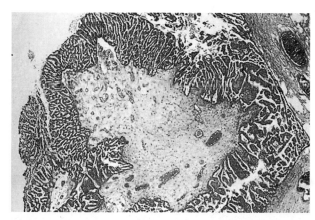

Fig. 10.5 An ovarian serous tumour of borderline malignancy, showing a pattern that has been considered to indicate that it should be regarded as a micropapillary serous adenocarcinoma (haematoxylin and eosin). (Kindly supplied by Dr R. J. Kurman, Baltimore, MD, USA; republished by kind permission of the editor and publishers of *Current Diagnostic Pathology*.)

and that these should be regarded as low-grade adenocarcinomas (micropapillary serous adenocarcinomas),[67,68,72] but this is still a matter for debate and far from proven.[73]

Mucinous tumours of borderline malignancy

There are two quite different types of ovarian mucinous tumour of borderline malignancy. In most such neoplasms the mucinous column-cell epithelium is of gastrointestinal type, but in a minority it is of endocervical type.[74] These two forms differ significantly from each other, both pathologically and clinically, but virtually the entire literature on mucinous borderline tumours relates solely to the intestinal type.

Intestinal type

The intestinal-type mucinous tumours of borderline malignancy usually present as large multilocular cysts. The cyst lining is generally smooth but there may be focal areas of thickening or nodularity. The epithelial component may show a complex glandular pattern, but is often characterized by short, papillary infoldings which give the epithelium a serrated appearance (Fig. 10.6). There are varying degrees of multilayering, loss of nuclear polarity, and cytological atypia, and mitotic figures are seen quite frequently. The outpouching of the epithelium and the formation of secondary glands in many borderline mucinous tumours of intestinal type make the assessment of stromal invasion more difficult than is the case with serous tumours (Fig. 10.7), but this is not usually an impossible task. Many of these neoplasms, like their serous counterparts, show a stereotyped pattern of non-invasive epithelial atypia throughout, but in a proportion there is a variety of patterns. Some show an admixture of benign and borderline areas, others borderline areas with foci of frankly invasive carcinoma, and yet others demonstrate the complete range of appearances, containing benign epithelium, areas of borderline malignancy, and focal adenocarcinoma. Therefore these neoplasms require extensive sampling.

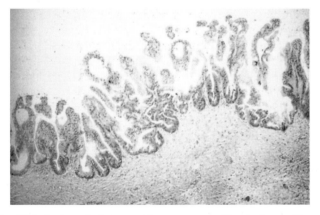

Fig. 10.6 An intestinal-type mucinous tumour of borderline malignancy (haematoxylin and eosin). (Republished by kind permission of the editor and publishers of *Current Diagnostic Pathology*.)

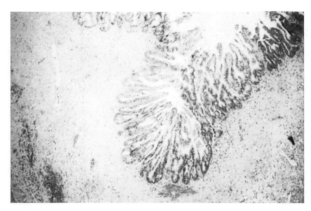

Fig. 10.7 An intestinal-type mucinous tumour of borderline malignancy. This has a complex glandular pattern which makes recognition of stromal invasion difficult. (Haematoxylin and eosin.) (Republished by kind permission of the editor and publishers of *Current Diagnostic Pathology*.)

Bilaterality of intestinal-type mucinous borderline tumours is uncommon and it has become increasingly evident that the long-term survival rate for women with stage I enteric-type mucinous ovarian tumours of borderline malignancy is extremely good; indeed, it is probable that the survival rate for thoroughly sampled and adequately staged tumours approaches 100%.[6,9,10,27,32,33,55,75–80]

Although the outlook for patients with stage I intestinal-type mucinous ovarian tumours of borderline malignancy is excellent, that for the rather small minority of women having such neoplasms but with apparent extraovarian spread is poor, largely because this takes the form of pseudomyxoma peritonei. The traditional view of the pathogenesis of this condition is that the accumulation of thick gelatinous mucoid material within the peritoneal cavity is due either to leakage of mucin or to seeding of mucin-secreting cells from the ovarian tumour. Most mucinous ovarian tumours associated with pseudomyxoma peritonei are, however, not overtly ruptured and it is now becoming apparent that pseudomyxoma peritonei rarely, if ever, occurs in the absence of a synchronous appendicular, or much less commonly, an intestinal neoplasm of low-grade malignancy.[81–83] It is currently still a matter for debate, but the balance of evidence favours the view that pseudomyxoma peritonei is usually, perhaps, invariably, secondary to a gastrointestinal neoplasm, and that the associated ovarian tumours are metastatic in origin despite their usually having an appearance of only borderline malignancy,[84,85] it thus being not surprising that they are associated with a poor prognosis.

Müllerian (endocervical) type

The Müllerian type of borderline mucinous neoplasm has more in common with borderline serous tumours than it does with enteric-type mucinous borderline neoplasms. Thus bilaterality is quite common, there is no association with pseudomyxoma peritonei, and although apparent extraovarian spread does occur this takes the form of endocervicosis, i.e. mucinous glands set in a fibrous stroma, which is considered to be analogous to endosalpingosis and, similarly, arises *in situ* within the secondary Müllerian system. Architecturally they also resemble serous borderline

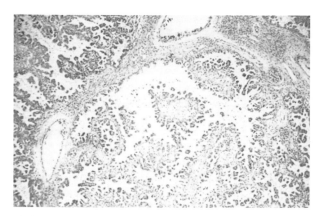

Fig. 10.8 A Müllerian-type mucinous tumour of borderline malignancy. This has a papillary pattern and architecturally closely resembles a papillary serous tumour of borderline malignancy. (Haematoxylin and eosin.) (Republished by kind permission of the editor and publishers of *Current Diagnostic Pathology*.)

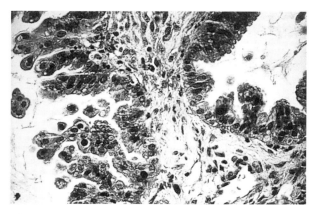

Fig. 10.9 A Müllerian-type mucinous tumour of borderline malignancy. The epithelium is of endocervical type and there is an inflammatory infiltrate of the stroma. (Haematoxylin and eosin.) (Republished by kind permission of the editor and publishers of *Current Diagnostic Pathology*.)

tumours, the only differences being that the papillae are covered by endocervical-type columnar epithelial cells (Fig. 10.8) and that the stroma almost invariably contains an acute inflammatory cell infiltrate (Fig. 10.9). Too little information is currently available about the natural history of this type of mucinous neoplasm to allow for any firm statement about its long-term prognosis, but so far all reported patients have remained well and symptom free after removal of their ovarian neoplasm.[17,74]

Prognostic features of borderline tumours

In ovarian epithelial tumours of borderline malignancy the most important prognostic factor is the nature of the extraovarian lesions, although the amount of residual disease may also have prognostic significance.[70,71,86] Nevertheless there have been many attempts to determine prognostic factors within the ovarian

neoplasm. It has been suggested that histological grading, in terms of the degree of budding, multilayering, and atypia, is of prognostic value,[10,75] but others have failed to confirm that such grading is of any predictive value.[25,87] Morphometric analysis appears to be of value in identifying those borderline tumours likely to pursue an unfavourable course,[88] but there has been quite marked disagreement about the prognostic value of flow cytometry: tumour aneuploidy has been found to be a highly significant prognostic indicator of a poor clinical outcome in some studies[32,89] but not in others.[33,90–92] Studies of oncogene expression and of tumour suppressor genes have not yielded any findings of prognostic value.

Comment

The main thrust of much recent work on ovarian tumours of borderline malignancy has been that most are associated with an excellent prognosis and should be regarded as benign, and that, by contrast, those that have pursued a malignant course are low-grade adenocarcinomas.[68] Thus there is an increasing tendency to negate both the concept and the diagnosis of 'borderline malignancy'.[93] Thus if all stage I serous tumours of borderline malignancy pursue, as they appear to do, a benign course, is there any point in separating them from serous cystadenomas and in retaining the term 'borderline malignancy'? It is currently being argued that those tumours showing a micropapillary pattern should be considered as low-grade carcinomas and that those showing the conventional pattern of borderline malignancy should be regarded as benign neoplasms showing an unusual histological pattern. It remains true, however, that stage I serous borderline tumours, unlike cystadenomas, require adequate surgical staging; that some recur; and that some are combined with, or later evolve into, a true adenocarcinoma. It would be prudent, therefore, to still put these tumours into a separate category, and if it is felt strongly that the term 'borderline malignancy' does convey an undue impression of cancer, a new form of nomenclature may eventually have to be sought.

As far as stage II or III serous borderline tumours are concerned, it has been suggested that those showing a micropapillary pattern are associated with invasive implants and should be regarded, and treated, as adenocarcinomas, and that tumours lacking a micropapillary pattern are benign and are usually associated with non-invasive peritoneal lesions not requiring treatment. It is further suggested that in the very rare cases in which invasive implants accompany an ovarian tumour lacking a micropapillary pattern the patient should be regarded as having a benign ovarian neoplasm with concomitant peritoneal serous carcinoma. This approach is not without merit, for there is no doubt that many women with non-invasive extraovarian lesions are overtreated. Doubts remain, however, as to whether non-invasive lesions can progress to become invasive, whether invasive peritoneal lesions really do behave as adenocarcinomas, and whether invasive lesions respond to chemotherapy. It is reasonable to suggest that whatever the ovarian neoplasm is called, the peritoneal lesions should still be described as 'invasive' and 'non-invasive' until these doubts are dispelled. The mucinous tumours of borderline malignancy pose a similar problem. If all stage I tumours pursue a benign course and all tumours with pseudomyxoma peritonei are actually metastases, is any point served in distinguishing between mucinous cystadenomas and stage I mucinous borderline tumours? Again, the borderline tumours do require surgical staging, whilst their potential for later development of an adenocarcinoma is currently unknown. These two factors do indicate that a useful purpose is still achieved by retaining 'mucinous tumours of borderline malignancy' as a discrete entity.

References

1. Fox, H. (1996). Ovarian tumours of borderine malignancy: time for a reappraisal? *Current Diagnost. Pathol.*, **3**, 143–51.
2. Serov, S.F., Scully, R.E., and Sobin, L.H. (1973). *International histological classification of tumours. No 9. Histological typing of ovarian tumours.* World Health Organization, Geneva.
3. Ovarian Tumour Panel of the Royal College of Obstetricians and Gynaecologists (1983). Ovarian epithelial tumours of borderline malignancy: pathological features and current status. *Br. J. Obstet. Gynaecol.*, **90**, 743–50.
4. Scully, R.E., Young, R.H., and Clement, P.B. (1998). *Tumors of the ovary, maldeveloped gonads, fallopian tube and broad ligament*, Atlas of tumor pathology, 3rd series, fascicle 23). Armed Forces Institute of Pathology, Washington, DC.
5. Bell, D.A., Rutgers, J.L., and Scully, R.E. (1989). Ovarian epithelial tumors of borderline malignancy. In *Progress in reproductive and urinary tract pathology, Vol. 1*, (ed. I. Damjanov, A. Cohen, S.E. Mills, and R.H. Young), pp. 1–30. Field and Wood, Philadelphia.
6. Hart, W.R. and Norris, H.J. (1973). Borderline and malignant mucinous tumors of the ovary. *Cancer*, **31**, 1031–45.
7. Hart, W.R. (1977). Ovarian epithelial tumors of borderline malignancy (carcinomas of low malignant potential) *Hum. Pathol.*, **8**, 541–9.
8. Hart, W.R. (1992). Pathology of malignant and borderline (low malignant potential) epithelial tumors of the ovary. In *Gynecologic oncology*, (2nd edn), (ed. M. Coppleson, J. Monaghan, C.P. Morrow, and M.R.N. Tattersall), pp. 863–87. Churchill Livingstone, Edinburgh.
9. Chaitin, B.A., Gershenson, D.M., and Evans, H.L. (1985). Mucinous tumors of the ovary: a clinicopathologic study of 70 cases. *Cancer*, **55**, 1958–62.
10. Sumithran, E., Susil, B.J., and Looi, L. (1988). The prognostic significance of grading in borderline mucinous tumors of the ovary. *Hum. Pathol.*, **19**, 15–18.
11. Watkin, W., Silva, E.G., and Gershenson, D.M. (1992). Mucinous carcinoma of the ovary: pathologic prognostic factors. *Cancer*, **69**, 208–12.
12. Russell, P. (1979). The pathological assessment of ovarian neoplasms. II. The proliferating epithelial tumours. *Pathology*, **11**, 251–82.
13. Russell, P. (1992). Ovarian epithelial tumours with atypical proliferation. In *Advances in gynaecological pathology*, (ed. D. Lowe and H. Fox), pp. 299–320. Churchill Livingstone, Edinburgh.
14. Russell, P. (1995). Surface epithelial–stromal tumours of the ovary. In *Haines and Taylor: textbook of obstetrical and gynaecological pathology*, (4th edn), (ed. H. Fox), pp. 743–821. Churchill Livingstone, New York.
15. Fox, H. (1989). The concept of borderline malignancy in ovarian tumours. *Curr. Topics Pathol.*, **78**, 111–34.
16. Fox, H. (1994). Ovarian tumours of borderline malignancy. In *Contributions to obstetrics and gynaecology*, Vol. 3, (ed. S.S. Ratnam, D.K. Sen, and S. Arulkumaran), pp. 327–41. Churchill Livingstone, Singapore.
17. Siriaunkgul, S., Robbins, K.M., McGowan, L., and Silverberg, S.G. (1995). Ovarian mucinous tumors of low malignant potential: a clinicopathologic study of 54 tumors of intestinal and Mullerian type. *Int. J. Gynecol. Pathol.*, **14**, 198–208.
18. Yoonessi, K., Crickard, K., Celic, C., and Yoonessi, S. (1988). Borderline epithelial tumors of the ovary: ovarian intraepithelial neoplasia. *Obstet. Gynecol. Survey*, **43**, 435–44.
19. Plaxe, S.C., Deligdisch, L., Dottino, P.R., and Cohen, C.J. (1990). Ovarian intraepithelial neoplasia demonstrated in patients with Stage I ovarian carcinoma. *Gynecol. Oncol.*, **38**, 367–72.
20. Tavassoli, F.A. (1988). Serous tumor of low malignant potential with early stromal invasion (serous LMP with microinvasion). *Mod. Pathol.*, **1**, 407–14.
21. Bell, D.A. and Scully, R.E. (1990). Ovarian serous borderline tumors with stromal microinvasion: a report of 21 cases. *Hum. Pathol.*, **21**, 397–403.
23. Purola E. (1963). Serous papillary ovarian tumours: a study of 233 cases with special reference to the histological type of tumour and its influence on prognosis. *Acta Obstet. Gynaecol. Scand.*, **42** (suppl. 3), 1–77.
24. Julian, C.G. and Woodruff, J.D. (1972). The biologic behaviour of low grade papillary serous carcinoma of the ovary. *Obstetrics and Gynecology*, **40**, 360–8.
25. Katzenstein, A.A., Mazur, M.T., Morgan, T.E., and Kao, G.F. (1978). Proliferative serous tumors of the ovary: histologic features and prognosis. *Am. J. Surg. Pathol.*, **2**, 339–55.
26. Tang, M., Lian, L., and Liu, T. (1980). The characteristics of ovarian serous tumors of borderline malignancy. *Chinese Med. J.*, **92**, 459–64.
27. Tasker, M. and Langley, F.A. (1985). The outlook for women with borderline epithelial tumours of the ovary. *Br. J. Obstet. Gynaecol.*, **92**, 969–73.
28. Tazelaar, H.D., Bostwick, D.G., Ballon, S.C. *et al.* (1985). Conservative treatment of borderline ovarian tumors. *Obstet. Gynecol.*, **66**, 417–22.
29. Kliman, L., Rome, R.M., and Fortune, D.W. (1986). Low malignant potential tumors of the ovary: a study of 76 cases. *Obstet. Gynecol.*, **68**, 338–44.
30. Nakashima, N., Nagasaka, T., Oiwa, N. *et al.* (1990). Ovarian epithelial tumors of borderline malignancy in Japan. *Gynecol. Oncol.*, **38**, 90–8.
31. Massad, L.S., Hunter, V.J., Szpakca, C.A. *et al.* (1991). Epithelial ovarian tumors of low malignant potential. *Obstet. Gynecol.*, **78**, 1027–32.
32. Kaern, J., Trope, C.G., and Abeler, V.M. (1993). A retrospective study of 370 ovarian borderline tumors treated at the Norwegian Radium Hospital from 1970 to 1982: a clinical and histopathological review. *Cancer*, **71**, 1810–20.
33. Sykes, P., Quinn, M., and Rome, R. (1997). Ovarian tumors of low malignant potential: a retrospective study of 234 patients. *Int. J. Gynecol. Cancer*, **7**, 218–26.
34. Aure, J.C., Hoeg, K., and Kolstad, P. (1971). Clinical and histologic studies of ovarian carcinoma: long term follow-up of 990 cases. *Obstet. Gynecol.*, **37**, 1–9.
35. Russell, P. (1984). Borderline epithelial tumours of the ovary: a conceptual dilemma. *Clin. Obstet. Gynaecol.*, **11**, 259–77.
36. Nikrui, N. (1981). Survey of clinical behaviour of patients with borderline epithelial tumors of the ovary. *Gynecol. Oncol.*, **12**, 107–19.
37. Gershenson, D.M. and Silva, E.G. (1990). Serous ovarian tumors of low malignant potential with peritoneal implants. *Cancer*, **65**, 578–85.
38. Trimble, C.L. and Trimble, E.L. (1994). Management of epithelial ovarian tumors of low malignant potential. *Gynecol. Oncol.*, **55**, 552–61.
39. McCaughey, W.T.E., Kirk, M.E., Lester, W., and Dardick, I. (1984). Peritoneal epithelial lesions associated with proliferative serous tumors of the ovary. *Histopathology*, **8**, 195–208.
40. Michel, H. and Roth, L.M. (1986). Invasive and non-invasive implants in ovarian serous tumors of low malignant potential. *Cancer*, **57**, 1240–7.
41. Bell, D.A., Weinstock, M.A., and Scully, R.E. (1988). Peritoneal implants of ovarian serous borderline tumors: histologic features and prognosis. *Cancer*, **62**, 2212–22.
42. Lauchlan, S.C. (1972). The secondary Mullerian system. *Obstet. Gynecol. Survey*, **27**, 133–46.
43. Lauchlan, S.C. (1994). The secondary Mullerian system revisited. *Int. J. Gynecol. Pathol.*, **13**, 73–9.

44. Segal, G.H. and Hart, W.R. (1992). Ovarian serous tumors of low malignant potential (serous borderline tumors): the relationship of exophytic surface tumor to peritoneal 'implants'. *Am. J. Surg. Pathol.*, **16**, 577–83.

45. Tutschka, B.G. and Lauchlan, S.C. (1980). Endosalpingiosis. *Obstet. Gynecol.*, **55**, 57s–60s.

46. Zinser, K.R. and Wheeler, J.E. (1982). Endosalpingiosis in the omentum: a study of autopsy and surgical material. *Am. J. Surg. Pathol.*, **6**, 109–17.

47. Bell, D.A. (1995). Pathology of the peritoneum and secondary Mullerian system. In *Haines and Taylor: Obstetrical and gynaecological pathology,* (4th edn), (ed. H. Fox), pp. 997–1014. Churchill Livingstone, New York.

48. Dallenbach-Hellweg, G. (1987). Atypical endosalpingiosis: a case report with consideration of the differential diagnosis of glandular subperitoneal inclusions. *Pathol. Res. Pract.*, **182**, 180–2.

49. Bell, D.A. and Scully, R.E. (1990) Serous borderline tumors of the peritoneum. *Am. J. Surg. Pathol.*, **14**, 230–9.

50. Biscotti, C.V. and Hart, W.R. (1992). Peritoneal serous micropapillomatosis of low malignant potential (serous borderline tumors of the peritoneum): a clinicopathologic study of 17 cases. *Am. J. Surg. Pathol.*, **16**, 467–75.

51. Farnsworth, H. and Russell, P. (1992). Extraovarian tumours of Mullerian type. In *Advances in gynaecological pathology*, (ed. D. Lowe and H. Fox), pp. 321–41. Churchill Livingstone, Edinburgh.

52. Lu, K.H., Bell, D.A., Welch, W.R., Berkowitz, R.S., and Mok, S.C. (1998). Evidence for the multifocal origin of bilateral and advanced serous borderline ovarian tumors. *Cancer Res.*, **58**, 2328–30.

53. Lim-Tan, S.K., Cagigas, H.A., and Scully, R.E. (1988). Ovarian cystectomy for serous borderline tumors: a follow-up study of 35 cases. *Obstet. Gynecol.*, **72**, 775–81.

54. Dgani, R., Blickstein, I., Stroham, Z. *et al.* (1990). Clinical aspects of ovarian tumors of low malignant potential. *Europ. J. Obstet. Gynecol. Reproduct. Biol.*, **35**, 251–8.

55. Rice, L.W., Berkowitz, R.S., Mark, S.D. *et al.* (1990). Ovarian epithelial tumors of borderline malignancy. *Gynecol. Oncol.*, **39**, 195–8.

56. Ayhan, A., Atakin, R., Develioglu, O. *et al.* (1991). Borderline epithelial tumours. *Aust. NZ J. Obstet. Gynaecol.*, **31**, 174–6.

57. Sawada, M., Yamasaki, M., Urabe, T. *et al.* (1991). Stage I epithelial ovarian tumors of low malignant potential. *Jap. J. Clin. Oncol.*, **21**, 30–4.

58. Manchul, L.A., Simm, J., Levin, W. *et al.* (1992). Borderline epithelial ovarian tumors: a review of 81 cases with an assessment of the impact of treatment. *Int. J. Radiat. Oncol. Biol. Phys.*, **22**, 867–74.

59. de Nictolis, M., Montironi, R., Tommasoni, S. *et al.* (1992). Serous borderline tumors of the ovary: a clinicopathologic, immunohistochemical, and quantitative study of 44 cases. *Cancer*, **70**, 152–60.

60. Piura, B., Dgani, R., Blickstein, I. *et al.* (1992) Epithelial ovarian tumors of borderline malignancy: a study of 50 cases. *Int. J. Gynecol. Cancer*, **2**, 189–97.

61. Kaern, J., Trope, C.G., Kristensen, G.B. *et al.* (1993). DNA ploidy: the most important prognostic factor in patients with borderline tumors of the ovary. *Int J Gynecol. Cancer*, **3**, 349–58.

62. Barnhill, D.R., Kurman, R.J., Brady, M.F. *et al.* (1995). Preliminary analysis of the behavior of stage I ovarian serous tumors of low malignant potential: a Gynecologic Oncology Group Study. *J. Clin. Oncol.*, **13**, 2752–6.

63. Buttini, M., Nicklin, J.L., and Crandon, A. (1997). Low malignant potential ovarian tumours: a review of 175 consecutive cases. *Aust. N.Z.J. Obstet. Gynaecol.*, **37**, 100–3.

64. Kurman, R.J. and Trimble, C.L. (1993). The behaviour of serous tumors of low malignant potential: are they ever malignant? *Int. J. Gynecol. Pathol.*, **12**, 120–7.

65. Silva, E.G., Tornos, C., Zhuang, Z. *et al.* (1998). Tumor recurrence in Stage I ovarian serous neoplasms of low malignant potential. *Int. J. Gynecol. Pathol.*, **17**, 1–6.

66. Silva, E.G., Tornos, C.S., Malpica, A., and Gershenson, D.M. (1997). Ovarian serous neoplasms of low malignant potential associated with focal areas of serous carcinoma. *Mod. Pathol.*, **10**, 663–7.

67. Burks, R.T., Sherman, M.E., and Kurman, R.J. (1996). Micropapillary serous carcinoma of the ovary and peritoneum: a distinctive low grade carcinoma related to serous borderline tumors. *Am. J. Surg. Pathol.*, **20**, 1319–30.

68. Seidman, J.D. and Kurman, R.J. (1996). Subclassification of serous borderline tumors of the ovary into benign and malignant types: a clinicopathologic study of 65 advanced stage cases. *Am. J. Surg. Pathol.*, **20**, 1331–45.

69. Padberg, P.C., Arps, H., Franke, U. *et al.* (1992). DNA cytophotometry and prognosis in ovarian tumors of borderline malignancy: a clinicopathological study of 80 cases. *Cancer*, **69**, 2510–14.

70. Gershenson, D.M., Silva, E.G., Levy, L. *et al.* (1998). Ovarian serous borderline tumors with invasive peritoneal implants. *Cancer*, **82**, 1096–103.

71. Gershenson, D.M., Silva, E.G., Tortolero-Luna, G. *et al.* (1998). Serous borderline tumors of the ovary with noninvasive peritoneal implants. *Cancer*, **83**, 2157–63.

72. Katabuchi, H., Tashiro, H., Cho, K.R. *et al.* (1998). Micropapillary serous carcinoma of the ovary: an immunohistochemical and mutational analysis of p53. *Int. J. Gynecol. Pathol.*, **17**, 54–60.

73. Eichhorn, J.H., Bell, D.A., Young, R.H., and Scully, R.E. (1999). Ovarian serous borderline tumors with micropapillary and cribiform patterns: a study of 40 cases and comparison with 44 cases without these patterns. *Am. J. Surg. Pathol.*, **23**, 397–409.

74. Rutgers, J.L. and Scully, R.E. (1988). Ovarian Mullerian mucinous papillary cystadenomas of borderline malignancy: a clinicopathologic analysis of 30 cases. *Cancer*, **61**, 340–8.

75. Russell, P. and Merkur, H. (1979). Proliferating ovarian 'epithelial' tumours: a clinicopathologic analysis of 144 cases. *Aust. NZ J. Obstet. Gynaecol.*, **19**, 45–51.

76. Barnhill, D., Heller, P., Brzozowski, P. *et al.* (1985). Epithelial ovarian carcinoma of low malignant potential *Obstet. Gynecol.*, **65**, 53–8.

77. Bostwick, D.G., Tazelaar, H.D., Ballon, S.C., Hendrickson, M.R., and Kempson, R.L. (1986). Ovarian epithelial tumors of borderline malignancy: a clinical and pathologic study of 109 cases. *Cancer*, **58**, 2052–65.

78. Nation, J.G. and Krepart, G.V. (1986). Ovarian carcinoma of low malignant potential: staging and treatment. *Am. J. Obstet. Gynecol.*, **154**, 290–3.

79. Guerriere, C., Hogberg, T., Wingren, S., Fristedt, S., Simonsen, E., and Boeryd, B. (1994). Mucinous borderline and malignant tumors of the ovary. *Cancer*, **74**, 2329–35.

80. de Nictolis, M., Montironi, R., Tommasoni, S. *et al.* (1994). Benign, borderline, and well differentiated malignant intestinal mucinous tumors of the ovary: a clinicopathologic, immunohistochemical, and nuclear quantitative study of 57 cases. *Int. J. Gynecol. Pathol.*, **13**, 10–21.

81. Young, R.H., Gilks, S.B., and Scully, R.E. (1991). Mucinous tumors of the appendix associated with mucinous tumors of the ovary and pseudomyxoma peritonei: a clinicopathological analysis of 22 cases. *Am. J. Surg. Pathol.*, **15**, 415–29.

82. Prayson, R.A., Hart, W.R., and Petras, R.E. (1994). Pseudomyxoma peritonei: a clinicopathologic study of 19 cases with emphasis on site of origin and nature of associated ovarian tumors. *Am. J. Surg. Pathol.*, **18**, 591–603.

83. Ronnett, B.M., Kurman, R.J., Zahn, C.M. *et al.* (1995). Pseudomyxoma peritonei in women: a clinicopathologic analysis of 30 cases with emphasis on site of origin, prognosis, and relationship to ovarian mucinous tumors of low malignant potential. *Hum. Pathol.*, **26**, 509–24.

84. Ronnett, B.M., Schmookler, B.M., Diener-West, M. *et al.* (1997). Immunohistochemical evidence supporting the appendiceal origin of pseudomyxoma peritonei. *Int. J. Gynecol. Pathol.*, **16**, 1–9.

85. Guerriere, C., Franlund, B., Fristedt, S. *et al.* (1997). Mucinous tumors of the vermiform appendix and ovary and pseudomyxoma peritonei: histogenetic implications of cytokeratin 7 expression. *Hum. Pathol.*, **28**, 1039–45.

86. Tamakoshi, K., Kikkawa, F., Nakashima, N. *et al.* (1997). Clinical behaviour of borderline ovarian tumors: a study of 150 cases. *J. Surg. Oncol.*, **64**, 147–152.

87. Fox, H. (1983). Ovarian tumors of borderline malignancy. In *Recent clinical developments in gynecological oncology*, (ed. C.P. Morrow, J. Bonnar, T.J. O'Brian, and W.E. Gibbons), pp. 137–50. Raven Press, New York.

88. Baak, J.P.A., Fox, H., Langley, F.A., and Buckley, C.H. (1985). The prognostic value of morphometry in ovarian epithelial tumors of borderline malignancy. *Int. J. Gynecol. Pathol.*, 4, 186–91.

89. Padberg, P.C., Stegner, H.E., von Sengbusch, S. *et al.* (1992). DNA cytophotometry and immunocytochemistry in ovarian tumours of borderline, malignancy and related peritoneal lesions. *Virchows Archiv A Pathol. Anat.*, 421, 497–503.

90. Harlow, B.L., Fuhr, J.E., McDonald, T.W. *et al.* (1995). Flow cytometry as a prognostic indicator in women with borderline epithelial ovarian tumors. *Gynecol. Oncol.*, 50, 305–9.

91. Kuoppala, T., Heinola, M., Aine, R. *et al.* (1996). Serous and mucinous borderline tumors of the ovary: a clinicopathologic and DNA-ploidy study of 102 cases. *Int. J. Gynecol. Cancer*, 6, 302–8.

92. Demirel, D., Laucirica, R., Fishman, A. *et al.* (1996). Ovarian tumors of low malignant potential: correlation of DNA index and S-phase fraction with histopathologic grade and clinical outcome. *Cancer*, 77, 1494–500.

93. Seidman, J.D., Rennett, B.M., and Kurman, K.J. (2000). Evaluation of the concept and terminology of borderline ovarian tumours. *Curr Diagn. Pathol.*, 6, 31–70.

11. Primary non-epithelial ovarian cancers

Naveena Singh and David Lowe

Primary ovarian cancers that are not of surface epithelial origin constitute approximately 20% of all ovarian cancers. These include malignancies of sex cord-stromal and germ cell derivation, sarcomas arising from non-specialized ovarian stroma, and some miscellaneous and unclassifiable tumours. A list of non-epithelial tumours based on the recent WHO classification is presented in Table 11.1.[1]

Table 11.1 Non-epithelial ovarian tumours

Sex cord-stromal tumours
  Granulosa-stromal cell tumours
    granulosa cell tumours
      adult
      juvenile
    tumours of thecoma-fibroma group
  Sertoli-stromal cell tumours; androblastoma
  Sex cord tumour with annular tubules
  Gynandroblastoma
  Unclassified
  Steroid cell tumours
Germ cell tumours
  Dysgerminoma
  Yolk sac tumour (endodermal sinus tumour)
  Embryonal carcinoma
  Polyembryoma
  Choriocarcinoma
  Teratoma
Germ cell-sex cord-stromal tumours
  Gonadoblastoma
  Germ cell-sex cord-stromal tumour of non-gonadoblastoma type
Tumours of uncertain origin
  Small cell carcinoma
  Tumour of probable Wolffian origin
  Hepatoid carcinoma
  Myxoma
  Others
Tumours of rete ovarii
  Adenoma and cystadenoma
  Adenocarcinoma
Mesothelial tumours
  Adenomatoid tumour
  Mesothelioma
Gestational trophoblastic diseases
Soft-tissue tumours not specific to ovary
Lymphoma and leukaemia
Unclassified tumours
Metastatic tumours

Sex cord–stromal tumours

This group comprises tumours of granulosa cells, theca cells, Sertoli cells, Leydig cells, and specialized stromal fibroblasts. These constituents may be present alone or in various combinations and in varying degrees of differentiation.[2,3] The sex-cord-derived components are granulosa and Sertoli cells, which tend to form structures resembling epithelial configurations in tumours, while theca, lutein, and Leydig cells are gonadal stromal derivatives. Granulosa cell tumours account for most clinically malignant sex cord–stromal tumours. These will be considered in detail.

Granulosa cell tumour

Granulosa cell tumours are defined as those in which at least 10% of the tumour is composed of granulosa cells; these constitute about 12% of all sex cord–stromal tumours and 70% of malignant subtypes.[2] There are two histopathological types: adult and juvenile, which have quite different clinical behaviour.

ADULT GRANULOSA CELL TUMOUR

General features
Ninety-five per cent of granulosa cell tumours are of adult type and these account for 1–2% of all ovarian tumours.[4,5] They may occur at any age but are most frequent in peri- and post-menopausal women.

Granulosa cell tumours are the most common ovarian tumours to have oestrogenic manifestations, which often account for the presenting symptoms. The typical effect of hyperoestrinism is simple endometrial hyperplasia. Complex and atypical hyperplasias may also occur, and well-differentiated endometrial adenocarcinoma has been reported in about 5% of cases, most often in postmenopausal patients.[6] Apart from uterine bleeding, hyperoestrinism may result in amenorrhoea or isosexual pseudoprecocity. Rarely, the endometrium may show features of progesterone stimulation with a secretory or decidual pattern. A small minority of tumours, typically those that have a thin-walled cystic structure, present with androgenic features of hirsutism of recent onset or other signs of virilization.[7] Most women also have symptoms related to the ovarian mass, such as abdominal pain and swelling, and up to 10% present with acute abdominal symptoms due to rupture of the tumour.

Granulosa cell tumours are typically associated with elevated serum levels of α-inhibin. This can serve as a useful tumour marker in the management of primary tumours and in detection of recurrences.[8] Inhibin is a dimeric glycoprotein hormone secreted by normal granulosa cells which suppresses pituitary gonadotrophin release. Neoplastic granulosa cells overexpress the α-subunit gene.[9] Inhibin production is also seen with other sex cord–stromal tumours and rarely in mucinous epithelial tumours.[10,11] Serum detection of Müllerian inhibiting substance, a hormone normally produced by the fetal testis that causes Müllerian duct regression, can also be used in the diagnosis and follow-up of these patients.[11,12]

Molecular events involved in the pathogenesis of these tumours are unknown. Non-random chromosomal abnormalities such as monosomy 22, trisomy 14, and trisomy 12 have been detected, of which the first two are considered to be early events in tumorigenesis.[13–15] Overexpression of the oncogene *erbB4* has been reported, with potential therapeutic as well as pathogenetic implications.[16]

Gross appearances

Adult granulosa cell tumours are characteristically unilateral, solid, hard, or rubbery tumours that vary from being microscopic to huge masses, with an average diameter of 12 cm. The outer surface is smooth and usually intact. The cut surface varies from solid and yellow or white to cystic with areas of haemorrhage and necrosis. The appearances depend on the relative proportions of granulosa and stromal cells. Some tumours are cystic, resembling cystadenomas, and these are often androgenic.

Microscopic features

These tumours exhibit a variety of histological patterns.[4,5] The tumour cells are round or polygonal with scanty cytoplasm, indistinct cell margins, and nuclei that are round or ovoid with typical longitudinal grooves ('coffee-bean' nuclei). The cells may form broad sheets, as in the diffuse (sarcomatoid) variant, parallel wavy rows (watered-silk pattern), or haphazard zigzag cords ('gyriform pattern'). In the best-differentiated tumours, the cells form follicles. In the microfollicular pattern, cells are arranged around small cavities containing eosinophilic material, nuclear debris, basement membrane material, or basophilic fluid. These microfollicular structures (Call–Exner bodies) simulate those seen in a normal maturing Graafian follicle. The macrofollicular pattern is characterized by large cysts lined by granulosa cells resting on theca cells.

Most tumours contain a mixture of different patterns of granulosa cells, or a combination of granulosa and stromal cells in trabecular or insular patterns. Mitotic activity varies but is typically low.[17] A reticulin stain is useful for delineating stromal areas (reticulin-rich) from diffuse granulosa cell areas (reticulin-poor with mostly perivascular reticulin).[1]

Other variations include luteinization of a proportion of the granulosa cells or the presence of Sertoli cells. Luteinization may occur in pregnancy[18] or otherwise, and may be associated with progesterone secretion.[19] A few tumours contain focal areas of cells with bizarre nuclei.[20]

The immunohistochemical profile of granulosa cells can be useful in difficult cases: α-inhibin and vimentin are usually positive, broad-spectrum cytokeratin staining may show punctate positivity, while cytokeratin 7 and epithelial membrane antigen (EMA) are negative.[21–24] Proliferative activity illustrated by Ki–67 staining is low and p53 protein is not detectable immunohistochemically.[25]

Differential diagnosis

The differential diagnosis of diffuse adult granulosa cell tumour includes undifferentiated carcinoma, small cell carcinoma, endometrial stromal sarcoma, and pure stromal tumours. Cystic tumours can occasionally be difficult to distinguish from cystic follicles. Well-differentiated microfollicular variants can resemble endometrioid tumours. These variants can also be confused with rare tumours such as carcinoids, sex cord tumours with annular tubules, or gonadoblastomas. Distinction from metastatic melanoma or breast carcinoma can also be a problem.

Clinical behaviour and prognosis

All adult-type granulosa cell tumours should be regarded as potentially malignant with a capacity for extraovarian spread and local recurrence. Recurrences or metastases tend to occur late, commonly after 5 years, with a median of 7.5 years, and occasionally 20 or more years postoperatively.[4,26,27]

Treatment for stage I disease is surgical, ideally total hysterectomy with bilateral salpingo-oophorectomy. Conservative surgery with removal of only the involved ovary may be considered if there is no evidence of extraovarian spread and careful follow-up, including monitoring of serum inhibin levels, is planned. Higher-stage disease and recurrences are treated more aggressively, with combinations of surgery, radiation, and chemotherapy.[28–33]

Survival figures vary with length of follow-up in various studies, and long-term survival is estimated at about 50%.[4] The strongest prognostic factors are stage, size of the tumour, and rupture during surgery.[34–36] The behaviour of granulosa cell tumours cannot be predicted from histological appearances. Of the various pathological parameters studied, only atypia and mitotic activity show weak correlation with early recurrence.[34,37] Studies relating aneuploidy to survival have shown conflicting results.[38–40]

JUVENILE GRANULOSA CELL TUMOUR

General features

These oestrogen-secreting neoplasms arise most commonly, but not invariably, in prepubertal girls who present with precocious puberty. Approximately 3% of cases arise after the third decade.[41–43] Trisomy 12 is a common cytogenetic abnormality present in these tumours.[14,44]

Gross and microscopic appearances

These tumours are unilateral with solid areas and cysts of various sizes. The solid areas are grey or yellow with areas of haemorrhage. Histologically, granulosa cells are typically arranged in nodules separated by oedematous fibrothecomatous stroma. Follicles lined by layers of granulosa cells may occur and a solid pattern may be seen. The granulosa cells in juvenile-type tumours differ from those in the adult type in having more rounded and hyperchromatic nuclei which lack longitudinal grooves, and in being more strikingly luteinized. Atypia and mitotic activity are also more conspicuous.

Clinical behaviour and prognosis

About 90% of cases present at stage I and bilaterality is exceedingly uncommon.[45,46] Only 5% of juvenile granulosa cell tumours behave in a malignant fashion. The prognosis is excellent for stage I tumours: removal of the involved ovary is curative. Haemoperitoneum and rupture during surgery are not necessarily indications for chemotherapy.[47] Prognosis is less favourable for higher-stage disease. The role of adjuvant therapy in such cases is controversial and treatment of the malignant forms has yet to be optimized.[45–50] Unlike in the adult type, recurrences in juvenile granulosa cell tumours tend to occur early, usually within 3 years.[41–43] Favourable prognostic factors are diagnosis at stage I, age less than 10 years, and the presence of precocious puberty.[46,47] Behaviour cannot be predicted from mitotic activity, atypia, ploidy, or S-phase fraction, although aneuploidy may be of prognostic significance in high-stage tumours.[51,52]

Fibrosarcoma and cellular fibroma

General features

Of the tumours of the thecoma–fibroma group, only fibrosarcomas behave in a clinically malignant fashion. These tumours are among the most common forms of ovarian sarcoma. They can occur at any age but are most frequent in the elderly.[53–55]

Gross and microscopic features

Fibrosarcomas are unilateral, bulky, fleshy masses typically with large areas of haemorrhage and necrosis. Microscopically they are cellular tumours with moderate to severe atypia and four or more mitotic figures per 10 high-power fields.

Clinical behaviour and prognosis

Fibrosarcomas are aggressive tumours that pursue a highly malignant course. Fibromas that are unduly cellular and mitotically active, with up to three mitoses per 10 high-power fields and no or minimal atypia, are designated cellular fibromas. These have a low malignant potential with a tendency for local recurrence if incompletely excised.[56] Rarely, fibrothecomas show malignant behaviour despite low mitotic activity.[57] Cytogenetic studies and proliferative indices are potentially useful in identifying malignant subtypes.[58]

Sertoli–stromal cell tumours; androblastoma

General features

These tumours are composed of Sertoli cells, Leydig cells, and rete epithelial cells, alone or in combination. They include the pure Sertoli cell tumour and the four major subtypes of Sertoli–Leydig cell tumours.[1] Sertoli cell tumours occur at an average age of 30 years and are generally non-functioning, although some are oestrogenic and occasionally androgenic. Only one malignant ovarian Sertoli cell tumour has been reported to date.[18]

Sertoli–Leydig cell tumours occur at an average age of 25 years, with 75% arising before the age of 30 and only 10% after the age

of 50.[59] These tumours account for less than 0.5% of ovarian tumours. The most characteristic presentation is with virilization, which is seen in about one-third of the cases. Fifty per cent of patients present with symptoms related to the pelvic mass and have no hormonal symptoms.

Gross appearances

Sertoli cell tumours are typically unilateral, solid, lobulated, yellow masses confined to the ovary. Sertoli–Leydig cell tumours are more variable in appearance and size, ranging from microscopic to huge masses. Most are unilateral and confined to the ovary. Rupture or capsular involvement is seen in 12% of cases at presentation.[59] The cut surface may be solid and yellow or have cystic and necrotic foci, depending on the constituent components.

Microscopic findings

Sertoli cell tumours are composed of nodules or hollow tubules of Sertoli cells within fibrous stroma containing few or no Leydig cells. Atypia and mitotic activity are unusual.

Sertoli–Leydig cell tumours are classified into well, intermediate and poorly differentiated, and retiform subtypes, which differ in their clinical behaviour.[59–61] Well-differentiated tumours are composed of Sertoli cells in tubules separated by fibrous tissue containing Leydig cells. Intermediate and poorly differentiated tumours lack this relatively orderly arrangement: Sertoli cells appear immature and arranged in short cords, loose aggregates, or diffuse sheets, the stroma appears sarcomatoid, and mitotic activity is conspicuous, particularly in poorly differentiated tumours. A variable degree of cystic change occurs, notably in the retiform variant that can resemble a cystadenoma.[60] Twenty per cent of Sertoli–Leydig cell tumours contain heterologous elements, which may be epithelial or stromal.[62,63]

Differential diagnosis

Due to marked variability in their histological appearances, these tumours can resemble a wide range of tumours. Positive staining for α-inhibin in Leydig and Sertoli cells can be extremely helpful in making a diagnosis of these tumours.[64]

Clinical behaviour and prognosis

Prognosis depends on histological features and stage. Well-differentiated tumours are benign and these and intermediate forms confined to the ovary are curable by unilateral salpingo-oophorectomy. Poorly differentiated and retiform tumours, and those with heterologous stromal elements, have a poor prognosis and need adjuvant therapy, as do intermediate-grade tumours complicated by rupture or extraovarian involvement. Unlike granulosa cell tumours, recurrences tend to occur early. These are usually confined to the pelvis but distant metastases can occur. Recurrences are frequently less differentiated than the original tumour and may resemble soft-tissue sarcomas.[59]

Sex cord tumour with annular tubules

These tumours have distinctive clinicopathological features and occur in young adults in the third or fourth decades of life. One-third of the cases occur in patients with Peutz–Jeghers syndrome

(PJS). In these cases the tumours are usually clinically silent and found incidentally at operation for some other indication, or at post-mortem examination. Such cases behave in a clinically benign fashion.[65]

Tumours occurring in patients without PJS present with hormonal, usually oestrogenic, manifestations and a palpable mass. These tumours are unilateral, large, solid masses with a yellow cut surface. Microscopically they are characterized by the presence of simple and complex annular tubules within a variable amount of stroma. The tubules are composed of cuboidal cells arranged peripherally around a central hyaline body with an intervening cytoplasmic zone. Areas of granulosa or Sertoli cell tumour, or both, may be present.

About 20% of the cases without PJS are clinically malignant with lymphatic spread and, usually late, local recurrences. Serum measurements of inhibin, Müllerian inhibiting substance, and progesterone have been useful in monitoring recurrences. Treatment is usually surgical; recurrent tumours may respond to chemotherapy.[66]

Gynandroblastoma

These tumours contain a mixture of granulosa and Sertoli–Leydig components. They occur in young adults and present with oestrogenic or androgenic manifestations. Most are clinically benign.[67]

Unclassified sex cord–stromal tumours

Up to 10% of sex cord–stromal tumours are difficult to assign to any specific category. This may be because of presentation during pregnancy, which results in massive oedema and luteinization and obscures the underlying features.[18,19,68,69] Their behaviour is reported to be similar to granulosa cell or Sertoli–Leydig tumours.[69]

Steroid cell tumours

These include three subtypes: stromal luteomas and pure Leydig cell tumours, which are benign, and steroid cell tumours not otherwise specified (NOS), a proportion of which are clinically malignant.[70]

Steroid cell tumours, NOS, occur at a mean age of 43 years and present with hormonal manifestations, most commonly androgenic or oestrogenic and rarely progestagenic or hypercortisolaemic (Cushingoid). The tumours are unilateral, large, lobulated and typically bright yellow. Histologically they are composed of polygonal cells with abundant granular, eosinophilic, or vacuolated cytoplasm. Atypia and mitotic activity are unusual. Staining for α-inhibin is positive as in other sex cord–stromal tumours.[23]

Treatment is primarily surgical. The proportion of malignant cases depends on the length of follow-up and is reported to be 43% in the largest series.[70] Adverse prognostic factors are age, presence of clinical Cushing's syndrome, large tumour size, necrosis, haemorrhage, cytological atypia, and two or more mitoses per 10 high-power fields.[70,71]

Germ cell tumours

Germ cell tumours as a group constitute about 30% of ovarian tumours, the majority of these being mature cystic teratomas.

Malignant germ cell tumours account for 1–3% of ovarian cancers in Western countries and two-thirds of ovarian cancers in the first two decades of life.[72,73] The proportion is much higher in Afro-Caribbean and Japanese populations because of a lower frequency of surface epithelial cancers.[1]

The most common malignant germ cell tumours are dysgerminoma (48%) and yolk-sac tumour (endodermal sinus tumour) (20%). Approximately 10% of the cases are composed of a mixture of different histological types.[74] The prognosis of these tumours in general is much better currently than in the pre-chemotherapy era. Owing to their preponderance in younger women, a conservative approach with preservation of fertility has to be balanced against achieving cure and minimizing the possibility of recurrence. In general, true stage 1A tumours are treated by conservative surgery (unilateral salpingo-oophorectomy), and adjuvant cisplatin-based chemotherapy is given in all other cases.[75–77] Serum levels of the tumour markers α-fetoprotein (AFP), the β-subunit of human chorionic gonadotrophin (βhGG), and lactate dehydrogenase (LDH) are useful in evaluating treatment and follow-up.

Dysgerminoma

General features

These tumours are composed of cells that resemble primordial germ cells. They are the ovarian equivalents of testicular seminomas. Dysgerminomas occur in patients in their second and third decades of life and account for 20–30% of ovarian cancers presenting during pregnancy.[78] They are the most common form of malignant tumour occurring in gonadal dysgenesis.

Clinical presentation is usually with mass-related signs and symptoms. About 3% of the tumours are associated with elevated βhCG levels, and these may present with oestrogenic or, very occasionally, androgenic symptoms. Ninety-five per cent of cases have raised LDH (isoenzymes 1 and 2) levels that are useful in follow-up.[79,80] Alkaline phosphatase and CA125 levels are sometimes elevated. Levels of AFP are normal in pure dysgerminomas, although exceptions have been reported.[79]

Gross appearances

Dysgerminomas are characteristically large masses with a smooth, bosselated outer surface and a solid, soft, grey or pink cut surface. Areas of cystic degeneration or haemorrhage may be present and should be sampled specifically to exclude other germ cell tumour elements. Twenty per cent of the cases are bilateral, although involvement of the second ovary is grossly apparent in only half of these cases.

Microscopic findings

These tumours are composed of a uniform population of large, rounded cells with clear glycogen-rich cytoplasm, distinct cell membranes, and central nuclei with coarse chromatin and prominent nucleoli. Mitotic activity is high. The tumour cells may be in solid sheets or cords and, typically, the intervening fibrous septa are infiltrated by mature lymphocytes. Occasionally a granulomatous reaction is seen.

In 3% of the cases there are scattered βhCG-reactive syncytial giant cells which are usually the source of elevated serum βhCG levels.[81] These do not constitute mixed germ cell tumours and are often associated with luteinized stromal cells within or adjacent to the tumour. The luteinized cells are believed to be the source of the excess oestrogen seen in some cases. All cases with raised serum βhCG, however, must be sampled extensively to exclude the presence of a choriocarcinoma or embryonal carcinoma component. Tumours showing marked pleomorphism and mitotic activity have been designated 'anaplastic' variants.[82] Dysgerminomas are positive for placental-like alkaline phosphatase (PLAP) and vimentin, may be positive for cytokeratin, and are negative for epithelial membrane antigen (EMA).[83] Syncytiotrophoblastic giant cells are positive for βhCG and cytokeratin.[81]

Differential diagnosis

Dysgerminomas can resemble other germ cell tumours, particularly yolk sac tumour and embryonal carcinoma. Ovarian clear cell carcinoma, lymphoma, metastatic melanoma, and poorly differentiated carcinoma are also potential mimics.

Clinical behaviour and prognosis

Disease confined to one ovary is treated by conservative surgery, and a surveillance policy has been advocated as in testicular germ cell tumours.[76] Chemotherapy is reserved for residual or recurrent disease, thereby minimizing the potential complications of infertility and leukaemias.[84,85] Although, like seminoma, dysgerminoma is particularly radiosensitive, radiotherapy is used only in the rare patients in whom chemotherapy has failed.[86] Prognosis is excellent and the only prognostic indicator is stage, with 5-year survival approaching 100% for stage I and 80–90% for higher stage and recurrent tumours.[84,85]

Yolk sac tumour

General features

These are primitive malignant germ cell tumours characterized by the presence of distinctive histological structures known as Schiller–Duval bodies. The resemblance of these to the yolk sac-derived 'endodermal sinuses' present in rat placentas was first noted by Teilum.[87] These account for 20% of all malignant germ cell tumours and are most frequent in the second and third decades of life. Typically, they present with abdominal pain of sudden onset, a large mass, and elevated serum AFP levels. Most patients are found to have involved retroperitoneal lymph nodes or peritoneal spread at laparotomy.[88]

Gross appearances

These tumours are unilateral, large masses with a smooth outer surface and a solid–cystic, soft, friable, yellow to grey cut surface. One-quarter of the cases have ruptured capsules. A dermoid cyst may be present in the same or contralateral ovary.

Microscopic findings

There is a wide variety of histological patterns, but the typical appearance is of a loose meshwork of channels lined by large cells with vacuolated cytoplasm and atypical, hyperchromatic nuclei. Schiller–Duval bodies are a characteristic feature: these are papillae with a fibrovascular core containing a central capillary, covered by a single layer of primitive columnar cells and lying within spaces lined by cuboidal, hobnail, or flattened cells. Eosinophilic hyaline droplets that are periodic acid–Schiff (PAS)-positive and diastase-resistant are commonly seen; these are composed predominantly of AFP. Macro- and microcystic areas occur in association with these usual patterns. There are three histological variants: polyvesicular–vitelline, hepatoid, and glandular.[1] Tumour cells from yolk sac tumour are always positive for AFP and cytokeratin, and negative for EMA.

Differential diagnosis

Yolk sac tumours can resemble a variety of primary and metastatic malignancies, the most common being clear cell carcinoma.

Clinical behaviour and prognosis

Treatment is with surgery and combination chemotherapy,[85,89,90] with survival of 70–90% of stage I and 30–50% higher-stage cases.[88,89] Prognosis depends on stage, with gross ascites and liver involvement being poor prognostic factors.[88] Histological patterns are not predictive of outcome, although the presence of a multiplicity of histological patterns has been reported to be associated with better prognosis.[91] Serum AFP levels are useful for monitoring treatment and detecting recurrences.[92,93]

Embryonal carcinoma

These tumours are rare in the ovary, as compared with the testis, accounting for approximately 3% of malignant germ cell tumours. They occur at a median age of 12 years and present as a pelvic mass. Approximately half of the patients have endocrine manifestations.[94,95] Serum levels of βhCG and AFP are raised[96] and the clinical presentation may mimic pregnancy.[94]

These are unilateral, large, solid masses with variegated cut surfaces due to foci of necrosis and haemorrhage as well as cystic areas. Extraovarian spread is grossly apparent in 40% of the cases.[94] Histologically these tumours are composed of large, primitive cells, which have abundant cytoplasm and distinct cell outlines. The nuclei are pleomorphic and vesicular with coarse chromatin and prominent nucleoli. The cells are arranged in solid sheets or papillary glandular structures. Syncytial giant cells are almost always present. Immunohistochemically there is consistent and strong positive staining for cytokeratin and PLAP, and negative staining for EMA. Staining for AFP may be positive. Syncytial giant cells are positive for βhCG. Treatment is with a combination of surgery and chemotherapy, with good results.[95,96]

Polyembryoma

These are exceptionally rare tumours, characterized by the formation of 'embryoid bodies', structures resembling developing embryos at various stages. Their presentation and behaviour is similar to that of other primitive germ cell tumours.[97]

Choriocarcinoma

Choriocarcinomas of the ovary can be of germ cell origin, a manifestation of primary or metastatic gestational trophoblastic disease or, very rarely and in old patients, of somatic surface epithelial origin.[98–100] It is not always possible to determine the origin in a given case, although the diagnosis of gestational choriocarcinoma has been made using DNA analysis.[101] Pure non-gestational ovarian choriocarcinomas are rare, accounting for less than 1% of primitive germ cell tumours. They are seen much more frequently as a component of mixed germ cell tumours.

Primary ovarian choriocarcinomas occur in children and young adults, presenting with a pelvic mass and hormonal symptoms due to raised βhCG levels. They are haemorrhagic and friable tumours composed of a mixture of cytotrophoblastic, intermediate trophoblastic, and syncytiotrophoblastic cells. They must be distinguished from germ cell tumours containing syncytiotrophoblastic giant cells and rare surface epithelial carcinomas with focal trophoblastic differentiation.

Treatment is with surgery and combination chemotherapy as for germ cell tumours (as opposed to the single-agent chemotherapy that is used for gestational choriocarcinoma).[98]

Mixed germ cell tumours

About 10% of germ cell tumours contain a mixture of two or, less commonly, more types of germ cell neoplasia.[74] In these tumours the components should be listed and quantified since the presence of a highly aggressive subtype occupying a large proportion of the tumour would be expected to dictate prognosis. In one large series, however, the presence and quantities of individual components did not correlate with survival in patients treated with postoperative chemotherapy.[102]

Teratoma

These tumours are composed of a variety of tissue types in which two or three of the germ layers are represented, i.e. endoderm, mesoderm, and ectoderm. The majority are mature cystic teratomas that are clinically benign. Malignant teratomas fall into two main categories: immature teratomas and dermoid cysts with secondary malignancies of adult type, accounting for 3% and 1%, respectively, of all teratomas. In addition, primary ovarian carcinoid tumours, classified as monodermal teratomas, are regarded as being of low malignant potential.

IMMATURE TERATOMA
General features
These are the third most common malignant germ cell tumours; they account for approximately 20% of primitive types and 1% of all ovarian cancers.[1] Patients who have had a dermoid cyst in the past, and those with multiple or ruptured dermoid cysts, may be at an increased risk of developing immature teratoma.[103,104]

These tumours occur in children and young adults, who present with symptoms of abdominal pain and a pelvic mass. Most patients have raised serum AFP levels, although these are not as high as with yolk sac tumour.[79,92] Other serum markers, such as βhCG, CA 125, CA 19–9, and carcino-embryonic antigen (CEA) may also be raised.[79] At presentation about one-third of the tumours show peritoneal deposits, lymph nodal metastases, and, rarely, evidence of haematogenous spread.[105]

Gross and microscopic appearances
Immature teratomas are large, solid encapsulated masses with a solid–cystic cut surface. Capsular rupture is present in half of the cases at laparotomy.

Usually the immature elements consist of primitive neuroectodermal derivatives forming rosettes and tubules. Immature mesenchymal tissues can also be seen. There is a variable admixture of other mature and immature tissues. The amount of immature neural or other tissues present forms the basis of histological grading systems.[105,106] Thorough sampling is therefore important. The peritoneal implants and nodal deposits are rarely composed of mature glial tissue alone (peritoneal gliomatosis).[107]

Clinical behaviour and prognosis
High cure rates are achieved by surgery and combination chemotherapy.[88,108,109] The presence of implants of exclusively mature tissue is not an indication for adjuvant chemotherapy, as the clinical course in such cases is usually benign.[109,110] Furthermore, such implants do not respond to chemotherapy and may even continue to grow.[109]

DERMOID CYSTS WITH SECONDARY MALIGNANT TUMOURS
Malignant transformation occurs in about 1–2% of mature teratomas. About 80% of the cases are squamous cell carcinomas, although a variety of other tumours have been reported.[111] They are usually seen in patients in their fifth or sixth decade of life.[112,113] Preoperative diagnosis is difficult. Features suggestive of squamous cell carcinoma arising in a dermoid cyst include: age over 45 years, size over 10 cm, elevated serum levels of squamous cell carcinoma antigen and CEA, and the presence of transmural extension and local invasion on magnetic resonance imaging (MRI).[114,115] The finding of an adherent cyst with foci of nodularity, necrosis, or haemorrhage should raise the suspicion of malignancy at laparotomy.[116] Treatment follows the general guidelines for ovarian cancer. Prognosis is generally poor and dependent on stage, histological grade, and other pathological features.[117]

MONODERMAL TERATOMA INCLUDING PRIMARY OVARIAN CARCINOID
Teratomas composed entirely or predominantly of a single tissue type include struma ovarii, various types of carcinoid tumour, and several rarer subtypes. Struma ovarii is a teratoma composed of thyroid tissue.[118] A small number of these may behave in a malignant fashion. Histological criteria for malignancy are not well defined, as most cases with foci of microscopically obvious papillary or follicular carcinoma follow a benign clinical course,[119] while occasional examples of struma ovarii showing extraovarian spread and local recurrence have been histologically benign. Thyroglobulin levels can be used to monitor completeness of removal, response to treatment, and detection of recurrences.[120] Iodine–131, alone or with recombinant human thyrotropin, has been used successfully for diagnosis and treatment of malignant struma ovarii.[121,122]

Carcinoids of the ovary occur in women in the third to sixth decades. Primary carcinoids are associated with other teratomatous elements in most cases, although carcinoid can be the sole component of an ovarian tumour. Ovarian carcinoids are most commonly of insular type, which resembles midgut carcinoids. One-third of these may be associated with clinical or laboratory evidence of carcinoid syndrome, even in the absence of liver metastases. Other variants are the trabecular type (resembling foregut or hindgut carcinoids), strumal carcinoid (a combination of trabecular or insular carcinoid with thyroid tissue), and goblet cell carcinoid (resembling equivalent tumours occurring in the appendix).[123-127] Distinction from metastatic carcinoid can be difficult in cases devoid of other teratomatous components. Metastases are usually from an ileal primary; these tend to be bilateral and multiple, are usually accompanied by peritoneal deposits, and have a poor prognosis.

The behaviour of primary ovarian carcinoids is generally that of ovarian cancers of low malignant potential, and conservative surgery is the treatment of choice for tumours confined to the ovaries. Urinary levels of 5-hydroxyindole acetic acid (5-HIAA) can be useful in the follow-up of cases associated with carcinoid syndrome.

Mixed germ cell–sex cord–stromal tumours

Tumours composed of a mixture of germ cell and sex cord-stromal derivatives fall into two subcategories: gonadoblastoma and a group of unclassified tumours.

Gonadoblastoma occurs almost exclusively in cases of pure or mixed gonadal dysgenesis with a karyotype containing Y-chromosome material.[1,128] These tumours are benign in pure form but contain an invasive germ cell tumour, usually dysgerminoma, in about 60% of cases. They therefore must be regarded as potential or *in situ* malignancies and treated with bilateral gonadectomy.[129,130]

The unclassified category consists of mixed germ cell–sex cord–stromal tumours that do not have the distinctive histological appearances of gonadoblastoma. These are extremely rare and occur in children with a normal karyotype. The behaviour is clinically benign.[1]

Miscellaneous primary ovarian malignancies

Small cell carcinoma of hypercalcaemic type

This is an undifferentiated carcinoma occurring in patients within a wide age range, with a mean age of 24 years at diagnosis. About two-thirds of the patients have associated hypercalcaemia.[131,132]

The tumours are solid, lobulated, fleshy, cream-coloured masses, about half of which are seen to show extraovarian involvement at laparotomy. Histologically they consist of sheets of uniform small cells with scanty cytoplasm and round or oval, dark nuclei with single small nucleoli. Larger cells may also be present. Mitotic activity is high. The differential diagnosis includes granulosa cell tumour and various other tumours composed of small, round cells that may involve the ovary. Tumour cells are invariably positive for vimentin, cytokeratin, and epithelial membrane antigen, and these, as well as other markers, may facilitate diagnosis. The presence of p53 protein has been demonstrated, suggesting a possible role of p53 gene mutation in pathogenesis.[68] Tumour cells have invariably been found to be diploid on DNA analysis, and it has been suggested that the diagnosis of small cell

carcinoma of hypercalcaemic type should be questioned in aneuploid tumours.[133]

The prognosis is extremely poor. Only one-third of stage IA patients were disease-free at an average follow-up of 5.7 years. The majority of these patients were over 30 years, had normal calcium levels preoperatively, and had tumours less than 10 cm in diameter. Treatment that included bilateral oophorectomy and postoperative radiotherapy was also associated with a favourable outcome in stage IA patients. Most higher-stage patients either have progressive disease or die from disease within 2 years.[132]

Small cell carcinoma of pulmonary type

This tumour is identical to small cell lung cancer and is rare as an ovarian primary. Metastasis from the lung has to be excluded. The undifferentiated cells in this tumour show immunohistochemical features of neuroendocrine differentiation, which distinguishes it from the hypercalcaemic type of small cell carcinoma. Prognosis is poor.[134]

Sarcomas

Many malignant stromal tumours have been reported to occur in the ovary, the most common being fibrosarcomas (see above) and leiomyosarcomas. These may arise *de novo* from ovarian stroma or within mixed mesodermal tumours, teratomas, or sex cord–stromal tumours with heterologous elements. The clinical presentation is usually with a rapidly enlarging pelvic mass. Diagnostic criteria for extraovarian equivalents generally apply. Criteria for defining malignancy in smooth muscle tumours are not as well established as for uterine tumours. Ovarian sarcomas are usually aggressive and associated with poor survival.[55]

Hepatoid carcinoma

This rare aggressive tumour, identical histologically to hepatocellular carcinoma, occurs in postmenopausal women. It must be distinguished from metastasis from a liver primary and hepatoid yolk sac tumour. Tumour cells are positive for AFP.[135,136]

References

1. Scully, R.E., Young, R.H., and Clement, P.B. (1998). *Tumours of the ovary, maldeveloped gonads, Fallopian tube and broad ligament*, (3rd edn).
2. Gee, D.C., and Russell, P. (1981). The pathological assessment of ovarian neoplasms. IV. The sex cord stromal tumors. *Pathology*, **13**, 235–255.
3. Young, R.H., and Scully, R.E. (1988). Ovarian sex cord-stromal tumors: problems in differential diagnosis. *Path. Ann.*, **23** (pt 1), 237–296.
4. Fox, H., Agrawal, K., and Langley, F.A. (1975). A clinicopathologic study of 92 cases of granulosa cell tumor of the ovary with special reference to the factors influencing prognosis. *Cancer*, **35**, 231–41.
5. Evans, A.T., Gaffey, T.A., Malkasian, G.D.J., and Annegers, J.F. (1980). Clinicopathologic review of 118 granulosa and 82 theca cell tumors. *Obstet. Gynecol.*, **55**, 231–8.
6. Gusberg, S.B. and Kardon, P. (1971). Proliferative endometrial response to theca-granulosa cell tumors. *Am. J. Obstet. Gynecol.*, **111**, 633–3.
7. Nakashima, N., Young, R.H., and Scully, R.E. (1984). Androgenic granulosa cell tumors of the ovary. A clinicopathologic analysis of 17 cases and review of the literature. *Arch. Pathol. Lab. Med.*, **108**, 786–91.

8. Jobling, T., Mamers, P., Healy, D.L. *et al.* (1994). A prospective study of inhibin in granulosa cell tumors of the ovary. *Gynecol. Oncol.*, **55**, 285–9.

9. Fuller, P.J., Chu, S., Jobling, T., Mamers, P., Healy, D.L., and Burger, H.G. (1999). Inhibin subunit gene expression in ovarian cancer. *Gynecol.Oncol.*, **73**, 273–9.

10. Yamashita *et al.* 1997.

11. Lane, A.H., Lee, M.M., Fuller, A.F.J., Kehas, D.J., Donahoe, P.K., and MacLaughlin, D.T. (1999). Diagnostic utility of Mullerian inhibiting substance determination in patients with primary and recurrent granulosa cell tumors. *Gynecol. Oncol.*, **73**, 51–5.

12. Rey, R.A., Lhomme, C., Marcillac, I. *et al.* (1996). Antimullerian hormone as a serum marker of granulosa cell tumorsof the ovary: comparative study with serum alpha-inhibin and estradiol. *Am. J. Obstet. Gynecol.*, **174**, 958–65.

13. Lindgren, V., Waggoner, S., and Rotmensch, J. (1996). Monosomy 22 in two ovarian granulosa cell tumors. *Cancer Genet. Cytogenet.*, **89**, 93–7.

14. Halperin, D., Visscher, D.W., Wallis, T., and Lawrence, W.D. (1995). Evaluation of chromosome 12 copy number in ovarian granulosa cell tumors using interphase cytogenetics. *Int. J. Gynecol. Pathol.*, **14**, 319–23.

15. Van, d.B., I., Dal Cin, P., De Groef, K., Michielssen, P., and Van den Berghe, H. (1999). Monosomy 22 and trisomy 14 may be early events in the tumorigenesis of adult granulosa cell tumor. *Cancer Genet. Cytogenet.*, **112**, 46–8.

16. Furger, C., Fiddes, R.J., Quinn, D.I., Bova, R.J., Daly, R.J., and Sutherland, R.L. (1998). Granulosa cell tumors express erbB4 and are sensitive to the cytotoxic action of heregulin-beta2/PE40. *Cancer Res.*, **58**, 1773–8.

17. Stenwig, J.T., Hazekamp, J.T., and Beecham, J.B. (1979). Granulosa cell tumors of the ovary. A clinicopathological study of 118 cases with long-term follow-up. *Gynecol. Oncol.*, **7**, 136–52.

18. Young, R.H., Dudley, A.G., and Scully, R.E. (1984). Granulosa cell, Sertoli–Leydig cell, and unclassified sex cord–stromal tumors associated with pregnancy: a clinicopathological analysis of thirty-six cases. *Gynecol. Oncol.*, **18**, 181–205.

19. Young, R.H., Oliva, E., and Scully, R.E. (1994). Luteinized adult granulosa cell tumors of the ovary: a report of four cases. *Int. J. Gynecol. Pathol.*, **13**, 302–10.

20. Young, R.H. and Scully, R.E. (1983). Ovarian sex cord–stromal tumors with bizarre nuclei: a clinicopathologic analysis of 17 cases. *Int. J. Gynecol. Pathol.*, **1**, 325–35.

21. Costa, M.J., DeRose, P.B., Roth, L.M., Brescia, R.J., Zaloudek, C.J., and Cohen, C. (1994). Immunohistochemical phenotype of ovarian granulosa cell tumors: absence of epithelial membrane antigen has diagnostic value. *Hum. Pathol.*, **25**, 60–6.

22. Otis, C.N., Powell, J.L., Barbuto, D., and Carcangiu, M.L. (1992). Intermediate filamentous proteins in adult granulosa cell tumors. An immunohistochemical study of 25 cases. *Am. J. Surg. Pathol.*, **16**, 962–8.

23. Rishi, M., Howard, L.N., Bratthauer, G.L., and Tavassoli, F.A. (1997). Use of monoclonal antibody against human inhibin as a marker for sex cord–stromal tumors of the ovary. *Am. J. Surg. Pathol.*, **21**, 583–9.

24. Hildebrandt, R.H., Rouse, R.V., and Longacre, T.A. (1997). Value of inhibin in the identification of granulosa cell tumors of the ovary. *Hum. Pathol.*, **28**, 1387–95.

25. Horny, H.P., Marx, L., Krober, S., Luttges, J., Kaiserling, E., and Dietl, J. (1999). Granulosa cell tumor of the ovary. Immunohistochemical evidence of low proliferative activity and virtual absence of mutation of the p53 tumor-suppressor gene. *Gynecol. Obstet. Invest.*, **47**, 133–8.

26. Kietlinska, Z., Pietrzak, K., and Drabik, M. (1993). The management of granulosa-cell tumors of the ovary based on long-term follow up. *Europ. J. Gynaecol. Oncol.*, **14** (suppl.), 118–27.

27. Hines, J.F., Khalifa, M.A., Moore, J.L., Fine, K.P., Lage, J.M., and Barnes, W.A. (1996). Recurrent granulosa cell tumor of the ovary 37 years after initial diagnosis: a case report and review of the literature. *Gynecol. Oncol.*, **60**, 484–8.

28. Segal, R., DePetrillo, A.D., and Thomas, G. (1995). Clinical review of adult granulosa cell tumors of the ovary. *Gynecol. Oncol.*, **56**, 338–44.

29. Gershenson, D.M., Morris, M., Burke, T.W., Levenback, C., Matthews, C.M., and Wharton, J.T. (1996). Treatment of poor-prognosis sex cord–stromal tumors of the ovary with the combination of bleomycin, etoposide, and cisplatin. *Obstet. Gynecol.*, **87**, 527–31.

30. Savage, P., Constenla, D., Fisher, C. *et al.* (1998). Granulosa cell tumours of the ovary: demographics, survival and the management of advanced disease. *Clin. Oncol.*, **10**, 242–5.

31. Homesley, H.D., Bundy, B.N., Hurteau, J.A., and Roth, L.M. (1999). Bleomycin, etoposide, and cisplatin combination therapy of ovarian granulosa cell tumors and other stromal malignancies: A Gynecologic Oncology Group study [see comments]. *Gynecol. Oncol.* **72**, 131–7.

32. Lee, I.W., Levin, W., Chapman, W., Goldberg, R.E., Murphy, K.J., and Milosevic, M. (1999). Radiotherapy for the treatment of metastatic granulosa cell tumor in the mediastinum: a case report. *Gynecol. Oncol.*, **73**, 455–60.

33. Wolf, J.K., Mullen, J., Eifel, P.J., Burke, T.W., Levenback, C., and Gershenson, D.M. (1999). Radiation treatment of advanced or recurrent granulosa cell tumor of the ovary. *Gynecol. Oncol.*, **73**, 35–41.

34. Miller, B.E., Barron, B.A., Wan, J.Y., Delmore, J.E., Silva, E.G., and Gershenson, D.M. (1997). Prognostic factors in adult granulosa cell tumor of the ovary. *Cancer*, **79**, 1951–5.

35. Fontanelli, R., Stefanon, B., Raspagliesi, F. *et al.* (1998). Adult granulosa cell tumor of the ovary: a clinico pathologic study of 35 cases. *Tumori*, **84**, 60–4.

36. Cronje, H.S., Niemand, I., Bam, R.H., and Woodruff, J.D. (1999). Review of the granulosa–theca cell tumors from the emil Novak ovarian tumor registry. *Am. J. Obstet. Gynecol.*, **180**, 323–7.

37. Malmstrom, H., Hogberg, T., Risberg, B., and Simonsen, E. (1994). Granulosa cell tumors of the ovary: prognostic factors and outcome. *Gynecol. Oncol.*, **52**, 50–5.

38. Haba, R., Miki, H., Kobayashi, S., and Ohmori, M. (1993). Combined analysis of flow cytometry and morphometry of ovarian granulosa cell tumor. *Cancer*, **72**, 3258–62.

39. Evans, M.P., Webb, M.J., Gaffey, T.A., Katzmann, J.A., Suman, V.J., and Hu, T.C. (1995). DNA ploidy of ovarian granulosa cell tumors. Lack of correlation between DNA index or proliferative index and outcome in 40 patients. *Cancer*, **75**, 2295–8.

40. Roush, G.R., el-Naggar, A.K., and Abdul-Karim, F.W.(1995). Granulosa cell tumor of ovary: a clinicopathologic and flow cytometric DNA analysis. *Gynecol. Oncol.*, **56**, 430–4.

41. Zaloudek, C. and Norris, H.J. (1982). Granulosa tumors of the ovary in children: a clinical and pathologic study of 32 cases. *Am. J. Surg. Pathol.*, **6**, 503–12.

42. Young, R.H., Dickersin, G.R., and Scully, R.E. (1984). Juvenile granulosa cell tumor of the ovary. A clinicopathological analysis of 125 cases. *Am. J. Surg. Pathol.*, **8**, 575–96.

43. Vassal, G., Flamant, F., Caillaud, J.M., Demeocq, F., Nihoul-Fekete, C., and Lemerle, J. (1988). Juvenile granulosa cell tumor of the ovary in children: a clinical study of 15 cases. *J. Clin. Oncol.*, **6**, 990–5.

44. Schofield, D.E. and Fletcher, J.A. (1992). Trisomy 12 in pediatric granulosa–stromal cell tumors. Demonstration by a modified method of fluorescence in situ hybridization on paraffin-embedded material. *Am. J. Pathol.*, **141**, 1265–9.

45. Bouffet, E., Basset, T., Chetail, N. *et al.* (1997). Juvenile granulosa cell tumor of the ovary in infants: a clinicopathologic study of three cases and review of the literature. *J. Pediatr. Surg.*, **32**, 762–5.

46. Cronje, H.S., Niemand, I., Bam, R.H., and Woodruff, J.D. (1998). Granulosa and theca cell tumors in children: a report of 17 cases and literature review. *Obstet. Gynecol. Surv.*, **53**, 240–7.

47. Plantaz, D., Flamant, F., Vassal, G. *et al.* (1992). Granulosa cell tumors of the ovary in children and adolescents. Multicenter retrospective study in 40 patients aged 7 months to 22 years [in French]. *Arch. Franc. Pediat.* **49**, 793–8.

48. Powell, J.L., Johnson, N.A., Bailey, C.L., and Otis, C.N. (1993). Management of advanced juvenile granulosa cell tumor of the ovary. *Gynecol.Oncol.*, **48**, 119–23.

49. Powell, J.L. and Otis, C.N. (1997). Management of advanced juvenile granulosa cell tumor of the ovary. *Gynecol. Oncol.*, **64**, 282–4.

50. Calaminus, G., Wessalowski, R., Harms, D., and Gobel, U. (1997). Juvenile granulosa cell tumors of the ovary in children and adolescents: results from 33 patients registered in a prospective cooperative study. *Gynecol. Oncol.*, **65**, 447–52.

51. Swanson, S.A., Norris, H.J., Kelsten, M.L., and Wheeler, J.E. (1990). DNA content of juvenile granulosa tumors determined by flow cytometry. *Int. J. Gynecol. Pathol.*, **9**, 101–9.

52. Jacoby, A.F., Young, R.H., Colvin, R.B., *et al.* (1992). DNA content in juvenile granulosa cell tumors of the ovary: a study of early- and advanced-stage disease. *Gynecol. Oncol.*, **46**, 97–103.

53. Azoury, R.S. and Woodruff, J.D. (1971). Primary ovarian sarcomas. Report of 43 cases from the Emil Novak Ovarian Tumor Registry. *Obstet. Gynecol.*, **37**, 920–41.

54. Miles, P.A., Kiley, K.C., and Mena, H. (1985). Giant fibrosarcoma of the ovary. *Int. J. Gynecol. Pathol.*, **4**, 83–7.

55. Anderson, B., Turner, D.A., and Benda, J. (1987). Ovarian sarcoma. *Gynecol. Oncol.*, **26**, 183–92.

56. Prat, J. and Scully, R.E. (1981). Cellular fibromas and fibrosarcomas of the ovary: a comparative clinicopathologic analysis of seventeen cases. *Cancer*, **47**, 2663–70.

57. McCluggage, W.G., Sloan, J.M., Boyle, D.D., and Toner, P.G. (1998). Malignant fibrothecomatous tumour of the ovary: diagnostic value of anti-inhibin immunostaining. *J. Clin. Pathol.*, **51**, 868–71.

58. Tsuji, T., Kawauchi, S., Utsunomiya, T., Nagata, Y., and Tsuneyoshi, M. (1997). Fibrosarcoma versus cellular fibroma of the ovary: a comparative study of their proliferative activity and chromosome aberrations using MIB–1 immunostaining, DNA flow cytometry, and fluorescence in situ hybridization [see comments]. *Am. J. Surg. Pathol.*, **21**, 52–9.

59. Young, R.H. and Scully, R.E. (1985). Ovarian Sertoli–Leydig cell tumors. A clinicopathological analysis of 207 cases. *Am. J. Surg. Pathol.*, **9**, 543–69.

60. Young, R.H. and Scully, R.E. (1983). Ovarian Sertoli–Leydig cell tumors with a retiform pattern: a problem in histopathologic diagnosis. A report of 25 cases. *Am. J. Surg. Pathol.*, **7**, 755–71.

61. Zaloudek, C. and Norris, H.J. (1984). Sertoli–Leydig tumors of the ovary. A clinicopathologic study of 64 intermediate and poorly differentiated neoplasms. *Am. J. Surg. Pathol.*, **8**, 405–18.

62. Young, R.H., Prat, J., and Scully, R.E. (1982). Ovarian Sertoli–Leydig cell tumors with heterologous elements. I. Gastrointestinal epithelium and carcinoid: a clinicopathologic analysis of thirty-six cases. *Cancer*, **50**, 2448–56.

63. Prat, J., Young, R.H., and Scully, R.E. (1982). Ovarian Sertoli–Leydig cell tumors with heterologous elements. II. Cartilage and skeletal muscle: a clinicopathologic analysis of twelve cases. *Cancer*, **50**, 2465–75.

64. Zheng, W., Sung, C.J., Hanna, I. *et al.* (1997). Alpha and beta subunits of inhibin/activin as sex cord-stromal differentiation markers. *Int. J. Gynecol. Pathol.*, **16**, 263–71.

65. Young, R.H., Welch, W.R., Dickersin, G.R., and Scully, R.E. (1982). Ovarian sex cord tumor with annular tubules: review of 74 cases including 27 with Peutz–Jeghers syndrome and four with adenoma malignum of the cervix. *Cancer*, **50**, 1384–1402.

66. Puls, L.E., Hamous, J., Morrow, M.S., Schneyer, A., MacLaughlin, D.T., and Castracane, V.D. (1994). Recurrent ovarian sex cord tumor with annular tubules: tumor marker and chemotherapy experience. *Gynecol. Oncol.*, **54**, 396–401.

67. Anderson, M.C. and Rees, D.A. (1975). Gynandroblastoma of the ovary. *Br. J. Obstet. Gynaecol.*, **82**, 68–73.

68. Seidman, J.D. (1995). Small cell carcinoma of the ovary of the hypercalcemic type: p53 protein accumulation and clinicopathologic features. *Gynecol. Oncol.*, **59**, 283–7.

69. Seidman, J.D. (1996). Unclassified ovarian gonadal stromal tumors. A clinicopathologic study of 32 cases. *Am. J. Surg. Pathol.*, **20**, 699–706.

70. Hayes, M.C. and Scully, R.E. (1987). Ovarian steroid cell tumors (not otherwise specified). A clinicopathological analysis of 63 cases. *Am. J. Surg. Pathol.*, **11**, 835–45.

71. Young, R.H. and Scully, R.E. (1987). Ovarian steroid cell tumors associated with Cushing's syndrome: a report of three cases. *Int. J. Gynecol. Pathol.*, **6**, 40–8.

72. Norris, H.J. and Jensen, R.D. (1972). Relative frequency of ovarian neoplasms in children and adolescents. *Cancer*, **30**, 713–19.

73. Lack, E.E., Young, R.H., and Scully, R.E. (1992). Pathology of ovarian neoplasms in childhood and adolescence. *Pathol. Annu.*, **27** (Pt 2), 281–356.

74. Kurman, R.J. and Norris, H.J. (1976). Malignant mixed germ cell tumors of the ovary. A clinical and pathologic analysis of 30 cases. *Obstet. Gynecol.*, **48**, 579–89.

75. Peccatori, F., Bonazzi, C., Chiari, S., Landoni, F., Colombo, N., and Mangioni, C. (1995). Surgical management of malignant ovarian germ-cell tumors: 10 years' experience of 129 patients. *Obstet. Gynecol.*, **86**, 367–72.

76. Dark, G.G., Bower, M., Newlands, E.S., Paradinas, F., and Rustin, G.J. (1997). Surveillance policy for stage I ovarian germ cell tumors. *J. Clin. Oncol.*, **15**, 620–4.

77. Culine, S., Lhomme, C., Kattan, J. *et al.* (1995). Cisplatin-based chemotherapy in dysgerminoma of the ovary: thirteen-year experience at the Institut Gustave Roussy. *Gynecol. Oncol.*, **58**, 344–8.

78. Gordon, A., Lipton, D., and Woodruff, J.D. (1981). Dysgerminoma: a review of 158 cases from the Emil Novak Ovarian Tumor Registry. *Obstet. Gynecol.*, **58**, 497–504.

79. Kawai, M., Kano, T., Kikkawa, F. *et al.* (1992). Seven tumor markers in benign and malignant germ cell tumors of the ovary. *Gynecol. Oncol.*, **45**, 248–53.

80. Pressley, R.H., Muntz, H.G., Falkenberry, S., and Rice, L.W. (1992). Serum lactic dehydrogenase as a tumor marker in dysgerminoma. *Gynecol. Oncol.*, **44**, 281–3.

81. Zaloudek, C.J., Tavassoli, F.A., and Norris, H.J. (1981). Dysgerminoma with syncytiotrophoblastic giant cells. A histologically and clinically distinctive subtype of dysgerminoma. *Am. J. Surg. Pathol.*, **5**, 361–7.

82. Gillespie, J.J. and Arnold, L.K. (1978). Anaplastic dysgerminoma. *Cancer*, **42**, 1886–9.

83. Lifschitz-Mercer, B., Walt, H., Kushnir, I. *et al.* (1995). Differentiation potential of ovarian dysgerminoma: an immunohistochemical study of 15 cases. *Hum. Pathol.*, **26**, 62–6.

84. Thomas, G.M., Dembo, A.J., Hacker, N.F., and Depetrillo, A.D. (1987). Current therapy for dysgerminoma of the ovary. *Obstet. Gynecol.*, **70**, 268–75.

85. Schwartz, P.E., Chambers, S.K., Chambers, J.T., Kohorn, E., and McIntosh, S. (1992). Ovarian germ cell malignancies: the Yale University experience. *Gynecol. Oncol.*, **45**, 26–31.

86. Gershenson, D.M. (1993). Update on malignant ovarian germ cell tumors. *Cancer*, **71**, 1581–90.

87. Teilum, G. (1959). Endodermal sinus tumours of the ovary and testis. Comparative morphogenesis of the so-called mesonephroma ovarii (Schiller) and extraembryonic (yolk sac-allantoic) structures of the rat's placenta. *Cancer*, **12**, 1092–105.

88. Kawai, M., Kano, T., Furuhashi, Y. *et al.* (1991). Prognostic factors in yolk sac tumors of the ovary. A clinicopathologic analysis of 29 cases. *Cancer*, **67**, 184–92.

89. Gershenson, D.M., Del Junco, G., Herson, J., and Rutledge, F.N. (1983). Endodermal sinus tumor of the ovary: the M.D. Anderson experience. *Obstet. Gynecol.*, **61**, 194–202.

90. Kawai, M., Kano, T., Furuhashi, Y. *et al.* (1991). Immature teratoma of the ovary. *Gynecol. Oncol.*, **40**, 133–7.

91. Sasaki, H., Furusato, M., Teshima, S. *et al.* (1994). Prognostic significance of histopathological subtypes in stage I pure yolk sac tumour of the ovary. *Br. J. Cancer*, **69**, 529–36.

92. Kawai, M., Furuhashi, Y., Kano, T. *et al.* (1990). Alpha-fetoprotein in malignant germ cell tumors of the ovary. *Gynecol. Oncol.*, **39**, 160–6.

93. Chow, S.N., Yang, J.H., Lin, Y.H., *et al.* (1996). Malignant ovarian germ cell tumors. *Int. J. Gynaecol. Obstet.*, **53**, 151–8.

94. Kurman, R.J. and Norris, H.J. (1976). Embryonal carcinoma of the ovary: a clinicopathologic entity distinct from endodermal sinus tumor resembling embryonal carcinoma of the adult testis. *Cancer,* **38**, 2420–33.

95. Nakakuma, K., Tashiro, S., Uemura, K., and Takayama, K. (1983). Alpha-fetoprotein and human chorionic gonadotropin in embryonal carcinoma of the ovary. An 8-year survival case. *Cancer*, **52**, 1470–2.

96. Ueda, G., Abe, Y., Yoshida, M., and Fujiwara, T. (1990). Embryonal carcinoma of the ovary: a six-year survival. *Int. J. Gynaecol. Obstet.*, **31**, 287–92.

97. Nakashima, N., Murakami, S., Fukatsu, T. *et al.* (1988). Characteristics of 'embryoid body' in human gonadal germ cell tumors. *Hum. Pathol.*, **19**, 1144–54.

98. Jacobs, A.J., Newland, J.R., and Green, R.K. (1982). Pure choriocarcinoma of the ovary. *Obstet. Gynecol. Surv.*, **37**, 603–9.

99. Axe, S.R., Klein, V.R., and Woodruff, J.D. (1985). Choriocarcinoma of the ovary. *Obstet. Gynecol.*, **66**, 111–14.

100. Oliva, E., Andrada, E., Pezzica, F., and Prat, J. (1993). Ovarian carcinomas with choriocarcinomatous differentiation. *Cancer*, **72**, 2441–6.

101. Lorigan, P.C., Grierson, A.J., Goepel, J.R., Coleman, R.E., and Goyns, M.H. (1996). Gestational choriocarcinoma of the ovary diagnosed by analysis of tumour DNA. *Cancer Lett.*, **104**, 27–30.

102. Gershenson, D.M., Del Junco, G., Copeland, L.J., and Rutledge, F.N. (1984). Mixed germ cell tumors of the ovary. *Obstet. Gynecol.*, **64**, 200–6.

103. Yanai-Inbar, I. and Scully, R.E. (1987). Relation of ovarian dermoid cysts and immature teratomas: an analysis of 350 cases of immature teratoma and 10 cases of dermoid cyst with microscopic foci of immature tissue. *Int. J. Gynecol. Pathol.*, **6**, 203–12.

104. Anteby, E.Y., Ron, M., Revel, A., Shimonovitz, S., Ariel, I., and Hurwitz, A. (1994). Germ cell tumors of the ovary arising after dermoid cyst resection: a long-term follow-up study. *Obstet. Gynecol.*, **83**, 605–8.

105. Norris, H.J., Zirkin, H.J., and Benson, W.L. (1976). Immature (malignant) teratoma of the ovary: a clinical and pathologic study of 58 cases. *Cancer*, **37**, 2359–72.

106. O'Connor, D.M. and Norris, H.J. (1994). The influence of grade on the outcome of stage I ovarian immature (malignant) teratomas and the reproducibility of grading. *Int. J. Gynecol. Pathol.*, **13**, 283–9.

107. Calder, C.J., Light, A.M., and Rollason, T.P. (1994). Immature ovarian teratoma with mature peritoneal metastatic deposits showing glial, epithelial, and endometrioid differentiation: a case report and review of the literature. *Int. J. Gynecol. Pathol.*, **13**, 279–82.

108. Koulos, J.P., Hoffman, J.S., and Steinhoff, M.M.(1989). Immature teratoma of the ovary. *Gynecol. Oncol.*, **34**, 46–9.

109. Bonazzi, C., Peccatori, F., Colombo, N., Lucchini, V., Cantu, M.G., and Mangioni, C. (1994). Pure ovarian immature teratoma, a unique and curable disease: 10 years' experience of 32 prospectively treated patients. *Obstet. Gynecol.*, **84**, 598–604.

110. Robboy, S.J. and Scully, R.E. (1970). Ovarian teratoma with glial implants on the peritoneum. An analysis of 12 cases. *Hum. Pathol.*, **1**, 643–53.

111. Comerci, J.T.J., Licciardi, F., Bergh, P.A., Gregori, C., and Breen, J.L. (1994). Mature cystic teratoma: a clinicopathologic evaluation of 517 cases and review of the literature. *Obstet. Gynecol.*, **84**, 22–8.

112. Pins, M.R., Young, R.H., Daly, W.J., and Scully, R.E. (1996). Primary squamous cell carcinoma of the ovary. Report of 37 cases. *Am. J. Surg. Pathol.*, **20**, 823–33.

113. Tseng, C.J., Chou, H.H., Huang, K.G. *et al.* (1996). Squamous cell carcinoma arising in mature cystic teratoma of the ovary. *Gynecol. Oncol.*, **63**, 364–70.

114. Kikkawa, F., Nawa, A., Tamakoshi, K. *et al.* (1998). Diagnosis of squamous cell carcinoma arising from mature cystic teratoma of the ovary. *Cancer*, **82**, 2249–55.

115. Kido, A., Togashi, K., Konishi, I. *et al.* (1999). Dermoid cysts of the ovary with malignant transformation: MR appearance *Am. J. Roentgenol.*, **172**, 445–9.

116. Curling, O.M., Potsides, P.N., and Hudson, C.N. (1979). Malignant change in benign cystic teratoma of the ovary. *Br. J. Obstet. Gynaecol.*, **86**, 399–402.

117. Kikkawa, F., Ishikawa, H., Tamakoshi, K., Nawa, A., Suganuma, N., and Tomoda, Y. (1997). Squamous cell carcinoma arising from mature cystic teratoma of the ovary: a clinicopathologic analysis. *Obstet. Gynecol.*, **89**, 1017–22.

118. Hasleton, P.S., Kelehan, P., Whittaker, J.S., Burslem, R.W., and Turner, L. (1978). Benign and malignant struma ovarii. *Arch. Pathol. Lab. Med.*, **102**, 180–4.

119. Devaney, K., Snyder, R., Norris, H.J., and Tavassoli, F.A. (1993). Proliferative and histologically malignant struma ovarii: a clinicopathologic study of 54 cases. *Int. J. Gynecol. Pathol.*, **12**, 333–43.

120. Rose, P.G., Arafah, B., and Abdul-Karim, F.W. (1998). Malignant struma ovarii: recurrence and response to treatment monitored by thyroglobulin levels. *Gynecol. Oncol.*, **70**, 425–7.

121. Brenner, W., Bohuslavizki, K.H., Wolf, H., Sippel, C., Clausen, M., and Henze, E. Radiotherapy with iodine–131 in recurrent malignant struma ovarii [see comments]. *Eur. J. Nucl. Med.*, **23**, 91–4.

122. Rotman-Pikielny, P., Reynolds, J.C., Barker, W.C., Yen, P.M., Skarulis, M.C., and Sarlis, N.J. (2000). Recombinant human thyrotropin for the diagnosis and treatment of a highly functional metastatic struma ovarii. *J. Clin. Endocrinol. Metab.*, **85**, 237–44.

123. Robboy, S.J., Scully, R.E., and Norris, H.J. (1977). Primary trabecular carcinoid of the ovary. *Obstet. Gynecol.*, **49**, 202–7.

124. Robboy, S.J. and Scully, R.E. (1980). Strumal carcinoid of the ovary: an analysis of 50 cases of a distinctive tumor composed of thyroid tissue and carcinoid. *Cancer*, **46**, 2019–34.

125. Robboy, S.J. (1984). Insular carcinoid of ovary associated with malignant mucinous tumors. *Cancer*, **54**, 2273–6.

126. Talerman, A. (1984). Carcinoid tumors of the ovary. *J. Cancer Res. Clin. Oncol.*, **107**, 125–35.

127. Alenghat, E., Okagaki, T., and Talerman, A. (1986). Primary mucinous carcinoid tumor of the ovary. *Cancer*, **58**, 777–83.

128. Mendes, J.R., Strufaldi, M.W., Delcelo, R. *et al.* (1999). Y-chromosome identification by PCR and gonadal histopathology in Turner's syndrome without overt Y-mosaicism. *Clin. Endocrinol.*, **50**, 19–26.

129. Scully, R.E. (1970). Gonadoblastoma. A review of 74 cases. *Cancer*, **25**, 1340–56.

130. Lo, K.W., Lam, S.K., Cheung, T.H., Wong, S.P., Chang, A., and Chow, J.H. (1996). Gonadoblastoma in patient with Turner's syndrome. *J. Obstet. Gynaecol. Res.*, **22**, 35–41.

131. Dickersin, G.R., Kline, I.W., and Scully, R.E. (1982). Small cell carcinoma of the ovary with hypercalcemia: a report of eleven cases. *Cancer*, **49**, 188–97.

132. Young, R.H., Oliva, E., and Scully, R.E. (1994). Small cell carcinoma of the ovary, hypercalcemic type. A clinicopathological analysis of 150 cases. *Am. J. Surg. Pathol.*, **18**, 1102–116.

133. Buono, J.P., Dechelotte, P., Glowaczower, E. *et al.* (1995). Ploidy analysis in a case of ovarian small cell carcinoma with hypercalcemia [in French]. *Ann. Pathol.*, **15**, 134–7.

134. Eichhorn, J.H., Young, R.H., and Scully, R.E. (1992). Primary ovarian small cell carcinoma of pulmonary type. A clinicopathologic, immunohistologic, and flow cytometric analysis of 11 cases. *Am. J. Surg. Pathol.*, **16**, 926–38.

135. Ishikura, H. and Scully, R.E. (1987). Hepatoid carcinoma of the ovary. A newly described tumor. *Cancer*, **60**, 2775–84.

136. Matsuta, M., Ishikura, H., Murakami, K., Kagabu, T., and Nishiya, I. (1991). Hepatoid carcinoma of the ovary: a case report. *Int. J. Gynecol. Pathol.*, **10**, 302–10.

12. Metastases in the ovary

Naveena Singh and David Lowe

Introduction

Tumours characteristically metastasize to the ovary late in the natural history of the primary malignancy. Metastatic tumour may be misdiagnosed, at least for a time until the parent tumour declares itself, as a primary ovarian tumour.[1,2] Women with metastatic ovarian disease are generally younger than women with primary ovarian cancer: the average age of women with a Krukenberg tumour is 45 years.[3] This is attributed to the fact that premenopausally the ovary is well vascularized and therefore likely to receive more tumour-laden blood, and also to the prevalence of breast and gastric cancer in women below the age of the menopause.

The routes of metastatic spread include direct spread from carcinoma of the Fallopian tube or colorectum; lymphatic and haematogenous spread; distant transcoelomic spread from the stomach or pancreaticobiliary system; transtubal spread of endometrial or tubal carcinoma with local transcoelomic spread to the surface of the ovary; and conceivably iatrogenic spread by implantation at laparoscopy or laparotomy.

Not all women with metastatic carcinoma in the ovary have a Krukenberg tumour as defined below. In 1896, Krukenberg[4] described a primary fibrosarcoma of the ovary that had mucinous elements. From the illustrations in his paper, it appears that he mistook the ovarian stromal reaction to the presence of metastatic signet ring cells for a primary ovarian neoplasm of connective tissue origin, a not unreasonable assumption as metastatic tumour cells may produce mitogenic agents that stimulate the ovarian stroma.[5] The term 'Krukenberg tumour' is best reserved for ovarian adenocarcinoma that has pleomorphic signet ring cells containing mucin surrounded by an excessive, reactive proliferation of ovarian stromal cells (irrespective of the site of the primary tumour, emphasizing the point that a 'true' Krukenberg tumour need not arise in the stomach, or large bowel, or any particular site) (Fig. 12.1). Tumours with these features account for 4–8% of all carcinomas metastatic to the ovary.[6,7] Women with Krukenberg tumours are usually premenopausal and have a poor prognosis.[3,8]

The primary carcinomas of most Krukenberg tumours arise in the gastrointestinal tract, and so the prevalence in a population depends on the prevalence of gastric and colorectal neoplasia. Diffuse or signet ring carcinoma of the stomach has a greater tendency to metastasize to the ovary than the intestinal variant.[9] Breast carcinoma metastasizes to the ovary in late cases but rarely produces a signet ring pattern with a stromal response.[10]

About three-quarters of women with Krukenberg tumours have pelvic symptoms, usually abdominal distension and pain. Gastric carcinoma may present much later than the metastases. Intestinal metastases can stimulate the stromal cells of the ovaries into secretion of oestrogens and androgens, so the patient may present with menstrual abnormalities or virilization.

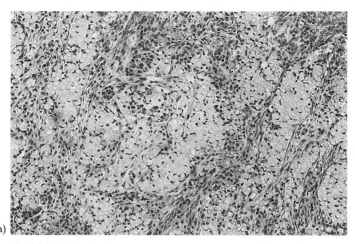
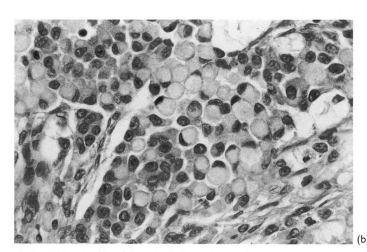

Fig. 12.1 (a) Krukenberg tumour composed of pale islands of tumour cells surrounded by a densely cellular stromal reaction (haematoxylin and eosin, ×100). (b) Signet ring cells in Krukenberg tumour (haematoxylin and eosin, ×400).

Ovarian tumours are bilateral in about one-third of cases. It is considered that borderline tumours that are bilateral or multifocal arise as separate primaries; this is based on analysis of loss of heterozygosity at several chromosomal sites,[11] the pattern of which is more in keeping with the development of individual primaries rather than metastasis from a single primary. In contrast, invasive carcinoma has been shown to be unifocal.[11] When bilateral invasive carcinoma is present, it is sometimes possible to be confident that one side is the metastasis of the other—surface malignancy alone without deep involvement is very suggestive of metastasis to the ovary from elsewhere. Endometrioid carcinoma of the ovary that is diagnosed synchronously or metachronously with endometrial carcinoma presents a similar problem. Again, with analysis of loss of heterozygosity it is possible to determine whether the ovarian and endometrial tumours are identical or not. When they are, it may still be possible on clinical grounds, and from the extent of ovarian involvement, to determine which represents the primary site of the tumour. Pragmatically this may not be a problem in management in any case, as aggressive surgical treatment with adjuvant chemotherapy has been advocated when a tumour involves adjacent tissues.[12]

Not all cases that are surgically assumed to be ovarian metastases are, in fact, neoplastic. Tamoxifen can cause necrosis of the ovaries and this can be mistaken for necrotic metastatic tumour;[13] the prevalence of ovarian metastases in breast cancer is unaffected by tamoxifen treatment.[14] Widespread involvement of the pelvic peritoneum by oxyuriasis can simulate metastatic carcinoma.[15]

Ovarian metastases from epithelial malignancies

Metastasis from breast carcinoma

The prevalence of ovarian involvement in patients with breast cancer depends on the population studied. In post-mortem examination studies before the introduction of tamoxifen the prevalence was about 40%.[16,17] Understandably, the prevalence in patients who had bilateral oophorectomy as part of the treatment of advanced disease was lower, at 20–30%[18] and when oophorectomy was prophylactic, in the absence of clinical evidence of ovarian metastases, was lower still, at 2–11%.[1] Involvement is characteristically bilateral.

The microscopical features generally reflect those of the parent primary. There may be trabecular, cribriform, and diffuse areas, and lobular carcinoma usually retains the characteristic 'Indian file' pattern of spread. Poorly differentiated examples may merge with the gonadal stroma and be relatively imperceptible, although on high-power magnification the pleomorphism and mitotic activity are apparent. A classical Krukenberg appearance with signet ring cells containing mucin is uncommon.

The differential diagnosis includes other primary and metastatic tumours with cribriform and trabecular growth patterns, such as carcinoid tumours, sex-cord stromal tumours, and pancreatic carcinoma. Poorly differentiated metastases can resemble poorly differentiated primary adenocarcinoma, especially serous adenocarcinoma. Metastases are not associated with benign elements (which are often found in some areas of a serous tumour), are usually solid rather than cystic, are bilateral with only surface involvement in early cases, and often have extensive lymphatic permeation.

Metastasis from primary carcinoma of the alimentary tract

Large bowel adenocarcinoma

The incidence of metastasis of carcinoma of the large bowel to the ovary depends on the stage of the primary tumour; in one series it was about 30%[19] and in others is much lower.[20] When the ovaries are removed at the time of the large bowel excision, about 10% are found to have metastatic colorectal carcinoma.[21] Rarely, a large bowel tumour may present as an apparently primary ovarian mass.[22] The prognosis is generally poor. It was considered that the prognosis could be improved by excision of the affected ovary or ovaries[23] but this is now disputed.[24]

Metastasis to the ovary from a primary adenocarcinoma of the appendix is rare as the primary lesion is rare, but is important as it may present as an apparently primary ovarian neoplasm.[25] Pseudomyxoma of the ovary, appendix, and peritoneum is considered by some to result from a low-grade primary carcinoma of the appendix,[26] but this is disputed in favour of separate ovarian and appendiceal neoplasms.[27] Ovarian involvement from the disseminated spread of the glandular variant of appendiceal carcinoid has also been described.[28]

Large bowel metastases in the ovary can closely resemble primary endometrioid or mucinous cystadenocarcinoma, both macroscopically and microscopically. Metastases tend to form large, variegated tumours with areas of mucin production, necrosis, and old and recent haemorrhage.[29] Primary ovarian tumours often have a benign or borderline component and may have squamous metaplasia or associated endometriosis that would be rare in relation to metastatic colorectal carcinoma. Metastases characteristically have more extensive necrosis, with collections of neoplastic glands around areas of necrosis.[29,30] Immunostaining for carcino-embryonic antigen (CEA) in tumours with an endometrioid growth pattern may be helpful, as it is strongly positive in intestinal tumours and negative in primary ovarian endometrioid carcinoma: when the tumour is mucinous both colorectal metastases and primary mucinous carcinoma of the ovary are positive.[31] Immunostaining for cytokeratins 7 and 20 can indicate whether an ovarian tumour is metastatic from the large bowel or primary endometrioid carcinoma: metastases tend to be 7-negative, 20-positive, while primary tumours are the reverse.[32]

Carcinoid tumour

Carcinoid tumour may be a primary or secondary ovarian tumour. Primary carcinoids are unilateral and usually associated with teratomatous elements; in rare cases a strumal carcinoid may be present with carcinoid tumour in association with thyroid follicles. They have an indolent natural history, rarely spread or recur, and are not associated with carcinoid in the small or large intestine. Secondary carcinoid tumours in the ovary are usually associated with widespread disease in the peritoneal cavity, are usually bilateral, are not associated with teratomatous elements and have a much more aggressive clinical course. Secondary carcinoid tumours of the ovary account for less than 2% of all ovarian secondaries.[18]

The ileum is the most common primary site, followed by the caecum, appendix, and pancreas (either as a carcinoid tumour with its usual histological characteristics or as an islet-cell tumour that secretes hormones as well as 5-hydroxytryptamine).[33] Metastasis from carcinoids of the jejunum and bronchus have also been reported.[30,33] The prognosis is generally poor, although it has been improved by use of MIBG (meta-iodobenzylguanidine), an adrenaline/serotonin analogue that is taken up into the neurosecretory granules of the carcinoid cells and can be labelled with ^{131}I to cause some degree of cell damage and so palliation.[34,35] Octreotide, a somatostatin analogue, can also be used but has distressing side-effects that some patients cannot tolerate.[35,36]

Secondary carcinoids are characteristically bilateral but of different sizes, with smooth surfaces that may adhere to adjacent structures. The cut surface is variegated with areas of degeneration (in contrast to primary carcinoids which have a homogeneous cut surface). Histologically the growth pattern is usually insular with peripheral palisading of nuclei and acinus formation. The cells stain for neuroendocrine markers such as chromogranin and NSE (neuron-specific enolase), and are usually positive for serotonin. Mucin-secreting carcinoid tumours from the appendix and elsewhere may metastasize to the ovary and have a typical Krukenberg appearance.[37,38]

The differential diagnosis includes sex-cord stromal tumour, Brenner tumour, and adenofibroma and adenocarcinoma that have trabecular or insular elements. Immunostaining in these is negative for chromogranin. The prognosis is generally poor for secondary carcinoid of the ovary.[33] There is some evidence that aggressive surgery with identification and resection of the primary tumour and bilateral salpingo-oophorectomy can result in a relatively favourable clinical outcome.[18]

Metastases from elsewhere in the alimentary system
Primary adenocarcinoma of the pancreas may metastasize to the ovary and closely resemble an ovarian primary.[2] Pancreatic and ovarian mucinous carcinomas can occur synchronously, and it is interesting that ovarian-type stroma and inhibin-containing cells have been found in a primary pancreatic adenocarcinoma.[39] Pancreatic carcinoids may metastasize to the ovary and be mistaken for primary ovarian tumours.[40] Biliary tract carcinoma is rare and only rarely metastasizes to the ovary.[41] A case of adenocarcinoma of the duodenum/jejunum with Krukenberg metastases to the ovaries has been described.[42]

Metastases to the ovary from neoplasms of the female genital system

Metastases to the ovary from endometrial adenocarcinoma are uncommon at the time of presentation, although they are much more common at post-mortem examination.[43] Synchronous and metachronous primaries in the endometrium and ovary are not uncommon. In most cases they can be shown to be different primaries, using restriction fragment length polymorphism studies.

Squamous cell carcinomas of the cervix, vagina, and vulva very rarely metastasize to the ovary; most squamous cell carcinomas in the ovary arise in cystic teratomas. Carcinoma of the Fallopian tube is a rare condition in its own right and so contributes only occasional examples of ovarian metastasis. Adenocarcinoma of the cervix metastasizes to the ovary in a stage-related way: involvement of the deep cervical stroma and the parametrium correlated with a tendency for ovarian metastases irrespective of lymph node status.[44]

Metastases to the ovary from, or ovarian involvement by, other malignancies

Metastases from rare epithelial tumours, sarcomas, and primitive or developmental tumours, such as blastomas and chordoma, are treated very well in standard texts.[20,45] For completeness they are listed, with references, in Tables 12.1–12.3.

Table 12.1 Rare epithelial metastases in the ovary

Primary neoplasm	References
Melanoma	5, 26, 46, 47
Renal cell carcinoma	10, 48, 49
Transitional cell carcinoma	30, 50, 51
Bronchial carcinoma	10, 52, 53
Hepatocellular carcinoma	53, 54
Thyroid carcinoma	16, 55
Adenoid cystic carcinoma	26
Small cell carcinoma	56

Table 12.2 Sarcomas metastatic to the ovary

Sarcoma	References
Leiomyosarcoma	57
Endometrial stromal sarcoma	57
Fibrosarcoma, haemangiosarcoma, chondrosarcoma	57
Osteosarcoma	57, 58
Rhabdomyosarcoma	10, 59, 60
Angiosarcoma	61, 62

Table 12.3 Metastases from blastomas and other developmental tumours

Tumour	Reference
Cerebellar medulloblastoma	63
Hepatoblastoma	64
Nephroblastoma	65
Neuroblastoma	60, 66, 67
Retinoblastoma	68
Ewing's sarcoma	55
Liposarcoma	5
Chordoma	69

References

1. Johansson, H. (1960). Clinical aspects of metastatic ovarian cancer of extragenital origin. *Acta Obstet. Gynecol. Scand.*, **39**, 681–97.

2. Young, R.H. and Hart, W.R. (1989). Metastases from carcinoma of the pancreas stimulating primary mucinous tumors of the ovary. A report of seven cases. *Am. J. Surg. Pathol.*, **13**, 748–56.

3. Holtz, F. and Hart, W.R. (1982). Krukenberg tumours of the ovary: a clinciopathologic analysis of 27 cases. *Cancer*, **50**, 2438–47.

4. Krukenberg, P. (1896). Ueben das Fibrosarcoma ovarii mucocellulari (carcinomases). *Archiv. Gynaecol.*, **50**, 287–321.

5. Russell, P. and Bannatyne, P. (1989). *Surgical pathology of the ovaries.* Churchill Livingstone, Edinburgh.

6. Soloway, I., Latour, J.P.A., and Young, M.H.V. (1956). Krukenberg tumors of the ovary. *Obstet. Gynecol.*, **8**, 636–8.

7. Metz, S.A., Karnei, R.F., Veach, S.R., and Hoskins, W.J. (1980). Krukenberg carcinoma of the ovary with bone marrow involvement; report of two cases and review of the literature. *Obstet. Gynecol.*, **55**, 99–104.

8. Webb, M.J., Decker, D.G., and Mussey, E. (1975). Cancer metastatic to the ovary; factors influencing survival. *Obstet. Gynecol.*, **45**, 391–6.

9. Duarte, I. and Llanos, O. (1981). Patterns of metastases in intestinal and diffuse types of carcinoma of the stomach. *Human Pathol.*, **12**, 237–42.

10. Mazur, M.T., Hsueh, S., and Gersell, D.J. (1984). Metastases to the female genital tract; analysis of 325 cases. *Cancer*, **53**, 1978–84.

11. Lu, K.H., Bell, D.A., Welch, W.R., Berkowitz, R.S., and Mok, S.C. (1998). Evidence for the multifocal origin of bilateral and advanced human serous borderline ovarian tumors. *Cancer Res.*, **58**, 2328–30.

12. Piura, B. and Glezerman, M. (1989). Synchronous carcinomas of endometrium and ovary. *Gynecol. Oncol.*, **33**, 261–4.

13. Jolles, C.J., Smotkin, D., Ford, K.L., and Jones, K.P. (1990). Cystic ovarian necrosis complicating tamoxifen therapy for breast cancer in a premenopausal woman. A case report. *J. Reprod. Med.*, **35**, 299–300.

14. McGonigle, K.F., Vasilev, S.A., Odom-Maryon, T., and Simpson, J.F. (1999). Ovarian histopathology in breast cancer patients receiving tamoxifen. *Gynecol. Oncol.*, **73**, 402–6.

15. FitzGerald, T.B., Mainwaring, A.R., and Ahmed, A. (1974). Pelvic peritoneal oxyuriasis simulating metastatic carcinoma. A case report. *J. Obstet. Gynaecol. Br. Commonw.*, **81**, 248–50.

16. Luisi, A. (1968). Metastatic ovarian tumors. In *Ovarian cancer*, UICC monograph series Vol 11, (ed. F. Gentil and A.C. Junqueira), pp. 87–104. Springer-Verlag, Berlin.

17. Harris, N.L. and Scully, R.E. (1984). Malignant lymphoma and granulocytic sarcoma of the uterus and vagina; a clinicopathologic analysis of 27 cases. *Cancer*, **53**, 2530–45.

18. Scully, R.E. (1979). *Tumours of the ovary and maldeveloped gonads.* Fascicle 16. Armed Forces Institute of Pathology, Washington.

19. Virieux, C. (1962). Untersuchungen uber Haufigkeit und Enstehungweise von Krebsmetastasen in den Eirstocken. *Gynaecologia (Basel)*, **153**, 209–24.

20. Scully, R.E., Young, R.H., and Clement, P.B. (1998). *Tumours of the ovary, maldeveloped gonads, Fallopian tube and broad ligament.* Fascicle 23. Armed Forces Institute of Pathology, Washington.

21. Graffner, H.O.L., Alm, P.O.R., and Oscarson, J.E.A. (1983). Prophylactic oophorectomy in colorectal cancer. *Am. J. Surg.*, **146**, 233–5.

22. Herrera-Ornelas, L., Natarajan N., Tsukada Y. *et al.* (1983). Adenocarcinoma of the colon masquerading as primary ovarian neoplasia: an analysis of ten cases. *Dis Colon Rectum*, **26**, 377–80.

23. Petru, E., Pickel, H., Heydarfadai, M. *et al.* (1992). Nongential cancer metastic to the ovary. *Gynecol. Oncol.*, **44**, 83–6.

24. Sielezneff *et al.* (1997).

25. Thorsen, P., Dybdahl, H., Sogaard, H., and Moller, B.R. (1991). Ovarian tumors caused by metastatic tumors of the appendix: two case reports. *Europ. J. Obstet. Gynecol. Reprod. Biol.*, **40**, 67–71.

26. Young, R.H. and Scully, R.E. (1991). Malignant melanoma metastatic to the ovary: a clinicopathologic analysis of 20 cases. *Am. J. Surg. Pathol.*, **15**, 849–60.

27. Seidman, J.D., Elsayed, A.M., Sobin, L.H., and Tavassoli, F.A. (1993). Association of mucinous tumours of the ovary and appendix: clinicopathologic study of 25 cases. *Am. J. Surg. Pathol.*, **17**, 85–90.

28. Tjalma, W.A., Schatteman, E., Goovaerts, G., Verkinderen, L., Van den Borre, F., and Keersmaekers, G. (2000). Adenocarcinoid of the appendix presenting as a disseminated ovarian carcinoma: report of a case. *Surg. Today*, **30**, 78–81.

29. Daya, D., Nazerali, L., and Frank, G.L. (1992). Metastatic ovarian carcinoma of large intestinal origin stimulating primary ovarian carcinoma: a clinicopathologic study of 25 cases. *Am. J. Clin. Pathol.*, **27**, 751–8.

30. Ulbright, T.M., Roth, L.M., and Stehman, F.B. (1984). Secondary ovarian neoplasia. A clinicopathologic study of 35 cases. *Cancer*, **53**, 1164–74.

31. Lash, R.H. and Hart, W.R. (1987). Intestinal adenocarcinomas metastatic to the ovaries: a clinicopathologic evaluation of 22 cases. *Am. J. Surg. Pathol.*, **11**, 114–21.

32. Loy, T.S., Calaluce, R.D., and Keeney, G.L.(1996). Cytokeratin immunostaining in differentiating primary ovarian carcinoma from metastatic colonic adenocarcinoma. *Mod. Pathol.*, **9**, 1040–4.

33. Robboy, S.J., Scully, R.E., and Norris, H.J. (1974). Carcinoid metastatic to the ovary: a clincopathologic analysis of 35 cases. *Cancer*, **33**, 798–811.

34. Halford, S. and Waxman, J. (1998). The management of carcinoid tumours. *Quart. J. Med.*, **91**, 795–8.

35. Zuetenhorst, H., Taal, B.G., Boot, H., Valdes Olmos, R., and Hoefnagel, C. (1999). Long-term palliation in metastatic carcinoid tumours with various applications of meta-iodobenzylguanidin (MIBG): pharmacological MIBG, ^{131}I-labelled MIBG and the combination. *Europ. J. Gastroenterol. Hepatol.*, **11**, 1157–64.

36. Caplin, M.E., Hodgson, H.J., Dhillon, A.P. *et al.* (1998). Multimodality treatment for gastric carcinoid tumor with liver metastases. *Am. J. Gastroenterol.*, **93**, 1945–8.

37. Paone, J.F., Bixler, T.J. 2nd, Imbembo, A.L. (1978). Primary mucinous adenocarcinoma of the appendix with bilateral Krukenberg ovarian tumors. *Johns Hopkins Med. J.*, **143**, 43–7.

38. Klein, E.A. and Rosen, M.H. (1996). Bilateral Krukenberg tumors due to appendiceal mucinous carcinoid. *Int. J. Gynaecol. Pathol.*, **15**, 85–8.

39. Ridder, G.J., Maschek, H., Flemming, P., Nashan, B., and Klempnauer, J. (1998). Ovarian-like stroma in an invasive mucinous cystadenocarcinoma of the pancreas positive for inhibin. A hint concerning its possible histogenesis. *Virch. Archiv.*, **432**, 451–4.

40. Serratoni, F.T. and Robboy, S.J. (1975). Ultrastructure of primary and metastatic ovarian carcinoids: analysis of 11 cases. *Cancer*, **36**, 157–60.

41. Young, R.H. and Scully, R.E. (1990). Ovarian metastases from carcinoma of the gallbladder and extrahepatic bile ducts stimulating primary tumours of the ovary: a report of six cases. *Int. J. Gynecol. Pathol.*, **9**, 60–72.

42. Loke, T.K., Lo, S.S., and Chan, C.S. (1997). Case report: Krukenberg tumours arising from a primary duodenojejunal adenocarcinoma. *Clin. Radiol.*, **52**(2), 154–155.

43. Beck, R.P., and Latour, J.P. (1963). Necropsy reports on 36 cases of endometrial carcinoma. *Am. J. Obstet. Gynecol.*, **85**, 307–311.

44. Natsume, N., Aoki, Y., Kase, H., Kashima, K., Sugaya, S., and Tanaka, K. (1999). Ovarian metastasis in stage IB and II cervical adenocarcinoma. *Gynecol. Oncol.*, **74**, 255–8.

45. Fox, H. (1995). Chapter 27: Metastatic tumours of the ovary. In: Fox, H. (ed) Obstetrical and Gynaecological Pathology. Fourth Edition. Churchill Livingstone, New York.

46. Fitzgibbons, P.L., Martin, S.E. and Simmons, T.J. (1987). Malignant melanoma metastatic to the ovary. *Am. J. Surg. Path.*, **11**, 959–964.

47. Nakano, J., Shimizu, T., Hirota, T., and Muto, M. (1998). An unusual female melanoma patient with late metastases to both skin and ovaries. *J. Dermatol.*, **25**(2), 126–128.

48. Buller, R.E., Braga, C.A., Tanagho, E.A., and Miller, T. (1983). Renal cell carcinoma metastatic to the ovary: a case report. *J. Reprod. Med.*, **28**, 217–20.

49. Young, R.H. and Hart, W.R. (1992). Renal cell carcinoma metastatic to the ovary: a report of three cases emphasizing possible confusion with ovarian clear cell adenocarcinoma. *Int. J. Gynecol. Pathol.*, **11**, 96–104.

50. Batata, M.A., Whitmore, W.F., Hilaris, B.S., Tokita, N., and Grabstald, H. (1975). Primary carcinoma of the ureter: a prognostic study. *Cancer*, **35**, 1616–32.

51. Young, R.H., and Scully, R.E. (1988). Urothelial and ovarian carcinomas of identical cell types: problems in interpretation. A report of three cases and review of the literature. *Int. J. Gynecol. Pathol.*, **7**, 197–211.

52. Malviya, V.K., Bansal, M., Chahinian, P., Deppe, G., Lauersen, N., and Gordon, R.E. (1982). Small cell anaplastic lung cancer presenting as an ovarian metastasis. *Int. J. Gynaecol. Obstet.*, **20**, 487–93.

53. Young, R.H. and Scully, R.E. (1985). Ovarian metastases from cancer of the lung: problems in interpretation: a report of seven cases. *Gynecol. Oncol.*, **21**, 337–50.

54. Young, R.H., Gersell, D.J., Clement, P.B., and Scully, R.E. (1992). Hepatocellular carcinoma metastatic to the ovary: a report of three cases discovered during life with discussion of the differential diagnosis of hepatoid tumors of the ovary. *Hum. Pathol.*, **23**, 574–80.

55. Woodruff, J.D., Murthy, Y.S., Bhaskar, T.N., Bordbar, F., and Tseng, S.S. (1970). Metastatic ovarian tumors. *Am. J. Obstet. Gynecol.*, **107**, 202–9.

56. Eichhorn, J.H., Young, R.H., and Scully, R.E. (1993). Non-pulmonary small cell carcinomas of extragenital origin metastatic to the ovary: a report of seven cases. *Cancer*, **71**, 177–86.

57. Young, R.H.and Scully, R.E. (1990). Sarcomas metastatic to the ovary; a report of 21 cases. *Int. J. Gynecol. Pathol.*, **9**, 231–52.

58. Eltabbakh, G.H., Piver, M.S., Werness, B.A. (1997). Primary peritoneal adenocarcinoma metastatic to the brain. *Gynecol Oncol.*, **66**(1), 160–3.

59. Young, R.H. and Scully, R.E. (1989). Alveolar rhabdomyosarcoma metastatic to the ovary: a report of two cases and discussion of the different diagnosis of small cell malignant tumors of the ovary. *Cancer*, **64**, 899–904.

60. Young, R.H., Kozakewich, H.P.W., and Scully, R.E. (1993). Metastatic ovarian tumors in children: a report of 14 cases and review of the literature. *Int. J. Gynecol. Pathol.*, **12**, 8–19.

61. Chen, K.T.K., Kirkegaard, D.D., and Bocian, J.J. (1980). Angiosarcoma of the breast. *Cancer*, **46**, 368–71.

62. Sedgely, M.G., ÷st˚r, A.G., and Fortune, D.W. (1985). Angiosarcoma of breast metastatic to the ovary and placenta. *Aust. NZ J. Obstet. Gynaecol.*, **25**, 299–302.

63. Paterson, E. (1961). Distant metastases from medulloblastoma of the cerebellum. *Brain*, **84**, 301–9.

64. Green, L.K. and Silva, E.G. (1989). Hepatoblastoma in an adult with metastasis to the ovaries. *Am. J. Clin. Pathol.*, **92**, 110–15.

65. Jereb, B., Golouh, R., and Havlicek, S. (1977). Ovarian cancer in children and adolescents: a review of 15 cases. *Med. Pediatr. Oncol.*, **3**, 339–43.

66. Meyer, W.H., Yu, G.W., Milvenan, E.S., Jeffs, R.D., and Kaizer, H. (1979). Ovarian involvement in neuroblastoma. *Med. Pediatr. Oncol.*, **7**, 49–54.

67. Sty, J.R., Kun, L.E., and Casper, J.T. (1980). Bone scintigraphy in neuroblastoma with ovarian metastasis. *Wisconsin Med. J.*, **79**, 28–9.

68. Moore, J.G., Schifrin, B.S., and Erez, S.(1967). Ovarian tumors in infancy, childhood and adolescence. *Am. J. Obstet. Gynaecol.*, **99**, 913–22.

69. Zukerberg, L.R. and Young, R.H. (1990). Chordoma metastatic to the ovary. *Arch. Pathol. Lab. Med.*, **114**, 208–10.

?? Morrow, M. and Enker, W.E. (1984). Late ovarian metastases in carcinoma of the colon and rectum. *Arch. Surg.*, **119**, 1385–8.

?? Robboy, S. J., Norris, H.J., and Scully, R.E. (1975). Insular carcinoid primary in the ovary. A clinicopathologic analysis of 48 cases. *Cancer*, **36**, 404–18.

13. Genetic analysis of putative precursors of ovarian cancer

Ian G. Campbell, Sarah J. Morland, Koshiro Obata, Phillippa J. Neville, and Nicola Thomas

Introduction

The poor prognosis associated with ovarian cancer is largely attributable to the fact that the majority of women present with late-stage disease. The relative rarity of early stage tumours and the absence of any histologically defined premalignant stages has led to speculation that ovarian cancer may arise predominantly *de novo* and not through benign or borderline precursors. The paradigm established by the colorectal tumorigenesis model[1] suggests that malignancies arise only after the accumulation of mutations in multiple tumour suppressor genes (TSGs), as a result of the clonal expansion of successively more genetically damaged cells. A *de novo* model for ovarian tumorigenesis would require that mutations in multiple TSGs occurred in rapid succession without significant clonal expansion of intermediate stages. On the other hand, the observation that histologically benign tumours are frequently observed adjacent to areas of invasive cancer, with many of these showing a direct transition from benign to invasive epithelium, supports a progression model.[2] In addition, ovarian cancers often contain areas of differing grades, again suggesting that high-grade tumours may arise by clonal expansion of low-grade tumours. Epidemiological studies have demonstrated that benign ovarian tumours are many times more common among first- and second-degree relatives of patients with ovarian cancer than controls, suggesting a biological link between the two types of tumour.[3]

Molecular genetic studies of benign epithelial ovarian tumours

Molecular genetic studies offer the best hope of obtaining a definitive answer about the biological relationship between benign and malignant ovarian tumours. If ovarian carcinomas do arise from benign tumours, we would expect to find genetic alterations common to both. Conversely, if benign tumours represent a distinct entity then we may expect to find alterations unique to the pathway that leads to benign neoplasms. To date there have been few molecular genetic studies of benign ovarian tumours and the total number of cases studied is quite small (Table 13.1). Some investigators have reported zero or very low frequencies of loss of heterozygosity (LOH) or *TP53* and *KRAS2* mutations, and therefore concluded that benign tumours represent distinct biological entities.[4,5] Other investigators who detected low frequencies of LOH, none of which were unique to benign tumours, concluded that the data were consistent with, but not proof of, a progression model for ovarian cancer development.[6] Zheng *et al.* [5] have provided the most compelling evidence for the malignant transformation of benign ovarian tumours by demonstrating concordant *TP53* mutations in benign epithelial cysts contiguous with ovarian carcinomas. Although the most obvious explanation for this was that the benign epithelium had undergone genetic alterations that led to malignant transformation, it was considered more likely that the histologically benign component was in fact a portion of

Table 13.1 Summary of reported *KRAS2* and *TP53* mutations and LOH in benign epithelial ovarian tumours[a]

| | Loss of heterozygosity on chromosome arm (reference numbers superscript) | | | | | | | | | | Somatic mutation | |
	2q[27]	6q[6,27]	7q[6]	9p[6,27,2]	9q[28]	11p[29]	11q[6,27]	17p[6,27]	17q[6,27]	X[6]	Kras2[6,3]	TP53[5,10]
				8							0	
LOH/Inf[b]	1/13	3/27	0/18	2/35	1/5	0/11	0/27	1/37	0/26	4/11	2/10	0/36
%	7	11	0	5	20	0	0	2	0	35	20	0

[a]This table presents a summary of selected studies of benign ovarian tumours and is not intended as a an exhaustive list of the such studies.
[b]Number of cases showing LOH, divided by the number of tumours informative for at least one marker on the indicated chromosome.

the carcinoma that had matured. Further genetic investigations of these cases, which could distinguish between these models, have to date not been reported. In an attempt to resolve the true relationship between benign ovarian tumours found in association with carcinomas, Wolf *et al.*[7] investigated 10 heterogeneous ovarian carcinomas using fluorescence *in situ* hybridization on chromosomes 8, 12, and 17. They demonstrated that the benign and borderline components harboured some, but not all, of the abnormalities present in the adjacent carcinoma. Their data clearly support a progression model for ovarian tumorigenesis and demonstrate that it is very unlikely that benign areas of heterogeneous carcinomas represent components of the carcinoma that have matured or differentiated.

Although such studies demonstrate that benign and borderline tumours may undergo malignant transformation, the low frequency of genetic alterations detected has led to suggestions that this occurs very rarely and therefore does not represent a major pathway for the development of ovarian cancers. However, even if benign tumours rarely transform, their overall contribution to ovarian cancer incidence will depend on their prevalence among asymptomatic women. In fact benign neoplasms are very common among postmenopausal asymptomatic women, possibly as high as 5%[8] and thus even a very low frequency of malignant transformation could account for the majority of ovarian carcinomas. Our goal has been to accumulate molecular genetic data for putative ovarian cancer precursor lesions in order to provide definitive data as to whether this is the case, and whether the aetiology of ovarian cancer conforms to a progression model or if the different biological subtypes of ovarian tumours arise via distinct pathways. In this chapter, data will be presented from our analysis of benign ovarian tumours and endometriosis, both of which may represent significant premalignant lesions.

Molecular genetic studies of serous and mucinous ovarian cystadenomas

We are currently investigating 77 serous and mucinous cystadenomas for genetic alterations, using LOH and *TP53* mutation analysis. A summary of some of our data is presented in Table 13.2. As the percentage of tumour tissue in such biopsies is low, ranging between 10 and 30%, tissue microdissection was performed in all cases to ensure minimal normal tissue contamination.[9] We estimate that all our tumour DNA extractions contain less than 25% stromal contamination and therefore our data will reflect more accurately the true incidence of somatic genetic alteration in benign tumours. In contrast to some previous studies, we detected LOH on the majority of chromosome arms, albeit at a low frequency. LOH was more common on chromosomes 6q, 7, 9p, and 11 which, interestingly, are the same sites of frequent LOH among low-grade/early stage ovarian carcinomas.[10] LOH on chromosome 7q was particularly frequent, with 23% (12/51) of the serous and mucinous cystadenomas showing LOH with at least one marker. Again, alterations on 7q are very common among ovarian and other epithelial cancers and are often implicated as an early event. We identified *TP53* mutations, without accompanying LOH of the wild-type allele, in 2/30 (6%) of benign tumours, which is in contrast to the absence of *TP53* mutations reported by others (Table 13.1). In total, 27/77 (35%) benign tumours showed LOH on at least one chromosome arm or harboured a *TP53* mutation, which is broadly similar to the frequency reported by Chenevix-Trench *et al.*[6] Of these 27 tumours, 19 showed LOH on only one chromosome arm, seven showed LOH on two arms, and one showed LOH on three arms. Compared to some published studies, our frequency of LOH detection is high and it is possible that some of these deletions may represent random non-pathological events. Even allowing for this possibility, our data are more consistent with a progression model for ovarian tumorigenesis rather than a *de novo* model.

Origin of endometrioid and clear cell ovarian tumours

Although the absolute frequency of LOH among benign tumours is low, there appear to be differences emerging between the serous and mucinous cystadenomas. We detected LOH on chromosome 6q in 5/19 (26%) of the mucinous cystadenomas but only 2/29 (7%) of the serous cystadenomas. Chenevix-Trench *et al.*[6] observed similar differences on chromosome 6, as well as LOH on chromosome Xq in 2/2 mucinous and only 2/8 serous cystadenomas. Distinct genetic alterations are also well recognized among their malignant counterparts, and it is becoming clear that the different histological subtypes of ovarian cancer arise through

Table 13.2 LOH data for benign epithelial ovarian tumours

	Loss of heterozygosity on chromosome arm[a]													TP53 mut.
	3p	5q	6q	7p	7q	8q	9p	10q	11p	11q	17p	17q	22q	
Serous	1/8	0/6	2/29	5/28	6/30	0/11	2/25	0/8	3/17	3/22	0/9	0/14	0/13	1/16
Mucinous	0/1	1/2	5/19	4/20	6/21	0/10	2/15	0/4	2/13	2/16	1/8	1/9	0/6	1/14
Total	1/9	1/8	7/48	9/48	12/51	0/21	4/40	0/13	5/30	5/38	1/17	1/23	0/19	2/30
(%)	(11)	(12)	(14)	(18)	(23)	(0)	(10)	(0)	(16)	(13)	(5)	(4)	(0)	(6)

[a] The top figure is the number of cases with LOH at any marker on the indicated chromosome over the total number of informative cases. The number in brackets is the percentage of informative cases showing LOH.

different developmental pathways. In particular, it has long been suspected that endometriosis may be the precursor of endometrioid and clear cell ovarian carcinomas.[11] Endometriosis is a condition in which endometrium proliferates at sites outside the uterine cavity. It is a very common gynaecological disease that may affect up to 10% of premenopausal women.[12,13] In the vast majority of cases, endometriosis follows a benign course but, paradoxically, it does exhibit some characteristics reminiscent of malignancy, including local invasion and metastases. However, despite the accumulation of some compelling data suggesting that endometriosis represents an ovarian cancer precursor, this hypothesis has been based largely on circumstantial evidence.

In the past few years, molecular genetic studies have revealed that alterations in oncogenes and tumour suppressor genes (TSGs) are central to the development of malignant tumours as well as the benign precursors of such malignancies. We and others have postulated that similar alterations could occur during the development and progression of endometriosis. However, few studies have addressed the genetic alterations that may be occurring in endometriosis. Ballouk et al.[14] provided some evidence for the involvement of genetic abnormalities in endometriotic cells by demonstrating DNA aneuploidy in cysts with severe atypia, and suggested that these cells represented the precursors of invasive malignancies that may arise in ovarian endometriotic cysts. In an immunohistochemical study, TP53 overexpression was observed in a poorly differentiated endometrioid carcinoma as well as in adjacent benign endometriotic tissue, suggesting that TP53 abnormalities may also contribute to malignant transformation of endometriosis.[15] In a multi-colour fluorescence in situ hybridization study, Shin et al.[16] observed monosomy of chromosome 16 and 17 as well as trisomy of chromosome 11 among some cases of severe/late-stage endometriosis. Our own studies have added support for a role of TSGs in the development of endometriosis by demonstrating LOH on chromosome arms 9p, 11q, and 22q in about 30% of ovarian endometriosis.[9] Nevertheless, no study was able to provide conclusive genetic evidence in support of a common lineage between endometriosis and ovarian carcinoma. To address this we applied molecular genetic techniques coupled with tissue microdissection to assess the relationship between endometriotic foci found adjacent to, or contiguous with, ovarian cancers.[17] We examined these cases for LOH on 12 chromosome arms to determine if they shared genetic alterations. In 4/4 of the cases where the carcinoma had arisen within endometriosis, and

in 5/7 cases where the carcinoma was adjacent to the endometriosis, common genetic lesions were detected, consistent with a common lineage. Our study provided the first direct evidence that endometrioid and clear cell ovarian carcinomas arise through malignant transformation of endometriotic lesions.

By way of illustration, the LOH frequency detected in endometriosis, with and without adjacent carcinoma, and endometrioid ovarian carcinoma are compared in Table 13.3. A striking trend is evident, with an increasing frequency of LOH as the disease progresses. The four chromosome arms showing LOH in solitary ovarian endometriosis (5q, 9p, 11q, and 22q) were also the ones most frequently lost in endometriosis synchronous with carcinoma, and each of these chromosome arms showed a high frequency of LOH in low-grade and early stage endometrioid ovarian cancer. While no LOH was observed on chromosome 6q in solitary endometriosis, it was detected in 27% of the endometriosis cases synchronous with carcinoma, indicating that 6q may play a role in malignant transformation.

Apart from linking endometriosis with ovarian cancer, our data reinforce the view that the major histological subtypes of ovarian cancer—serous, mucinous, and endometrioid—arise through fundamentally different developmental pathways. If this is true, it raises the possibility that important insights into the development of ovarian cancer may previously have been overlooked when the histological differentiation was considered to be a relatively inconsequential developmental variation of the same disease pathway.

PTEN gene mutation analysis in ovarian cancer

Recently the tumour suppressor gene PTEN/MMAC on chromosome 10q23 has been shown to be mutated somatically in a wide range of tumours, including brain, prostate, breast, and thyroid.[18,19] PTEN mutations are particularly common in endometrial tumours but are found predominantly in those of endometrioid histology and not in the more aggressive serous histological subtype.[20] Since 10q23 LOH has been observed in ovarian cancers, it was an attractive candidate as an ovarian TSG as well. However, in four separate studies[21–24] no mutations were identified in a total of 88 primary ovarian cancers and 14 ovarian cancer cell lines, and it was concluded that PTEN was of no

Table 13.3 LOH in solitary endometriosis, endometriosis synchronous with ovarian cancer, and endometrioid carcinoma

| | Number analysed | LOH on chromosome arms: | | | | | | | | | | | |
		2q	4q	5p	5q	6q	7p	9p	11q	17p	17q	22q	Xq
Solitary E[a]	40	0	0	0	6	0	0	17	18	0	0	15	0
E with EC	14	0	8	0	25	27	0	31	20	0	0	31	0
EC	31	40	29	14	46	29	28	54	37	42	46	47	38

[a]Abbreviations: E, endometriosis; EC, endometrioid ovarian cancer.

relevance in ovarian tumorigenesis. Considering the histological subtype distribution of *PTEN* mutations in endometrial cancers, we reasoned that a similar bias may occur for endometrioid ovarian cancers and that the failure of previous studies to identify *PTEN* mutations may simply have been due to a bias toward analysis of the more common serous ovarian tumours. Furthermore, if endometrioid ovarian tumours are derived from endometriosis, then, in a sense, they are of endometrial rather than ovarian origin, providing a plausible developmental link between the two tumour types. Consequently we analysed 81 ovarian tumours, including 34 endometrioid and 10 mucinous tumours, for LOH on 10q23 and for mutations in all nine coding exons of *PTEN*. LOH was common among the endometrioid (43%) and serous (28%) tumours, but infrequent among the other histological subtypes (Table 13.4). A total of eight tumours were identified with somatic *PTEN* mutations, and all but one of these was of endometrioid differentiation. The only non-endometrioid tumour with a *PTEN* mutation had an overall mucinous histological appearance but it appeared atypical and contained foci of endometrioid differentiation. No *PTEN* mutations were found among the serous or clear cell tumours.

The identification of TSGs with critical roles in the development of ovarian cancer is at a very early stage and only *TP53* is known to be mutated in the majority of serous ovarian cancers and less than 15%[17,25] of endometrioid ovarian cancers. Our finding of *PTEN* mutations in about 20% of all endometrioid ovarian tumours and 50% of those with 10q LOH makes this the most common mutation so far described in this histological subtype. The absence of *PTEN* mutation in any of the 29 serous tumours examined is consistent with previous studies of ovarian tumours and suggests that, at best, *PTEN* is rarely involved in this histological subtype.

The majority of tumours with *PTEN* mutations were grade 1 and/or stage 1, suggesting that inactivation of *PTEN* is an early event in ovarian tumorigenesis. The hallmark of Cowden disease is the development of multiple hamartomas which are composed of disorganized cell masses, and has led to suggestions that one of the functions of *PTEN* is to control cellular proliferation and organization.[26] Our data show that inactivation is an early event in endometrioid ovarian tumorigenesis, suggesting that it is the cellular proliferation function of *PTEN* which is most relevant in the development of this tumour type. This is consistent with the idea that endometrioid ovarian cancers arise from endometriosis, which essentially results from the inappropriate proliferation of ectopic endometrial implants.

Conclusions

Technical advances in the analysis of molecular genetic alterations, when coupled with microdissection techniques and ready access to large cohorts of archival tissues, will continue to revolutionize our understanding of the aetiology and pathogenesis of gynaecological malignancies. Using these techniques we have been able to demonstrate conclusively that endometriosis is a precursor of endometrioid ovarian cancer. Based on this knowledge we have been able to demonstrate that the *PTEN* tumour suppressor gene has a major role in the aetiology of endometrioid but not serous ovarian cancers. This finding contrasts with other studies which concluded that *PTEN* had no role in the development of ovarian cancers, and is a poignant demonstration of the utility of viewing the different histological subtypes as distinct diseases.

Our data for benign and mucinous cystadenomas are less advanced, and currently there is insufficient data to provide unequivocal support for either a *de novo* or progression model for the development of serous and mucinous carcinomas. Nevertheless our view is that the bulk of genetic, epidemiological, and histological data are more consistent with a progression model.

References

1. Fearon, E.R. and Vogelstein, B.A. (1990). A genetic model for colorectal tumorigenesis. *Cell*, **61**, 759–67.
2. Puls, L.E., Powell, D.E., De Priest, P. D. *et al.* (1992). Transition from benign to malignant epithelium in mucinous and serous ovarian cystadenocarcinoma. *Gynecol. Oncol.*, **47**, 53–7.
3. Bourne, T.H., Whitehead, M.I., Campbell, S. *et al.* (1991). Ultrasound screening for familial ovarian cancer. *Gynecol. Oncol.*, **43**, 92–7.
4. Cheng, P.C., Gosewehr, J.A., Kim, T. M. *et al.* (1996). Potential role of the inactivated X-chromosome in ovarian epithelial tumor-development. *J. Natl Cancer Inst.*, **88**, 510–18.
5. Zheng, J.P., Benedict, W.F., Xu, H. J. *et al.* (1995). Genetic disparity between morphologically benign cysts contiguous to ovarian carcinomas acid solitary cystadenomas. *J. Natl Cancer Inst.*, **87**, 1146–53.
6. Chenevix-Trench, G., Kerr, J., Hurst, T. *et al.* (1997). Analysis of loss of heterozygosity and KRAS2 mutations in ovarian neoplasms: Clinicopathological correlations. *Genes Chrom. Cancer*, **18**, 75–83.
7. Wolf, N.G., Abdulkarim, F.W., Schork, N. J., and Schwartz, S. (1996). Origins of heterogeneous ovarian carcinomas—a molecular cytogenetic analysis of histologically benign, low malignant potential, and fully malignant components. *Am. J. Pathol.*, **149**, 511–20.
8. Bailey, C.L., Ueland, F.R., Land, G. L. *et al.* (1998). The malignant potential of small cystic ovarian tumors in women over 50 years of age. *Gynecol. Oncol.*, **69**, 3–7.
9. Jiang, X., Hitchcock, A., Bryan, E. J. *et al.* (1996). Microsatellite analysis of endometriosis reveals loss of heterozygosity at candidate ovarian tumor-suppressor gene loci. *Cancer Res.*, **56**, 3534–9.

Table 13.4 Summary of 10q23 LOH and *PTEN* mutations in ovarian tumours

Histological subtype	Number analysed	10q LOH[a]	*PTEN* mutation
Endometrioid	34	13/30 (43%)	7/34
Serous[b]	29	7/25 (28%)	0/29
Clear cell	8	1/7 (14%)	0/8
Mucinous[c]	10	1/10 (10%)	1/10

[a]Number of tumours showing LOH with any 10q23 microsatellite marker divided by the total number of tumours informative for at least one microsatellite marker. Percentage of cases with LOH is shown in brackets.
[b]Two of these tumours were of borderline malignancy. Neither showed 10q23 LOH.
[c]Four tumours were of borderline malignancy, none of which showed 10q23 LOH. One tumour, case 144, was classified as mucinous but was atypical and contained foci of endometrioid differentiation.

10. Watson, R.H., Neville, P.J., Roy, W. J. *et al.* (1998). Loss of heterozygosity on chromosomes 7p, 7q, 9p and 11q is an early event in ovarian tumorigenesis. *Oncogene*, **17**, 207–12.

11. De la Cuesta, R.S., Eichhorn, J.H., Rice, L. W. *et al.* (1996). Histologic transformation of benign endometriosis to early epithelial ovarian cancer. *Gynecol. Oncol.*, **60**, 238–44.

12. Brincat, M., Galea, R., and Buhagiar, A. (1994). Polycystic ovaries and endometriosis: a possible connection. *Br. J. Obstet. Gynaecol.*, **101**, 346–8.

13. Mahmood, T.A. and Templeton, A. (1991). Prevalence and genesis of endometriosis. *Hum. Reprod.*, **6**, 544–9.

14. Ballouk, F., Ross, J.S., and Wolf, B. C. (1994). Ovarian endometriotic cysts; an analysis of cytologic atypia and DNA ploidy. *Am. J. Clin. Pathol.*, **102**, 415–19.

15. Kupryjanczyk, J., Thor, A.D., Beauchamp, R. *et al.* (1993). p53 gene mutations and protein accumulation in human ovarian cancer. *Proc. Natl Acad. Sci. USA*, **90**, 4961–5.

16. Shin, J.C., Ross, H.L., Elias, S. *et al.* (1997). Detection of chromosomal aneuploidy in endometriosis by multi-color fluorescence in situ hybridization (FISH). *Hum. Genet.*, **100**, 401–6.

17. Jiang, X., Morland, S.J., Hitchcock, A. *et al.* (1998). Allelotyping of endometriosis with adjacent ovarian carcinoma reveals evidence of a common lineage. *Cancer Res.*, **58**, 1707–12.

18. Steck, P.A., Pershouse, M.A., Jasser, S.A. *et al.* (1997). Identification of a candidate tumour suppressor gene, MMAC1, at chromosome 10q23.3 that is mutated in multiple advanced cancers. *Nature Genet.*, **15**, 356–62.

19. Li, J., Yen, C., Liaw, D. *et al.* (1997). *PTEN*, a putative protein tyrosine phosphatase gene mutated in human brain, breast, and prostate cancer. *Science*, **275**, 1943–7.

20. Risinger, J.I., Hayes, K., Maxwell, G.L. *et al.* (1998). *PTEN* mutation in endometrial cancers is associated with favorable clinical and pathologic characteristics. *Clin. Cancer Res.*, **4**, 3005–10.

21. Maxwell, G.L., Risinger, J.I., Tong, B. *et al.* (1998). Mutation of the *PTEN* tumor suppressor gene is not a feature of ovarian cancers. *Gynecol. Oncol.*, **70**, 13–16.

22. Tashiro, H., Blazes, M.S., Wu, R. *et al.* (1997). Mutations in PTEN are frequent in endometrial carcinoma but rare in other common gynecological malignancies. *Cancer Res.*, **57**, 3935–40.

23. Teng, D. H.F., Hu, R., Lin, H. *et al.* (1997). MMAC1/PTEN mutations in primary tumor specimens and tumor cell lines. *Cancer Res.*, **57**, 5221–5.

24. Sakurada, A., Suzuki, A., Sato, M. *et al.* (1997). Infrequent genetic alterations of the *PTEN/MMAC1* gene in Japanese patients with primary cancers of the breast, lung, pancreas, kidney, and ovary. *Jap. J. Cancer Res.*, **88**, 1025–8.

25. Milner, B.J., Allan, L.A., Eccles, D.M. *et al.* (1993). p53 mutation is a common genetic event in ovarian carcinoma. *Cancer Res.*, **53**, 2128–32.

26. Liaw, D., Marsh, D.J., Li, J. *et al.* (1997). Germline mutations of the PTEN gene in Cowden disease, an inherited breast and thyroid cancer syndrome. *Nature Genet.*, **16**, 64–7.

27. Saretzki, G., Hoffmann, U., Rohlke, P. *et al.* (1997). Identification of allelic losses in benign, borderline, and invasive epithelial ovarian tumors and correlation with clinical outcome. *Cancer*, **80**, 1241–9.

28. Schultz, D.C., Vanderveer, L., Buetow, K.H. *et al.* (1995). Characterization of chromosome–9 in human ovarian neoplasia identifies frequent genetic imbalance on 9q and rare alterations involving 9p, including cdkn2. *Cancer Res.*, **55**, 2150–7.

29. Zheng, J.P., Wan, M.H., Zweizig, S. *et al.* (1993). Histologically benign or low grade malignant tumors adjacent to high grade ovarian carcinomas contain molecular characteristics of high grade carcinomas. *Cancer Res.*, **53**, 4138–42.

30. Teneriello, M.G., Ebina, M., Linnoila, R.I. *et al.* (1993). P53 and ki-ras gene-mutations in epithelial ovarian neoplasms. *Cancer Res.*, **53**, 3103 8.

14. Molecular pathogenesis of borderline and invasive ovarian tumors

Samuel C. Mok, Karen H. Lu, Shu-wing Ng, Gary K. Yiu, William R. Welch, Debra A. Bell, and Ross S. Berkowitz

Introduction

Epithelial ovarian neoplasms comprise 97% of ovarian tumor cases. They are classified into three main groups: benign, borderline, and invasive. Each group includes several histological subtypes: serous, mucinous, endometrioid, clear cell, undifferentiated, and mixed. Serous and mucinous subtypes comprise 50% and 30% of all tumor types, respectively. Hereditary predisposition and the involvement of the *BRCA1* gene are involved in the development of about 10% of cases of epithelial ovarian carcinoma,[1-3] but the specific genetic pathways for the development of epithelial ovarian tumors are largely unknown. It is unclear whether different histological subtypes of ovarian tumors have different pathogenetic pathways. Using a molecular genetic approach, Campbell *et al.* demonstrated that endometriosis may be the precursor of the majority of endometrioid and clear cell ovarian carcinomas.[4] In addition, Obata *et al.* recently showed frequent *PTEN/MMAC* mutations in endometrioid, but not serous or mucinous epithelial ovarian tumors.[5] These data suggest that tumors with different histological subtypes may arise through distinct developmental pathways.

The pathogenetic pathways of serous and mucinous tumors remain largely unknown and precursors of these tumors have not been identified. However, there are several uncommon histopathological features identified in early stage ovarian tumors, as shown in Fig. 14.1, which may give us insight into the pathogenesis of epithelial ovarian tumor development. First, benign, borderline, and invasive-appearing areas are frequently seen coexisting in low-grade mucinous ovarian carcinomas. In contrast, benign, borderline, and invasive-appearing areas are seen only in a small percentage of low-grade serous ovarian carcinomas. Secondly, incidental microscopic serous carcinomas, which are high grade, can be identified in grossly normal ovaries.[6] Thirdly, high-grade serous carcinoma can be found on the surface of the ovary with little or no stromal invasion.[7] Based on the histopathological findings and the prevalence of each histological subtype, we developed a working hypothesis for serous and mucinous ovarian tumor development (Fig. 14.2). A majority of ovarian tumors may develop from ovarian inclusion cysts which arise from ovarian surface epithelium invaginated into the cortex of the ovary. The epithelial lining of the cyst may develop into a mucinous or serous cystadenoma through distinct pathogenetic pathways. Mucinous cystadenoma may give rise to mucinous borderline ovarian tumors (BOTs). A subset of these tumors may progress to invasive low-grade mucinous carcinoma and subsequently into high-grade carcinoma.

Serous cystadenoma may give rise to serous BOTs; however, a majority of serous BOTs may develop directly from ovarian inclusion cysts, i.e. without the intervening stage of cystadenoma. In contrast to mucinous BOTs, only a small percentage of serous BOTs may progress to low-grade carcinoma and subsequently to high-grade carcinoma. We hypothesize that a majority of high-grade serous carcinomas derive *de novo* from ovarian cysts. Furthermore, serous carcinomas may also develop on the surface of the ovary directly from the ovarian surface epithelial cells.

We have attempted to test this working hypothesis by using several approaches. First, X-chromosome inactivation studies were used to determine whether bilateral and late-stage borderline and invasive ovarian tumors are unifocal or multifocal in origin. Secondly, mutation analysis of specific oncogenes, such as K-*ras*, and tumor suppressor genes, such as *p53*, was performed on borderline and invasive serous and mucinous tumors. Thirdly, loss of heterozygosity patterns in different histological subtypes were studied. Finally, the expression pattern of differentially expressed genes identified by RNA fingerprinting, reverse transcriptase polymerase chain reaction (RT-PCR), and immunohistochemistry were also compared among BOTs and invasive tumors.

Focality studies on borderline and invasive ovarian tumors

While the majority of borderline tumors are confined to a single ovary at the time of diagnosis, 30–40% will present as bilateral or late-stage disease. Whether bilateral or late-stage BOTs are derived from a single ovarian tumor that metastasizes or 'seeds' the other ovary and peritoneum, or is the result of a 'field defect' that causes

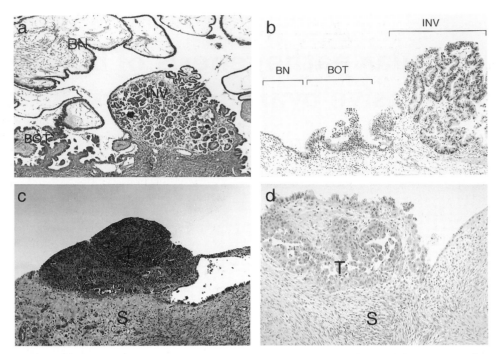

Fig. 14.1 (a) Stage I serous adenocarcinoma with benign (BN), borderline (BOT), and invasive (INV) epithelial components (hematoxylin and eosin, ×125). (b) Stage I mucinous adenocarcinoma with benign (BN), borderline (BOT), and invasive (INV) epithelial components (hematoxylin and eosin, ×125). (c) Surface serous adenocarcinoma (T) with minimal stromal invasion (S) (hematoxylin and eosin, ×125). (d) Microscopic high-grade serous adenocarcinoma (T) located near the surface of the ovary (hematoxylin and eosin, ×250).

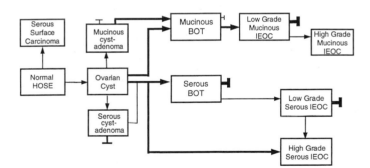

Fig. 14.2 A working hypothesis for ovarian tumor development. HOSE, normal ovarian surface epithelium; BOT, borderline ovarian tumor; IEOC, invasive epithelial ovarian tumor.

multiple primary tumors to occur simultaneously, is unknown. We used the pattern of X-chromosome inactivation to address this question in bilateral and advanced-stage serous BOTs. *Hpa*II restriction endonuclease digestion, followed by PCR amplification of the androgen receptor (AR) locus located on chromosome Xq11–12, was used to differentiate the active from the inactive X chromosome. In two of six patients, the left and right ovarian tumor sites had different AR alleles inactivated, indicating that the bilateral tumors originated independently. In a third patient, the X-inactivation pattern in the left ovarian tumor differed from the two peritoneal implants, suggesting that the implants were separate primary tumors, and not metastatic from the left ovarian tumor.[8] The remaining three patients had the same pattern of X

inactivation. These results suggest that bilateral and advanced-stage serous BOTs may be multifocal in origin, which is in contrast to invasive epithelial ovarian cancer, which has been shown to be unifocal in origin.[9,10]

Mutation analysis on K-*ras* and *p53* genes

Using single-strand conformation polymorphism (SSCP) analysis, K-*ras* mutations have been found in borderline ovarian tumors, especially those of the mucinous subtype. We found that K-*ras* mutations were present in 63% of mucinous BOTs and 75% of invasive mucinous ovarian cancers.[11] These data suggest that K-*ras* mutations are involved in the development of mucinous BOTs and support the notion that mucinous BOTs may represent a pathological continuum between benign and frankly malignant mucinous cancers. In contrast to mucinous tumors, both serous BOTs and serous invasive ovarian cancers demonstrated a lower K-*ras* mutation rate. Serous BOTs showed a significantly higher K-*ras* mutation rate than serous invasive cancers (36% versus 6%, $P = 0.0008$). These data suggest that serous BOTs and invasive carcinomas may have different pathogenesis pathways, and only a small percentage of BOTs may progress to invasive cancers.

SSCP analysis was also performed on BOTs and invasive ovarian cancers using primers flanking exon 2 to 11 of the *p53* gene. The results are summarized in Fig. 14.3. *p53* gene mutations are uncommon in BOTs. In our study, none of the 32 serous BOTs

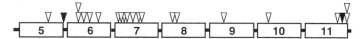

Fig. 14.3 Spectrum of *p53* mutations in borderline (▼) and invasive ovarian tumors ({open inverted triangle}) along exon 5 to exon 11 of the *p53* gene.

demonstrated mutations in the *p53* gene. This is in contrast to invasive serous ovarian tumors, which demonstrated a *p53* mutation rate of 60%. Among mucinous tumors, 2 of 15 (13%) BOTs had mutations in *p53*, compared to 40% of the invasive mucinous cancers.[12] This further suggests that mucinous BOTs and mucinous invasive carcinomas may represent a continuum.

Loss of heterozygosity on multiple chromosome arms

Loss of heterozygosity has been used widely to define minimally deleted regions where tumor suppressor genes may reside. Using 105 microsatellite markers to perform detailed deletion mapping on chromosomes 1, 3, 6, 7, 9, 11, 17, and X in BOTs, invasive ovarian cancers, and serous surface carcinoma of the ovary (SSC), we identified several common loss regions. The results are summarized in Table 14.1. Besides the androgen receptor (AR) locus on the X chromosome,[13] BOTs showed significantly lower LOH rates (0–18%) in all loci screened, suggesting that LOH at autosomes is less significant in the development of BOTs. Significance in LOH at the AR locus in BOTs and invasive cancers remains to be determined.

LOH at the *p73* locus on 1p36 was found in both high-and low-grade ovarian carcinomas as well as in the surface serous carcinomas, but not in borderline ovarian tumors. LOH rates at 3p25, 6q25.1–26, and 7q31.3 were significantly higher in high-grade serous carcinomas, as compared to low-grade serous carcinomas, mucinous carcinomas, and borderline tumors.[14–16] LOH rates at a 9 cM region on 6q23–24 were significantly higher in surface serous carcinoma than in serous ovarian tumors.[17] LOH at a 4 cM region on chromosome 11p15.1 and an 11 cM region on chromosome 11p15.5 was found only in serous invasive tumors. Furthermore, LOH rates in these two regions were significantly higher in high-grade serous tumors than in low-grade serous tumors.[18] Multiple, minimally deleted regions have been identified on chromosome 17. Significantly higher LOH rates were identified at the *p53* locus on 17p13.1 and the *NF1* locus on 17q11.1 in high-grade serous carcinomas, as compared to low-grade and borderline serous tumors and all mucinous tumors.[19] LOH at the region between THRA1 and D17S1327, including the *BRCA1* locus on 17q21, was found exclusively in high-grade serous tumors.[20] The finding of significantly higher LOH rates at multiple chromosomal sites in serous compared to mucinous subtypes suggests that serous and mucinous tumors may have different pathogenetic pathways.

Differential expression patterns of novel and known genes

Using RNA fingerprinting, reverse transcriptase polymerase chain reaction (RT-PCR), Northern blot analysis, Western blot analysis, and immunohistochemistry, we have identified several novel and known genes that are expressed differentially among normal ovarian surface epithelial cells, the epithelial lining of benign ovarian cysts, serous and mucinous BOTs, and invasive ovarian cancers. The results are summarized in Table 14.2.

Using RNA fingerprinting, several differentially expressed sequences which are downregulated in ovarian cancer cells have been identified.[21,22] Subsequent cloning and sequencing showed that one of them corresponds to an extracellular matrix protein, osteonectin (SPARC). SPARC has been demonstrated to suppress ovarian carcinoma cell growth *in vitro* and *in vivo*.[23] Immunohistochemistry has been performed to evaluate the differential expression patterns of SPARC in normal ovary, and benign, borderline, and invasive ovarian tumor tissues. High levels of SPARC expression were observed in normal ovarian surface epithelium and in the epithelial lining of benign cysts and cystadenomas. In comparison, both serous and mucinous BOTs had a lower expression, and serous and mucinous invasive carcinomas had an even lower expression.

Another differentially expressed gene that has been identified and characterized is a novel gene named *DOC-2/hDAB2*.[24] This gene encodes a 105 kDa signal transduction protein which contains a phosphotyrosine interacting domain (PID) and multiple SH3 binding motifs. *In situ* immunohistochemistry was performed on normal ovaries, benign ovarian cysts and cystadenomas, BOTs, and invasive serous and mucinous ovarian cancers. The results showed that the surface epithelium of the ovaries and the epithelial lining of benign cysts and cystadenomas demonstrated high levels of *DOC-2/hDAB2* expression. A significantly lower level of expression was identified in both high-grade and low-grade serous invasive carcinomas. In contrast, both mucinous BOTs and invasive carcinomas showed high levels of *DOC-2/hDAB2* expression.[24] When *DOC-2/hDAB2* was transfected into the ovarian carcinoma cell line which has been shown to downregulate *DOC-2/hDAB2*, the stable transfectants showed significantly reduced growth rate and diminished ability to form tumors in nude mice. These data suggest that downregulation of *DOC-2/hDAB2* may play an important role in the development of serous ovarian tumors. They also imply that serous and mucinous ovarian tumors may have different pathogenetic pathways.

Expression of several hormone receptor genes, including estrogen receptor-alpha (ER-α), estrogen receptor-beta (ER-β), androgen receptor (AR), and progesterone receptor (PR) has also been examined in normal ovaries, benign cysts, and cystadenomas, and invasive carcinomas by RT-PCR and immunohistochemistry. Both ER-α and ER-β are expressed at high levels in the surface epithelium of normal ovaries, in the epithelial lining of benign tumors, in BOTs and invasive carcinomas.[25] In contrast, AR was expressed at significantly lower levels in invasive carcinomas than in borderline and benign tumors, and PR was expressed at significantly lower levels in both BOTs and invasive carcinomas. These results

Table 14.1 Percentage of loss of heterozygosity at different sites in serous (S) and mucicus (M) borderline tumors (BOT); low-grade (L) and high-grade (H) invasive epithelial ovarian tumors (IEOC); and surface serous carcinomas (SSC)

Chromosome sites	Flanking loci	Physical/genetic distance	BOT S	BOT M	IEOC S L	IEOC S H	IEOC M L	IEOC M H	SSC	Reference
1p36	p73				▲	▲			▲	
					▲	▲	▲	?	▲	
3p25	D3S1038–THRB					▲				
			▲			▲	▲	▲	?	14
						▲				
6q25.1–26	D6S473–D6S448	4 cM				▲			▲	
			▲	▲	▲	▲	▲	?	▲	15
6q23–24	D6S250–ESR	9 cM							▲	
			▲	▲	▲	▲	▲	?	▲	17
7q31.3	D7S655–D7S480	1300 kb				▲				
					▲	▲	▲			16
11p15.1	D11S926–D11S899	4 cM	▲	▲	▲	▲	▲	?	?	
						▲				18
					▲	▲			?	
11p15.5	D11S2071–D11S988	11 cM				▲				
					▲	▲			?	18
17p13.1	p53					▲				
					▲	▲			▲	19
			▲	▲	▲	▲	▲	?	▲	
17q11.1	CHRNB1–D17S250					▲				
					▲	▲				19
					▲	▲			?	
17q21	D17S1320–D17S1328	400 kb			▲	▲	▲			
					▲	▲	▲			20
					▲	▲	▲			
17q21	THRA1–D17S1327					▲		▲		
						▲		▲		19
					▲	?	?	▲		
17q21	D17S1327–D17S588					▲				
					▲	▲	▲	▲		19
Xq11.2–q12	D11S926–D11S899	1 cM	▲	▲	▲	▲	▲	?	▲	
			▲	▲		▲				13
			▲	▲	▲	▲	?	?	?	

▲, 1–25% ▲, 26–50% ▲ 51–75%

suggest that downregulation of AR may be important for the development of invasive carcinomas and downregulation of PR may be important for the development of both BOTs and invasive carcinomas.

Several genes that are overexpressed in ovarian tumors have been identified. Using RNA fingerprinting, we isolated a novel cDNA which is highly expressed in ovarian cancer cells.[26] The encoded protein is highly homologous to trypsin and members of

Table 14.2 Levels of expression of multiple genes in normal ovarian surface epittelium (HOSE), epithelial lining of benign cysts and cystadenomas, serous (S) and mucinos (M) borderline ovarian tumors (BOT), low-grade (L) and high-grade (H) invasive epithelial ovarian tumors (IEOC)

Gene name	Normal HOSE	Benign cyst	BOT S	BOT M	IEOC S L	IEOC S H	IEOC M L	IEOC M H	Reference
SPARC Osteonectin	▲▲▲▲	▲▲▲▲	▲▲	▲▲	▲▲	▲	▲▲	▲	22
DOC-2/ hDAB2	▲▲▲▲	▲▲▲▲	▲▲	▲▲▲▲	▲		▲▲▲▲	▲▲▲	23
Bcl-2	▲▲▲▲	▲▲▲▲	▲▲▲	▲▲▲	▲▲	▲▲	▲▲	▲▲	
AR	▲▲▲▲	▲▲▲▲	▲▲▲	▲▲▲	▲▲	▲▲	▲▲	▲▲	
PR	▲▲▲▲	▲▲▲▲	▲▲	▲▲	▲	▲	▲	▲	
Protease M			▲▲	▲	▲▲▲▲	▲▲▲▲	▲▲▲▲	?	25,26
p53					▲▲	▲▲▲	▲▲	▲▲	18
p73		?	▲▲▲	▲▲	▲▲▲▲	▲▲▲	▲▲▲	?	
HER-2/neu	▲	▲▲	▲▲	▲▲	▲▲▲	▲▲▲	▲▲▲	▲▲▲	27

Percentage of positive staining cells/levels of expression:
▲, 1–25%; ▲, 26–50% ▲, 51–75% ▲, 76–100%

the kallikrein protease family. The novel protease, named Protease M, was demonstrated by RT-PCR and Western blot analysis to be highly expressed in more than 90% of ovarian tumors, particularly in invasive carcinomas. High levels of expression were also detected in a majority of Stage I tumors. In addition, Protease M has been shown to be secreted and detectable in the conditioned media culturing the tumor cells.[27] These findings suggest that Protease M may have a great potential as a serum marker for both early detection of ovarian cancer and for monitoring response of ovarian cancer patients, similar to the use of another kallikrein member, prostate-specific antigen (PSA), in prostate cancer management.

Expression of *p53* and *HER-2/neu* was also examined in normal ovaries, benign ovarian cysts and cystadenomas, borderline and invasive ovarian tumors by immunohistochemistry and Western blot analysis. Overexpression of *p53* was detected in 60% of high-grade invasive carcinomas and in 40% of low-grade invasive carcinomas. In contrast, overexpression of *p53* was not observed in any of the borderline tumors, benign tumors, or normal ovaries. Overexpression of *HER-2/neu* has been described in ovarian cancers and has been shown to correlate with poor prognosis of the disease.[28] Using an *anti-HER-2/neu* polyclonal antibody (Dako, Carpinteria, California, USA), *HER-2/neu* overexpression was detected in 10% of benign ovarian tumors, 18% of BOTs, and 52% of invasive ovarian carcinomas.[29] These findings suggest that overexpression of *HER-2/neu* may be an early event in the development of a subset of ovarian tumors.

p73 is a gene that exhibits high sequence homology and similar gene structure to the tumor suppressor gene *p53* . *p73* shares 29% amino-acid identity in the N-terminal transactivation domain of *p53*, 63% identity in the specific DNA-binding region, and 38% identity in the oligomerization domain.[30] When overexpressed in transfection systems, *p73* can transactivate *p53*-responsive genes and induce apoptosis. However, unlike *p53*, *p73* is not induced by radiation-mediated DNA damage. *p73* resides on chromosome 1p36.33, a region where frequent abnormalities have been detected in ovarian carcinomas. We analyzed this gene in a group of ovarian cancer cell lines and ovarian tumor tissues. Preliminary data showed a 50% loss of heterozygosity rate at the *p73* locus in invasive ovarian cancers, but not in borderline ovarian tumors. However, mutation of the *p73* gene was not identified. RT-PCR and Western blot analysis showed that borderline and invasive ovarian tumors have significantly higher levels of *p73* expression than normal ovarian surface epithelial cells. These findings suggest that upregulation of *p73* may be involved in the development of borderline and invasive ovarian tumors.

Conclusion and future directions

Data from our genetic studies suggest that in the mucinous subtype of ovarian tumors, progression may occur from benign to borderline and to invasive tumors. In the serous subtype, we believe that borderline and invasive tumors may have different pathogenesis pathways. By using new technologies such laser capture microdissection,[31] we can study these specimens in which benign, borderline and invasive components coexist. Furthermore, we can study those microscopic high-grade serous tumors that lack evidence for a pre-malignant phenotype. Identifying specific genetic changes in each component may aid in establishing pathways for ovarian carcinogenesis. Ultimately, we hope that findings from these studies will add to our knowledge of the very early events in the development of epithelial ovarian cancer, and provide markers for early diagnosis of this disease.

References

1. Greggi, S., Genuardi, M., Benedetti-Panici, P. *et al.* (1990). Analysis of 138 consecutive ovarian cancer patients; incidence and characteristics of familial cases. *Gynecol. Oncol.*, **39**, 300–4.
2. Houlston, R.S., Collins, A., Slack, J. *et al.* (1991). Genetic epidemiology of ovarian cancer: segration analysis. *Ann. Hum. Genet.*, **55**, 291–9.
3. Narod, S.A., Madlensky, L., Bradley, L. *et al.* (1994). Hereditary and familial ovarian cancer in Southern Ontario. *Cancer*, **74**, 2341–6.
4. Campbell, I.G., Morland, S., Hitchcock, A. *et al.* (1998). Endometriosis and the relationship with ovarian cancer. In *Ovarian cancer 5*, (eds. F. Sharp, T. Blackett, J. Derek, and R. Bast), pp. 159–70. ISIS Medical Media Ltd, Oxford.
5. Obata, K., Morland, S.J., Watson, R.H. *et al.* (1998). Frequent PTEN/MMAC mutations in endometrioid but not serous or mucinous epithelial ovarian tumors. *Cancer Res.*, **58**, 2059–97.
6. Bell, D.A. and Scully, R.E. (1994). Early de novo ovarian carcinoma. *Cancer*, **73**, 1859–64.
7. Schorge, J. and Mok, S.C. (1999). Understanding the pathogenesis of primary peritoneal carcinoma: involvement of the BRCA1 and p53 genes. *Hum. Pathol*, **30**, 115–16.
8. Lu, K.H., Bell, D.A., Welch, W.R. *et al.* (1998). Evidence for the multifocal origin of bilateral and advanced human serous borderline ovarian tumors. *Cancer Res.*, **58**, 2328–30.
9. Jacobs, I.J., Kohler, M.F., Wiseman, R.W. *et al.* (1992). Clonal origin of epithelial ovarian carcinoma: analysis by loss of heterozygosity, p53 mutation, and X chromosome inactivation. *J. Natl Cancer Inst.*, **84**, 298–300.
10. Mok, C.H., Tsao, S.W., Knapp, R.C. *et al.* (1992). Unifocal origin of advanced human epithelial ovarian cancers. *Cancer Res*, **52**, 5119–22.
11. Mok, S.C., Bell, D.A., Knapp, R.C. *et al.* (1993). Mutation of K-ras protooncogene in human ovarian epithelial tumors of borderline malignancy. *Cancer Res.*, **53**, 1489–92.
12. Wertheim, I., Muto, M.G., Welch, W.R. *et al.* (1994). p53 gene mutation in human borderline epithelial ovarian tumors. *J. Natl Cancer Inst.*, **86**, 1549–51.
13. Edelson, M.I., Lau, C.C., Colitti, C.V. *et al.* (1998). A one centimorgan deletion unit on chromosome Xq12 is commonly lost in borderline and invasive epithelial ovarian tumors. *Oncogene*, **16**, 197–202.
14. Tangir, J., Loughridge, N.S., Berkowitz, R.S. *et al.* (1996). Frequent microsatellite instability in epithelial borderline ovarian tumors. *Cancer Res.*, **56**, 2501–5.
15. Colitti, C.V., Rodabaugh, K.J., Welch, W.R. *et al.* (1998). A novel 4 cM minimal deletion unit on chromosome 6q25.1–q25.2 associated with high grade invasive epithelial ovarian carcinomas. *Oncogene*, **16**, 555–9.
16. Edelson, M.I., Scherer, S.W., Tsui, L.C. *et al.* (1997). Identification of a 1300 kilobase deletion unit on chromosome 7q31.3 in invasive epithelial ovarian carcinomas. *Oncogene*, **14**, 2979–84.
17. Huang, L.W., Garrett, A.P., Schorge, J.O. *et al.* (1999). Detailed mapping of chromosome 6q in papillary serous carcinoma of the peritoneum compared with high grade late stage invasive serous epithelial ovarian carcinomas. *Proc. Am. Assoc. Cancer Res.*, **40**, 543–4.
18. Lu, K.H., Weitzel, J.N., Srilatha, K. *et al.* (1997). A novel 4-cM minimally deleted region on chromosome 11p15.1 associated with high grade nonmucinous epithelial ovarian carcinomas. *Cancer Res.*, **57**, 387–90.
19. Wertheim, I., Tangir, J., Muto, M.G. *et al.* (1996). Loss of heterozygosity of chromosome 17 in human borderline and invasive epithelial ovarian tumors. *Oncogene*, **12**, 2147–53.
20. Tangir, J., Muto, M.G., Berkowitz, R.S. *et al.* (1996). A 400 kb novel deletion unit centromeric to the BRCA1 gene in sporadic epithelial ovarian cancer. *Oncogene*, **12**, 735–40.
21. Mok, S.C., Wong, K.K., Chan, R.K.W. *et al.* (1994). Molecular cloning of differentially expressed genes in human epithelial ovarian cancer. *Gynecol. Oncol.*, **52**, 247–52.

22. Welsh, J., Chada, K., Dalal, S.S. *et al.* (1992). Arbitrarily primed PCR fingerprinting of RNA. *Nucleic Acids Res.*, **20**, 7213–18.

23. Mok, S.C., Chan, W.Y., Wong, K.K. *et al.* (1996). SPARC, an extracellular matrix protein with tumor-suppressing activity in human ovarian epithelial cells. *Oncogene*, **12**, 1895–901.

24. Mok, S.C., Chan, W.Y., Wong, K.K. *et al.* (1996). DOC-2, a candidate tumor suppressor gene in human epithelial ovarian cancer. *Oncogene*, **16**, 2381–7.

25. Lau, K.M., Mok, S.C. and Ho, S.M. (1999). Expression of human estrogen receptor-α and -β, progesterone receptor, and androgen receptor mRNA in normal and malignant ovarian epithelial cells. *Proc. Natl Acad. Sci. USA*, in press.

26. Anisowicz, A., Sotiropoulou, G., Stenman, G. *et al.* (1996). A novel protease homolog differentially expressed in breast and ovarian cancer. *Mol. Med.*, **2**, 624–36.

27. Colitti, C.V., Yiu, G.K., Ng, S.W. *et al.* (1998). Identification of a novel protease gene overexpressed in invasive ovarian carcinomas. *Proc. Am. Assoc. Cancer Res.*, **39**, 118.

28. Tanner, B., Kreutz, E., Weikel, W. *et al.* (1996). Prognostic significance of c-erbB-2 mRNA in ovarian carcinoma. *Gynecol. Oncol.*, **62**, 268–77.

29. Schorge, J.O., Su, A.L., Colitti, C.V. *et al.* (1999). EGF family protein expression in patients with papillary serous carcinoma of the peritoneum. *Proc. Am. Assoc. Cancer Res.*, **40**, 377.

30. Kaghad, M., Bonnet, H., Yang, A. *et al.* (1997). Monoallelically expressed gene related to p53 at 1p36, a region frequently deleted in neuroblastoma and other human cancers. *Cell*, **90**, 809–19.

31. Bonner, R.F., Emmert-Buck, M., Cole, K. *et al.* (1997). Laser capture microdissection: Molecular analysis of tissue. *Science*, **278**, 1481–3.

Part 3
Tumour biology

15. The application of novel technology to the study of ovarian cancer

Monica R. Brown, Michael Emmert-Buck, David B. Krizman, Emmanuel Petricoin, Lance A. Liotta, and Elise C. Kohn

Introduction

Advances in technology are yielding new directions for studying the molecular mechanisms of ovarian carcinogenesis. To date, this information has been gained through examination of cultured cells and through the use of animal models. One of the limitations of molecular analysis from cells grown in culture is the difficulty in determining the contribution of the surrounding stroma to the malignant phenotype.[1] Analysis of ovarian epithelial cell populations as they exist in their native tissue environment may provide insight into genes, proteins, and signal transduction pathways critical to ovarian cancer development and progression. Several technologies have been developed that may aid in the simultaneous molecular assessment of multiple genes and proteins from tissue-derived cells. The generation of genetic and protein profiles specifically from epithelial ovarian cells may guide the development of therapeutic targets and biomarkers focused to ovarian cancer. We have applied recent advances in technology to improve the sensitivity of a traditional genomic assay, and to define genetic and proteomic profiles in epithelial ovarian cancer.

Microdissection

Ovarian neoplasms are histologically and biologically heterogeneous. In addition to neoplastic cells, histologic sections also contain fibroblasts, inflammatory, vascular, and occasionally non-malignant epithelial cells. It has been demonstrated that molecular interactions between cancer cells and their surrounding stroma contribute to the malignant phenotype. Thus, studying ovarian epithelial cells and their surrounding stromal cells *in situ* may provide insight into these interactions. Various microdissection techniques have been used for the acquisition of selected cell populations to investigate the contribution of these cells to the neoplastic phenotype. Hand microdissection, one of the earliest forms of microdissection, requires a sterile glass pipette tip or needle to obtain desired cells under direct microscopic visualization.[2] Although select cell populations are removed with this technique, fragments of microdissected cells frequently contaminate surrounding cells. This contamination may limit the sensitivity and specificity of assay results.

Hand microdissection has been made more precise by micromanipulator instrumentation; however, the limitations of adjacent cell contamination remain.[3] As the use of lasers in medicine and science has increased, the adaptation of laser technology to microdissection has improved the precision of mechanical microdissection. Ultraviolet ablation of undesired cells, as initially described by Shibata *et al.*,[4] is a two-step process, in which the desired cells are delineated by a protective pigment, and the unwanted cells are subsequently ablated by an ultraviolet laser. The remaining cells are microdissected manually as described previously. This technique adds an element of specificity to microdissection and reduces the risk of contamination. Adjacent epithelium is, however, destroyed and therefore unavailable for later analysis.

Our laboratory has developed and applied a low-energy infrared laser as a tool for selective cell procurement from tissue sections. Laser capture microdissection (LCM) utilizes a microfuge tube cap that has been modified by placement of a thermoplastic film on its undersurface. The cells of interest are visualized microscopically and the cap is placed in direct opposition to the cells. The desired cells become fused to the thermoplastic film upon activation of the laser.[5] Captured cells are suspended in extraction buffer for further downstream molecular applications. A homogeneous population is obtained in a single step, without contamination of adjacent tissue. The surrounding histological architecture is maintained and available for future microdissections. The current LCM prototype uses 30–60 μm laser diameters that are particularly suited for microdissection of 10–15 μm epithelial ovarian cells (Fig. 15.1). We have used LCM-derived ovarian tissues for genomic, genetic, and proteomic applications. Our goal is the identification of genes and proteins specific for ovarian cancers.

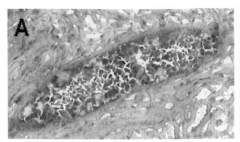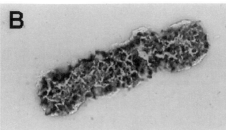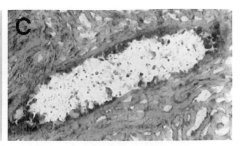

Fig. 15.1 Laser capture microdissection of invasive ovarian epithelial cancer cells. Digitalized images of an invasive, poorly differentiated epithelial ovarian cancer. (A) Ovarian epithelial cancer cells with surrounding stroma as visualized prior to microdissection; (B) cap image of procured tumor cells adherent to the thermoplastic transfer film; (C) surrounding stroma after removal of the tumor focus.

Genomics

Ovarian cancers occur as a result of multiple genetic alterations. Mutations in tumor suppressor genes such as p53 and oncogenes such as *AKT2* have been demonstrated.[6,7] Amplification of c-erbB2 and PIK3CA, the latter of which encodes the catalytic subunit of phosphatidylinositol 3-kinase, has also been shown to occur in ovarian cancers.[8,9] The identification of putative tumor suppressor gene loci has been facilitated by loss of heterozygosity analysis (LOH). LOH analysis utilizes microsatellite repeats that map to specific chromosomal loci to identify minimal genomic deletion regions. LOH frequency of greater than 35% in a defined study population is considered to exceed the rates of random genomic instability and thereby suggests the presence of a tumor suppressor gene(s) at a particular chromosomal locus.[10]

Ovarian cancers have been shown to exhibit allelic loss at many chromosomal loci, including 6q27, 9p21, 11p15, 14q12, 17p13.3, and 17q12–25 among others.[11–16] Few studies have examined the frequency of allelic loss on chromosome 8. We were interested in this chromosome, particularly the region of 8p12–21, because we have recently demonstrated LOH in 7 of 9 ovarian cancer patients with known *BRCA1* mutations.[17] We hypothesized that this event may also occur in sporadic forms of ovarian cancer and examined 45 unselected ovarian tumors for LOH in this region.

DNA was isolated from 1500 microdissected normal and stromal cells and amplified with microsatellite markers spanning the region of 8p12–22. Fifty-eight per cent of the cases exhibited LOH in this region. The highest frequency of loss, 15 of 30 informative cases (50%), was demonstrated at marker D8S136 which maps to 8p21 (Fig. 15.2).[18] A previous study, which used bulk tissues for DNA isolation, reported an LOH frequency of 31% at this locus.[19] This confirms the added sensitivity for detecting LOH achieved from microdissection of ovarian tumors and suggests a tumor suppressor gene at this locus. Efforts to further refine the minimal interval and identify the gene are under way.

Genetics

In addition to genomic studies, expression technologies have advanced our understanding of ovarian cancer genetics. For example, differential display, an RNA-based method, was used by Yu *et al.* to clone NOEY2.[20] This gene was shown to be absent in breast and ovarian cancers and present in their normal counterparts, supporting its role as a putative tumor suppressor gene for these cancers. Differential display and other classical techniques, such as subtractive hybridization, have been useful tools for identifying single genes that may participate in cancer development. More recent cDNA library construction techniques coupled with high throughput automated sequencing has facilitated the identification of multiple genes or gene profiles in several human cancers.[21] cDNA libraries contain genes or gene fragments (expressed sequence tags) that are expressed in a given cell population. cDNA libraries developed from homogeneous cell populations have the advantage of selective gene representation for that particular cell type. We hypothesize that the construction of cDNA libraries from microdissected ovarian samples may lead to the identification of novel genes or gene profiles specific for ovarian cancer.[22, 23]

To investigate this hypothesis, we constructed cDNA libraries from 10 000 LCM-derived ovarian epithelial cells. Total RNA was isolated from these cells and primed with oligo-dT and strand switch primers to create single-stranded cDNA. The second-strand cDNA was created by PCR amplification of the first strand with selected primers. PCR products above 300 bp were selected and inserted into a unidirectional cloning vector.[23]

The clones were submitted to the Cancer Genome Anatomy Project (CGAP), an initiative of the National Cancer Institute committed to the identification of the genes expressed in cancer progression. Through this initiative, cDNA libraries are being created for normal, pre-malignant, malignant, and metastatic cell populations, where available. The five tumor types targeted include breast, prostate, colon, lung, and ovary cancers. The clones are arrayed and sequenced by extramural collaborators after the libraries are constructed, and the sequences are returned to CGAP. In addition to making the sequences available to the general public through the CGAP website (http://www.ncbi.nlm.nih.gov/ncicgap) they are arranged into unigene clusters based on sequence homology at the 3' end of the transcripts.

We were interested in the unigene clusters specific for microdissected ovary libraries. At the time of our analysis, four invasive ovarian cancer libraries, and three low malignant potential (LMP) ovarian tumor libraries were available. All the libraries analyzed

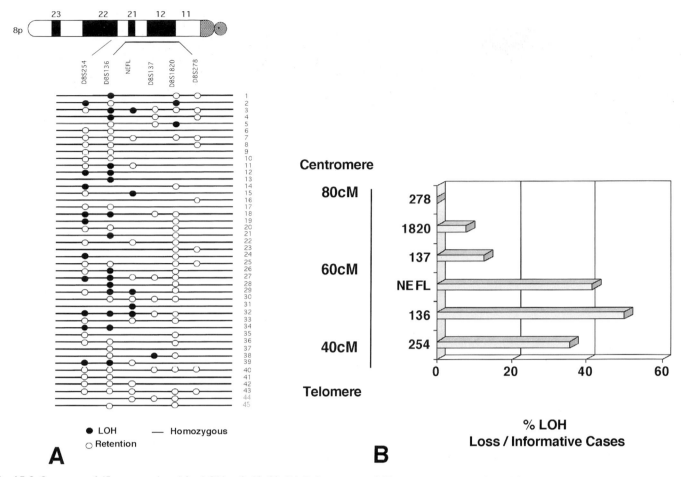

Fig. 15.2 Summary of 45 cases analyzed for LOH at 8p12–22. (A) Deletion map of 45 ovarian tumors evaluated for LOH on chromosome 8p. Cases 1–40 are ovarian tumors. Cases 41–45 are low malignant potential tumors. Microsatellite marker location is shown at the top of the figure. Closed circles represent allelic loss in the tumor, open circles represent allelic retention, and a straight line represents homozygous cases. (B) Histogram showing allelic loss frequency at each of the microsatellite markers evaluated, as well as their estimated location (in centimorgans) from the centromere of chromosome 8.

were of papillary serous histology, and all libraries, except one, were from cases at an advanced stage. Approximately 7000 sequences in total were read from the seven libraries analyzed. We examined the CGAP database for genes and/or expressed sequence tags (ESTs) exclusive to the microdissected ovarian cancer libraries. This preliminary analysis generated 801 unigenes, half of which segregated to the LMP libraries and half to invasive libraries. We next asked how many unigenes were present in microdissected ovary cancer libraries and absent in all other libraries in the database. This represented a comparison of 7000 sequences from the microdissected ovarian cancer libraries with over 500 000 sequences within the CGAP database. This generated 107 unigenes, 69 of which were unknown or novel ESTs. A similar analysis was performed by Vasmatzis *et al.* for prostate cDNA libraries, and 15 novel transcripts were identified and determined to be prostate specific.[21] Our analysis of the ovarian cancer libraries is ongoing and validation of our findings is under way. Identifying ovary-specific transcripts may provide useful candidates for genetic markers for this cancer.

Proteomics

Biomarkers specific for ovarian cancer are needed, in addition to genetic marker development, for diagnosis, disease progression determination, and to follow patient outcome. Many of the currently available markers were developed from antibodies raised to antigens on ovarian cancer cell lines.[24] Several obstacles have challenged ovarian cancer-specific tumor marker development. The limited resource of normal ovarian tissues and early stage tumors has made the identification of proteins and protein profiles unique to ovarian cancer patients difficult.

LCM has been coupled with two-dimensional polyacrylamide gel electrophoresis (2-D PAGE) and surface-enhanced laser desorption and ionization (SELDI) analysis to overcome some of the above limitations. 2-D PAGE permits the separation of proteins by charge in the first electrophoretic dimension and by molecular weight in the second dimension. The first dimension separates proteins along a pH gradient until they reach a position of neutral

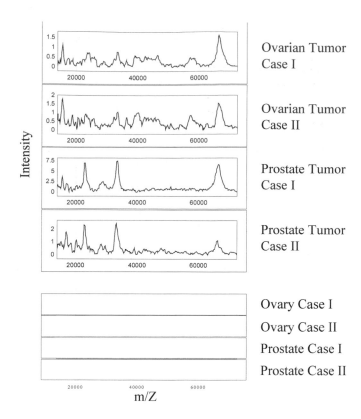

Ovarian Tumor Case I

Ovarian Tumor Case II

Prostate Tumor Case I

Prostate Tumor Case II

Ovary Case I

Ovary Case II

Prostate Case I

Prostate Case II

m/Z

Fig. 15.3 SELDI analysis of two ovarian and two prostate carcinomas. The data generated from SELDI analysis of cell lysates may be viewed by direct mass map (top panel) or by a gel view (bottom panel). The laser intensity required to generate a mass map for the proteins within a population of cells is plotted against the molecular weight. The similarities and differences in protein fingerprints between and within tumors may be appreciated.

charge called the isoelectric point. After isoelectric focusing is complete, the proteins are separated by molecular weight using sodium dodecyl sulfate polyacrylamide gel electrophoresis (SDS-PAGE) followed by silver nitrate staining.[25] Staining of two-dimensional gels with special stains, such as zinc imidizole, permits removal of peptides directly from the gel for mass spectroscopy analysis and protein identification. These gels are analyzed to generate a fingerprint for a particular cell population. This application requires 50 000 microdissected cells or 10 000 laser shots. The sensitivity of 2-D PAGE declines for proteins of 7000 Da or less. Although 2-D PAGE is limited by its requirement for a large number of cells and decreased sensitivity for small molecular weight proteins, the ability to microsequence proteins directly from these gels is an important advantage of this technique.

Recently we have used SELDI analysis to generate protein profiles from as few as 200–300 microdissected cells. The lysates of these cells are applied to an aluminum chip containing 1–2 mm foci of chemical 'bait'. The composition of the chemical bait is based upon the chemical nature of the protein class that is being targeted. For example, hydrophobic, hydrophilc, aliphatic, and aromatic chips may be used to evaluate proteins of comparable chemical composition. After the cell lysate is applied to the foci of

chemical bait, washing conditions designed to optimize the formation of protein-to-chip complexes are used. Laser activation promotes desorption and ionization of bound peptides from the matrix. A mass detector senses the time of flight of bound proteins from the chip and a mass map is generated (Fig. 15.3). Although this technique is not strictly quantitative and lacks the ability to identify specific proteins, it is capable of detecting protein concentrations in the attamole concentration range (10^{-18} moles) and can discriminate protein mass within 100 Da. We are currently using SELDI to define protein fingerprints for breast, prostate, colon, and ovarian cancers.[26] SELDI analysis of microdissected tumors may be used to create protein profiles that, after analysis, may reveal unique protein patterns specific for a given tumor type. This technique may aid the determination of specific disease states.

Conclusions

We have demonstrated how novel technologies may be used for the genomic, genetic, and proteomic study of ovarian cancer. Using these new approaches we have identified a putative tumor suppressor gene locus at 8p21, generated ovary-specific ESTs, and are now developing protein fingerprints specific for ovarian cancer. Molecular analysis from tissue-derived samples may provide insight into molecular events specific to ovarian cancer. This information should be useful for the generation of ovary-specific genetic and serum biomarkers. Rational therapeutic targets and diagnostics may translate into improved morbidity and mortality for patients with ovarian cancer.

References

1. Price, J.T., Bonovich, M.T., and Kohn, E.C. (1997). The biochemistry of cancer dissemination. *Crit. Rev. Biochem. Mol. Biol.*, **32**, 175–253.
2. Zhuang, Z., Bertheau, P., Emmert-Buck, M.R. *et al.* (1995). A microdissection technique for archival DNA analysis of specific cell populations in lesions less that one millimeter in size. *Am. J. Pathol.*, **146**, 620–5.
3. Going, J. and Lamb, R.F. (1996). Practical histologic microdissection for PCR analysis. *J. Pathol.*, **179**, 121–4.
4. Shibata, D., Hawes, D., and Li, Z.H. (1992). Specific genetic analysis of microscopic tissue after selective ultraviolet radiation, fractionation, and polymerase chain reaction. *Am. J. Pathol.*, **141**, 539–43.
5. Emmert-Buck, M.R., Bonner, R.F., Smith, P.D. *et al.* (1996). Laser capture microdissection. *Science*, **274**, 998–1001.
6. Marks, J.R., Davidoff, A.M., Kerns, B.J. *et al.* (1991). Overexpression and mutation of p53 in epithelial ovarian cancer. *Cancer Res.*, **51**, 2979–84.
7. Bellacosa, A., de Feo, D., Godwin, A.K. *et al.* (1995). Molecular alterations of the AKT2 oncogene in ovarian and breast carcinomas. *Int. J. Cancer*, **64**, 280–5.
8. Slamon, D.J., Godolphin, W., Jones, L.A. *et al.* (1989). Studies of HER–2/neu proto-oncogene in human breast and ovarian cancer. *Science*, **244**, 707–12.
9. Shayesteh, L., Lu, Y., Kuo, W.L. *et al.* (1999). PIK3CA is implicated as an oncogene in ovarian cancer. *Nature Genet.*, **21**, 99–102.
10. Cliby, W., Ritland, S., Hartman, L. *et al.* (1993). Human epithelial cancer allelotype. *Cancer Res.*, **53**, 2393–8.
11. Saito, S., Sirahama, S., Matsushima, M. *et al.* (1996). Definition of a commonly deleted region in ovarian cancers to a 300 kb segment of chromosome 6q27. *Cancer Res.*, **56**, 5586–9.

12. Cooke, I.E., Shelling, A.N., Le Meuth, V.G. *et al.* (1996). Allele loss on chromosome arm 6q and fine mapping of the region at 6q27 in epithelial ovarian cancer. *Gen. Chrom. Cancer*, **15**, 223–33.

13. Rodabaugh, K.J., Qureshi, J.A., Barrett, A.J. *et al.* (1995). Detailed deletion mapping of chromosome 9p and p16 gene alterations in human borderline and invasive epithelial ovarian tumors. *Oncogene*, **11**, 1249–54.

14. Lu, K.H., Weitzel, J.N., Kodali, S. *et al.* (1997). A novel 4-cM minimally deleted region on chromosome 11p15.1 associated with high grade nonmucinous epithelial ovarian carcinomas. *Cancer Res.*, **57**, 387–90.

15. Tangir, J., Muto, M.G., Berkowitz, R.S. *et al.* (1996). A 400 kb novel deletion unit centromeric to the BRCA1 gene in sporadic epithelial ovarian cancer. *Oncogene*, **12**, 735–40.

16. Phillips, N.J., Ziegler, M.R., Radford, D.M. *et al.* (1996). Allelic deletion on chromosome 17p13.3 in early cancer. *Cancer Res.*, **56**, 606–11.

17. Emmert-Buck, M.R., Weiss, R., DiFranco, E. *et al.* (1998). Allelic loss on chromosome 8p in BRCA1 mutation positive breast/ovarian cancers. *Breast J.*, **4**, 9–12.

18. Brown, M.R., Chuaqui, R., Vocke, C.D. *et al.* (1999). Allelic loss on chromosome arm 8p: Analysis of low malignant potential and invasive epithelial ovarian tumors. *Gynecol. Oncol.*, **74**, 98–102.

19. Wright, K., Wilson, P.J., Kerr, J. *et al.* (1998). Frequent loss of heterozygosity and three critical regions on the short arm of chromosome 8 in ovarian adenocarcinomas. *Oncogene*, **17**, 2715–19.

20. Yu, U., Xu, F., Peng, H. *et al.* (1999). NOEY2 (ARHI), an imprinted putative tumor suppressor gene in ovarian and breast carcinomas. *Proc. Natl Acad. Sci. USA*, **96**, 214–19.

21. Vasmatzi, G., Essand, M., Brinkmann, U. *et al.* (1998). Discovery of three genes specifically expressed in human prostate by expressed sequence tag database analysis. *Proc. Natl Acad. Sci. USA*, **95**, 300–4.

22. Krizman, D., Chuaqui, R., Meltzer, P.S. *et al.* (1996). Construction of a representative cDNA library from prostatic intraepithelial neoplasia (PIN). *Cancer Res.*, **56**, 5380–3.

23. Peterson, L.A., Brown, M.R., Carlisle, A.J. *et al.* (1998). An improved method for construction of directionally cloned cDNA libraries from microdissected cells. *Cancer Res.*, **58**, 5326–8.

24. Bast, R.C., Klug, T.L., St. John, E. *et al.* (1981). Reactivity of a monoclonal antibody with human ovarian carcinoma. *J. Clin. Invest.*, **68**, 1331–7.

25. Dunbar, B.S., Kimura, H., and Timmons, T.M. (1990). Protein analysis using high resolution two-dimensional polyacrylamide gel electrophoresis. *Meth. Enzymol.*, **182**, 29.

26. Paweletz, C.P., Gillespie, J.W., Ornstein, D.K. *et al.* (2000). Rapid protein display profiling of cancer progression directly from human tissue using a protein biochip. *Drug Devel. Res.*, **49**, 34–42.

16. The biology of the ovarian surface epithelium

Rudi Bao, Abbas Abdollahi, and Thomas C. Hamilton

Introduction

Although tumors originate from most every cell type present in the ovary, approximately 90% of cancers originating in this organ are referred to as common epithelial tumors. As early as 1872, Sir Spencer Wells suggested that these tumors originated from the cells covering the ovarian surface. Much observational data have accumulated during the intervening period in support of this early notion. As such, efforts have been made over the years to understand the biology of the surface epithelium in the hope that such information might explain the propensity of these relatively rare ovarian cells to undergo malignant transformation. In the following sections, we will present some of this information in the hope that it will provide a point from which readers may conceptualize experiments that may shed additional light on how to prevent, more effectively diagnose, and treat this frequently fatal disease.

General information

The ovarian surface epithelial cells are modified peritoneal mesothelial cells and are contiguous with those cells that line the peritoneal cavity. It is of interest that the surface epithelial cells, even in their normal surface context, are often more 'lush'-appearing than the peritoneal mesothelium. This may well be due to the proximity of these cells to the hormone- and growth factor-producing components of the ovary for which they have receptors (see below) and is clearly evident when they become entrapped in the ovarian cortex and form inclusion cysts.[1] Embryologically, ovarian surface epithelium is related to other gynecological tissues as well as the peritoneal mesothelium, since these cells originate from the coelomic epithelium which overlies the gonadal ridge.[2] It is therefore of mesodermal origin, and developmentally closely related to the underlying stromal fibroblasts. The coelomic epithelium gives rise to the Müllerian ducts which are the primordia for the epithelia of the Fallopian tube, uterus, and endocervix. Thus, the embryonic coelomic epithelium in the urogenital region is competent to develop along many different pathways. The re-expression of this capacity upon the malignant transformation of the surface epithelium is likely to be the basis for the striking variety of phenotypes found among ovarian surface epithelial cell-derived carcinomas. These tumors frequently differentiate along the lines of Müllerian duct derivatives, such that their histological features are reminiscent of the architecture and epithelial cells of the endocervix in the case of mucinous tumors, the endometrium in the case of endometrioid tumors, and the Fallopian tube in the case of the most common serous tumors.[3,4]

Histological study of the surface epithelium

Numerous investigators have examined the surface epithelium at the histological and ultrastructural level. A series of very detailed examinations was conducted in the rabbit, where the appearance of the surface epithelium was examined in the context of ovulation.[5] These studies provided very strong circumstantial evidence that, in the rabbit at least, the surface epithelium actively participates in ovulation, with changes suggesting that the cells secrete proteolytic enzymes from their basal surface and aid in the breakdown of the tunica albuginea and follicular rupture. Several other investigators have performed less detailed studies in other species[6] and these generally support the work done on the rabbit. What is apparent from these studies is that the surface epithelium must be under paracrine or endocrine control in order for it to participate coordinately in the ovulatory process. Additional studies in the rabbit clearly support the notion that the rabbit surface epithelium is responsive to hormones. For example, it has been shown that chronic treatment of rabbits with estrogen or gonadotropins results in marked proliferation of the surface epithelium, which creates complex papillary structures.[7] In summary, these data support the idea that the surface epithelium is responsive to paracrine or endocrine factors. More direct experimental data on those factors to which the surface epithelium may respond will be presented below.

Other histological studies of the ovary have attempted to determine if there are identifiable changes that precede overt malignancy. Many of the original studies evaluated the contralateral 'normal' ovary of women with unilateral ovarian cancer and detected a range of changes.[8–11] In a recent study, we have taken a slightly different approach. We evaluated ovaries removed from women at an inherited increased risk of ovarian cancer.[1] This investigation revealed that cancer-prone ovaries contained two or more, or three or more, of the following histological features: surface epithelial pseudostratification, surface epithelial papillomatosis, deep cortical invaginations of the surface epithelium, epithelial inclusion cysts, and increased stromal activity in 85% and 75% of cases ($n = 20$), respectively.[1] These changes were observed far less frequently (and were less intense) in ovaries from women in the general population (two or more in 30% of cases and three or more in 10% of cases). These differences were statistically significant ($P = 0.001$ and $P < 0.001$). We suggest that these changes are an identifiable pre-neoplastic phenotype that is a fertile environment from which ovarian cancer may arise. The notion that HOSE cells from ovarian cancer-prone individuals have developed a distinct phenotype prior to the development of overt malignancy is also supported by work on the cultured cells which we have performed in collaboration with others. For example, the HOSE cells from cancer-prone individuals, in comparison to normal-risk individuals, are more stable with regard to epithelial morphology and CA125 production.[12] Furthermore, the suggestion of increased mitotic activity by the histological studies described above is supported by recent evidence that telomere length is shorter and rate of loss greater in the cells from the ovarian cancer-prone individuals.[13]

Growth regulation of the surface epithelium

As noted above, histological studies suggest that the growth and function of ovarian surface epithelial cells is regulated by paracrine or endocrine pathways and many investigations have begun to clarify which hormones and growth factors might be involved. Based on the finding some years ago that malignant ovarian tumors contain estrogen receptors,[14] we investigated whether this was the result of a signaling pathway present in normal cells being retained in some cancers, or whether expression coincided with differentiation of the tumors along Müllerian lines. Using isolated rat ovarian surface epithelial cells in tissue culture, we detected estrogen binding with the affinity and specificity of estrogen receptors,[15] and others have subsequently shown the presence of estrogen receptors in the human ovarian surface epithelium.[16] Although we have clearly shown estrogen to be a mitogen in some human ovarian cancer cell lines,[17] it has been problematic to demonstrate such an effect in normal ovarian surface epithelial cells in tissue culture. Hence, the question remains to be answered as to what role the interaction of estrogen with its receptor might have in the normal surface epithelium.

With regard to peptide growth factors and gonadotropins, data on the former are extensive, but in the case of the latter it has only recently been shown that the surface epithelium has receptors for follicle stimulating hormone (FSH). There are, however, no clear data on the effects of interaction of FSH with its receptor in this cell type. In the case of peptide growth factors, extensive studies

have investigated the role of epidermal growth factor receptor (EGFR) signaling in both normal and malignant ovarian surface epithelial cells (see ref. 18 for a general review).

Peptide growth factors, including EGF/transforming growth factor-α(TGF-α), are ubiquitous proteins that stimulate proliferation or differentiation of a variety of cell types by binding to specific membrane receptors.[19] Unlike peptide hormones, such as gonadotropins (luteinizing hormone (LH), FSH) which are synthesized by well-defined cells within specific glands and released into the circulation, peptide growth factors are commonly found to be produced by a variety of cells and act locally in the body via autocrine or paracrine mechanisms. Treatment of EGF/TGF-α—responsive cells with the growth factor results in binding of the ligand to the EGFR. This receptor–ligand interaction results in the variable activation of at least two signal transduction cascades, i.e. Ras (or Ras-related)/MEK and phosphoinositol 3-kinase (PI3 kinase) pathways. This initiates a process which causes quiescent cells to advance into the first gap phase (G_1) of the cell cycle, traverse the G_1 phase, and then become committed to DNA synthesis or S phase.[19,20] EGF/TGF-α responsive cells require sustained exposure to the growth factor for at least 6–8 h before they are committed to DNA synthesis and transition through the G_1 phase.[21–24] Binding of the ligand to the EGFR results in activation of the receptor's kinase activity and leads to autophosphorylation of several tyrosines in the receptor protein.[25] This is followed by induction of Ras signaling due to the association of the Shc–Grb2–SOS complex with the activated EGFR. Active, guanosine triphosphate (GTP)-bound Ras then binds the serine/threonine kinase, Raf. These initial events trigger a phosphorylation cascade utilizing mitogen-activated protein kinases (MAPKs).[19,26] These MAPKs (also called extracellular signal-regulated kinases, or ERKs) are themselves activated by phosphorylation by the MAPK-activating enzymes (MAPK/ERK kinases, or MEKs).[19,26,27] They, in turn, phosphorylate a number of additional kinases and transcription factors which then affect cellular responses following growth factor stimulation. The Ras/MAPK pathway may crosstalk with an alternate signaling pathway of EGFR, i.e. PI3 kinase/AKT2. Data are emerging that ovarian cancers may have increased amounts of PI3 kinase[28] as well as AKT2.[29]

Alterations in EGFR family signaling have perhaps been among the most frequently implicated effectors of human oncogenesis.[19] We have had a long-standing view, and experimental and correlative data support this, that perturbations in EGFR signaling could also be a frequent contributor to ovarian surface epithelial oncogenesis. Our view has its origins in the fact that DNA replication is a weak mutagen, and the finding that follicular fluid contains EGF, which is a mitogen to normal ovarian surface epithelial cells.[30,31] The notion is bolstered further by several studies in ovarian cancer. In cultured human ovarian cancer cells, the mitogenic response to EGFR ligands was found to be variable.[32–35] Of interest, we have similarly found variations in the responsiveness of our individual transformed rat ovarian surface epithelial cell lines to EGF.[36,37] Additionally, we have reported that in estrogen-responsive ovarian cancer[38] at least a part of the mitogenic effect utilizes the EGFR ligand, TGF-α, as an autocrine second messenger.[17] Furthermore, neutralization of TGF-α in ovarian cancer cells in tissue culture with a monoclonal antibody results in inhibition of proliferation, most probably by blocking a TGF-α/EGFR autocrine loop.[39] When mitogenic responsiveness to EGF is lost, it is not often due to decreased receptor expression. Therefore, the attenuated response may be due to alterations in the downstream signals generated after receptor and ligand interaction, such that proliferation does not require growth factor. This could occur in a variety of ways, including constitutive activation of some component along the EGFR signaling cascades,[19] or elimination of a growth inhibitory signal in the absence of growth factor, such as inactivation of a growth/tumor suppressor gene.

Several additional studies suggest the involvement of EGFR signaling in the clinical features of ovarian cancer. Laboratory studies have suggested that TGF-α might contribute to an aggressive tumor phenotype.[40] Clinical correlative studies would seem to support this concept since several authors have reported that EGF receptor expression in ovarian cancer is associated with a poor prognosis.[41–46] Additionally, clinical investigations have found that while TGF-α was not detectable in normal pre- and post-menopausal ovaries, the majority of malignant epithelial tumors of the ovary did express this EGFR ligand.[47] Transforming growth factor activity has also been found in effusions from ovarian cancer patients[42,43] and EGF-like factors were present in ovarian tumors.[48,49] Another recent report indicated that serum TGF-α was detected in a greater proportion (62%) of patients with ovarian cancer compared to those with benign ovarian tumors (28%).[20] The TGF-α levels were even higher in serous and endometrioid ovarian cancers, 71 and 70%, respectively. In summary, the above data suggest the frequent involvement of EGF/TGF-α signal transduction pathways in many aspects of the biology of ovarian cancer.

Other studies have found additional evidence of strategies used by ovarian cancer cells to escape the need for growth factors in order to proliferate. For example, Ras activation was found in 50% of ovarian cancers tested, mostly resulting in constitutive activation of MAPK.[28] Mutations of the Ras oncoprotein have been observed frequently in mucinous ovarian cancers and in about 20–50% of borderline epithelial ovarian tumors.[50] Very recently, a gene homologous to Ras and Rap G proteins, namely *NOEY2*, was discovered during an effort to find genes expressed in normal human ovary but not ovarian cancer. The report indicates lack of *NOEY2* message in about 90% of ovarian cancer cell lines.[28] In an independent study with similar intent, *DOC2* was discovered. It is a *mDab2* homologue and the gene product was suggested to bind Grb2, preventing docking of SOS which is required as an early event for tyrosine kinase-linked receptor signaling.[51]

The concept of how and why malignant transformation of the surface epithelium occurs

Data outlined above suggest that the ovarian surface epithelium actively participates in the ovulatory process. In addition, it is abundantly clear that, after ovulation, return to continuity of the ovarian surface is achieved by the growth of these cells to repair the ovulatory wound. This observation, coupled with epidemio-

logical data showing that factors that limit ovulations decrease ovarian cancer risk and, conversely, those that are associated with increased ovulations increase risk, contributed many years ago to the development by M.F. Fathalla of the incessant ovulation hypothesis of ovarian cancer etiology.[52] Briefly, he hypothesized that the repeated rupture/wounding of the ovarian surface followed by rapid proliferation of surface epithelial cells, as occurs with repetitious ovulation, somehow drives the transformation of these cells. Over the years since its inception the incessant ovulation hypothesis has been embellished in many ways and is often stated as dogma in reviews which cover the subject of ovarian cancer etiology.[53,54] However, not until recently have experimental data to support this idea been presented.[36,37] These data will be summarized in a subsequent section. Another issue related to this hypothesis derives from a recent provocative preliminary report describing the histological analysis of the ovaries of cynomolgus monkeys treated for 2 years with an oral contraceptive containing the synthetic estrogen and progestin ethinyl estradiol and levonorgestrel, respectively, or the individual components.[55] The authors noted a marked increase in apoptosis of surface epithelial cells from animals treated with the combination contraceptive or the synthetic progestin component. An important issue to be reconciled if these data are confirmed is why such a high percentage of cells (14–25%) are undergoing apoptosis. It would seem counterproductive for the occurrence of apoptosis in genetically normal cells. Hence, it is tempting to speculate that the progestin is initiating apoptosis in surface epithelial cells that contain genetic damage. This idea is consistent with the notion that ovarian surface epithelial cells may be prone to genetic damage which is not repaired. Notably, these cells have not been under strong evolutionary pressure to develop the capacity for repeated wound repair since, in the Darwinian sense, repetitious ovulation is a recent event. In summary, there is abundant evidence to suggest that some aspect of repeated ovulation drives the process of malignant transformation of the ovarian surface epithelium. Recent preliminary data, however, suggest that multiparity and oral contraceptives may be exerting their protective effects by different routes.

Experimental malignant transformation of the surface epithelium

The studies described above are providing important leads toward understanding how ovarian cancer develops. To provide an additional tool to aid in unraveling this process, we have recently attempted to utilize the concepts put forward in the 'incessant ovulation' hypothesis of ovarian cancer etiology to create an experimental model of ovarian cancer.[52] Using the idea that repeated growth of surface epithelial cells might cause mutations leading to malignant transformation, surface epithelial cells from rat ovaries were isolated and subjected to the repetitious requirement for growth *in vitro* by repeated subculture. This strategy resulted in malignant transformation as assessed by tumorigenicity in 10 out of 39 independent attempts.[37] Furthermore, cytogenetic analysis revealed that karyotypic complexity was increased in undifferentiated tumors,[37] although the complexity seen was far less than that characteristic of clinical ovarian cancer. This suggests to us that perhaps the majority of changes seen might be directly related to transformation. Furthermore, this system provided a situation where independent events leading to malignant transformation occurred in cells which originally had the same genetic constitution. This not only provided related normal/tumor cell pairs, which is an important asset when molecular biological techniques are applied to uncover genetic differences associated with malignant versus normal cells, but also provided the opportunity to determine the frequency of the same genetic event in multiple independent transformants.

Using this rat ovarian surface epithelial cell transformation model system we have discovered a growth suppressor gene *LOT1*[56] which is part of the EGFR signaling pathway and is likely involved in human ovarian cancer.[57] Additionally, we have used the technique of genome scanning to isolate a portion of an amplicon inferred to be present in one of the transformed cell lines by a homogeneously staining chromosomal region (hsr). This allowed us to initiate chromosomal walking, with the end result being the discovery that cathepsin B is amplified in the hsr-containing cell line and is frequently overexpressed in other transformed rat ovarian surface epithelial cell lines.[58] Cathepsin B is a peptidyl peptide hydrolase endopeptidase that has been found to be a prognostic factor in many solid tumors.[59] Our current efforts in this model revolve around a comprehensive analysis of the genes consistently disregulated during transformation.

Conclusions

Progress in unraveling the biology of the surface epithelium and how this may contribute to its propensity for malignant transformation has been slow. This has been caused by several factors, including the limited number of investigators with a sustained effort in the field, the difficulty of working with cells so limited in number, and the lack of well-characterized animal models of the disease. None the less, momentum is building and, with the rapid advances in technologies which may be brought to bear on the problem, there should be optimism that the pace of progress in the next millennium will be more rapid than in the one just ending.

References

1. Salazar, H., Godwin, A., Daly, M. *et al.* (1996). Microscopic benign and invasive malignant neoplasms and preoplastic phenotype in prophylactic oophorectomies. *J. Natl Cancer Inst.*, **88**, 1810–20.
2. Cormack, D. (1987). *Ham's Histology,* (9th edn). Lippincott, Philadelphia.
3. Scully, R., Bell, D., and Abu-Jawdeh, G. (1995). Update on early ovarian cancer and cancer developing in benign ovarian tumors. In *Ovarian cancer 3,* (ed. F. Sharp, P. Mason, T. Blackett, and J. Berek), pp. 139–44. Chapman & Hall, London.
4. Fox, H. (1993). Pathology of early malignant change in the ovary. *Int. J. Gyn. Path.*, **12**, 153–5.
5. Bjersing, L. and Cajander, S. (1975). Ovulation and the role of the ovarian surface epithelium. *Experientia*, **31**, 605–8.
6. Motta, P., Van Blerkom, J., and Makabe, S. (1980). Changes in the surface morphology of the ovarian 'germinal' epithelium during the reproductive cycle and in some pathological conditions. *J. Submicro. Cytol.*, **12**, 407–25.
7. Nicosia, S. and Nicosia, R. (1988). Neoplasms of the ovarian mesothelium. In *Pathology of human neoplasms,* (ed. H. Azar), pp. 435–86. Raven Press, New York.
8. Deligdisch, L., Einstein, A., Guera, D., and Gil, J. (1995). Ovarian dysplasia in epithelial inclusion cysts. *Cancer*, **76**, 1027–34.
9. Mittal, K., Zeleniuch-Jacquette, A., Cooper, J., and Demopoulos, R. (1993). Contralateral ovary in unilateral ovarian carcinoma: a search for preneoplastic lesions. *Int. J. Gyn. Path.*, **12**, 59–63.
10. Resta, L., Russo, S., Colucci, G., and Prat, J. (1993). Morphologic precursors of ovarian epithelial tumors. *Obstet. Gynecol.*, **82**, 181–6.
11. Tresserra, F., Grases, P., Labastida, R., and Ubeda, A. (1998). Histological features of the contralateral ovary in patients with unilateral ovarian cancer: A case control study. *Gynecol. Oncol.*, **71**, 437–41.
12. Auersperg, N., Maines-Bandiera, S., Booth, J. *et al.* (1995). Expression of two mucin antigens in cultured human ovarian surface epithelium: influence of a family history of ovarian cancer. *Am. J. Obstet. Gynecol.*, **173**, 558–65.
13. Kruk, P., Godwin, A., Hamilton, T., and Auersperg, N. (1999). Telomeric instability and reduced proliferative potential in ovarian surface epithelial cells from women with a family history of ovarian cancer. *Gynecol. Oncol.*, in press.
14. Hamilton, T., Davies, P., and Griffith, K. (1981). Androgen and oestrogen binding of cytosols of human ovarian tumors. *J. Endocrinol.*, **??**, 421–31.
15. Hamilton, T., Davies, P., and Griffiths K. (1982). Oestrogen receptor-like binding in the surface epithelium of the rat ovary. *J. Endocrinol.*, **95**, 377–85.
16. Karlan, B., Jones, J., Greenwald, M., and Lagasse, L. (1995). Steroid hormone effects on the proliferation of human ovarian surface epithelium *in vitro. Am. J. Obstet. Gynecol.*, **173**, 97–104.
17. Nash, J., Ozols, R., Smith, J., and Hamilton, T. (1989). Estrogen and anti-estrogen effects on the growth of human epithelial ovarian cancer *in vitro. Obstet. Gynecol.*, **73**, 1009–16.
18. Berchuck, A. and Carney, M. (1997). Human ovarian cancer of the surface epithelium. *Biochem. Pharm.*, **54**, 541–4.
19. Aaronson, S. (1991). Growth factors and cancer. *Science*, **254**, 1146–53.
20. Chien, C.-H., Huang, C.-C., Lin, Y.-H. *et al.* (1997). Detection of serum transforming growth factor-α in patients of primary epithelial ovarian cancers by enzyme immunoassay. *Gynecol. Oncol.*, **66**, 405–10.
21. Shechter, Y., Hernaez, L., and Cuatrecasas, P. (1978). Epidermal growth factor: Biological activity requires persistent occupation of high-affinity cell surface receptors. *Proc. Natl Acad. Sci. USA*, **75**, 5788–91.
22. Aharonov, A., Pruss, R., and Herschman, H. (1978). Epidermal growth factor. Relationship between receptor regulation and mitogenesis in 3T3 cells. *J. Biol. Chem.*, **253**, 3970–7.
23. Carpenter, G. and Carpenter, S.C. (1976). Human epidermal growth factor and the proliferation of human fibroblasts. *J. Cell Physiol.* **88**, 227–38.
24. Weinberg, R. (1991). Tumor suppressor genes. *Science*, **254**, 1138–46.
25. Schlessinger, J. and Ullrich, A. (1992). Growth factor signaling by receptor tyrosine kinases. *Neuron*, **9**, 383–91.
26. Ahn, N., Weiel, J., Chan, C., and Krebs, E. (1990). Identification of multiple epidermal growth factor-stimulated protein serine/threonine kinases from Swiss 3T3 cells. *J. Biol. Chem.*, **265**, 11487–94.
27. Zheng, C.-F. and Guan, K. (1993). Cloning and characterization of two distinct human extracellular signal-related kinase activator kinases, MEK1 and MEK2. *J. Biol. Chem.*, **268**, 11435–9.
28. Bast, R. Jr, Xu, F., Yu, Y. *et al.* (1998) Overview—The molecular biology of ovarian cancer. In *Ovarian cancer 5,* (ed. F. Sharp, T. Blackett, J. Berek, and R. Bast), pp. 87–97. Isis Medical Media, Oxford, UK.
29. Bellacosa, A., de Feo, D., Godwin, A. *et al.* (1995). Molecular alterations of the AKT2 oncogene in ovarian and breast carcinomas. *Int. J. Cancer*, **64**, 280–5.

30. Skinner, M., Lobb, D., and Dorrington, J. (1987). Ovarian thecal/interstitial cells produce an epidermal growth factor-like substance. *Endocrinology*, **121**, 1892–9.

31. Skinner, M., Keski-oja, J., Osteen, K., and Moses, H. (1987). Ovarian thecal cells produce transforming growth factor-β which can regulate granulosa cell growth. *Endocrinology*, **121**, 786.

32. Berchuck, A., Olt, G., Everitt, L. *et al.* (1990). The role of peptide growth factors in epithelial ovarian cancer. *Obstet. Gynecol.*, **75**, 255–62.

33. Singletary, S., Baker, F., Spitzer, G. *et al.* (1987). Biological effect of epidermal growth factor on the *in vitro* growth of human tumors. *Cancer Res.*, **47**, 403–6.

34. Crew, A., Langdon, S., Miller, E., and Miller, W. (1992). Mitogenic effects of epidermal growth factor and transforming growth factor-α on EGF-receptor positive human ovarian carcinoma cell lines. *Eur. J. Cancer*, **28**, 337–41.

35. Zhou, L. and Leung, B. (1992). Growth regulation of ovarian cancer cells by epidermal growth factor and transforming growth factors α and β-1 *Biochim. Biophysic. Acta*, **1180**, 130.

36. Godwin, A., Testa, J., Handel, L. *et al.* (1992). Spontaneous transformation of rat ovarian surface epithelial cells implicates repeated ovulation in ovarian cancer etiology and is associated with clonal cytogenetic changes. *J. Natl Cancer Inst.*, **84**, 592–601.

37. Testa, J., Getts, L., Salazar, H. *et al.* (1994). Spontaneous transformation of rat ovarian surface epithelial cells results in well to poorly differentiated tumors with a parallel range of cytogenetic complexity. *Cancer Res.*, **54**, 2778–84.

38. Nash, J., Hall, L., and Ozols, R. (1989). Estrogenic regulation and growth factor expression in human ovarian cancer *in vitro*. *Am. Assoc. Cancer Res.*, **30**, 299.

39. Stromberg, K., Collins, T., Gordon, A, *et al.* (1992). Transforming growth factor-α acts as an autocrine growth factor in ovarian carcinoma cell lines. *Cancer Res.*, **52**, 341–7.

40. Morishige, K., Kurachi, H., Amemiya, K. *et al.* (1991). Evidence for the involvement of transforming growth factor-α and epidermal growth factor receptor autocrine growth mechanism in primary human ovarian cancers *in vitro*. *Cancer Res.*, **51**, 5322–8.

41. Berchuck, A., Rodriguez, G., Kamel, A. *et al.* (1991). Epidermal growth factor receptor expression in normal ovarian epithelium and ovarian cancer. I. Correlation of receptor expression with prognostic factors in patients with ovarian cancer. *Am. J. Obstet. Gynecol.*, **164**, 669–74.

42. Arteaga, C., Hanauske, A., Clark, G. *et al.* (1988). Immunoreactive α transforming growth factor activity in effusions from cancer patients as a marker of tumor burden and patient prognosis. *Cancer Res.*, **48**, 5023–8.

43. Hanauske, A., Arteaga, C., Clark, G. *et al.* (1988). Determination of transforming growth factor activity in effusions from cancer patients. *Cancer*, **61**, 1832–7.

44. Kohler, M., Janz, I., and Wintzer, H. (1989). The expression of EGF receptors, EGF-like factors and c-*myc* in ovarian and cervical carcinomas and their potential clinical significance. *Anticancer Res.*, **9**, 1537–47.

45. Sainsbury, J., Farndon, J., and Needham, G. (1987). Epidermal-growth-factor receptor status as predictor of early recurrence of and death from breast cancer. *Lancet*, **1**, 1398–402.

46. Scambia, G., Benedetti-Panici, P., Ferrandina, G. *et al.* (1995). Epidermal growth factor, oestrogen and progesterone receptor expression in primary ovarian cancer: correlation with clinical outcome and response to chemotherapy. *Br. J. Cancer*, **72**, 361–6.

47. Kommoss, F., Wintzer, H., Von Kleist, S. *et al.* (1990). *In situ* distribution of transforming growth factor-α in normal human tissues and in malignant tumours of the ovary. *J. Pathol.* **162**, 223–30.

48. Bauknecht, T., Kiechle, M., Bauer, G., and Siebers, J. (1986). Characterization of growth factors in human ovarian carcinomas. *Cancer Res.*, **46**, 2614–18.

49. Bauknecht, T., Kohler, M., Janz, I., and Pffeiderer, A. (1989). The occurrence of epidermal growth factor receptors and the characterization of EGF-like factors in human ovarian, endometrial, cervical and breast cancer. *J. Cancer Res. Clin. Oncol.*, **115**, 193–9.

50. Mok, S.-H., Bell, D., Knapp, R. *et al.* (1993). Mutation of K-*ras* protooncogene in human ovarian epithelial tumors of borderline malignancy. *Cancer Res.*, **53**, 1489–92.

51. Mok, S., Chan, W., Wong, K. *et al.* (1998). DOC–2, a candidate tumor suppressor gene in human epithelial ovarian cancer. *Oncogene*, **16**, 2381–7.

52. Fathalla, M. (1971). Incessant ovulation—a factor in ovarian neoplasia. *Lancet*, ii, 163.

53. Brinton, L. and Hoover, R. (1992). Epidemiology of gynecologic cancers. In *Gynecologic oncology: principles and practice*, (ed. W. Hoskins, C. Perez, and R. Young), pp. 3–26. Lippincott, Philadelphia,

54. Lingeman, C. (1983). Environmental factors in the etiology of carcinoma of the human ovary: a review. *Am. J. Ind. Med.*, **4**, 365–79.

55. Rodriguez, G., Walmer, D., Lessey, B. *et al.* (1997). The effect of contraceptive progestins on the ovarian epithelium: Cancer prevention through apoptosis. *J Soc. Gynecol. Invest.* **4** (**suppl**), 79A.

56. Abdollahi, A., Roberts, D., Godwin, A. *et al.* (1997). Identification of a zinc-finger gene at 6q25: a chromosomal region implicated in development of many solid tumors. *Oncogene*, **14**, 1973–9.

57. Abdollahi, A., Godwin, A., Miller, P. *et al.* (1997). Identification of a gene containing zinc-finger motifs based on lost expression in malignantly transformed rat ovarian surface epithelial cells. *Cancer Res.*, **57**, 2029–34.

58. Abdollahi, A., Getts, L., Sonoda, G. *et al.* (1999). Genome scanning detects amplification of the cathepsin B gene (*CstB*) in transformed rat ovarian surface epithelial cells. *J. Soc. Gynecol. Invest.*, **6**, 32–40.

59. Keppler, D. and Sloane, B.F. (1996). Multiple enzyme forms from a single gene and its relation to cancer. *Enzyme Prot*, **49**, 94–105.

17. The tumour microenvironment of epithelial ovarian cancer

Frances Burke, Chris Scotton, Kate Scott, Robert Moore, Caroline Arnott, and Fran Balkwill

Many novel cancer treatments target the relationship between a tumour and its supporting stroma. However our knowledge of individual components of the tumour microenvironment and their regulation is far from complete. This chapter will review the work of our laboratory in defining the tumour microenvironment of epithelial ovarian cancer with particular emphasis on the cells; the cytokines used in intercellular communication, and the matrix metalloprotcases involved in tissue remodelling and cell migration. We will also discuss some therapeutic implications of our results.

The cells of epithelial ovarian cancer

In a study of 20 biopsies of human epithelial ovarian cancer we identified the major cellular components as tumour cells, fibroblasts, endothelial cells, CD68+ macrophages and T lymphocytes (predominantly of a CD8/CD45RO cytotoxic memory phenotype).[1] We have not yet characterized dendritic cells but B cells, natural killer (NK) cells, mast cells, and polymorphonuclear leucocytes (PMNs) were generally sparse. The importance of the stroma as a genetically stable target is emphasized by the fact that stromal elements occupied a median of 37% of the area in the tumour. The tumour cells themselves occupied 43%, necrotic areas 4%, and the remaining area was space (real or artefactual).[1]

Infiltrating macrophages and lymphocytes were found in both tumour and stromal areas and macrophages also clustered in areas of necrosis. As described below, hypoxia has a dual influence on macrophage migration, which may explain their presence in areas of necrosis. Apart from the macrophage clusters, most of the infiltrating cells were found singly, although some lymphocyte clusters were found in stromal areas. There was great variability in numbers of infiltrating cells in different biopsies. For instance, a median of 2200 CD3 cells/mm^3 (range 50–40 300) and a median of 3700 CD68+ cells/mm^3 (range 600–15 200) were counted in a survey of 20 biopsies.

The cytokine network of ovarian cancer

Cytokines are soluble mediators of intercellular communication. They contribute to a chemical signalling language that regulates development, tissue repair, haematopoiesis, inflammation, and the immune response. Potent cytokine polypeptides have pleiotropic activities and functional redundancy. They act in a complex network where one cytokine can influence the production of, and response to, many other cytokines. The pathophysiology of infectious, autoimmune, and malignant disease can be partially explained by the induction of cytokines and the subsequent cellular response.

The cytokine context of a tumour can influence many aspects of tumour biology, especially communication between tumour and host cells. Cytokines may control the tumour microenvironment, providing the appropriate environment for the tumour to grow and spread.

As assessed by reverse transcriptase polymerase chain reaction (RT-PCR) analysis, the cytokine network of epithelial ovarian cancer is rich in growth factors, inflammatory cytokines, and chemoattractant cytokines (chemokines) but lacking lymphocyte-associated cytokines that might facilitate tumour-specific immune responses.[2] In a published study, we determined the expression of 22 cytokine and 11 cytokine receptor mRNAs in malignant and normal ovary, ovarian cancer cell lines, and xenografts. The profile was almost identical in normal and malignant biopsies, with 13 of 22 cytokines (IL–1α, IL–6, IL–8, IL–10, TNF-α, LT, MCP–1, RANTES, M-CSF, PDGF-A, PDGF-B, IGF-I, and TGF-β) expressed by a majority of samples. Nine of these were also expressed by a majority of cell lines. The profile was more varied in xenografts, suggesting that murine cytokines may provide some of the necessary context. Potential autocrine loops existed for IL–1, IGF-I, M-CSF, GM-CSF, and TNF, with mRNA for both receptors and ligand present. IL–4 and IFN-γ receptors were expressed in the absence of their ligand. RANTES was expressed in all the biopsies, but was absent from the cell lines and xenografts. T-cell cytokines IL–2, IL–4, IL–7, and IFN-γ were expressed infrequently in the biopsies.

These data, taken with previously published information, suggest that genetic and environmental changes render tumour cells capable of producing stromal cytokines, especially in advanced tumours and in cell lines selected by tissue culture or nude mouse transplantation. RT-PCR is not a quantitative technique, and it is not yet known whether cytokine production is increased in malignant tissues. However, one cytokine that was expressed abundantly in the epithelial tumour islands of ovarian cancer, was the pro-inflammatory cytokine tumour necrosis factor-α(TNF-α).[3] As described below, we have evidence that this is a pivotal cytokine in the ovarian tumour microenvironment, and one of its potential roles is in chemokine induction.

The chemokine profile of ovarian cancer

Chemokines are a large subfamily of cytokines, characterized by the presence of a conserved cysteine motif adjacent to the N-terminus.[4] They can be divided into CC- and CXC-chemokines, in which the first two cysteine residues are either adjacent, or separated by one amino acid, respectively. There are two additional subfamilies, the CX$_3$C- and C-chemokines, but only one example of each has been identified (fractalkine and lymphotactin, respectively).

Chemokines induce the directional migration and activation of specific leucocyte subsets. CXC-chemokines act predominantly on neutrophils, while CC-chemokines attract macrophages, monocytes, lymphocytes, dendritic cells, eosinophils, NK cells, and basophils. Certain chemokines may also regulate stem-cell growth, haematopoiesis, lymphopoiesis, and angiogenesis (for review, see ref. 4).

Chemokines act as ligands for seven-transmembrane, G-protein-coupled receptors. There are 10 receptors for the CC-chemokines (CCR1–10), five for the CXC-chemokines (CXCR1–5), and receptors for the C- and CX$_3$C-chemokines have been identified recently.[5,6] Chemokines bind to the extracellular N-terminus of the chemokine receptor, leading to phosphorylation of serine/threonine residues on the cytoplasmic C-terminus, signalling, and receptor desensitization. There is an apparent redundancy in the system, in that each receptor can respond to more than one chemokine, and each chemokine can use more than one receptor. Moreover, each leucocyte subset may express several different receptors. Despite this, a deficiency in any one chemokine or receptor can lead to a distinctive phenotype, as indicated by studies in knockout mice.[7,8]

The interplay between chemokines and their receptors is involved in many pathological states, such as the accumulation of macrophages during atherosclerosis and pulmonary fibrosis. As discussed above, leucocytes also infiltrate many solid malignant tumours, including those of the ovary, and a number of chemotactic factors have been isolated from tumours.

Our laboratory has been studying chemokines in human ovarian cancer, particularly their role in host cell infiltration of the tumour. Initial studies focused on the CC-chemokine, monocyte chemoattractant protein–1 (MCP–1). This chemokine was expressed by both tumour and stromal cells in ovarian cancer biopsies and expression levels in individual tumours correlated with the extent of the lymphocyte and macrophage infiltrate, which, as stated above, showed considerable variability in individual samples.[1,9] We also identified TNF-α as being a potent inducer of the chemokine in ovarian tumour cells.[10]

We have now conducted a more extensive survey of CC-chemokine and receptor expression in ovarian cancer using RT-PCR and RNase protection assays (RPA) (Scotton *et al.*, submitted for publication). Experiments so far suggest that a range of CC-chemokines are expressed but that expression of chemokine receptors is more restricted. RT-PCR analysis of 25 ovarian cancer biopsies showed that CC-chemokine receptors CCR1 and CCR4 were expressed in a majority (approximately 70%) but CCR2a, CCR2b, CCR3, and CCR5 were infrequently or never expressed. In contrast, all of the chemokines investigated were expressed at high levels (>80% of biopsies). RPA was used to further analyse expression of CCR1, CCR2, CCR2a, CCR2b, CCR3, CCR4, CCR5, and CCR8 quantitatively in 24 of the 25 biopsy samples used for the RT-PCR screen.

The results obtained for CCR1 agreed with the RT-PCR, but no CCR4 expression was seen. This suggests that the level of CCR4 expression in the tumours is very low, below the level of detection of the RPA assay. In only one biopsy was another chemokine receptor, CCR8, expressed.

In situ hybridization (ISH) was performed on nine ovarian cancer biopsies from the RT-PCR screen, using ^{35}S-labelled riboprobes. CCR1 was expressed in 8/9 biopsies, while CCR4 was found in 4/9 biopsies. The ISH to CCR1 was much stronger than that for CCR4, which agreed with the results of the RPA. It appears that CCR4 is expressed on very few cells within the tumour. The distribution of cells expressing CCR1 and CCR4 suggested that these cells were infiltrating cells, rather than tumour cells.

Our current hypothesis is that there may be a multistep process for leucocyte trafficking in ovarian cancer. Peripheral leucocytes expressing the MCP–1 receptor CCR2b are attracted to the tumour by MCP–1, where this receptor is downregulated by pro-inflammatory cytokines. Movement within the tumour could then be controlled by the CCR1 receptor in response to other chemokines, such as macrophage inflammatory protein –1α(MIP–1α) and RANTES. Thus, chemokine-directed leucocyte migration is controlled at the level of chemokine receptors, and the cytokine/chemokine profile in the majority of the ovarian cancer biopsies may favour expression of CCR1.

Hypoxia, chemokine gradients, and macrophage accumulation at sites of necrosis

As described above, the chemokine MCP–1 plays a role in regulating the lymphocyte and macrophage infiltrate in ovarian cancer, but macrophages also accumulate in necrotic areas of the tumours where there is little MCP–1 expression.[1] The necrotic regions in the ovarian cancer microenvironment are likely to be hypoxic. We have recently found that hypoxia inhibited MCP–1-induced migration of THP–1 monocytic cells and human macrophages.[11] In contrast, lymphocytes from peripheral blood migrate normally to an MCP–1 gradient in hypoxic conditions. The inhibition of monocyte migration by hypoxia was rapid and reversible. At the exposure times studied (30–90 min) hypoxia did not affect expression of the MCP–1 receptor CCR2b and cells exposed to hypoxia still responded to MCP–1 with an elevation of intracellular calcium. Although hypoxia is known to modulate gene expression, its inhibition of migration was not due to the production of soluble factors, and mRNA expression of macrophage migration inhibitory factor was unchanged.

Hypoxia-induced inhibition of chemotaxis was not limited to MCP–1. Hypoxia also inhibited the chemotactic response to MIP–1α, RANTES, and the chemoattractant fMLP, but hypoxic cells were still able to phagocytose opsonized red blood cells. We do not yet know whether hypoxia influences CCR1 expression.

We conclude that inhibition of migration by hypoxia is not due to gene regulation but is a reflection of metabolic changes in the cell. This could explain the high density of macrophages in areas of necrosis in the ovarian tumour microenvironment, even in the presence of a chemokine gradient. We suggest that macrophages migrate in response to chemokine gradients throughout the tumour until they encounter a necrotic region where they accumulate and function as phagocytes, clearing up cell debris.

Another possible reason for macrophage accumulation in areas of necrosis is regulation of chemokine synthesis by hypoxia. As stated above, TNF-α is a potent stimulus of ovarian tumour cell production of MCP–1, but we have found that this induction is reversibly abrogated in cells incubated under hypoxic conditions.[10]

Matrix metalloproteases in the tumour microenvironment

The major route of ovarian tumour spread is via detachment of cells from the primary tumour and implantation into the peritoneal cavity, with subsequent invasion of the peritoneal wall. Matrix metalloproteases are one group of proteolytic enzymes that may be involved in this process. In situ hybridization studies in our laboratory have localized MMP–2 expression and its specific inhibitor TIMP–2 to stromal areas of ovarian tumour tissue, and MMP–9 mRNA correlated with the presence of infiltrating macrophages.[12] In co-culture studies we have also defined soluble and cell membrane associated induction of stromal MMPs by ovarian tumour cells.[13,14] In order to obtain a more comprehensive picture of MMPs in the ovarian tumour microenvironment we studied MMP and TIMP mRNA expression by RT-PCR, MMP–2 and MMP–9 levels by zymography, and the total collagenolytic activity of tumour lysates.

MMP and TIMP mRNA expression was studied in 7 normal ovaries, 10 ovaries with benign disease, 11 carcinomas, and 5 metastatic tumours, a total of 33 samples. The analysis showed

that a variety of MMPs and TIMPs were expressed in ovarian tissues (Scott *et al.*, manuscript submitted). TIMP–1, TIMP–2, and TIMP–3 mRNA were present in nearly all tissues examined (33/33, 31/33, and 30/33 respectively). MMP–2 (72 kDa gelatinase) mRNA was found in every sample analysed and its activator MT-MMP–1 was also present in high frequency (30/33). However, MMP–9 (92 kDa gelatinase), the other MMP responsible for degradation of basement membrane, was not expressed in all ovarian tissues studied (14/33). mRNAs for MMP–1 and MMP–13, which both degrade type I collagen, were present in 8/33 and 11/33 samples, respectively. In the stromelysin family of enzymes, MMP–11 (stromelysin–3) was expressed in 33/33 samples but MMP–3 (stromelysin–1) was only found in 6/33 samples. Matrilysin (MMP–7), another member of the stromelysin subgroup, was expressed in many of the samples analysed (25/33) but MMP–10 (stromelysin–2) was found in very low frequency (2/33). MT-MMP–2 was not present in any of the samples analysed. Six MMPs or TIMPs were always expressed in normal ovary (TIMP–1, TIMP–2, TIMP–3, MT-MMP–1, MMP–2, and MMP–11). Thus tissue turnover in the ovary appears to require the degradative ability of at least one gelatinase (MMP–2) and one stromelysin (MMP–11). MT-MMP–2 is presumably expressed to activate proMMP–2 protein and allow localized proteolysis at the cell surface.

The malignant tissues expressed a wider range of MMPs (Fig. 17.1). For example, the interstitial collagenases MMP–1 and MMP–13 were expressed in 2/17 and 3/17 non-malignant tissues as compared with 6/16 and 8/16 malignant tissues, respectively.

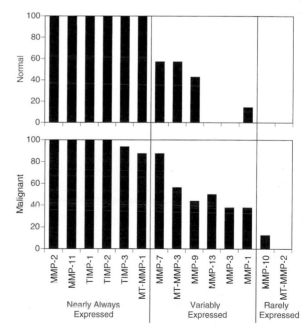

Fig. 17.1 RT-PCR screen of ovarian tissues for MMP and TIMP mRNA. Total RNA was isolated from 7 normal ovarian tissues and 16 carcinoma samples. Five micrograms of total RNA was reversed transcribed and subjected to PCR using primers designed to measure different MMP and TIMP mRNAs. PCR products were analysed by agarose gel electrophoresis. The bar charts show the percentage frequency of expression in the two different types of tissue.

MMP–1 and MMP–13 were never expressed together in normal or benign tissues but were co-expressed in 4/16 malignant tissues. MMP–7 mRNA was detected in every metastatic sample analysed (5/5). MMP–3 appeared to be tumour specific. It was not expressed in any normal or benign samples (0/17) but was found in 8/16 malignant tissues. Thus malignancy within the ovary resulted in a greater proportion of the MMP family being expressed, either by the tumour epithelial cells, stromal cells, or the inflammatory cells recruited to the site. A wider range of gelatinases and stromelysins were present (MMP–9, MMP–7, and MMP–3) perhaps to allow degradation of the rapidly changing tumour environment.

Gelatinolytic zymography was used to measure proMMP–9, proMMP–2, and active MMP–2 protein in 5 normal ovaries, 10 ovaries with benign disease, 10 carcinomas, and 5 metastatic tissues. ProMMP–2 was present in every sample analysed (30/30) which confirmed the RT-PCR results. Active MMP–2 was found in 1/5 normal samples analysed but was detected in higher frequency in benign (5/10) and carcinoma (5/10) tissues. All metastatic samples were positive for active MMP–2 (5/5). ProMMP–9 was only present in 1/5 normal samples. ProMMP–9 was detected in increasing frequency in benign (5/10), carcinoma (7/10), and metastatic samples (3/5), which again correlated with the RT-PCR results. These results are summarized in Table 17.1.

The amount of each gelatinase species in the tumour samples was analysed by quantitative gelatin zymography. The mean level of proMMP–9 was low in normal samples. Benign tissues had twofold higher levels of proMMP–9 compared to normal. Malignant samples displayed significantly higher mean levels of proMMP–9, with carcinoma tissues containing threefold and metastasis samples having eightfold the level of normal tissues ($P = 0.05$). ProMMP–2 levels were highest in normal and benign samples and the amount of proMMP–2 protein was approximately 50% lower in carcinoma and metastasis tissues ($P = 0.02$). Active MMP–2 levels were low or non-existent in normal tissue samples. Active MMP–2 levels were increased approximately twofold in benign, carcinoma, and metastatic samples. Statistical analysis revealed that an increase in active MMP–2 with disease progression was not significant ($P = 0.2$) but, as stated earlier, the metastasis sample group was the only group in which all samples were positive for active MMP–2. In normal tissues the majority of MMP–2 was present as proMMP–2. However, malignant tissues displayed a fourfold higher ratio of active to pro-enzyme, indicating that the amount of active MMP–2 present was much higher.

Table 17.1 Presence of proMMP-9, proMMP-2, and active MMP-2 in tissue samples

Sample	ProMMP-9	ProMMP-2	Active MMP-2
Normal	1/5	5/5	2/5
Malignant	7/10	10/10	5/10

Soluble protein was isolated from ovarian tissue specimens by Triton X-114 extraction. Presence of MMP-2 and MMP-9 activity was analysed in 5 normal and 10 carcinoma samples by gelatin zymography.

Thus the decreased levels of proMMP–2 observed in carcinoma and metastasis samples was probably due to an increase in active MMP–2 species.

In conclusion, during the transition from benign to malignant disease, MMP and TIMP expression in the tumour microenvironment became more complex, and levels of at least two MMPs increased. Some MMPs also showed tumour-specific expression. However, the activity of individual enzymes appears to be tightly controlled by tumour–stroma interactions and natural inhibitors. Highly localized and transient activation of minute quantities of these enzymes at the membrane of individual cells is probably central to their action.

Therapeutic implications of ovarian cancer microenvironment

Interferon-γ as a cytostatic/cytotoxic agent

One striking observation from our microenvironment studies was that mRNA for IFN-γ was never detected in any ovarian tumour sample, although components of the IFN-γ receptor were always detected, whether in tumour biopsies or tumour cell lines. As there is some evidence that intraperitoneal IFN-γ has anti-tumour activity in ovarian cancer patients,[15] we studied the ability of this cytokine to act directly on ovarian tumour cells.

Clinically achievable doses of IFN-γ have cytostatic and generally apoptotic effects on approximately 75% of ovarian cancer cell lines and freshly isolated tumour cells from ascites (Wall *et al.*, manuscript in preparation).[16,17] This effect is superior to similar concentrations of IFN-α. Comparable doses of IFN-γ increase survival of mice bearing intraperitoneal xenografts of human ovarian cancer and induce apotosis *in vivo*. Experiments in tissue culture and in nude mice indicate that prolonged exposure (2–3 days *in vitro*, 7–14 days *in vivo*) is crucial for this apoptotic activity with a critical 'point of no return' at 2–3 days. IFN-γ signalling was confirmed by stat–1 activation, even if there was no apoptotic response, and several IFN-γ- inducible genes were upregulated *in vitro* and *in vivo*. In a comparison between two cell lines, one killed by IFN-γ, the other resistant, prolonged upregulation of the transcription factor IRF–1 and the cyclin dependent kinase inhibitor p21 was associated with cell death.

Although the effects of IFN-γ on the immune system (e.g. upregulation of MHC and activation of macrophages) may be involved in anti-tumour activity *in vivo*, our results suggest that long-term exposure to moderate doses of this cytokine might have direct destructive effects on ovarian tumour cells. Pilot clinical studies to study the apoptotic effects of IFN-γ are currently being planned.

TNF-α and the tumour microenvironment

Our studies have implicated TNF-α as a pivotal cytokine in the pathophysiology of human ovarian carcinoma. This cytokine is expressed in the epithelial tumour islands, where it may play a role in tumour–stroma interactions, the level of TNF-α expression increasing with severity of disease in a study of 40 ovarian cancer biopsies.[3] In ovarian tumour biopsies, TNF-α co-localizes with MMP–9 in tumour-associated macrophages,[12] and the combination of autocrine TNF-α and a soluble tumour cell-derived factor upregulates production of this MMP.[13] As described above, TNF-α also induces tumour cell production of the chemokine MCP–1, which is produced in the ovarian tumour microenvironment, and may control the extent and distribution of the host-cell infiltrate.[1,9] Further evidence for the involvement of TNF-α in ovarian malignancies comes from human tumour xenograft models where TNF-α injection converts ascitic free-floating tumour to solid tumours with well-developed stroma.[18] These actions of TNF-α in the tumour microenvironment of ovarian cancer are summarized in Fig. 17.2.

A role for TNF-α in promoting development of tumour stroma and controlling host/tumour interactions, may be analogous to its roles in inflammatory disease. High doses of TNF-α delivered locally to the tumour site cause disruption of the tumour vasculature followed by tumour necrosis.[19] These destructive actions of TNF can also be seen in some acute inflammatory situations. However, lower doses of endogenous TNF-α can promote tissue repair via stimulation of fibroblasts and neovasculature.[20–22] The actions of TNF-α in the tumour microenvironment may be similar, except that TNF-α produced chronically in the tumour microenvironment does not lead to resolution of the lesion.

Direct proof of the importance of TNF-α to the development of tumours comes from experiments in mice deficient in this cytokine. We studied the susceptibility of these mice to skin carcinogenesis. TNF-α –/– mice were resistant to development of benign and malignant skin tumours, whether induced by DMBA initiation/12-O-tetradecanoylphorbol–13 acetate (TPA) promotion or repeated DMBA dosing.[23] Ten- to twentyfold fewer tumours developed in TNF-α –/– compared with wild-type (wt) mice during initiation/promotion and fourfold fewer after repeated carcinogen. TNF-α is a pleiotropic cytokine that could influence tumour–stromal interactions in early and late stages of tumour development. Early stages of tumour promotion are characterized by keratinocyte hyperproliferation and inflammation. These were diminished in TNF-α –/– mice. TNF-α was induced extensively in epidermis, but not dermis, of TPA-treated wt skin, suggesting that dermal inflammation is controlled by keratinocyte TNF-α production. These data provide evidence that a pro-inflammatory cytokine is required for de novo carcinogenesis and that TNF-α is important for the early stages of tumour promotion.

There are two clinical implications from our studies on TNF-α in the tumour microenvironment in human and murine cancer. First, therapeutic strategies that neutralize TNF-α may be useful in cancer treatment. There is already evidence for their utility in chronic inflammatory diseases such as Crohn's disease and rheumatoid arthritis.[24] Secondly, functional polymorphisms of inflammatory cytokine genes may influence risk or outcome of malignancy.[25] It was reported recently that possession of high-producer alleles of the TNF locus are an independent risk factor for progression-free survival in patients with non-Hodgkin's lymphoma.[26] A case-controlled study of inflammatory cytokine polymorphisms in 1000 women with epithelial ovarian cancer is currently under way.

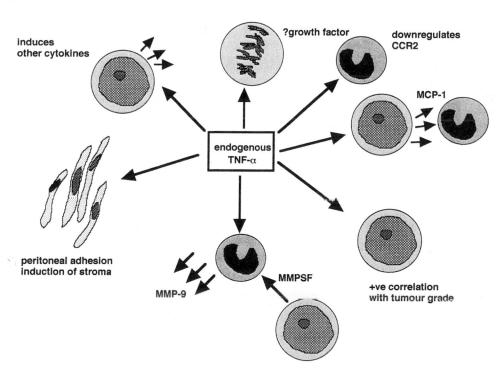

Fig. 17.2 The many ways in which endogenous TNF-α may influence the tumour microenvironment (see refs 1,2,3,9,13,18). MCP-1, monocyte chemoattractant protein-1; CCR2, chemokine receptor for MCP-1; MMP-9, matrix metalloprotease-9; MMPSF, putative MMP regulatory factor made by ovarian cancer cells.

Chemokines and MMPs

While the multiplicity of chemokines in the ovarian tumour microenvironment makes them an unlikely target for therapy, the limited expression of chemokine receptors, described above, is of interest. The infiltrating lymphocytes and macrophages may be important for the growth and spread of ovarian tumours. It is possible that antagonizing CCR1 and decreasing the cellular infiltrate could result in retarded tumour growth. This will be tested in an appropriate animal tumour model.

Our MMP results to date provide further rationale for using broad-spectrum MMP inhibitors, although the apparent tumour specificity of MMP–3 expression warrants further study.

Conclusions

We have begun to define some elements of the tumour microenvironment in human epithelial ovarian cancer. While this complex environment has many cellular and molecular components, we have been able to identify some therapeutic targets and suggest novel uses for existing biological therapies.

References

1. Negus, R.P.M., Stamp, G.W., Naylor, M.S. *et al.* (1997). A quantitative assessment of the leucocyte infiltrate in ovarian cancer and its relationship to the expression of c-c chemokines. *Am. J. Pathol.*, **150**, 1723–34.
2. Burke, F., Relf, M., Negus, R. *et al.* (1996). A cytokine profile of normal and malignant ovary. *Cytokine*, **8**, 578–85.
3. Naylor, M.S., Stamp, G.W.H., Foulkes, W.D. *et al.* (1993). Tumor necrosis factor and its receptors in human ovarian cancer. *J. Clin. Invest.*, **91**, 2194–206.
4. Rollins, B.J. (1997). Chemokines. *Blood*, **90**, 909–28.
5. Imai, T., Hieshima, K., Haskell, C. *et al.* (1997). Identification and molecular characterization of fractalkine receptor CX3CR1, which mediates both leukocyte migration and adhesion. *Cell*, **91**, 521–30.
6. Yoshida, T., Imai, T., Kakizaki, M. *et al.* (1998). Identification of single c-motif–1 lymphotactin receptor xcr1. *J. Biol. Chem.*, **273**, 16551–4.
7. Lu, B., Ebensperger, C., Dembic, Z. *et al.* (1998). Targeted disruption of the interferon-γ receptor 2 gene results in severe immune defects in mice. *Proc. Natl Acad. Sci. USA*, **95**, 8233–8.
8. Gao, J.-L., Wynn, T.A., Chang, Y. *et al.* (1997). Impaired host defense, hematopoiesis, granulomatous inflammation and type 1-type 2 cytokine balance in mice lacking CC chemokine receptor 1. *J. Exp. Med.*, **185**, 1959–68.
9. Negus, R.P.M., Stamp, G.W.H., Relf, M.G. *et al.* (1995). The detection and localization of monocyte chemoattractant protein–1 (MCP–1) in human ovarian cancer. *J. Clin. Invest.*, **95**, 2391–6.
10. Negus, R.P.M., Turner, L., Burke, F. *et al.* (1998). Hypoxia down-regulates MCP–1 expression: implications for macrophage distribution in tumors. *J. Leukoc. Biol.*, **63**, 758–65.
11. Turner, L., Scotton, C., Negus, R. *et al.* (1999). Hypoxia inhibits macrophage migration. *Eur. J. Immunol.*, in press.
12. Naylor, M.S., Stamp, G.W., Davies, B.D. *et al.* (1994). Expression and activity of MMPs and their regulators in ovarian cancer. *Int. J. Cancer*, **58**, 50–6.
13. Leber, T.M. and Balkwill, F.R. (1998). Regulation of moncyte MMP–9 production by TNF-α and a tumour-derived soluble factor (MMPSF). *Br. J. Cancer*, **78**, 724–32.
14. Boyd, R. and Balkwill, F.R. (1999). Release and activation in ovarian carcinoma: the role of fibroblasts. *Br. J. Cancer.*, in press.
15. Pujade-Lauraine, E., Guastalla, J.-P., Colombo, N. *et al.* (1996). Intraperitoneal recombinant interferon gamma in ovarian cancer patients with residual disease at second-look laparotomy. *J. Clin. Oncol.*, **14**, 343–50.
16. Burke, F.R., East, N., Upton, C. *et al.* (1997). Interferon-gamma induces cell cycle arrest and apoptosis in a model of ovarian cancer: enhancement of effect by Batimastat. *Eur. J. Cancer*, **33**, 1114–21.
17. Burke, F., Smith, P.D., Crompton, M.R. *et al.* (1999). The response of ovarian cancer cells to interferon gamma. *Br J Cancer*, **80**, 1236–44.
18. Malik, S.T.A., Griffin, D.B., Fiers, W. *et al.* (1989). Paradoxical effects of tumour necrosis factor in experimental ovarian cancer. *Int. J. Cancer*, **44**, 918–25.
19. Ruegg, C., Yilmaz, A., Bieler, G. *et al.* (1998). Evidence for the involvement of endothelial cell integrin αVβ3 in the disruption of the tumor vasculature induced by TNF and IFN-γ. *Nature Med.*, **4**, 408–14.
20. Gordon, H.M., Kucera, G., Salvo, R. *et al.* (1992). Tumor necrosis factor induces genes involved in inflammation, cellular and tissue repair, and metabolism in murine fibroblasts. *J. Immunol.*, **148**, 4021–7.
21. Piguet, P.F., Grau, G.E., and Vassalili, P. (1990). Subcutaneous perfusion of tumor necrosis factor induces local proliferation of fibroblasts, capillaries, and epidermal cells, or massive tissue necrosis. *Am. J. Pathol.*, **136**, 103–10.
22. Montrucchio, G., Lupia, E., Battaglia, E. *et al.* (1994). Tumor Necrosis Factor α-induced angiogenesis depends on *in situ* platelet-activating factor biosynthesis. *J. Exp. Med.*, **180**, 377–82.
23. Moore, R., Owens, D., Stamp, G. *et al.* (1999). Tumour necrosis factor-α deficient mice are resistant to skin carcinogenesis. *Nature Med.*, in press.
24. Feldmann, M., Elliott, M.J., Woody, J.N. *et al.* (1997). Anti-tumor necrosis factor-α therapy of rheumatoid arthritis. *Adv. Immunol.*, **64**, 283–349.
25. Wilson, A.G., Symons, J.A., McDowell, T.L. *et al.* (1997). Effects of a polymorphism in the human tumor necrosis factor α promoter on transcriptional activation. *Proc. Natl Acad. Sci. USA*, **94**, 3195–9.
26. Warzocha, K., Ribeiro, P., Bienvenu, J. *et al.* (1998). Genetic polymorphisms in the tumor necrosis factor locus influence non-Hodgkin's lymphoma outcome. *Blood*, **91**, 3574–81.

18. *ARHI (NOEY2)*, a novel imprinted tumor suppressor gene in ovarian cancer

Yinhua Yu, Fengji Xu, Hongqi Peng, Xianjun Fang, Shulei Zhao, Weiya Xia, Wen-lin Kuo, Joe W. Gray, Michael Siciliano, David Hogg, Andrew Berchuck, Kelly Hunt, Gordon B. Mills, and Robert C. Bast, Jr

Introduction

The expression and function of several tumor suppressor genes has been evaluated in epithelial ovarian cancer (Table 18.1). Abnormalities can occur in RB, WT and VHL, but loss of function is uncommon.[2,3] Mutations of p53 have been observed in more than 50% of ovarian cancers in advanced stages, but in only 15% of lesions limited to the ovary.[4] Consequently, loss of p53 function may correlate with the metastatic phenotype.

Early studies of tumor suppressor genes in ovarian cancer have concerned genes discovered in studying other tumor types. Over the past 3 years, functional inactivation of several novel putative suppressor genes has been observed, primarily in ovarian cancer. Tumor suppressor candidates have been identified by positional cloning or by differential gene expression, comparing normal and malignant ovarian epithelial cells. Candidates include a calcium-binding matrix protein (SPARC),[5] a GRB2-binding protein upstream of RAS (DOC2),[6] a phosphoinositol 3-phosphatase (MMAC1/PTEN),[7] a probable transcription factor (LOT-1),[8] and a protein without known function (OVCA1).[9]

Over the past 5 years, we have utilized differential display PCR to identify additional genes that are expressed regularly in normal ovarian epithelial cells, but not in ovarian cancer cells. One of the most interesting genes to emerge from this screen is *NOEY2*, which has been designated *ARHI* (RAS homology member I) by the Human Gene Nomenclature Committee.[10]

Cloning and characterization of *ARHI*

ARHI bears homology to Ras and Rap

Normal ovarian surface epithelial cells (OSE) were grown using the techniques developed by Nellie Auersperg.[11] RNA was extracted from normal OSE and from multiple ovarian cancer cell lines grown under similar conditions. Using differential display PCR, several gene segments were identified that were expressed by three specimens of OSE, but not by six different ovarian cancer cell lines. One of these sequences, *ARHI*, was extended using rapid amplification of cDNA ends. A cDNA library from OSE cells was screened using the extended *ARHI* cDNA as a probe. The full-

Table 18.1 Putative tumor suppressor genes in epithelial ovarian cancer[1]

Gene	Chromosome	Function
SPARC	5q31	Matrix
DOC2	5p13	Binds grb2
MMAC1 (PTEN)	10q23	Phosphatase
ARHI (NOEY2)	1p31	Induces p21[WAFICIPI]
		Inhibits cyclin D1
p53	17p13	DNA stability
		Apoptosis
LOT-1	6q25	Zinc finger
OVCA1	17p13	Unknown

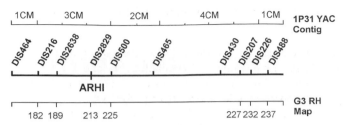

Fig. 18.1 Chromosome 1p31 physical map. The order of 10 microsatellite markers and *ARHI* at 1p31 is shown on the central scale. The upper and lower scales include the 1p31 yeast artificial chromosome (YAC) contig map and the G3 RH map for each marker.[15]

length *ARHI* sequence included an open reading frame of 687 bp that encoded a 1.9 kb message and a 26 kDa protein of 229 amino acids.[10] ARHI is a member of the Ras/Rap superfamily of small G proteins. Starting from its N-terminal amino acid 35, ARHI shares 56% amino-acid homology with Rap1A, 56% with Rap1B, 58% with Rap2A, 62% with Rap2B, 59% with K-Ras, and 54% with H-Ras.[10] The ARHI protein contains three motifs typical of the Ras family, including GTP-binding domains, a putative effector domain, and a membrane localizing CAAX motif. The sequence of the effector domain, YLPTIENTY, differs from the effector motif found in Ras and Rap family members, YDPTIEDSY.

Decreased expression of ARHI in ovarian and breast cancers

On Northern analysis, a 1.9 kb message was found in all 17 primary cultures of OSE and in all 14 cultures of breast epithelial cells, but in only 1 of 9 ovarian cancer cell lines and 1 of 8 breast cancer cell lines.[10] In those cancer cell lines where *ARHI* message could be detected (CaOv3 and MDA-MB–468), expression was reduced relative to normal epithelial cells. More precise measurement of *ARHI* mRNA was attained using Taqman real-time PCR. Nine cultures of normal OSE expressed $4.2 \pm 1.2 \times 10^4$ copies *ARHI*/100 ng cDNA, whereas 8 ovarian cancer cell lines expressed $5.1 \pm 6.5 \times 10^2$ copies/100 ng cDNA ($P < 0.05$). CaOV3 expressed 3.9×10^4 copies/100 ng cDNA. *ARHI* message could not be detected by Northern blotting in tumor cells purified from the ascites fluid of nine ovarian cancer patients[10]. When 16 different normal tissues were studied, *ARHI* message was detected in heart, liver, pancreas, and brain, but the highest level of expression was found in normal ovary.

Murine monoclonal antibodies were prepared against an ARHI–glutathione-*S*-transferase fusion protein. On Western analysis, these antibodies detected a protein of 26 kDa in normal OSE and breast epithelial cells, but not in the ovarian or breast cancer cell lines tested.[10] The same antibodies were used to detect *ARHI* expression in normal OSE, but not in the ovarian stroma by histochemical analysis. Among eight ovarian cancers, staining was not detected in five and less intense expression was detected in three.

Localization of ARHI to chromosome 1p31 at a site of frequent LOH

Many tumor suppressor genes can be mapped to sites of loss of heterozygosity (LOH). A P1 genomic library was screened using primers that encompassed the coding and 3' untranslated regions of *ARHI*. Positive clones were mapped to 1p31 by fluorescence *in situ* hybridization (FISH). LOH in this region had been reported in breast cancers,[12–14] but had not been described in ovarian cancers. Using an intragenic TA repeat marker within *ARHI*, LOH was found in 9 of 22 informative cases of ovarian cancer (41%).[10]

In subsequent studies, the gene was localized with greater precision using radiation hybrid mapping.[15] A detailed 1p31 physical map is provided in Fig. 18.1. One intragenic TA repeat marker and six flanking 1p31 microsatellite markers were also used for 1p31 deletion mapping by PCR-LOH analysis in 49 ovarian and breast cancers. Among the polymorphic markers studied, the highest frequency of LOH occurred in *ARHI* and in its linked marker D1S2829 (41% and 42%, respectively). These data support the hypothesis that *ARHI* is a tumor suppressor gene at 1p31. Two other discrete regions of LOH were found centered on D1S207 and D1S488, consistent with the possibility that other suppressor genes might be linked to *ARHI*.

Genomic structure and sequence abnormalities

As loss of function for a tumor suppressor gene requires inactivation of both alleles, sequence abnormalities were sought in 18 ovarian and breast cancer cell lines. Possible polymorphisms were evaluated in 110 normal DNA samples. The genomic sequence of *ARHI* was obtained, including 2.0 kb upstream of the transcription start site region. The *ARHI* gene contains two exons and one intron (Fig. 18.2). Three polymorphisms have been detected:

(1) a TA repeat polymorphism in the intron;
(2) a G to A substitution at coding +231; and
(3) an A to G substitution at –750 in the promoter region.

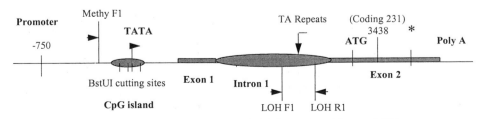

Fig. 18.2 Genomic structure of *ARHI*. (Reproduced from ref. 10.)

When tumor tissue and normal tissue from the same individual have been compared, only a single acquired mutation has been found (C to G at position −19) in the promoter region and no mutations have been found in the coding region. Consequently, it appeared unlikely that the decreased expression of *ARHI* resulted from mutational events of the normal allele in most ovarian and breast cancers.

Methylation and monoallelic expression of ARHI

Methylation has been implicated in silencing several growth regulatory genes.[16,17] Hypermethylation of the *ARHI* promoter region near the TATA box was found in 2 of 8 breast cancer cell lines, suggesting a mechanism by which expression of the gene could be downregulated. Hypomethylation was observed in 3 of 8 breast cancer cell lines and partial methylation was exhibited in all normal cells and in most cancer cell lines, consistent with monoallelic expression. To test this possibility directly, four specimens were identified that were heterozygous for a coding +231 polymorphism that eliminates a *Hha*I restriction site. In each specimen, only the G allele or the A allele was expressed.[10]

Maternal imprinting and loss of the functional allele

In studies of lymphocyte DNA from four informative families with TA repeat or −750 A/G polymorphisms, only the maternal alleles could be amplified after genomic DNA was digested with the methylation-sensitive restriction enzyme *Bst*UI.[10] Consequently, the *ARHI* gene appeared to be maternally imprinted, and loss of its expression in a fraction of breast and ovarian cancers could result from deletion of the non-imprinted allele. Among nine informative cases in which both LOH and imprinting could be evaluated in normal and tumor DNA, the retained allele was methylated and presumably silenced in seven.

Transcriptional regulation of ARHI expression

To assess whether transcriptional regulation of *ARHI* could contribute to decreased expression, the *ARHI* promoter was linked to a luciferase reporter and transfected into normal OSE or ovarian cancer cells (SKOv3, Hey). Relative to transfection of an SV40 promoter linked to a luciferase reporter, *ARHI* promoter activity was 50–100% in normal OSE and less than 10% in the two cancer cell lines. When promoter segments of different lengths were compared, optimal promoter activity was observed with a promoter of 1.5 kb. Thus, transcriptional regulation may contribute to decreased ARHI expression.

Inhibition of cancer cell growth with ARHI

Sense and antisense constructs of *ARHI* were transfected into breast and ovarian cancer cell lines that did not express the gene and into a lung cancer cell line (A–549) that expressed *ARHI*. The sense, but not the antisense, construct suppressed clonogenic growth in each of the cell lines that failed to express endogenous *ARHI*, but did not inhibit growth of the A–549 lung cancer cells that expressed the gene (Fig. 18.3a).

Effect of ARHI on expression of p21$^{WAF1/CIP1}$ and cyclin D1

Growth stimulation of normal OSE and breast epithelial cells was associated with downregulation of both *ARHI* and p21$^{WAF1/CIP1}$ by Northern analysis. To test the possible interaction of the two genes, a construct was prepared fusing *ARHI* with a triple hemagglutinin repeat (ARHI–HA). When this construct was transfected into NIH3T3 cells, p21$^{WAF1/CIP1}$ was induced. Induction of p21$^{WAF1/CIP1}$ was not observed when similar cells were transfected with an Erk2–HA construct.[10] An *ARHI* sense construct, but not an antisense construct, strongly inhibited cyclin D1 promoter activity when co-transfected with a construct that linked the cyclin D1 promoter with luciferase (Fig. 18.3b). Consequently, expression of the *ARHI* gene was associated with induction of p21$^{WAF1/CIP1}$ and downregulation of cyclin D1, alterations that could produce a cell cycle arrest at G_1–S.

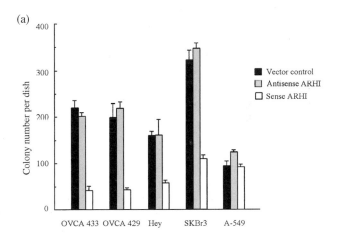

(a)

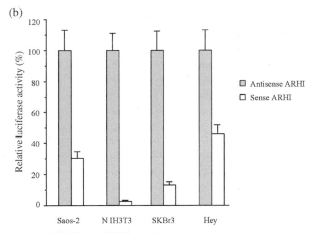

(b)

Fig. 18.3 *ARHI*-induced growth inhibition of ovarian and breast cancer cell lines. (a) Colony formation after *ARHI* cDNA transfection. *ARHI* in the sense orientation inhibited growth of OVCA433, OVCA429, Hey, and SKBr3 (*P* < 0.001) relative to vector alone or antisense controls. (b) Inhibition of cyclin D1 promoter activity in Saos-2, NIH3T3, SKBr3, and Hey cells. Luciferase activity in cells transfected with the sense construct was expressed as a percentage of the activity in cells transfected with the antisense vector. The results are from representative experiments performed in triplicate. (Reproduced from ref. 10.)

Phenotype of mice bearing the *ARHI* transgene

The *ARHI* gene was linked to a cytomegalovirus (CMV) promoter (5') and to a BGH polyadenylation sequence (3'). The construct was microinjected into individual pro-nuclei of one-cell stage FVB/N mouse embryos that were implanted in pseudopregnant ICR mice. Five founders were obtained from 33 newborn mice. From these founders, 413 litters have been screened and 197 of them were PCR positive for the human *ARHI* gene. The transgene was expressed in most organs, with the highest levels in heart, muscle, kidney, brain, and lung.[18]

Mice that overexpressed ARHI were smaller than non-transgenic littermates with a decrease of 10–40% in body weight. Small size has also been observed in cyclin D1 knockout mice,[19] consistent with downregualtion of cyclin D1 observed in tumor cells after the introduction of *ARHI*.

Female mice bearing the transgene have been unable to nurse and have lacked the histologic changes in mammary tissue associated with lactation. Circulating progesterone levels have been reduced, as has the expression of estrogen receptor (ER), progesterone receptor (PR), and prolactin in the mammary epithelial cells. Atrophy has been observed in testis and ovary. In mice with strong transgene expression and sterility, seminiferous tubules have contained very few Sertoli cells and have had markedly reduced spermatogenesis. Thymic atrophy has been observed in mice bearing the *ARHI* transgene, with a 30% decrease in thymocytes. Loss of CA1 and CA2 neurons has been found in the hippocampus, and loss of Purkinje cells has been documented in the cerebellum of transgenic animals. Alterations in the CNS have been associated with spontaneous twirling behavior.

Discussion

Taken together, our data suggest that *ARHI* may serve as a growth inhibitory tumor suppressor gene, the function of which is downregulated or lost in a majority of ovarian and breast cancers. Loss of expression can occur through several different mechanisms. As *ARHI* is a maternally imprinted gene, each normal cell can express only one allele. Deletion of the remaining functional allele can occur through LOH that has been observed at this locus in approximately 40% of breast[12–14] and ovarian cancers.[10] To our knowledge, this is the first imprinted tumor suppressor gene to be implicated in an adult cancer. Among the pediatric neoplasms, the *WT1* gene associated with Wilms tumor is part of an imprinted cluster on chromosome 11p.[20] Expression of *ARHI* can also be lost through transcriptional regulation, and we are currently attempting to identify relevant transcription factors with differing expression between normal and transformed ovarian epithelial cells.

Transfection of the *ARHI* gene induces p21[WAF1/CIP1] and downregulates cyclin D1, associated with inhibition of clonogenic growth. Cyclin D1 expression is upregulated in 25–30% of ovarian cancers in the absence of gene amplification.[21] Whether this correlates precisely with loss of *ARHI* expression has not yet been evaluated. Increased apoptosis has been observed in thymocytes from transgenic mice, but it is not yet clear whether induction of apoptosis is the primary mechanism by which *ARHI* inhibits tumor growth. Recent development of an adenoviral vector containing *ARHI* should facilitate studies of signal transduction and of apoptosis. The A–549 lung cancer cell line continued to express endogenous *ARHI* and was not affected by transfection of the gene. This observation raises the possibility that a therapeutic index might be attained using *ARHI* for gene therapy.

Acknowledgement

This work was supported in part by a grant CA 79003 from the National Cancer Institute and by the Ovarian Cancer research Fund at UT M.D. Anderson Cancer Center.

References

1. Bast, R.C. Jr and Mills, G.B. (2000). The molecular pathogenesis of ovarian cancer. In *The molecular basis of cancer*, (2nd edn), (ed. J. Mendelsohn, P. Howley, M. Israel and L. Liotta), in press.
2. Kim, T.M., Benedict, W.F., Xu, H.J. *et al.* (1994). Loss of heterozygosity on chromosome 13 is common only in the biologically more aggressive subtypes of ovarian epithelial tumors and is associated with normal retinoblastoma gene expression. *Cancer Res.*, **54** (3), 605–9.
3. Dodson, M.K., Cliby, W.A., Xu, H.J. *et al.* (1994). Evidence of functional RB protein in epithelial ovarian carcinomas despite loss of heterozygosity at the RB locus. *Cancer Res.*, **54** (3), 610–13.
4. Marks, J.R., Davidoff, A.M., Kerns, B.J.M. *et al.* (1991). Overexpression and mutation of p53 in epithelial ovarian cancer. *Cancer Res.*, **51**, 2979–84.
5. Mok, S.C., Chan, W.Y., Wong, K.K. *et al.* (1996). SPARC, an extracellular matrix protein with tumor-suppressing activity in human ovarian epithelial cells. *Oncogene*, **12**, 1895–901.
6. Mok, S.C., Wong, K.K., Chan, R.K. *et al.* (1994). Molecular cloning of differentially expressed genes in human epithelial ovarian cancer. *Gynecol. Oncol.*, **52**, 247–52.
7. Steck, P.A., Pershouse, M.A., Jasser, S.A. *et al.* (1997). Identification of a candidate tumor suppressor gene, MMAC1, at chromosome 10q23.3 that is mutated in multiple advanced cancers. *Nature Gen.*, **15**, 356–62.
8. Abdollahi, A., Godwin, A.K., Miller, P.D. *et al.* (1997). Indentification of a gene containing zinc finger motifs based on lost expression in malignantly transformed rat ovarian surface epithelial cells. *Cancer Res.*, **57**, 2029–34.
9. Schultz, D.C., Vandeweer, L., Berman, D.B. *et al.* (1996). Identification of two candidate tumor suppressor genes on chromosome 17p13.3. *Cancer Res.*, **56**, 1997–2002.
10. Yu, Y., Xu, F., Peng, H. *et al.* (1999). NOEY2 (ARHI), an imprinted putative tumor suppressor gene in ovarian and breast carcinomas. *Proc. Natl Acad. Sci. USA*, **96**, 214–19.
11. Zheng, J.P., Robinson, W.R., Ehlen, T. *et al.* (1991). Distinction of low grade from high grade human ovarian carcinomas on the basis of losses of heterozygosity on chromosomes 3, 6, and 11 and HER–2/neu gene amplification. *Cancer Res.*, **51** (15), 4045–51.
12. Nagai, H., Negrini, M., Carter, S.L. *et al.* (1995). Detection and cloning of a common region of loss of heterozygosity at chromosome 1p in breast cancer. *Cancer Res.*, **55**, 1752–7.
13. Loupart, M.L., Armour, J., Walker, R. *et al.* (1995). Allelic imbalance on chromosome 1 in human breast cancer. I. Minisatellite and RLFP analysis. *Gene. Chrom. Cancer*, **12**, 16–23.
14. Hoggard, N., Brintnell, B., Howell, A. *et al.* (1995). Allelic imbalance on chromosome 1 in human breast cancer. II. Microsatellite repeat analysis. *Gene. Chrom. Cancer*, **12**, 24–31.

15. Peng, H.Q., Xu, F.J., Pershad, R. *et al.* (2000). The functional allele of ARHI (NOEY2), an imprinted tumor suppressor gene, is deleted in ovarian and breast cancers. Submitted for publication.

16. Ohtani-Fujita, N., Fujita, T., Aoike, A. *et al.* (1993). CpG methylation inactives the promoter activity of the human retinoblastoma tumor-suppressor gene. *Oncogene*, **8** (4), 1063–7.

17. Myohanen, S.K., Baylin, S.B., and Herman, J.G. (1998). Hypermethylation can selectively silence individual p16ink4A alleles in neoplasia. *Cancer Res.*, **58** (4), 591–3.

18. Xu, F.-J., Xia, W., Zhao, S. *et al.* (1995). ARHI acts as a growth inhibitor in transgenic mice. Submitted for publication.

19. Fant, V., Stamp, G., Aneheus, A. *et al.* (1995). Mice lacking cyclin D1 are small and show defects in eye and mammarian gland development. *Genes and Dev.*, **9**, 2364–72.

20. Zhang, Y.H., Shields, T., Crenshaw, T., *et al.* (1993). Imprinting of human H19: allele-specific CpG methylation, loss of the active allele in Wilms tumor and potential for somatic allele switching. *Am. J. Hum. Genet.*, **53**, 113–24.

21. Worsley, S.D., Ponder, B.A.J., and Davies, B.R. (1997). Overexpression of cyclin D1 in epithelial ovarian cancers. *Gynecol. Oncol.*, **64**, 189–95.

19. Regulation of angiogenesis in ovarian cancer: role of p53, vascular endothelial growth factor, and hypoxia

E. Ferreux, C.E. Lewis, C.W. Perrett, and M. Wells

Introduction

Angiogenesis (the development of a new blood supply from existing blood vessels) plays an important part in the growth and metastasis of solid tumours. The cytokine, vascular endothelial growth factor (VEGF) is a potent and specific mitogen for endothelial cells, and stimulates tumour angiogenesis *in vivo*. Moreover, increased expression of VEGF by tumour cells has been closely correlated with increased tumour angiogenesis and reduced patient survival in various types of solid tumour, including early stage ovarian carcinoma.[1]

Mutations in the tumour suppressor gene *p53* and transient tumour hypoxia, such as that occurring in poorly vascularized areas of tumours, have both been implicated in the upregulation of VEGF gene expression in many human tumours. Mutations in *p53* are present in up to 50% of epithelial ovarian tumours, and recent studies have suggested that this may be an early molecular event in the pathogenesis of ovarian cancer.[2] A systematic correlative study of *p53* status, VEGF expression and angiogenesis in ovarian epithelial neoplasia has yet to be undertaken. In this chapter we will discuss the role of *p53* and hypoxia in the regulation of VEGF expression in ovarian cancer and their relationship to histological type. It is envisaged that a better understanding of these aspects of tumour biology will provide insight into the factors involved in tumour progression and potentially lead us to new therapeutic strategies.

Angiogenesis in ovarian cancer: the expression of vascular endothelial growth factor

Angiogenesis is a crucial factor in various physiological and pathological processes such as embryogenesis, wound healing, inflammation, and tumour growth.[3] Excessive angiogenesis is implicated in such diverse diseases as cancer, chronic inflammatory conditions, and diabetic retinopathy. In contrast, inadequate angiogenesis may impair wound healing and organ repair.

Ovarian cancer in its advanced stages is characterized by the rapid growth of solid intraperitoneal tumour cells, creating large areas of hypoxia and large volumes of ascitic fluid.[4] Angiogenesis has been correlated with poor prognosis in patients with advanced ovarian cancer.[5,6] In diagnostic terms, angiogenesis plays an important role in the detection of, and distinction between, benign and malignant ovarian neoplasms by transvaginal ultrasonography and colour Doppler imaging.[7]

VEGF is a multifunctional cytokine that is expressed in a wide variety of human malignancies and is considered to be an important mediator of angiogenesis, especially in epithelial ovarian cancer.[8] This protein is an endothelial cell mitogen and a modulator of microvascular permeability, all of which contribute to tumour growth and metastasis.[9] VEGF is generally expressed as four isoforms through alternative splicing, two small ones (121 and 165 amino acids), which are secreted, and two larger ones (189 and 206 amino acids), which are membrane bound.[10]

VEGF has been linked in a number of human tumours (e.g. breast cancer) to vascular density and to the degree of malignancy of the tumour. In epithelial ovarian cancer, VEGF appears to be a prognostic factor[2] as well as helping to monitor the clinical course of the disease.[11] Patients with disseminated cancer have higher serum levels of VEGF compared to patients with localized disease and healthy controls.[12] Mesiano *et al.* have shown higher levels of VEGF in the ascitic fluid of patients with high-stage tumours.[4] Barton *et al.* reported an increased concentration of VEGF in ascitic fluid and serum.[13] These workers also showed that the concentration of VEGF was higher in poorly differentiated tumours. The formation of ascites in human ovarian cancer seems to be directly associated with VEGF expression.[14] *In vivo* studies have shown that antibodies to VEGF effectively inhibit neovascularization in ovarian cancer cell lines by binding to VEGF itself and preventing the cytokine binding to its receptor.[15,16] VEGF mRNA has been found in the majority of epithelial ovarian cancers in the malignant cells but not in the normal stroma, although the protein does accumulate in the stromal matrix.[17] The protein was found to be expressed by neoplastic cells in all malignant cases

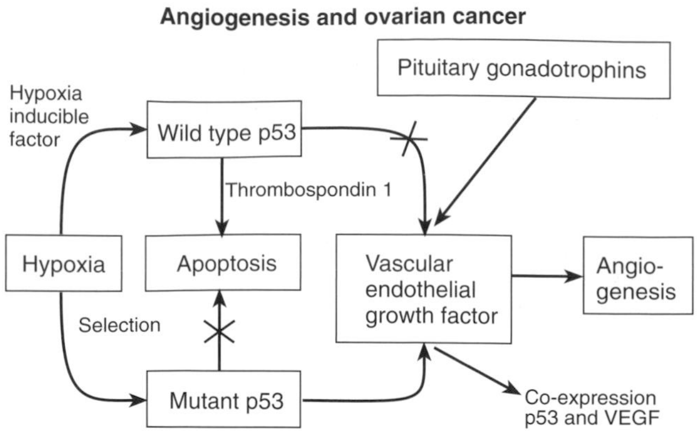

Angiogenesis and ovarian cancer

Fig. 19.1 Suggested interrelationships regulating angiogenesis in ovarian cancer.

studied, but no expression was found in the normal ovarian cortex or benign tumours.[9]

Hypoxia is a common feature of all solid tumours, occurring as a transient stress throughout the neoplastic tissue. In tumours, hypoxia has been correlated with areas of apoptosis as well as necrosis.[18] Hypoxic tumour cells are often found to be resistant to chemotherapeutic agents. Hypoxia has also been implicated in the selection of cells bearing mutations for *p53*.[18] Hypoxia-inducible factor (HIF) is a nuclear protein which acts as a transcription factor and is constantly transcribed but rapidly degraded under normoxia and stabilized under hypoxia. Hypoxic stress induces HIF DNA-binding activity through cognate recognition sequences (hypoxia response elements, or HREs) stimulating the expression of other factors which counteract the effect of hypoxia, such as VEGF.[19] HIF is at the centre of a complex interaction between *p53* and VEGF although its full molecular pathway remains to be elucidated (Fig. 19.1).

Although these data suggest a strong relationship between angiogenesis in ovarian cancer and VEGF, the actual mechanism of solid tumour angiogenesis and its regulation at the molecular level is not well understood, and the relationship that may exist between tumour suppressor gene-dependent gene transcription and hypoxia in such solid tumours is not well defined.

p53 in ovarian cancer

p53 is a 53 kDa nuclear phosphoprotein transcribed from the *p53* gene situated on the short arm of chromosome 17, at a position close to the *BRCA1* gene. Wild-type p53 protein regulates cell-cycle inhibition and apoptosis in response to DNA damage and cellular stress by acting, via p21, on the cell-cycle kinases to cause cell-cycle arrest at the G_1/S phase. It promotes either repair of the mistake or apoptosis by inducing transcription of the Bcl-2 protein.[20] The C-terminus of the protein is postulated to be a damage recognition region, based on its ability to bind to DNA ends and single-strand mismatches.[21] p53 protein is then degraded in the cytoplasm by the proteosome ubiquitin pathway, after being re-located from the nucleus by binding to MDM2.[22,23]

This mechanism is so rapid that, under physiological conditions, the protein is not visible due to its short half-life, but some mutations lead to an increased half-life. Point mutations of the *p53* tumour suppressor gene leading to overexpression of mutant p53 protein are the most common molecular alterations described in human cancers to date.[24]

One hypothesis for the cause of epithelial ovarian cancer is that of 'incessant ovulation', which is based on neoplastic transformation arising through serial damage to epithelial cells covering the serosal surface of the ovary as a consequence of ovulation.[25] The greater the frequency of ovulation, the more surface epithelial cells need to undergo repair and thus the greater chance that genetic abnormalities will occur. The protective effect of pregnancy and the contraceptive pill in the development of ovarian cancer is consistent with this hypothesis. The neoplastic process may be initiated by the selection of mutated cells due to their resistance to local stress and loss of the apoptotic pathway. A recent paper on the relationship between the number of ovulatory cycles and the expression of mutant *p53* expression in epithelial ovarian cancer has lent further support to this hypothesis.[26]

There are three main pathways by which p53 may be implicated in neoplastic progression:

(1) overexpression of mutant p53 (loss of wild-type function sometimes associated with acquisition of a new function, e.g. cells becoming more resistant to hypoxia);
(2) overexpression and stabilization of wild-type p53;
(3) mutation of another oncogene or tumour suppressor gene (or viral gene).

In most solid human cancers, the *p53* gene is mutated in the highly conserved region which is the specific DNA-sequence binding domain. *p53* mutations in ovarian cancer are mainly localized between exons 5–8 of the gene, with a few on exon 4.[27] Most recent publications concerned with ovarian cancer have studied overexpression of the p53 protein by immunohistochemistry and loss of heterozygosity. The overall percentage of tumours overexpressing p53 ranges from 29% to 60%, depending on whether antigen retrieval was used.[28,29] The protein has been found to be overexpressed mainly in malignant tumours, although benign lesions show expression of the protein in the absence of mutation. On the other hand, no expression at all has been found in ovaries from normal, age-matched patients or in normal ovaries removed from cancer patients.[30]

It seems that *p53* mutation is, in most ovarian cancers, a key pathogenetic event. It has been shown to act as a transcription factor, stimulating the expression of other genes, but its interaction under hypoxic stress in solid tumours has yet to be properly defined.

The relation between p53 status and VEGF expression in human cancer

Angiogenesis is an essential component of the growth and spread of solid tumours. p53 has been implicated in this phenomenon, particularly in the upregulation of VEGF that occurs in specific areas of such tissues. Hypoxia is present in distinct areas of vascular collapse or inadequate supply in most tumours, and often co-localizes with focal areas of both necrosis and increased expression of p53 and VEGF protein by tumour cells. This is illustrated by the recent reports showing that hypoxia upregulates HIF-1α, which causes p53 protein stabilization in tumour cells *in vitro*[31] independently of p53 status.[32] However, contradictory results have shown that hypoxia may, of itself, be insufficient.[33] It may help to enhance the survival of tumour cells expressing mutant, but not wild-type, p53. Hypoxia has also been shown to stimulate the expression of VEGF by tumour cells *in vivo* and *in vitro*.[34,35]

In 1994, Kieser *et al.* showed by transient transfection experiments that specific *p53* mutations (mouse form of Ala 135→Val) induced VEGF mRNA expression and potentiated TPA (12-O-tetradecanoylphorbol-13 acetate)-stimulated VEGF mRNA expression via the activation of protein kinase C.[36] They also showed that TPA-dependent VEGF expression was enhanced by human *p53* mutation at amino acid 175. Dameron *et al.* showed that the control of angiogenesis in cultured fibroblasts from Li–Fraumeni patients, who have lost the *p53* wild-type allele, resulted in a reduction in expression of thrombospondin-1 (TSP-1), a potent inhibitor of angiogenesis.[37] Furthermore, wild-type p53 downregulated endogenous VEGF mRNA, as well as VEGF promoter activation, in a dose-dependent manner, whereas the mutant form of p53 had no effect. Agani *et al.* have shown that p53 does not repress hypoxia-induced transcription of the VEGF gene.[38]

In lung cancer an association between the expression of p53, Bcl-2, and VEGF has been shown,[39,40] whereas in gastric cancer a recent study failed to show any relationship between p53 and VEGF.[41] Nevertheless, an association between VEGF and clinicopathological variables was shown, and the authors concluded that the progression of gastric cancer may be promoted by VEGF expression.[41] Most recently, attention has focused on the relationship between p53 and hypoxia-inducible factor (HIF). HIF-1α has been shown to stabilize wild-type p53,[42] whereas wild-type p53 inhibits HIF-1α-stimulated transcription.[43] These two findings provide evidence for the existence of an auto-loop between HIF and p53. Transcription is regulated by hypoxia, which appears to be a requirement for the formation of a multiprotein conformation formed by HIF-1α and p300/CREB (cyclic AMP response element binding protein).[44]

Experimental study

The aim of the first part of our study was to investigate the relationship between *p53* status (exons 5 and 7) and VEGF expression in 43 epithelial ovarian cancers; 26 serous, 9 mucinous, 2 clear cell, and 6 endometrioid. To do this we combined VEGF/p53 immunohistochemistry with tissue microdissection and DNA sequencing to compare immunoreactive VEGF with *p53* gene status and p53 protein expression in the same areas of the tumours. Two microdissected areas, one positive and one negative for VEGF were analysed for each tissue section (Fig. 19.2).

Twenty-two samples (51%) were found to overexpress p53; 34 samples (79%) expressed VEGF and 17 samples expressed both

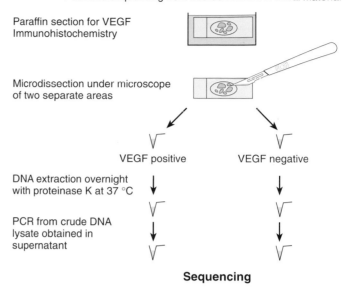

Method I

PCR and sequencing from microdissected archival material

Paraffin section for VEGF Immunohistochemistry

Microdissection under microscope of two separate areas

VEGF positive   VEGF negative

DNA extraction overnight with proteinase K at 37 °C

PCR from crude DNA lysate obtained in supernatant

Sequencing

Fig. 19.2 Summary of the methods employed in the first part of the experimental study.

p53 and VEGF (39.5%). VEGF expression was localized in the stroma as well as in the tumour cells, while p53 protein was found specifically in the nucleus of the tumour cells. Unexpectedly, we found no significant correlation (chi squared test $P > 0.05$)

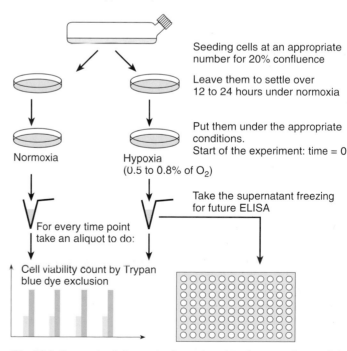

Method II

Hypoxia experiments on tissue cultures

Seeding cells at an appropriate number for 20% confluence

Leave them to settle over 12 to 24 hours under normoxia

Put them under the appropriate conditions.
Start of the experiment: time = 0

Normoxia   Hypoxia (0.5 to 0.8% of O$_2$)

Take the supernatant freezing for future ELISA

For every time point take an aliquot to do:

Cell viability count by Trypan blue dye exclusion

Fig. 19.3 Summary of the methods employed in the second part of the experimental study.

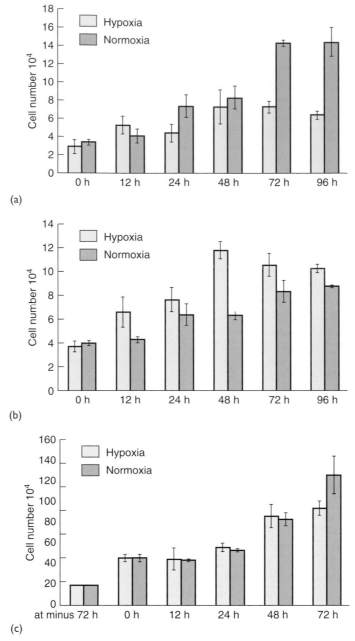

Fig. 19.4 Growth response to hypoxic and normoxic conditions in three different cell lines: *p53* null (a), *p53* mutated on exon 5 (b), and *p53* mutated on exon 7 (c).

between *p53* mutational status and VEGF expression, either between cases or between different microdissected regions within the same tumour; the *p53* gene status usually being uniform throughout the tumour irrespective of VEGF expression. However, there was a significant positive correlation (chi squared test $0.01 < P < 0.05$) between histological tumour type and *p53* gene status, with serous tumours containing higher levels of mutations in exon 7 than mucinous tumours. We have, at present, only sequenced exons 5 and 7. Nine samples were mutated (three on exon 5 and six on exon 7). Eight of the nine mutants (88.9%) showed strong expression of both VEGF and p53 protein by immunohistochemistry. All six tumours showing a mutation on exon 7 were of serous type (Table 19.1).

It is known that secreted as well as membrane-bound VEGF is expressed in ovarian cancer, unlike in breast cancer where only the membrane-bound form is found. Therefore, the VEGF expression seen by immunohistochemistry may be due to antigen diffusion and may not necessarily imply expression by the immediately adjacent neoplastic epithelial cells. There is also a growing awareness that p53 protein overexpression does not necessarily correlate with *p53* gene mutation.[45]

The second part of our study investigated the effect of *p53* gene status on the survival of three human ovarian tumour cell lines (which were either *p53* null or mutated at exon 5 or 7) in response to hypoxic stress *in vitro* (Fig. 19.3). The null *p53* cell line was unable to grow/function after 48 hours of hypoxia (0.5% oxygen)

Table 19.1 p53 and VEGF expression and *tp53* mutations in epithelial ovarian cancer (*n* = 43)

Immunostaining		tp53 gene status		
p53	VEGF	Exon 5	Exon 7	Tumour type
++++	++	Wt	Wt	Serous
+++	++++	Wt	Mut 248	Serous
–	++++	Wt	Mut 236	Serous
++++	++	Wt	Mut 226	Serous
+/–	++++	Wt	Wt	Serous
–	–	Wt	Wt	Serous
++++	–	Wt	Wt	Serous
++	+	Wt	Wt	Serous
++++	+/–	Wt	Mut 226	Serous
+/–	+++	Wt	Wt	Serous
++	+	Wt	Wt	Serous
+++	–	Wt	Wt	Serous
++/+++	++	Wt	Mut 245	Serous
++/+++	+/++	Wt	Mut 251	Serous
–	+	Wt	Wt	Serous
–	++	Wt	Wt	Serous
+	+/–	Wt	Wt	Serous
–	+	Wt	ND	Serous
+++	+/–	Wt	Wt	Serous
–	+	Wt	Wt	Serous
+++	++	ND	ND	Serous
–	+/++	Wt	ND	Serous with necrosis
–	+	ND	Wt	Serous with necrosis
+++	+++	Wt	Wt	Serous with necrosis
++++	+++	Mut 184	Wt	Serous with necrosis
++++	+	Mut 127	ND	Serous with necrosis
–	++	Wt	Wt	Endometrioid/serous
–	++	Wt	Wt	Enodmetroid
++++	++	Mut 163*	Wt	Endometrioid
–	+++	Wt	Wt	Endometrioid
–	+	Wt	Wt	Endometrioid
+/–	+++	Wt	ND	Endometrioid
+++	+	Wt	Wt	Mucinous
++++	+++	ND	Wt	Mucinous
–	+/–	Wt	Wt	Mucinous
+	++	ND	Wt	Mucinous
++++	++	ND	Wt	Mucinous
–	+++	Wt	Wt	Mucinous
–	++/+++	Wt	Wt	Mucinous
–	+/–	Wt	Wt	Mucinous
+/–	+++	Wt	Wt	Mucinous
+++	++++	Wt	Wt	Clear cell
+/–	++	ND	Wt	Clear cell

* The corresponding VEGF-negative area is wild type.

–, Negative; +/–, less than 5% cells positive; +, 6–24%; ++, 25–49%; +++, 50–74%; and ++++, 74–100% cells positive.

Wt, wild type; Mut, mutation; ND, not determined.

(Fig. 19.4a). The cell line bearing a mutation on exon 5 grew better under hypoxia than normoxia (Fig. 19.4b), whereas the cell line mutated on exon 7 grew equally well under normoxia and hypoxia (Fig. 19.4c). These results suggest that the type and localization of mutation may imbue the cells with a different level of resistance to hypoxic stress, or may merely reflect other genetic differences between the donors of these cells. Therefore the next step is to transfect a *p53* null cell line with different *p53* mutations

to study its resistance to apoptosis under hypoxia and its VEGF expression level by enzyme-linked immunosorbent assay (ELISA).

Conclusions

From these findings we deduce that there may be at least two main pathways regulating VEGF expression in ovarian cancer; one that is *p53*-dependent and one *p53*-independent, perhaps relying more on the HIF pathway to stimulate VEGF expression regardless of *p53* status. The *in vitro* results support the concept that hypoxia may contribute to the selection of *p53* mutated cell clones, more resistant to stress and probably lacking the apoptotic pathway.

References

1. Paley, P.J., Staskus, K.A., Gebhard, K. *et al.* (1997). Vascular endothelial growth factor expression in early stage ovarian carcinoma. *Cancer*, **80**, 98–106.
2. DiCioccio, R.A., Werness, B.A., Peng, R. *et al.* (1998). Correlation of TP53 mutations and p53 expression in ovarian tumors. *Cancer Genet. Cytogenet.*, **105**, 93–102.
3. Tempfer, C., Obermair, A., Hefler, L. *et al.* (1998). Vascular endothelial growth factor serum concentrations in ovarian cancer. *Obstet. Gynecol.*, **92**, 360–3.
4. Mesiano, S., Ferrara, N., and Jaffe, R.B. (1998). Role of vascular endothelial growth factor in ovarian cancer: inhibition of ascites formation by immunoneutralization. *Am. J. Pathol.*, **153**, 1249–56.
5. Hollingsworth, H.C., Kohn, E.C., Steinberg, S.M. *et al.* (1995). Tumor angiogenesis in advanced stage ovarian carcinoma. *Am. J. Pathol.*, **147**, 33–41.
6. Van Diest, P.J., Zevering, J.P., Zevering, L.C., and Baak, J.P. (1995). Prognostic value of microvessel quantitation in cisplastin treated FIGO 3 and 4 ovarian cancer patients. *Pathol. Res. Pract.*, **191**, 25–30.
7. Wu, C.C., Lee, C.N., Chen, T.M. *et al.* (1994). Incremental angiogenesis assessed by color Doppler ultrasound in the tumorigenesis of ovarian neoplasms. *Cancer*, **73**, 1251–6.
8. Nakanishi, Y., Kodama, J., Yoshinouchi, M. *et al.* (1997). The expression of vascular endothelial growth factor and transforming growth factor-β associates with angiogenesis in epithelial ovarian cancer. *Int. J. Gynecol. Pathol.*, **16**, 256–62.
9. Abu-Jawdeh, G.M., Faix, J.D., Niloff, J. *et al.* (1996). Strong expression of vascular permeability factor (vascular endothelial growth factor) and its receptors in ovarian borderline and malignant neoplasms. *Lab. Invest.*, **74**, 1105–15.
10. Ferrara, N. and Davis-Smyth, T. (1997). The biology of vascular endothelial growth factor. *Endocrine Rev.*, **18**, 4–23.
11. Yamamoto, S., Konishi, I., Mandai, M. *et al.* (1997). Expression of vascular endothelial growth factor (VEGF) in epithelial ovarian neoplasms: correlation with clinicopathology and patient survival, and analysis of serum VEGF levels. *Br. J. Cancer*, **76**, 1221–7.
12. Salven, P., Maenpaa, H., Orpana, A. *et al.* (1997). Serum vascular endothelial growth factor is often elevated in disseminated cancer. *Clin. Cancer Res.* **3**, 647–51.
13. Barton, D.P.J., Cai, A., Wendt, K. *et al.* (1997). Angiogenic protein expression in advanced epithelial ovarian cancer. *Clin. Cancer Res.*, **3**, 1579–86.
14. Yoneda, J., Kuniyasu, H., Crispens, M.A. *et al.* (1998). Expression of angiogenesis-related genes and progression of human ovarian carcinomas in nude mice. *J. Natl. Cancer Inst.*, **90**, 447–54.
15. Borgstrom, P., Hillan, K.J., Sriramarao, P., and Ferrara, N. (1996). Complete inhibition of angiogenesis and growth of microtumors by anti-

vascular endothelial growth factor neutralizing antibody: Novel concepts of angiostatic therapy from intravital videomicroscopy. *Cancer Res.*, **56**, 4032–9.

16. Mu, J., Abe, Y., Tsutsui, T. *et al.* (1996). Inhibition of growth and metastasis of ovarian carcinoma by administering a drug capable of interfering with vascular endothelial growth factor activity. *Jap. J. Cancer Res.*, **87**, 963–71.

17. Boocock, C.A., Charnock-Jones, S., Sharkey, A.M. *et al.* (1995). Expression of vascular endothelial growth factor and its receptors fit and KDR in ovarian carcinoma. *J. Natl. Cancer Inst.*, **87**, 506–16.

18. Graeber, T.G., Osmanian, C., Jacks, T. *et al.* (1996). Hypoxia-mediated selection of cells with diminished apoptotic potential in solid tumours. *Nature*, **379**, 88–91.

19. Wang, G.I. and Semenza, G.L. (1993). General involvement of hypoxia-inducible factor 1 in transcriptional response to hypoxia. *Proc. Natl. Acad. Sci. USA*, **90**, 4304–8.

20. Tang, H., Zhao, K., Pizzolato, J.F. *et al.* (1998). Constitutive expression of the cyclin-dependent kinase inhibitor p21 Is transcriptionally regulated by the tumor suppressor protein p53. *J. Biol. Chem.*, **273**, 29156–63.

21. Prives, C. and Hall, P.A. (1999). The p53 pathway. *J. Pathol.*, **187**, 112–6.

22. Haupt, Y., Maya, R., Kazaz, A., and Oren, M. (1997). Mdm2 promotes the rapid degradation of p53. *Nature*, **387**, 296–9.

23. An, W.G., Chuman, Y., Fojo, T., and Blagosklonny, M.V. (1998). Inhibitors of transcription, proteasome inhibitors, and DNA-damaging drugs differentially affect feedback of p53 degradation. *Exp. Cell Res.*, **244**, 54–60.

24. Greenblatt, M.S., Bennett, W.P., Hollstein, M., and Harris, C.C. (1994). Mutations in the p53 tumor suppressor gene: clues to cancer etiology and molecular pathogenesis. *Cancer Res.*, **54**, 4855–78.

25. Fathalla, M.F. (1971). Incessant ovulation: a factor in ovarian neoplasia? *Lancet*, **2**, 163.

26. Webb, P.M., Green, A., Cummings, M.C. *et al.* (1998). Relationship between number of ovulatory cycles and accumulation of mutant p53 in epithelial ovarian cancer. *J. Natl. Cancer Inst.*, **90**, 1729–34.

27. Hollstein, M., Sidransky, D., Vogelstein, B., and Harris, C.C. (1991). p53 mutations in human cancers. *Science*, **253**, 49–53.

28. Kohler, M.F., Kerns B.M., Humphrey, P.A. *et al.* (1993). Mutation and overexpression of p53 in early-stage epithelial ovarian cancer. *Obstet. Gynecol.*, **81**, 643–50.

29. Kiyokawa, T. (1994). Alteration of p53 in ovarian cancer: its occurence and maintenance in tumor progression. *Int. J. Gynecol. Pathol.*, **13**, 311–18.

30. Naito, M., Satake, M., Sakai, E. *et al.* (1992). Detection of p53 gene mutations in human ovarian and endometrial cancers by polymerase chain reaction-single strand conformation polymorphism analysis. *Jap. J. Cancer Res.* **83**, 1030–6.

31. An, W.G., Kanekal, M., Simon, C.M. *et al.* (1998). Stabilization of wild-type p53 by hypoxia-inducible factor 1α. *Nature*, **392**, 405–8.

32. Graeber, T.G., Osmanian, C., Jacks, T. *et al.* (1996). Hypoxia-mediated selection of cells with diminished apoptotic potential in solid tumours. *Nature*, **379**, 88–91.

33. Wenger, R.H., Camenisch, G., Desbaillets, I. *et al.* (1998) Up-regulation of hypoxia-inducible factor-1α Is not sufficient for hypoxic/anoxic p53 induction. *Cancer Res.*, **58**, 5678–80.

34. Waleh, N.S., Brody, M.D., Knapp, M.A. *et al.* (1995). Mapping of the vascular endothelial growth factor-producing hypoxic cells in multicellular tumor spheroids using a hypoxia-specific marker. *Cancer Res.*, **55**, 6222–6.

35. Stein, I., Neeman, M., Shweiki, D. *et al.* (1995). Stabilization of vascular endothelial growth factor mRNA by hypoxia and hypoglycemia and coregulation with other ischemia-induced genes. *Mol. Cell. Biol.*, **15**, 5363–8.

36. Kieser, A., Weich, H.A., Brandner, G. *et al.* (1994). Mutant p53 potentiates protein kinase C induction of vascular endothelial growth factor expression. *Oncogene*, **9**, 963–9.

37. Dameron, K.M., Volpert, O.V., Tainsky, M.A., and Bouck, N. (1994). Control of angiogenesis in fibroblasts by p53 regulation of thrombospondin-1. *Science*, **265**, 1582–4.

38. Agani, F., Kirsch, D.G., Friedman, S.L. *et al.* (1997). p53 does not repress hypoxia-induced transcription of the vascular endothelial growth factor gene. *Cancer Res.* **57**, 4474–7.

39. Fontanini, G., Vignati, S., Lucchi, M. *et al.* (1997). Neoangiogenesis and p53 protein in lung cancer: their prognostic role and their relation with vascular endothelial growth factor (VEGF) expression. *Br. J. Cancer*, **75**, 1295–301.

40. Fontanini, G., Boldrini, L., Vignati, S. *et al.* (1998). Bcl-2 and p53 regulate vascular endothelial growth factor (VEGF)-mediated angiogenesis in non-small cell lung carcinoma. *Europ. J. Cancer*, **34**, 718–23.

41. Baba, M., Konno, H., Maruo, Y. *et al.* (1997). Relationship of p53 and vascular endothelial growth factor expression to clinicopathological factors in human scirrhous gastric cancer. *Europ. Surg. Res.*, **30**, 130–7.

42. An, W.G., Kanekal, M., Simon, M.C. *et al.* (1998). Stabilization of wild-type p53 by hypoxia-inducible factor-1α. *Nature*, **392**, 405–8.

43. Blagosklonny, M.V., An, W.G., Romanova, L.Y. *et al.* (1998). p53 Inhibits hypoxia-inducible factor-stimulated transcription. *J. Biol. Chem.*, **273**, 11995–8.

44. Ebert, B.L. and Bunn, H.F. (1998). Regulation of transription by hypoxia requires a multiprotein complex that includes hypoxia-inducible factor-1, and adjacent transcription factor, and p300/CREB binding protein. *Mol. Cell. Biol.*, **18**, 4089–96.

45. Stewart, R.L., Royds, J.A., Burton, J.L. *et al.* (1998). Direct sequencing of the p53 gene shows absence of mutations in endometrioid endometrial adenocarcinomas expressing p53 protein. *Histopathology*, **33**, 440–5.

20. Role of Fas/FasL in the control of human ovary cancer growth and progression

Delia Mezzanzanica, Alessandra Mazzoni, Donatella R.M. Negri, Mariangela Figini, Maria I. Colnaghi, and Silvana Canevari

Introduction

Ovarian cancer is the most frequent cause of cancer death in women with gynecological neoplasms in Europe. As an alternative to classical chemotherapy, we recently investigated the efficacy of antibody-targeted treatment of ovarian carcinoma patients.[1,2] In particular we developed a model of adoptive immunotherapy based on the re-targeting of activated T lymphocytes by a bispecific antibody directed against the CD3 molecule of lymphocytes and a glycoprotein marker of tumor cells, the α-folate receptor (αFR), that is overexpressed on the majority of ovarian carcinomas.[3,4] After proving of the concept of specific T-cell re-targeting in an experimental model,[5,6] our phase II study indicated tumor regression in 27% of ovarian carcinoma patients at advanced stages of the disease.[2] These results, which are similar or slightly superior to the complete response rates obtained with second-line chemotherapy, could represent a great advance in the curability of ovarian carcinoma. In fact, humoral and cellular immunological approaches are effective on drug-resistant tumors and have low toxicity and side-effects, with consequent improvement of quality of life, unlike chemotherapy.

Like many other tumors, ovarian carcinomas use a vaste array of different molecules to promote proliferation and have evolved multiple mechanisms to evade the immune system. These range from the passive failure to express co-stimulatory and major histocompatibility complex molecules,[7] to active strategies such as the production of immunosuppressive cytokines and other factors.[8] Passive and active processes are also involved in the most recently discovered mechanism by which tumors may evade the immune system: the Fas counterattack.[9] The Fas receptor (Fas, APO-1/CD95) and its ligand (FasL), are both transmembrane proteins belonging to the tumor necrosis factor family of receptors and ligands. Engagement of Fas by FasL triggers a cascade of subcellular events that result in programmed cell death (apoptosis). Fas-mediated apoptosis plays a key role in many physiological mechanisms, including cytotoxic T cell (CTL)-mediated cytotoxicity and downregulation of the immune response.[10] Although FasL was initially thought to be expressed only in cells of the lymphoid/myeloid series, it has now been shown to be expressed by non-lymphoid cells, where it contributes to immune privilege by inducing apoptosis in infiltrating pro-inflammatory immunocytes.[11] Evidence that some non-lymphoid tumor cells express FasL raised the intriguing possibility that cancer cells might also be sites of immune privilege, representing a novel mechanism of immunoevasion.[12–18] Tumor-cell resistance to Fas-mediated apoptosis is a crucial component of the Fas counterattack. For tumor cells, in fact, the expression of Fas is a necessary, but not sufficient trait, for sensitivity to Fas-induced apoptosis; there is mounting evidence suggesting that defective or disrupted apoptotic pathways may be involved in tumor progression and may confer resistance to therapy.[19]

We started to study the Fas/FasL system on both ovarian carcinoma cells and normal ovary surface epithelium (OSE), the pelvic modified mesothelium that overlies the ovary. OSE cells are the source of ovary epithelial tumors, which constitute 80–90% of all ovarian tumors. The proliferation of OSE cells in physiological conditions is tightly controlled, and several hormones and growth factors have been suggested to contribute to proliferative stimulation or inhibition. The Fas/FasL interaction has been postulated as one of the mechanisms of growth control in hormone-regulated tissues such as mammary gland,[20] but no data, to date, on Fas/FasL expression on OSE are available. Analysis of the mechanism(s) of Fas resistance and of the functional activity of FasL could contribute to a better understanding of the alterations in the growth control in ovarian carcinoma cells and of their escape to the host immune system. To test this hypothesis, we analyzed Fas/FasL expression and functional activity in OSE cells and in ovarian carcinoma cells also in relation to tumor development and progression.

OSE cells do express Fas but lack expression of FasL

After isolation from the surface of normal ovaries, OSE cells were kept in culture for a maximum of 5–6 passages.[21,22] During this period they were characterized by analyzing different epithelial markers, including Fas and FasL. Figure 20.1 shows a typical cytofluorometric profile that we obtained on OSE cells for Fas expression. The Jurkat cell line or activated PBMC, used as positive controls, showed an expression of Fas three times higher than that obtained on OSE cells (data not shown). The expression of FasL could not be detected by fluorescence-activated cell sorter (FACS), therefore the analysis was carried out by reverse transcriptase polymerase chain reaction (RT-PCR), results are shown in the inset of Fig. 20.1. Activated PBMC were used as a positive control for both Fas and FasL expression (lane 4). The transcript for Fas could be amplified in all OSE cell preparations (lanes 2 and 3), whereas the transcript for FasL was not detectable (lanes 2 and 3). After three passages of culture, OSE cells were tested for sensitivity to Fas-mediated apoptosis using an agonistic anti-Fas monoclonal antibody (CH-11). Cells were incubated for different periods of time with CH-11 or with an isotype-matched control Ab, and cell viability was measured by a colorimetric MTT assay.[6] Figure 20.2 shows the results obtained on four different preparations of OSE cells in comparison with the Jurkat cell line used as positive control for Fas sensitivity. On Jurkat, we repeatedly obtained a cytotoxicity of approximately 50% after 24 hours of incubation with CH-11. This cytotoxicity did not increase by prolonging the incubation time. The sensitivity of OSE cells was very low, even after 48 hours of incubation; a moderate level of cytotoxicity was obtained only after 72 hours of incubation, indicating a partial resistance of OSE cells to Fas-mediated apoptosis.

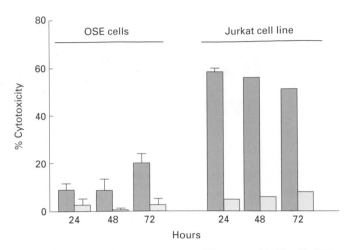

Fig. 20.2 Kinetics of cytotoxicity on anti-Fas-treated OSE cells. OSE cells and the Jurkat cell line were incubated with 300 ng/ml of agonistic anti-Fas antibody (dark gray) or isotype-matched control antibody (light gray) and cell viability was measured by a colorimetric MTT assay after 24, 48, and 72 hours. Columns represent the mean of 1–4 experiments for each cell line ± SD.

Expression of FasL could be detected on some ovarian carcinoma surgical specimens

The expression of Fas and FasL was evaluated, at RNA level, also on ovarian carcinoma surgical specimens obtained at different stages of the disease from eight different patients. For five patients (BD, CG, BL, PV, and BM) we could analyze both the primary and the metastatic tumor. The analysis was carried out by RT-PCR and the results are shown in Fig. 20.3. The transcript for Fas was present in all the tested samples, as we originally observed in OSE cells. This was in contrast with FasL, which was not expressed on OSE cells yet was evident in 4 out of 8 patients (Fig. 20.3, panel B). The appearance of FasL did not correlate with the stage of the disease. In fact, for patients PV and BM both primary (lanes 9 and 11) and metastatic tumor (lanes 10 and 12) expressed FasL. For patient CG we found positivity only for the primary tumor (lane 5), but this is probably due to a difference in RNA quantity. A borderline tumor (lane 13) also expressed FasL.

Since the RNA was extracted from surgical specimens, it was possible that it could be contaminated with RNA from tumor-infiltrating lymphocytes (TIL) that are known to express both Fas and FasL. To check the possible level of contamination of our preparations, we amplified the ϵ-chain of the CD3 molecule. A very faint band was evident only in samples 11 and 13, thus excluding the possibility of heavy TIL contamination (data not shown). The data obtained from patients' RNA could not provide information on the functional activity of Fas and FasL in ovarian carcinoma. We then used ovarian carcinoma cell lines to test Fas-mediated apoptosis and the ability of the expressed FasL to induce apoptosis on Fas-sensitive cell lines such as Jurkat.

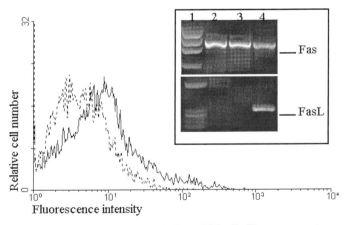

Fig. 20.1 Expression of Fas and FasL on OSE cells. Flow cytometric analysis of cell-surface Fas expression: OSE cells were stained with FITC-labeled anti-CD95 antibody (solid line) or with control antibody (dotted line). The inset shows an RT-PCR of Fas and FasL. cDNAs were amplified with primers specific for Fas and FasL and the resulting products were electrophoresed in a 1.8% ethidium bromide-stained agarose gel. Lane 1, marker is ΦX174/*Hae*III digest; lanes 2,3, two different preparations of OSE cells; lane 4, activated PBMC.

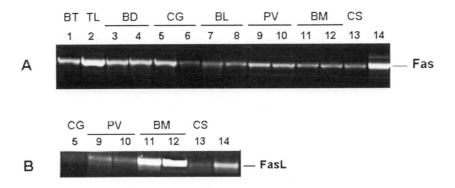

Fig. 20.3 RT-PCR for Fas and FasL. RNA from ovarian carcinoma surgical specimens was reverse transcribed and the resulting cDNA was amplified using specific primers for Fas (panel A) and FasL (panel B). Lanes 1–13 represent samples from different surgical specimens of ovarian carcinoma obtained from eight patients at different stages of the disease. The 13 samples analyzed derived from: two borderline tumors (lanes 2 and 13), four primary tumors (lanes 3, 5, 9, 11), four metastatic solid tumors (lanes 4, 6, 8, 12), and three ascites (lanes 1, 7, 10). Lines over the numbers indicate specimens at different stages of the disease obtained from the same patient whose initials are reported over the lanes. Lane 14 corresponds to activated PBMC, used as a positive control.

Most of the ovarian carcinoma cell lines are resistant to Fas-mediated apoptosis

Eight ovarian carcinoma cell lines were tested for expression of Fas by flow cytometry and for sensitivity to Fas-mediated apoptosis. As reported in Fig. 20.4, the expression of Fas on the cell surface is a condition necessary, but not sufficient, for Fas sensitivity. OAW42, which expresses twice the amount of Fas compared to Jurkat, is much less sensitive to Fas-mediated apoptosis. On the contrary, INTOV1, with a very low expression of Fas, can be con-

sidered slightly sensitive. In the attempt to evaluate the behavior of ovarian carcinoma cell lines, we tested their sensitivity by prolonging the incubation time with the agonistic anti-Fas antibody CH-11. On the basis of the results obtained, we could divide the cell lines in three groups. Group A including OAW42 and INTOV1, which eventually became sensitive to CH-11 treatment, reaching at 72 hours of incubation the levels of cytotoxicity observed on Jurkat (60–80% cytotoxicity). Group B included two cell lines (IGROV1 and INTOV2) and also the OSE cells, showing moderate sensitivity to anti-Fas treatment only after 72 hours of incubation (20–30% of cytotoxicity). Group C included all the remaining cell lines (SW626, OVCAR3, OCVA432, and SKOv3) that could not be induced to apoptosis even after 72 hours of incubation with CH-11. All the attempts to up-modulate Fas expression or Fas sensitivity by treatment with interferon-γ or tumor necrosis factor-α (TNF-α) failed (data not shown).

The expression of FasL in ovarian carcinoma cell lines was tested by RT-PCR. Only one cell line, SW626, expressed a level of FasL comparable to that observed in activated PBMC used as the positive control.

Protein synthesis inhibitors in some cases can revert resistance to apoptosis

Protein synthesis inhibitors, such as cycloheximide (CHX), can increase Fas-mediated apoptosis as previously reported.[23] Accordingly, we tested the effect of anti-Fas antibody in combination with CHX on both ovarian carcinoma cell lines and on OSE cells (Table 20.1). We observed that cells belonging to group A, which eventually became sensitive to CH-11 treatment after 72 hours of incubation, greatly increased their sensitivity to apoptosis after 24 hours of incubation by the addition of CHX (sensitive cells). Cells belonging to group B, showing a moderate sensitivity to anti-Fas treatment only after 72 hours of incubation, could be

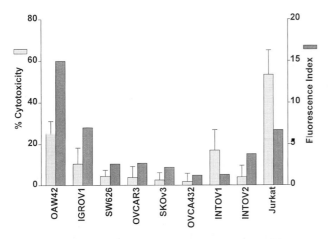

Fig. 20.4 Fas-mediated apoptosis of ovarian carcinoma cell lines in relation to Fas membrane expression. Left y-axis refers to cytotoxicity measured by the MTT assay after 24 hours of incubation with 300 ng/ml of agonistic anti-Fas antibody CH-11. Columns represent the mean of 2–7 experiments for each cell line ± SD. Right y-axis refers to membrane expression of Fas evaluated by flow cytometry. Columns represent the fluorescence index, evaluated as the ratio of mean fluorescence intensity (MFI) of cells treated with fluorescinated anti-CD95 antibody versus MFI of cells treated with fluorescinated control antibody.

Table 20.1 Protein synthesis inhibitors can revert resistance to apoptosis

Cells Ab+CHX	Group[b]	CH-11	CH-11+CHX	Cont
		% of cytotoxicity (SD) mediated by[a]		
OAW42	A	25 (5.9)	**56** (11)	11 (1.5)
INTOV1	A	17 (9.8)	**67** (5)	4.5 (3.5)
IGROV1	B	10.4 (7.7)	**37** (11)	11.8 (7.6)
INTOV2	B	4 (5.6)	**30** (14)	7 (4.2)
OSE	B	9 (5.2)	**45** (16)	13.5 (4.6)
SW626	C	**4.4** (3)	13.5 (8.4)	9.8 (2.6)
OVCAR3	C	3.8 (5.4)	7 (6.3)	5.8 (6.6)
SKOv3	C	2.6 (3.5)	17.5 (7.6)	11.2 (5.9)
OVCA432	C	1.8 (4)	3.6 (3)	2.8 (4.7)

[a] Cells were incubated with 300 ng/ml of agonistic anti-Fas antibody (CH-11) or isotype-matched control antibody in the presence or absence of 1 μg/ml of cycloheximide (CHX). Cell viability was measured by the MTT assay after 24 hours. Numbers represent the mean of 2–7 experiments for each cell line (SD).

[b] Groups are defined on the basis of sensitivity to Fas-mediated apoptosis evaluated by MTT assay after 24, 48, and 72 hours of incubation. Group A, sensitive cells; group B, inducible cells; group C, resistant cells.

Number in bold are significantly increased percentages of cytotoxicity compared to the control.

induced to apoptosis after 24 hours by the addition of CHX (inducible cells). The resistance of cells belonging to group C could not be overcome even under these conditions (resistant cells).

To check whether the cytotoxicity observed in the MTT assay was indeed the effect of an apoptotic phenomenon, ovarian carcinoma cell lines were tested for DNA fragmentation. In sensitive cell lines, belonging to group A, we observed DNA fragmentation with CH-11 alone (as we observed for Jurkat cells). Inducible cell lines and OSE cells underwent DNA fragmentation only when CHX was added to the assay. In all the other cases we could not obtain any DNA fragmentation (data not shown).

Mechanisms of resistance to Fas-mediated apoptosis

Apoptotic resistance in Fas-expressing malignant cells has already been reported.[24] Potential mechanisms for apoptotic resistance include: (1) alteration of the Fas molecule; (2) alteration of Fas intracellular signaling pathways; (3) overexpression of Bcl-2 family proteins; (4) overexpression of the Fas-associated phosphatase-1 (FAP-1).

One of the alterations of the Fas molecule responsible for Fas-mediated apoptosis resistance is the expression of a truncated Fas receptor lacking the intracellular death-signaling domain (FasExo8Del).[25] Resistance might also be due to the presence of soluble forms of Fas, which are produced by alternative splicing and do not contain the trans-membrane (TM) domain (FasΔTM).[26–28] To determine whether FasExo8Del and FasΔTM forms of the Fas receptor were expressed in ovarian carcinoma and in OSE cells, mRNA transcripts were analyzed by RT-PCR using primers flanking exon 8 and exon 6, respectively. None of the samples analyzed, irrespective of their origin, showed the presence of the band corresponding to the exon 8 deleted form of Fas

(data not shown). Concerning exon 6, all the cell lines showed the presence of a faint band corresponding to the FasΔTM. The ratio of FasΔTM to FasTM, evaluated using a phosphoImager, was comparable, in all cell lines, to that obtained in Jurkat and in activated PBMC used as controls. The only exception was observed in one preparation of OSE cells, in which we obtained a band of FasΔTM giving a higher ratio. Using the RNA from surgical specimens, we observed in five cases a ratio of FasΔTM to FasTM exceeding that of controls (Fig. 20.5).

Concerning the possible alteration of Fas intracellular signaling pathways, at present we have only analyzed by RT-PCR the presence of transcripts for Fas-associated death domain protein (FADD) and for FADD-like ICE (FLICE). FADD is recruited to Fas upon its activation[29] and binds to Fas via interactions between the death domains. FADD is then responsible for downstream

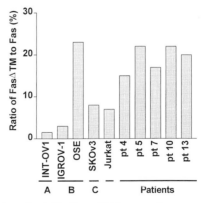

Fig. 20.5 Evaluation of soluble Fas. mRNA transcripts were analyzed by RT-PCR using primers flanking exon 6 and amplifying a band corresponding to the intact form of Fas, and, when present a 69 bp shorter band corresponding to FasΔTM. Columns represent the ratio of FasΔTM to Fas obtained by measuring the bands with a PhosphorImager. Jurkat is reported as a control. For patient description, see Fig. 20.3.

signal transduction. FLICE, or caspase-8,[30] is the signaling molecule downstream of FADD. The oligomerization of FLICE may result in self-activation of proteolytic activity and trigger the ICE protease cascade.[10] Both FADD and FLICE are present, at least at the molecular level, in all the samples tested, irrespective of their origin. Experiments are in progress to test their biological activity in OSE cells and in the carcinoma cell lines.

The overexpression of Bcl-2 family members, such as Bcl-2 itself or Bcl-X_L, can block apoptosis triggered by a number of different stimuli, such as factor deprivation, irradiation, anti-cancer drugs, and Fas-mediated apoptosis.[10] The expression of Bcl-2 and Bcl-X_L was analyzed by RT-PCR in OSE cells, carcinoma cell lines, and RNA from surgical specimens (Table 20.2). As a positive control for overexpression we used the Raji cell line. None of the seven preparations of OSE cells was found to be positive for the Bcl-2 transcript; whereas Bcl-X_L was expressed in all OSE cell preparations. Concerning the cell lines, we found an expression of Bcl-2 greater than that of Raji only in OVCA432, which is a resistant cell line. Traces of Bcl-2 transcript were also found in INTOV1 (sensitive cell line), IGROV1 and INTOV2 (inducible cell lines), and OVCAR3 (resistant cell line). The only two cell lines that gave negative results were SW626 and SKOv3, which are resistant to Fas-mediated apoptosis. Transcripts for Bcl-X_L were found in all cell lines but SKOv3. In INTOV2, OVCAR3, and OVCA432, the level of Bcl-X_L expression was greater than that observed in Raji. Concerning the samples derived from patients, traces of Bcl-2 were expressed in 1 out of 2 borderline tumors and in all primary tumors. All the solid metastatic tumors but one, and all the ascites were definitively positive for Bcl-2 expression. Bcl-X_L was found in 1 borderline tumor, 2 out of 4 primary tumors, 2 out of 4 metastatic solid tumors and 2 out of 3 ascites (Table 20.2).

FAP-1 has been reported to inhibit Fas-mediated apoptosis by interacting with a suppressive domain of Fas.[31] FAP-1 mRNA expression was absent in OAWA2 (sensitive cell line), SW626 and SKOv3 (resistant cell lines). INTOV1 (sensitive cell line) and IGROV1 (inducible cell line) expressed a low level of FAP-1, whereas INTOV2 (inducible cell line), OVCAR3 and OVCA432 (resistant cell lines), and OSE cells expressed a high level of transcript. Among patients, the transcript for FAP-1 was found in one borderline, one primary, two metastatic solid tumors, and one ascite (Table 20.2).

The FasL expressed on the SW626 cell line is functionally active

The functional activity of FasL expressed by SW626 was tested as its ability to induce DNA fragmentation of the Fas-sensitive Jurkat cell line. Adherent SW626 cells were incubated with Jurkat cells at an effector to target ratio of 10:1. After 7 hours of incubation Jurkat cells were harvested and DNA was analyzed by agarose gel electrophoresis. As shown in Fig. 20.6, the typical ladder due to apoptotic DNA fragmentation was present in Jurkat cells incubated with SW626 (lane 1) but not in untreated cells (lane 2).

Conclusions

In this chapter we have shown that OSE cells, the source of ovary epithelial tumors, express Fas and are inducible to Fas-mediated apoptosis, yet do not express FasL. In contrast to this, ovarian carcinoma cells lines, although expressing Fas, have different sensitivity to Fas-mediated apoptosis. In fact, 50% of the ovarian carcinoma cell lines tested were resistant to Fas-mediated apoptosis. Furthermore, FasL expressed by one of these cell lines was functionally active. We were not able to identify one specific mechanism used by ovarian carcinoma cell lines to resist Fas-mediated apoptosis. In fact, Bcl-2 was found to be overexpressed in only one of the resistant cell lines analyzed (OVCA432) and

Table 20.2 Overepression of Bcl-2 family members and overepression of FAP-1[a]

Samples	Group	Bcl-2	Bcl-X_L	FAP-1
OAW42	Sensitive	−	+/−	−
INTOV1	Sensitive	+/−	+	+
IGROV1	Inducible	+/−	+	+
INTOV2	Inducible	+/−	++	++
OSE	Inducible	−	+	++
SW626	Resistant	−	+	−
OVCAR3	Resistant	+/−	++	++
SKOv3	Resistant	−	−	−
OVCA432	Resistant	++	++	++
Borderline tumors (2)		+/− (1/2)	+ (1/2)	+/−
Primary tumors (4)		+/− (4/4)	+ (2/4)	+ (1/4)
Metastatic solid tumors (4)		+ (3/4)	+ (2/4)	+ (2/4)
Ascites (3)		+ (3/3)	+ (2/3)	+ (1/3)

[a] The overexpression was evaluated by RT-PCR using Raji cells as the positive control for Bcl-2 and Bcl-X_L, and activated PBMC as the positive control for FAP-1.

−, Absence of transcript; +/−, level of transcript lower than positive control; +, level of transcript equal to positive control; ++, level of transcript greater than positive control.

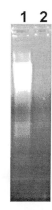

Fig. 20.6 DNA fragmentation induced in Jurkat cells by SW626 FasL. SW626 cells (5×10^6) were incubated overnight to allow cell adherence. Jurkat cells (5×10^3) were then added and incubated for 7 hours. The DNA of Jurkat cells was extracted and analyzed for the presence of the typical ladder by ethidium bromide-stained agarose gel. Lane 1, Jurkat cells incubated with SW626; lane 2, untreated cells.

Bcl-X$_L$ in only two resistant cell lines (OVCAR3 and OVCA432) and in one inducible cell line (INTOV2). Furthermore, two other resistant cell lines (SKOv3 and SW626) failed to express both transcripts. As already reported by others,[24] we failed to find a correlation between Bcl-2 levels and Fas-mediated apoptosis in solid tumors. Also in the case of FAP-1 we can not assume a general mechanism of inhibition. We are evaluating at present whether the treatment of cells with transcription inhibitors, such as actinomycin D, reduces the level of FAP-1 mRNA without affecting β-actin, Bcl-2, and Fas mRNA, thus suggesting a possible direct correlation of FAP-1 with Fas resistance.

In keeping with observations made in other solid tumors, several mechanisms in ovarian carcinoma may be considered responsible for resistance to Fas-mediated apoptosis. Additional studies examining the sensitization of ovarian cancer cells to Fas-mediated apoptosis *in vivo*, should provide a new therapeutic approach in the treatment of ovarian carcinoma.

In August 1999, a short communication appeared in *J. Natl. Cancer Inst.*, **91**, 1327–8, showing evidence for the colonic origin of ovarian cancer cell line SW626.

Acknowledgements

We are grateful to Dr Rosanna Fontanelli of the Surgery Branch for providing normal ovaries (source of OSE cells) obtained from women with pathological disease other than ovarian tumors. We thank Fabio Turatti for his help in reviewing the manuscript, Miss Elena Luison and Mrs Paola Alberti for excellent technical help, and Miss Laura Mameli for manuscript preparation. This work was supported partially by Associazione Italiana per la Ricerca sul Cancro.

References

1. Crippa, F., Bolis, G., Seregni, E. *et al.* (1995). Single dose intraperitoneal radioimmunotherapy with the murine monoclonal antibody ^{131}I-MOv18: clinical results in patients with minimal residual disease of ovarian cancer. *Eur. J. Cancer*, **31A**, 686–90.

2. Canevari, S., Stoter, G., Arienti, F. *et al.* (1995). Regression of advanced ovarian carcinoma by intraperitoneal treatment with autologous T-lymphocytes retargeted by a bispecific monoclonal antibody. *J. Natl Cancer Inst.*, **87**, 1463–9.

3. Miotti, S., Canevari, S., Ménard, S. *et al.* (1987). Characterization of human ovarian carcinoma-associated antigens defined by novel monoclonal antibodies with tumor-restricted specificity. *Int. J. Cancer*, **39**, 297–303.

4. Coney, L.R., Tomassetti, A., Carayannopoulos, L. *et al.* (1991). Cloning of a tumor-associated antigen: MOv18 and MOv19 antibodies recognize a folate-binding protein. *Cancer Res.*, **51**, 6125–32.

5. Mezzanzanica, D., Garrido, M.A., Neblock, D.S. *et al.* (1991). Human T-lymphocytes targeted against an established human ovarian carcinoma with a bispecific F(ab')$_2$ antibody prolong host survival in a murine xenograft model. *Cancer Res.*, **51**, 5716–21.

6. Mazzoni, A., Mezzanzanica, D., Jung, G. *et al.* (1996). CD3-CD28 costimulation as a means to avoiding T cell preactivation in bispecific monoclonal antibody-based treatment of ovarian carcinoma *Cancer Res.*, **56**, 5443–9.

7. Chen, L., Linsley, P.S., and Hellstrom, K.E. (1993). Costimulation of T cells for tumor immunity. *Immunol. Today*, **14**, 483–6.

8. Chouaib, S., Asselin-Paturel, C., Mami-Chouaib, F. *et al.* (1997). The host–tumor immune conflict: from immunosuppression to resistance and destruction. *Immunol. Today*, **18**, 493–7.

9. O'Connel, J., Bennett, M.W., O'Sullivan, G.C. *et al.* (1999). The Fas counterattack: cancer as a site of immune privilege. *Immunol. Today*, **20**, 46–52.

10. Nagata, S. (1997). Apoptosis by death factor. *Cell*, **88**, 355–65.

11. Griffith, T.S. and Ferguson, T.A. (1997). The role of FasL-induced apoptosis in immune privilege. *Immunol. Today*, **18**, 240–4.

12. O'Connell, J., O'Sullivan, G.C., Collins, J.K. *et al.* (1996). The Fas counterattack: Fas-mediated T cell killing by colon cancer cells expressing Fas ligand. *J. Exp. Med.*, **184**, 1075–82.

13. Hahne, M., Rimoldi, D., Schroter, M. *et al.* (1996). Melanoma cell expression of Fas(Apo-1/CD95) ligand: implications for tumor immune escape. *Science*, **274**, 1363–6.

14. Strand, S., Hofmann, W.J., Hug, H. *et al.* (1996). Lymphocyte apoptosis induced by CD95 (APO-1/Fas) ligand-expressing tumor cells. A mechanism of immune evasion? *Nature Med.*, **2**, 1361–6.

15. Saas, P., Walker, P.R., Hahne, M. *et al.* (1997). Fas ligand expression by astrocytoma *in vivo*: maintaining immune privilege in the brain? *J. Clin. Invest.*, **99**, 1173–8.

16. Niehans, G.A., Brunner, T., Frizelle, S.P. *et al.* (1997). Human lung carcinomas express Fas ligand. *Cancer Res.*, **57**, 1007–12.

17. Shiraki, K., Tsuji, N., Shioda, T. *et al.* (1997). Expression of Fas ligand in liver metastases of human colonic adenocarcinomas. *Proc. Natl. Acad. Sci. USA*, **94**, 6420–5.

18. Walker, P.R., Saas, P., and Dietrich, P.-Y. (1997). Role of Fas ligand (CD95L) in immune escape. The tumor cell strikes back. *J. Immunol.*, **158**, 4521–4.

19. O'Connell, J., Bennett, M.W., O'Sullivan, G.C. *et al.* (1997). The Fas counterattack: a molecular mechanism of tumor immune privilege. *Mol. Med.*, **3**, 294–300.

20. Leithauser, F., Dhein, J., Mechtersheimer, G. *et al.* (1993). Constitutive and induced expression of APO-1, a new member of the nerve growth factor/tumor necrosis factor receptor superfamily, in normal and neoplastic cells. *Lab. Invest.*, **69**, 415–29.

21. Van Niekerk, C.C., Ramaekers, F.C.S., Hanselaar, A.G.J.M. *et al.* (1993). Changes in expression of differentiation markers between normal ovarian cells and derived tumors. *Am. J. Pathol.*, **142**, 157–77.

22. Auersperg, N., Maines-Bandiera, S.L., Dyck, H.G. *et al.* (1994). Characterization of cultured human ovarian surface epithelial cells: Phenotypic plasticity and premalignant changes. *Lab. Invest.*, **71**, 510–18.

23. Yonehara, S., Ishii, A., and Yonehara, M. (1989). A cell-killing monoclonal antibody (anti-Fas) to a cell surface antigen co-downregulated with the receptor of tumor necrosis factor. *J. Exp. Med.*, **169**, 1747–56.

24. Owen-Schaub, L.B., Radinsky, R., Kruzel, E. *et al.* (1994). Anti-Fas on non-hematopoietic tumors: levels of Fas/APO-1 and bcl-2 are not predictive of biological response. *Cancer Res.*, **54**, 1580–6.

25. Cascino, I., Papoff, G., De Maria, R. *et al.* (1996). Fas/APO-1 (CD95) receptor lacking the intracytoplastic signaling domain protects tumor cells from Fas-mediated apoptosis. *J. Immunol.*, **156**, 13–17.

26. Cheng, J., Zhou, T., Liu, C. *et al.* (1994). Protection from Fas-mediated apoptosis by a soluble form of the Fas molecule. *Science*, **263**, 1759–62.

27. Cascino, I., Fiucci, G., Papoff, G. *et al.* (1995). Three functional soluble forms of the human apoptosis-inducing Fas molecule are produced by alternative splicing. *J. Immunol.*, **154**, 2706–13.

28. Papoff, G., Cascino, I., Eramo, A. *et al.* (1996). An N-terminal domain shared by Fas/Apo-1 (CD95) soluble variants prevents cell death *in vitro*. *J. Immunol.*, **156**, 4622–30.

29. Kischkel, F.C., Hellbardt, S., Behrmann, I. *et al.* (1995). Cytotoxicity-dependent APO-1 (Fas/CD95)-associated proteins form a death-inducing signaling complex (DISC) with the receptor. *EMBO J.*, **14**, 5579–88.

30. Alnemri, E.S., Livingston, D.J., Nicholson, D.W. *et al.* (1996). Human ICE/CED-3 protease nomenclature. *Cell*, **87**, 171.

31. Sato, T., Irie, S., Kitada, S. *et al.* (1995). FAP-1: a protein tyrosine phosphatase that associates with Fas. *Science*, **268**, 411–14..

Part 4

Prevention and screening

21.   The surgical prevention of ovarian cancer

David H. Oram

Introduction

It has been suggested that the clinical practice of gonad removal is influenced by an underlying attitude that 'an ovary is not good enough to be saved, whereas a testis is not bad enough to be removed'. Although these two situations are not analogous in surgical, or indeed other terms, one can easily identify with the philosophy. Nevertheless, the only real reason to consider the removal of apparently healthy ovaries at the time of hysterectomy for benign disease is as prophylaxis against the subsequent development of epithelial ovarian cancer. Re-operation for benign pathology in conserved ovaries is necessary in 1–5% of cases,[1] and perhaps should not be dismissed with the alacrity suggested in the previous sentence, but it is not really a major determinant in clinical decision making. If ovaries are obviously diseased, e.g. involved in endometriosis, then the issue is entirely different and is not really part of the underlying theme this chapter.

Whatever the rights and wrongs of prophylactic oophorectomy, there is no doubt that an increasing number of these operations are being performed. Thirty years ago bilateral salpingo-oophorectomy accompanied total abdominal hysterectomy in 26% of cases; the most recent data indicate that this figure has now risen to 48% With increasing confidence in long-term hormone replacement therapy (HRT) as well as wider usage of laparoscopic surgery, the age limits at which gynaecologists are prepared to consider prophylactic oophorectomy are progressively reducing, and the numbers of such procedures are unquestionably set to rise even further. Support is lent to this prediction by a survey of UK gynecologists conducted in 1988, in which Jacobs and Oram[2] reported that only 2.4% of Fellows and Members of the Royal College of Gynaecologists (RCOG) routinely removed ovaries at the time of hysterectomy in women under the age of 45 years. This figure only rose to 20% in women aged between 45 and 49 years, and clinical practice only really changed when post-menopausal status had been attained, at which stage 85% of respondents were prepared to perform oophorectomy. It was significant that this study identified that the more senior the clinician (as measured by years since passing the MRCOG examination) the less likely he or she was to remove ovaries prophylactically. Nearly 10 years on, it is not unreasonable to

assume that as this subset of gynaecologists passes into retirement a less conservative practice will ensue. Impressions have been gained on teaching ward rounds and at scientific meetings that the practice of prophylactic oophorectomy by younger gynaecologists is considerably more aggressive. However, more recent data to support this speculation are limited and the only evidence to endorse this opinion comes from a small survey of Alaskan gynaecologists published in 1996, by Conklin *et al.*[3] In this study they found that 40% of their members would perform oophorectomy in women with normal ovaries, and 81% for patients between the ages of 45 and 49 years. In the light of this, it was decided to repeat the 1988 survey in almost identical form, 10 years on, to assess how practice had changed during a course of a decade. The results are presented in Tables 21.1 and 21.2. They demonstrate a far greater tendency to remove ovaries prophylactically in all the age groups, with the most striking change demonstrated in the 45–49-year group, where opinion regarding the wisdom of opportunistic oophorectomy has increased more than threefold. Interestingly, no difference in clinical practice was observed between male and female gynaecologists. Once again, a more aggressive approach to oophorectomy was demonstrated by younger gynaecologists.

Table 21.1 Numbers of oophaectomies performed in 1988 and 1998 (survey of UK gynaecologists)

Age of patient	Yes in 1988	Yes in 1998
35–39	4 (0.4%)	20 (1.3%)
40–44	27 (2%)	148 (9.4%)
45–49	234 (20%)	1009 (64%)
>49	585 (51%)	1350 (86%)
Postmenopausal	974 (85%)	1488 (94.4%)

Table 21.2 Numbers of oophorectomies performed by surveyed male and female UK gynaecologists)

Age of patient	Yes (male)	Yes (female)
35–39	17 (1.6%)	3 (0.6%)
40–44	109 (10%)	40 (8.5%)
45–49	701 (64.4%)	301 (64.3%)
>49	931 (85.5%)	408 (87.2%)
Postmenopausal	1031 (94.7%)	441 (94.2%)

The reasons behind this significant change in practice can only be the subject of speculation, but it would not be unreasonable to assume that factors such as the expansion of knowledge of all aspects of ovarian cancer, increased confidence in the long-term use of HRT, greater acceptance of the role of oophorectomy in the prevention of ovarian cancer, and the improvement in information available to women themselves are contributory. Although this study demonstrated a trend to a more enthusiastic approach to prophylactic oophorectomy, attitudes among currently practising clinicians in the UK, however, still vary between ultra-conservative and positively cavalier.

This range of opinion and practice reflects the paucity of data, in particular the absence of long-term prospective studies assessing the value of prophylactic oophorectomy in the prevention of ovarian cancer. As a result, this issue, which forms part of our weekly decision-making, is devoid of guidelines and continues to be managed in a completely arbitrary fashion. Implicit in the decision-making process is the patient herself, and while not wishing to diminish the importance of her contribution, it is naive to think that her wishes are paramount, because her decision is often based on the advice she is given and most importantly the way that it is presented to her (see below). So what is the correct advice?

Prophylactic oophorectomy: the case for

Ovarian cancer – the problem

This is addressed comprehensively throughout this book and it will suffice in the context of this chapter merely to state that epithelial ovarian cancer is the most commonest gynaecological cancer in the United Kingdom, and the largest cause of mortality from gynaecological malignancy. The vast majority of cases. Familial or hereditary ovarian cancer accounts for a tiny proportion of cases and should be considered as a separate issue (see below). The advent of platinum-based chemotherapy in the lates 1970s and 1980s, and paclitaxel (taxol) in the 1990s has had a striking effect on medium-term survival figures, but long-term cures remain elusive. The benefits of screening and early diagnosis are as yet unproven and this subject is still very much within the realms of research. For as long as this is the case, the concept of prevention is of relevance.

Medical prevention

Medical prevention with the oral contraceptive pill is of enormous importance. Pill usage appears to afford a sustained reduction in the risk of the subsequent development of ovarian cancer. Ovulation inhibition with the pill is associated with a 40% reduction in risk, compared to the risk in those who have never used it,[4] and with prolonged usage (>10 years) the risk reduction might be as high as 80%.[5] The evidence for the protective effect of the pill is sufficiently strong that many groups are recommending it for prophylaxis in women with strong family histories and confirmed mutations,[6] although no studies have been performed which

demonstrate this. Widespread long-term pill usage in women in their forties, however, might not be considered to be appropriate, and it is in this group that the issue of surgical prevention of ovarian cancer becomes relevant.

Surgical prevention

Prophylactic oophorectomy works. It is an effective method of preventing ovarian cancer. It has been estimated that approximately 12% of ovarian cancers are already prevented by the current practice of bilateral salpingo-oophorectomy at the time of hysterectomy.[7] Several studies have examined the frequency of the 'missed opportunity'. Sightler et al. (1991)[8] examined all cases of ovarian cancer in their institution over a 14-year period. They found that 12.6% had previously undergone hysterectomy with conservation of one or both ovaries, 7.9% had undergone hysterectomy after the age of 40 years. They calculated that 60 cases of ovarian cancer could have been prevented if prophylactic oophorectomy had been practised routinely in women over the age of 40 years. Several other studies support this theory[9,10] (see also Table 21.3, refs 11–21).

The consensus from these reports is that a further 10–15% of ovarian cancers could be prevented if a more aggressive approach to prophylactic oophorectomy was adopted. In UK terms, this represents 500–800 cases per year.

Re-operation for benign disease and ovarian longevity

There are two other arguments that can be used to support the practice of prophylactic oophorectomy. First, re-operation for benign disease is a requirement in approximately 1–5% of cases. Secondly, there is some evidence to suggest that ovarian function and longevity is compromised post-hysterectomy. Interestingly, this is not borne out by recent work, which examined ovarian function following radical hysterectomy.[22] The showed that whereas 58% of women over 40 years had gonadotrophins in the

Table 21.3 Reported incidence of previous surgery in women subsequently developing ovarian cancer

Author	Year	Surgery	
		Abdominal hysterectomy	Pelvic operation
Speert[12]	1949	9/260 (3.5)	52/260 (20)
Golub[13]	1953	16/210 (7.6)	n.a.
Counsellor[14P]	1955	67/1500 (4.5)**	
Fagan[15]	1956	2/172 (1.2)	8/172 (4.7)
Bloom[16]	1962	14/141 (9.9)	n.a.
Terz[17]	1967	27/624 (4.3)	50/624 (8.0)
Gibbs[18]	1971	21/236 (8.9)	38/236 (16.1)
Kofler[19]	1972	45/556 (8.1)	66/556 (11.9)
Grundsell[20]	1981	N/A	21/352 (6.0)
Jacobs and Oram[21]	1986	28/407 (6.9)	37/407 (9.1)
Total		229/4106 (5.6)	272/2607 (10.4)

* Percentages in parentheses.
** Number of abdominal and vaginal hysterectomies not specified
n.a., not assessed

menopausal range within 2 years of hysterectomy, only 3% of women who were less than 40 years had compromised ovarian function within this time scale. Four years following surgery the difference between the two groups is maintained, 73% compared with 13%.

Prophylactic oophorectomy: the case against

Long-term hormone replacement therapy

It is axiomatic that if the ovaries are removed from a premenopausal woman, then hormone replacement therapy is indicated on a long-term basis. The risk–benefit analysis of prophylactic oophorectomy and long-term HRT versus ovarian conservation has been reported by Speroff et al.[23] They demonstrated that in order for an improvement in life expectancy to be achieved, long-term compliance with HRT was essential. Viewed another way, if a woman is not prepared to take HRT on a long-term basis, she would be better served if her ovaries were left *in situ* (Fig. 21.1). The variables involved in such risk–benefit calculations centre around the balance between the decrease in mortality from ovarian cancer and the increased morbidity and mortality associated with osteoporosis and cardiovascular disease in the absence of oestrogen. For the balance in terms of improved life expectancy to change in favour of prophylactic surgery, long-term

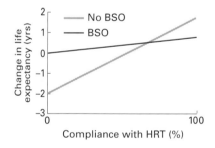

Fig. 21.1 Risk-benefit analysis for bilateral Salpingo-Oöphorectomy (BSO) in a premenopausal women aged 40 years—no BSO;—BSO. (from ref. 23)

compliance with HRT is required in 70–80% of any given population. Such long-term use of HRT and subsequent increased risk of breast cancer has been of major concern for those considering premenopausal oophorectomy. Recent data suggest that the risk of having breast cancer diagnosed is increased in women having used HRT, this risk increasing with increasing duration of use. This effect stops when HRT is stopped and no significant excess in risk was seen 5 years after cessation.[74] It should be noted, however, that these studies were performed on postmenopausal women and that although the incidence of breast cancer was increased, there was no increase in mortality, and therefore when considering survival and mortality it should not be a factor (unlike osteoporosis). There are no data on what effect HRT has on breast cancer risk among women carrying *BRCA1* or *BRCA2* mutations.

Psychological sequelae

The psychological sequelae associated with gonad removal are difficult to quantify but are of undoubted relevance and obvious to all in clinical practice. Nevertheless they are easily and all too frequently underestimated.

The number of oophorectomies required

Although, as already stated, the diligent practice of prophylactic oophorectomy at the time of hysterectomy might prevent 15% of ovarian cancers, the counter argument is that ovarian cancer is in fact a relatively rare disease, and a very large number of oophorectomies have to be performed in order to prevent a single case. Because of the lack of long-term follow-up in the studies that have addressed the frequency with which ovarian cancer occurs in conserved ovaries, the exact ratio of prophylactic oophorectomies to ovarian cancer is unknown.[25–31] (Table 21.4)

Failure of prevention

It is an extremely rare, but none the less well-known fact, that in certain genetically exposed high-risk individuals oophorectomy fails to prevent intraperitoneal carcinomatosis. This was initially described by Tobacman et al. (1982)[32] who reported the results of prophylactic oophorectomy in 28 female members of 16 families at high risk of ovarian cancer. Three of these women subsequently

Table 21.4 Incidence of ovarian cancer in ovaries retained at surgery for benign gynaecological disorders

Author	Year	Length of follow-up	Cases of ovarian cancer	Total no. of patients
Grogan[25]	1957	1.2 years average	0	391
Whitelaw[26]	1959	Min 1, max 28 years	0	1215
Randall[27]	1963	20 years average	2	915
Randall[28]	1962	15 years average	4	345*
De Neef[29]	1966	Min 3 weeks, max 21 years	0	207
McKenzie[30]	1968	n.a.	0	252
Ranney[31]	1977	7.5 years average	4	1265
Total			10 (0.2%)	4590

*Unilateral oöphorectomy for benign tumor of contralateral ovary
n.a., not assessed.

developed disseminated intra-abdominal malignancy of uncertain origin, which was histologically indistinguishable from ovarian cancer. This report questioned the ability of prophylactic oophorectomy to reduce the risk of ovarian cancer to zero, and in high-risk women with a genetic susceptibility any tissue derived from the coelomic epithelium may potentially undergo malignant transformation. Further reports[33–36] also illustrate the possible development of intraperitoneal carcinomatosis occurring between 1 and 27 years after oophorectomy, either because of an individual's genetic propensity or, in a small number of cases, because microscopic malignancy was present but unidentified at the time of oophorectomy[37] or because a small amount of ovarian tissue was inadvertently left behind at the time of surgery. Salazar *et al.* (1996)[38] reported the findings of a comparison of the histological features of the ovaries of women at increased risk of ovarian cancer with women whose ovaries were removed for reasons unrelated to cancer risk. They suggested that there were certain histological charactcristics associated with the 'high-risk' ovaries (two cases were found to have microscopic or near-microscopic malignant neoplasms). The need for thorough examination of the abdominal cavity, and even formal staging, in these high-risk women becomes apparent. It is important to stress that these cases, although well known, are in fact extremely rare even in the family history group and, as such, should not command undue emphasis in clinical decision-making.

What is correct clinical practice?

Against this background of conflicting argument it is readily apparent that individual assessment and counselling is the only rational practice. Any woman's decision-making, as mentioned above, is influenced not only by her fears of the development of ovarian cancer or the apprehension of losing her ovaries but also by the way in which the facts are presented to her. This is regularly demonstrated by the author by laying undue emphasis on one or other argument to successive groups of medical students and then asking for a vote on what constitutes correct clinical practice. The results can vary between abhorrence at the mere contemplation of gonad removal to the view that castration is a woman's right and should not be denied!

In calculating an individual's risk, factors such as age, parity, pill usage, ovulation stimulation, and a past history of breast cancer are all relevant. Perhaps the overriding factor in the mix, however, is the presence of a positive family history of ovarian cancer.

The influence of family history

After the age of 40 any woman's lifetime risk of developing ovarian cancer is 1.6%. With one first-degree relative with the disease, this lifetime risk increases to approximately 5%. If a woman has two first-degree relatives with ovarian cancer there is a 66% risk that an autosomal dominant predisposing gene is in the family; there is therefore a 33% chance that the woman has inherited the gene. The penetrance of the gene, however, is incomplete (around 40%) and so the risk to the individual woman of developing the disease is about 15%. These figures need to be viewed in the context of any woman's lifetime risk of developing breast cancer being approximately 8% (and the fact that there is no rush for prophylactic mastectomies!). Any family history is an influence as far as opportunistic prophylactic oophorectomy is concerned. Primary prophylaxis (i.e. prophylactic oophorectomy as a primary surgical procedure) is not justifiable with one family member with the disease; it is justifiable with two histologically proven family members and it is justifiable following genetic testing and the proven inheritance of *BRCA1* and *BRCA2* mutations. In both groups, such advice is given only after very detailed personal risk assessment and counselling, and only on the completion of childbearing.[39] Kerlikowske *et al.* (1992)[6] suggest that among women with one relative with ovarian cancer, the lifetime probability of ovarian cancer is not sufficiently great to recommend oophorectomy as a primary surgical procedure, but would be an influential factor of some significance should that patient require hysterectomy. They also suggest that in womcn with hereditary ovarian cancer syndromes with pedigrees suggesting an autosomal dominant mode of inheritance, the lifetime risk of ovarian cancer is high enough to outweigh the risks of oophorectomy. Despite this most groups prefer to advocate more intense surveillance.[6,39]

The removal of ovaries as a primary surgical procedure is therefore only justifiable in a very small cohort of women, following careful counselling and individual risk assessment based on a verified history and possible genetic testing to demonstrate *BRCA1* or *BRCA2* mutations. For women who are at increased, but not very high, risk of ovarian cancer, in whom primary prophylaxis is not justifiable, the opportunity for prevention afforded by incidental pelvic surgery, including hysterectomy, should of course be taken.

The influence of other factors

Age

The single biggest risk factor for ovarian cancer is age. There is a progressive increase in incidence into the sixth decade, with a small decline thereafter.[40] This knowledge is not, however, of great value in decision-making in Western countries, as it must be assumed that all women will reach the high-risk age group. It is of more use in women from families with hereditary ovarian cancer syndromes who tend to be 7–14 years younger at diagnosis than the general population.[41] With regard to age as an influencing factor for oophorectomy at the time of hysterectomy in a premenopausal woman, obviously the decision-making is more straightforward the older she is. Perhaps it would not be too controversial to recommend oophorectomy at the time of hysterectomy for all women over the age of 45 years.

Ovulation interruption

One of the leading theories in the aetiology of ovarian cancer is the 'incessant ovulation' theory.[42,43] The protective effect of the pill has already been mentioned. The association between number of pregnancies and decreased risk of ovarian cancer is well established. Risk decreases with increasing parity among parous women and each additional pregnancy appears to be associated with a percentage risk reduction. Lactation, in the same way, incurs protection.[44]

Ovulation stimulation

There has been much debate on the issue of the use of fertility drugs and the risk of ovarian cancer. In keeping with theory that repeated ovulations disrupt the surface epithelium of the ovary, increasing the risk of malignant transformation, the use of drugs which result in multiple ovulations in one cycle, could potentially increase the risk of ovarian cancer. The same has been postulated for the use of gonadotrophins. Whittemore *et al.* in 1992[44] in their analysis of 12 US case-control studies, found an increased risk in women who had used fertility drugs (OR = 2.8) relative to women with no history of infertility, whereas women with infertility who had not used these drugs showed no increase in risk (OR = 0.91). This risk was greatest in women who had taken clomiphene (clomifene) for more than 10 cycles without achieving a pregnancy. It was later stressed by Whittemore (1994)[45] that the data did not allow for the separation of treatment effects from abnormalities of ovulation, which may themselves increase a woman's risk of ovarian cancer. She also commented that the lifetime risk, therefore, in women having used fertility drugs would be about 4–5%, less than that of breast cancer. Rossing *et al.* in 1994,[46] in a study of 3837 women who had been evaluated for infertility, also found a positive association between the use of clomiphene and ovarian cancer and, in particular, borderline tumours, if taken for more than a 12 month period. There are still insufficient data to prove a causal link.

Past history of breast cancer

A past history of premenopausal breast cancer increases an individual's propensity to develop ovarian cancer.[47] If such an individual were to undergo hysterectomy, this would provide a basis for recommending removal of the ovaries at the time of surgery. This advice, however, has to be tempered by the knowledge that HRT in these circumstances carries its own problems. The decision-making is inevitably influenced by discussion, not only with the patient herself, but also with her breast cancer surgeon. Increasingly, HRT is used in such patients and a compromise may be a combination of oestrogen, progesterone, and tamoxifen given concurrently, although it must be acknowledged that the data in support of such therapeutic manoeuvring are non-existent.

Racial and cultural considerations

When assessing an individual's risk of ovarian cancer, certain racial and cultural factors are of importance. Ovarian cancer is a disease of industrialized societies and there are marked differences in geographical incidence rates: the highest rates being seen in Scandinavia, notably Sweden, followed closely by Germany, the United Kingdom, and the United States; the lowest incidence rates are seen in Asia and Africa.[48] Interestingly, immigration studies have shown that this racial difference is not sustained when Asians and Africans migrate to Western countries.[49] The incidence is higher for professional groups rather than the unskilled.[50] Certain ethnic groups are at particular risk of ovarian cancer, which is the most common gynaecological cancer to be diagnosed amongst Israeli Jewish women, with familial aggregation occurring within this population.[51]

When counselling a woman for prophylactic oophorectomy, it is important to take into account her cultural beliefs and under-standing. Organ removal, especially gonad removal, may well be against a woman's cultural beliefs and have considerable social and psychological sequelae. It is important that when a language barrier exists, an advocate is available who not only understands the language but also the woman's beliefs. The presence or absence of certain family members may also be of importance during the consultation.

Conclusions and recommended practice

Past advocacy of an individualized approach to this controversial subject has been greeted not so much by an appreciation of balance and fairness as by accusations of fence sitting. Lest this chapter be branded similarly indecisive, the author suggests a schema for clinical practice. He does so in the knowledge that in the absence of firm scientific data in many areas, his recommendations are open to criticism for not being 'evidence based'. (You can't win!)

Oophorectomy as a primary surgical procedure

This procedure is advocated in women with a strong family history of disease. Primary prophylaxis on completion of childbearing in women with two family members with the disease or with proven genetic mutations is justifiable, following careful risk assessment and detailed counselling. The reports of primary peritoneal carcinomatosis, although of concern, are in fact rare, even in these very high-risk women, and should not detract from the value of oophorectomy, nor deter the clinician from recommending prophylactic surgery. If prophylactic oophorectomy is performed in this high-risk group, careful surgical staging should be undertaken, and thorough histological examination should be performed to rule out microscopic malignancy.

Oophorectomy at the time of pelvic surgery

Opportunistic secondary oophorectomy should be offered to all women undergoing hysterectomy who are over the age of 40 years, and should be positively recommended to all women over the age of 45 years. Such a recommendation is strengthened if there is any family history of ovarian cancer, or if there is a past history of

Table 21.5 Recommended practice for prophylactic oöphorectomy

Prophylactic oöphorectomy	Suitable patients
Primary Secondary	• Defined very-high-risk groups[*] • Offer to all >40 years • Recommended to all >45 years[**] • Consider at vaginal hysterectomy • Involve surgical colleagues

[*] Two or more proven first-degree relatives with disease.
[**] Particularly those with one relative with disease or a past history of ovulation stimulation.

ovarian stimulation. Greater consideration should be given to the possibility of oophorectomy at the time of vaginal hysterectomy. The feasibility and safety of this procedure has been demonstrated by Sheth and Malpani.[52] Laparoscopic assistance for this procedure may be chosen by some.

Finally, general surgical colleagues, when operating in the pelvis of postmenopausal women, might be encouraged to consider the possibility of opportunistic bilateral oophorectomy (Table 21.5).

References

1. Randall, C.L., Hall, D.W., Armenia, C.S. (1962). Pathology in the preserved ovary after unilateral oophorectomy. *Am. J. Obstet. Gynecol.*, **84**, 1233.

2. Jacobs, I., Oram, D. (1989). Prevention of ovarian cancer: a survey of the practice of prophylactic oophorectomy by fellows and members of the Royal College of Obstetricians and Gynaecologists. *Br. J. Obstet. Gynaecol.*, **96**(5), 510–515.

3. Conklin, B.H., McGuire, P.A., Weiler, P.L., Webb, D.I. (1996). A survey of the practice of prophylactic oophorectomy by gynecologists in the state of Alaska. *Alaska. Med.*, **38**(2), 71–74.

4. The Cancer and Steroid Hormone Study of the Centers for Disease Control and the National Institute of Child Health and Human Development. The reduction in risk of ovarian cancer associated with oral contraceptive use. (1987). *N. Engl. J. Med.*, **316**(11), 650–655.

5. Vessey, M., Metcalf, A., Well, C. *et al.* (1987). Ovarian neoplasms, functional ovarian cysts and oral contraceptives. *Br. Med. J.*, **294**, 1518–1520.

6. Kerlikowske, K., Brown, J.S., Grady, D.G. (1992). Should women with familial ovarian cancer undergo prophylactic oophorectomy? *Obstet. Gynecol.*, **80**(4), 700–707.

7. Howe, H.L. (1984). Age specific hysterectomy and oophorectomy prevalence rates and the risks for cancer of the reproductive system. *Am. J. Public Health*, **74**(6), 560–563.

8. Sightler, S.E., Boike, G.M., Estape, R.E., Averette, H.E. (1991). Ovarian cancer in women with prior hysterectomy: a 14-year experience at the University of Miami. *Obstet. Gynecol.*, **78**(4), 681–684.

9. Jacobs, I., Oram, D. (1987). Prophylactic oophorectomy. *Br. J. Hosp. Med.*, **38**(5), 440–449.

10. Kontoravdis, A., Kaligirou, D., Antoniou, G. *et al.* (1996). Prophylactic oophorectomy in ovarian cancer prevention. *Int. J. Gynaecol. Obstet.*, **54**(3), 257–262.

11. Jacobs, I.J., Oram, D.H. (1988). Oöphorectomy and prevention of ovarian cancer. In: Chamberlain G (ed) Contemporary obstetrics and gynaecology. London: Butterworths, 397–408.

12. Speert, H. Prophylaxis of ovarian cancer. (1949). *Ann. Surg.*, **129**, 468

13. Golub, L.J. (1953). The diagnosis of ovarian cancer. *Am. J. Obstet. Gynecol.*, **66**, 169–177.

14. Counsellor, V.S., Hunt, W., Haigler, F.H. (1955). Carcinoma of the ovary following hysterectomy. *Am. J. Obstet. Gynecol.*, **69**, 538–542.

15. Fagan, G.E., Allen, E.D., Klawans, A.H. (1956). Ovarian neoplasms and repeat pelvic surgery. *Obstet. Gynecol.*, **2**, 418–421.

16. Bloom, M.L. (1950–1959). Certain observations based on a study of 141 cases of primary adenocarcinoma of the ovaries. *South Afr. Med. J.*, **36**, 714

17. Terz, J.J., Barber, H.R.K., Brunschwiz, A. (1967). Incidence of carcinoma in the retained ovary. *Am. J. Surg.*, **113**, 511

18. Gibbs, E.K. (1971). Suggested prophylaxis for ovarian cancer. *Am. J. Obstet. Gynecol.*, **111**, 756–765.

19. Kofler, E. (1972). The incidence of previous hysterectomies and/or unilateral oophorectomies in women with malignant ovarian tumours. *Geburtshilfe und Frauenheilkunde*, **32**, 873–881.

20. Grundsell, H., Ekman, G., Gullberg, B. *et al.* (1981). Some aspects of prophylactic oophorectomy and ovarian carcinoma. *Ann. Chir. Gynaecol.*, **70**, 36–42.

21. Jacobs, I.J., Oram, D.H. (1987). Prophylactic oophorectomy. *Br. J. Hosp. Med.*, **38**, 440–444.

22. Stillwell, S., Houdmont, M., Paterson, M.E.L. (1997). Ovarian function after radical hysterectomy for carcinoma of the cervix. *Int. J. Gynecol. Cancer*, **7**, 49–56.

23. Speroff, T., Dawson, N.V., Speroff, L., Haber, R.J. (1991). A risk-benefit analysis of elective bilateral oophorectomy: effect of changes in compliance with estrogen therapy an outcome. *Am. J. Obstet. Gynecol.*, **164**, 165–174.

24. Collaborative Group on Hormonal Factors in Breast Cancer. (1997). Breast Cancer and Hormone Replacement Therapy: collaborative reanalysis of data from 51 epidemiological studies of 52705 women with breast cancer and 105411 women without breast cancer. *Lancet*, **350**, 1047–1059.

25. Grogan, R.H. (1967). Reappraisal of residual ovaries. *Am. J. Obstet. Gynecol.*, **97**, 124–129.

26. Whitelaw, R.G. (1959). Pathology and the conserved ovary. *J. Obstet. Gynaecol. Br. Empire*, **66**, 413–416.

27. Randall, C.L. (1963). Ovarian conservation. In: Progress in Gynecology. Volume 4. New York: Grune and Stratton, 457.

28. Randall, C.L., Hall, D.W., Armenia, C.S. (1962). Pathology in the preserved ovary after unilateral oophorectomy. *Am. J. Obstet. Gynecol.*, **84**, 1233

29. De Neef, J.C., Hollenbeck, Z.J.R. (1966). The fate of ovaries preserved at the time of hysterectomy. *Am. J. Obstet. Gynecol.*, **96**, 1088–1097.

30. McKenzie, L.L. (1968). Discussion of the frequency of oophorectomy at the time of hysterectomy. *Am. J. Obstet. Gynecol.*, **100**, 626–634.

31. Ranney, B., Abu-Ghazaleh, S. (1977). The future function and fortune of ovarian tissue which is retained *in vivo* during hysterectomy. *Am. J. Obstet. Gynecol.*, **128**, 626–634.

32. Tobacman, J.K., Tucker, M.A., Kase, R. *et al.* (1982). Intra-abdominal carcinomatosis after prophylactic oophorectomy in ovarian cancer prone families. *Lancet*, **ii**, 795.

33. Weber, A.M., Hewett, W.J., Gajewski, W.H., Curry, S.L. (1992). Serous carcinoma of the peritoneum after oophorectomy. *Obstet. Gynecol.*, **80**(3 Pt 2), 558–560.

34. Piver, M.S., Tishi, M.F., Tsukada, Y., Naraz, G. (1993). Primary peritoneal carcinomatosis with prophylactic oophorectomy in women with a family history of ovarian cancer. *Cancer*, **71**(8), 2751–2755.

35. Kemp, G.M., Hsiu, J.G., Andrews, M.C. (1992). Papillary peritoneal carcinomatosis after prophylactic oophorectomy. *Gynecol. Oncol.*, **47**(3), 395–397.

36. Struewing, J.P., Watson, P., Easton, D.F. *et al.* (1995). Prophylactic oophorectomy in inherited breast/ovarian cancer families. *Natl. Cancer. Inst. Monogr.*, 17. Bethesda: NCI, 33–35.

37. Chen, K.T.K., Schooley, J.L., Flam, M.S. (1985). Peritoneal carcinomatosis after prophylactic oophorectomy in familial ovarian cancer syndrome. *Obstet. Gynecol.*, **66**(3), 935–945.

38. Salazar, H., Godwin, A.K., Daly, M.B. *et al.* (1996). Microscopic benign and malignant neoplasms and a cancer-prone phenotype in prophylactic oophorectomies. *J. Natl. Cancer. Inst.*, **88**(24), 1810–1820.

39. Burke, W., Daly, M., Garber, J. *et al.* (1997). Recommendations for follow-up care of individuals with an inherited predisposition to cancer. II: BRCA1 and BRCA2. *JAMA*, **277**(12), 997.

40. Yancik, R., Ries, L.G., Yates, J.W. (1986). An analysis of surveillance, epidemiology, and end results program data. *Am. J. Obstet. Gynecol.*, **154**, 639–647.

41. Lynch, H.T., Watson, P., Bewtra, C. *et al.* (1991). Hereditary ovarian cancer: heterogeneity in age at diagnosis. *Cancer*, **67**, 1460–1466.

42. Fathalla, M.F. (1971). Incessant ovulation—a factor in ovarian neoplasia? *Lancet*, **ii**, 163.

43. La Vecchia, C., Franceschi, S., Gallus, G. et al. (1983). Incessant ovulation and ovarian cancer: a critical approach. *Int. J. Epidemiol.*, **12**, 161–164.

44. Whittemore, A.S., Harris, R., Itnyre, J. (1992). Characteristics relating to ovarian cancer risk: collaborative analysis of 12 U.S. case–control studies. II. Invasive epithelial ovarian cancers in white women. Collaborative Ovarian Cancer Group. *Am. J. Epidemiol.*, **136**(10), 1184–1203.

45. Whittemore, A.S. (1994). Characteristics relating to ovarian cancer risk: implications for prevention and detection. *Gynecol. Oncol.*, **55**(3 Pt 2), S15–19.

46. Rossing, M.A., Daling, S.R., Weiss, N.S. *et al.* (1994). Ovarian tumours in a cohort of infertile women. *N. Engl. J. Med.*, **331**(12), 771–774.

47. Prior, P., Waterhouse, J.A.H. (1981). Multiple primary cancers of the breast and ovary. *Br. J. Cancer*, **44**, 628–636.

48. International Agency for Research on Cancer (1976). Cancer incidence in five continents, Vol 3. IARC Scientific Publication No. 15. Lyon: IARC.

49. Weiss, N.S., Homonchuck, T., Young, J.L. Jr. (1977). Incidence of the histologic types of ovarian cancer: the US Third National Cancer Survey 1969–1971. *Gynecol. Oncol.*, **5**, 161–167.

50. Beral, V., Fraser, P., Chilvers, C. (1978). Does pregnancy protect against ovarian cancer? *Lancet*, **1**, 1083–1087.

51. Menczer, J., Ben-Baruch, G. (1991). Familial ovarian cancer in Israeli Jewish women. *Obstet. Gynecol.*, **77**(2), 276–277.

52. Sheth, S., Malpani, A. (1992). Routine prophylactic oophorectomy at the time of vaginal hysterectomy in postmenopausal women. *Arch. Gynecol. Obstet.*, **251**(2), 87–91.

22. Chemoprevention of ovarian cancer

Christine E. Szarka, Thomas C. Hamilton, Andres J.P. Klein-Szanto, and Robert F. Ozols

Introduction

Ovarian cancer is the most common cause of death from gynecologic cancer among women of all ages in the United States.[1] Because ovarian cancer generally presents in advanced stages, efforts to improve survival have been focused on early diagnosis and cancer prevention. Transvaginal ultrasound, Doppler color flow study, and serum CA–125 have demonstrated some potential benefit as screening tools; however, screening has not been proven to be cost effective. Prophylactic oophorectomy remains the only effective method of ovarian cancer prevention.

Very little is known about ovarian carcinogenesis due to the difficulty in obtaining ovarian tissue at various time points during the process. The development of a clinical model whereby drug effects on ovarian tissue can be determined is crucial to advancing ovarian cancer prevention in high-risk populations. Scientific endeavors evaluating promising chemopreventive agents in women who have agreed to undergo a prophylactic oophorectomy for medical reasons related to cancer risk allows the establishment of a clinical prevention research system. In this system, not only can ovarian tissue be obtained from high-risk women to elucidate ovarian carcinogenesis, but drug effects can be determined as well.

Agents such as fenretinide and progestin currently have the most scientific evidence to suggest a cancer preventive role in ovarian cancer and would be investigated in this model first. As their modulating and clinical effects are determined, a combination of the two agents may be explored. As ovarian carcinogenesis and biomarker modulation is elucidated, new agents with novel targets will likely be developed.

Prophylactic oophorectomy

From an epidemiologic viewpoint, it is undeniable that prophylactic oophorectomy can prevent a large number of ovarian cancer cases.[2–4] For women with a family history of ovarian cancer, prophylactic oophorectomy could effectively reduce the lifetime risk of ovarian cancer from 5–50% to near zero.[5] In addition to ovarian cancer prevention, another major benefit of prophylactic oophorectomy may be protection from breast cancer.

There are disadvantages to prophylactic oophorectomy, including the psychological impact of losing the ovaries, and the risks associated with the induction of surgical menopause. These patients require prolonged estrogen-replacement therapy to alleviate the problems of surgical menopause, such as vasomotor instability, hot flashes, atrophic changes of the breast and genital tissues, osteoporosis, and cardiovascular disease.[6–8] In addition, a prophylactic oophorectomy does not eliminate the risk of peritoneal carcinoma, which can develop in high-risk women after surgical removal of their ovaries. Whether this results from the shedding of malignant or premalignant cells from the ovary prior to oophorectomy remains to be determined. There is great interest in finding an alternative method of providing protection to women with an increased risk for ovarian cancer.

Ovarian cancer chemoprevention

Cancer chemoprevention is defined as the use of specific chemical compounds to prevent, inhibit, or reverse carcinogenesis. Chemoprevention is intended to be a long-term treatment, conceivably up to a lifetime in high-risk subjects. A consequence of this extended treatment period is a requirement for agents with very low toxicity.

Truly high-risk women, i.e. members of autosomal dominant breast–ovarian cancer site-specific ovarian cancer families and *BRCA1* and *BRCA2* gene carriers are the optimal population for screening and prevention trials.[9] Although a randomized clinical trial between prophylactic oophorectomy versus screening or prevention measures in high-risk women seems ideal, such a study may have ethical limitations. Since prophylactic oophorectomy is the only established method to prevent ovarian cancer in high-risk women, there is substantial concern about randomly assigning these women on a no surgery arm. An alternative study design would be to randomize a high-risk individual to a preventive intervention or no intervention for a period of time prior to a prophylactic oophorectomy.

A critical feature of chemoprevention is that it intervenes at the early stages of carcinogenesis when normal cell order and function are partially preserved. Chemoprevention strategies can be designed to target these preserved pathways before they are lost during the process that terminates in uncontrolled growth of malignant cells. An important aspect of chemoprevention is the selection of appropriate endpoints for intervention trials. Cancer incidence generally is not a feasible endpoint for the evaluation of chemopreventive drugs because of the long time needed for carcinogenesis (5–20 years) and the relatively low incidence of cancer, even in high-risk populations. Many clinical chemoprevention studies have used well-recognized precancerous lesions or indicators of cell proliferation and/or apoptosis as surrogate endpoints or biomarkers of cancer.

Ovarian cancer biomarkers

Precancerous lesions have not been well defined for ovarian cancer, in part due to the difficulty in obtaining ovarian tissue from high-risk subjects at multiple time points. Histologic changes identified in ovaries removed from women undergoing prophylactic oophorectomy because of a high familial risk for ovarian cancer may be precursors for malignant changes. These histological markers may serve as a novel target for chemoprevention trials. In addition, other potential surrogate markers include Mib–1 and apoptosis.

These potential surrogate biomarkers of ovarian carcinogenesis and the effects of promising chemopreventive agents could be evaluated by asking high-risk women who are planning to undergo an advocated prophylactic oophorectomy to delay their surgery for 4–6 months and allow randomization to drug treatment versus placebo during this time period. By performing histologic and histochemical analyses on the ovarian tissue post-treatment, significant knowledge regarding biomarkers for ovarian cancer and the potential preventive effect of drugs are likely to be obtained. This trial design has been accepted as part of a peer-reviewed funded United States Department of Defense grant.

Histopathological biomarkers

Hamilton *et al.*[10] addressed the issue of whether a pre-neoplastic lesion precedes the development of ovarian cancer by studying individuals with an inherited predisposition for ovarian cancer. This Mendelian dominant inheritance of risk provides a subset of individuals at sufficiently high risk for development of the disease that oophorectomy for prophylaxis is often performed. The histological features of the ovaries from such individuals were compared to ovaries from individuals at no increased risk for ovarian cancer.

This study revealed two important findings.[10] First, examination of the ovaries from 20 high-risk individuals revealed two unanticipated near-microscopic malignant common epithelial tumors. This creates a remarkably high incidence, i.e. 10% of malignant neoplasms, and underscores the importance of thorough histopathological evaluation of ovaries removed from ovarian cancer-prone individuals. The second finding in this study relates to the histological features of the ovaries in which cancer is likely to develop.

The cancer-prone ovaries contained a range of histological features not usually seen in such magnitude, combination, and complexity in control ovaries. A significant number of cases (70% of high-risk ovaries versus 20% of the control group of ovaries, $P = 0.005$) presented multifocal surface papillomatosis ranging from a few foci to markedly extensive. These projections were usually short and stubby, with a fibrous core covered by cuboidal or pseudostratified epithelium. These superficial papillae are similar to those commonly seen in association with the deep surface invaginations. The features of these ovaries, including papillomatosis and deep invaginations, often resulted in 'lesions' which, except for size, fit the criteria to be designated as benign papillary cystadenomas. For example, a frequently observed change, seen in 19 of 20 high-risk ovaries, was the presence of invaginations of the surface epithelial cells into the stroma, usually associated with short papillary excrescences. These invaginations were often very deep into the cortex, sometimes with bifurcations or branches. Similar, but fewer and less deep, invaginations were also observed in 11 of 20 control ovaries. The difference is statistically significant, $P = 0.00038$.

In the cancer-prone ovaries, the minute papillary cystic lesions were often formed at the end of the deep invaginations of the surface epithelium, with distention of the deepest portion and papillary proliferation within the lumen. The papillae were of various sizes and presented with a fibrovascular core lined by a single layer of columnar or cuboidal epithelial cells, but did not show hyperplasia, tufting, atypia, or any suggestion of invasiveness. Furthermore, as suggested above, the epithelium often could be seen to be continuous, via the deep invaginations, with the cells covering the ovarian surface.

Another frequent finding in the cancer-prone ovaries was the presence of cortical superficial 'inclusion' cysts in 70% of high-risk cases, against 25% of controls ($P = 0.00619$). The cysts have the appearance of 'disturbed glands'. They are of variable size and shape, usually lined by a pseudostratified epithelium of 'serous' or tubal type, and usually devoid of any contents within the space. In some cases, groups of the cysts of varying complexity occur, creating the appearance of microscopic cystadenomas or adenofibromas. Occasionally, a solid epithelial connection with the surface is seen. Although epithelial hyperplasia and papillomatosis were present in several cases, no mitoses or atypia were observed in any of the 'lesions' credited to this category.

Occasional mitoses, as well as shrunk, degenerated, apoptotic cells, were observed in the surface epithelium of cancer-prone ovaries associated with an increase in height and pseudostratification of the tall columnar cells. A significantly increased number of cells or real hyperplasia, however, was not detected, but the surface epithelial cells of these ovaries appeared to be 'active'. This term is used to denote the apparent activation of some functional capability, such as secretion. For example, the cells were often enlarged, tall, columnar, and pseudostratified, with elongated or ovoid nuclei containing dispersed or dense chromatin and occasional small nucleoli, and increased granular cytoplasm, as compared with the smaller, cuboidal, or flat ordinary superficial cells, with small, round nuclei and scant cytoplasm.

Table 22.1 Histological features of surrogate endpoint biomarkers in ovaries from women with and without significant risk for ovarian cancer

	High-risk ovaries (n = 20)	Control ovaries (n = 20)	
Papillomatosis	70%	20%	P = 0.005
Invaginations	95%	55%	P = 0.00038
Inclusion cysts	70%	25%	P = 0.00619
Stromal activity	75%	10%	P = 0.000147

In addition to described differences in the appearance and growth pattern of the cells which may become malignant if cancer develops in a cancer-prone ovary, the stroma of these organs also appears to be uncharacteristically active or hyperplastic. Activity as defined below is noted in 75% of high-risk ovaries, against only 10% of controls ($P = 0.000147$). A range of alterations was often present which may generally be described as stromal hyperplasia. These changes included increased follicular activity, stromal hyperthecosis and luteinization, hylar cell hyperplasia, as well as corpus luteum hyperplasia.[10] Considered together, these histological features (Table 22.1) permit strong differentiation between control and high-risk ovaries on the basis of statistical analysis.[10]

In addition to the study of high-risk ovaries at the histological level, we have also studied the surface epithelial cells from these and control ovaries in tissue culture. We have found that the cells from individuals with a high risk of ovarian cancer transfected with SV40 antigens had a tendency to undergo malignant transformation as assessed by tumorigenicity in immunocompromised mice (unpublished data). Further studies showed that cells from the cancer-prone individuals had a decreased tendency for epithelial to mesenchymal conversion compared to control cells. This was based on morphological as well as immunohistochemical criteria.[11,12] These studies clearly indicate that surface epithelial cells from cancer-prone individuals are not only different in their growth pattern *in situ* but also *in vitro*, and that these changes precede overt malignancy.

Proliferation and apoptosis

Several putative markers of cancer susceptibility have also been identified. Among those that are relevant to evaluate the effects of a chemopreventive agent, two groups have been identified: (1) cell cycle progression markers, and (2) apoptosis markers. Expression of Mib–1 is useful for the first purpose in that it is an epitope of the Ki–67 antigen that is expressed in all cells actively cycling.[13] Numerous studies have indicated its utility as a marker of human cell proliferation in premalignant and malignant lesions.[13–15]

Dysregulation of apoptosis may contribute to tumor formation and malignant progression by allowing the accumulation of proliferating cell populations and obstructing the elimination of cells with genetic abnormalities conferring an enhanced malignant potential.[16,17] Thus, it is not surprising that apoptotic indices are altered as cells move toward malignant transformation. Hence, markers of apoptosis within neoplastic or premalignant lesions have often been utilized to evaluate the efficacy of cancer chemoprevention agents.[18–23]

Morphologically, apoptosis is evaluated by light microscopy by observation of nuclear and cytoplasmic condensation, formation of apoptotic bodies from condensed nuclear and cytoplasmic material, and the absence of inflammatory reaction adjacent to the apoptosing cells.[18,19] This approach permits a semiquantitative evaluation of apoptosis by the pathologists. A more in-depth quantitative study establishes an apoptotic index using *in situ* detection techniques.

The TUNEL technique entails a non-isotopic *in situ* end-labeling of fragmented DNA, characteristically produced by non-random nucleosomal fragmentation during programmed cell death.[24] This procedure will be performed using a commercial kit with digoxigenin-dUDP and terminal deoxynucleotidyl transferase (Apoptag, Oncor, Gaithersburg, MD, USA).[25] The quantitation of positive cells will result in apoptotic indices reflecting the percentage of cells in apoptosis.

An alternative technique that is rapidly gaining acceptance because it is more specific for apoptosis and does not stain necrotic cells, utilizes an anti-single-stranded DNA antibody using a commercially available immunohistochemical kit (Apopstain, Miami, FL, USA).[26] Similarly, an apoptotic index is calculated that reflects the percentage of apoptotic cells.

The protein encoded by the *bcl–2* gene is a potent blocker of apoptosis.[27] Overexpression of this gene occurs in a large variety of human cancers and has been associated with malignant cell expansion by tilting the balance in favor of cell proliferation through the inhibition of programmed cell death. Conversely, another gene of the same family, called *bax*, promotes apoptosis. Both genes have been shown to have a role in ovarian cell biology and in human ovarian cancer cells.[28,29] These proteins can be detected using immunohistochemical techniques.[30] The evaluation of *bcl–2* and *bax* expression could be of great value as surrogate endpoint biomarkers. Antibodies are commercially available and can be detected in paraffin-embedded material.[30,31] Staining intensity is evaluated semiquantitatively using the grading system described by Krajewska *et al.*[30]

Candidate ovarian chemopreventive drugs

Fenretinide

Retinoids are the natural derivatives and synthetic analogues of vitamin A. They are particularly interesting as chemopreventive agents because of their ability to inhibit cellular proliferation, differentiation induction, cytostatic activity, ability to inhibit growth factor synthesis, and ability to affect immunity and extracellular matrix formation. The use of vitamin A analogues is limited by the requirement for large pharmacological doses in order to reach therapeutic efficacy. High doses of naturally occurring retinoids produce significant side-effects.

By modifying the basic retinoid structure, analogues with reduced toxicity have been developed. Fenretinide, N-(4-hydroxyphenyl)retinamide, a retinamide derivative of vitamin A, is an extremely promising chemopreventive compound with therapeutic efficacy in a variety of carcinogenesis models. It is currently being evaluated in clinical trials as a chemopreventive agent for oral leukoplakia, breast, lung, and ovarian cancer.

There is evidence for a significant role of retinol and its derivatives in ovary growth and functions. Vitamin A is essential for the maintenance of normal reproductive functions in both female and male rats,[32] and retinal and retinoic acid modulate follicle-stimulating hormone action on ovarian cells.[33] Of the human organs studied, the ovary has the highest concentration of cellular retinol binding protein[34] and expresses nuclear retinoic acid receptor β.[35] There is some evidence to suggest that the growth inhibitory effect of retinoids is mediated by induction of secretion of specific isoforms of transforming growth factor-β (TGF-β).[36] However, the mechanisms for anti-tumor effects have not been fully determined.

Formelli *et al.*[37] reported for the first time that a synthetic retinoid, fenretinide, has a therapeutic effect against a human ovarian carcinoma cell line. The anti-tumor activity of fenretinide against ascitic growing IGROV–1 tumor, a human epithelial ovarian adenocarcinoma cell line, was tested by administering the drug orally or intraperitoneally to Swiss *nu/nu* mice. Groups of six mice were inoculated intraperitoneally with 2.5×10^6 tumor cells. Drug treatment was initiated 1 day after inoculation. Fenretinide was administered intraperitoneally (daily doses of 60 or 120 mg/kg) or orally (daily doses of 60, 120, or 240 mg/kg) for 5 days per week until the onset of ascitic tumor in 2–3 treated mice per group. There was no evidence of local or systemic toxicity after either mode of treatment. Benefit was seen with the intraperitoneal administration, with a significant increase in the survival time ($P > 0.05$) at both doses. The orally administered fenretinide neither increased survival time nor produced long-term survivors. The lack of activity of fenretinide when given orally may be related to the fenretinide levels needed in the peritoneum for cell death, which are achieved only after intracavitary administration.

Supino[38] further studied the effects of fenretinide on ovarian carcinoma cell lines A2780, IGROV–1, SW626, and OVCA432 to investigate the mechanisms of the antiproliferative activity of the retinoid. When exposed to fenretinide, all four cell lines showed a marked dose-dependent growth inhibition. The A2780 cells after exposure to fenretinide showed a 50% growth inhibition and changes typical of apoptosis. Nuclear condensation, hypodiploid DNA, and chromatin cleavage into oligonucleosome-sized fragments, all hallmarks of apoptosis, were clearly seen in cells which became detached from the substrate following fenretinide treatment. The plate-adherent cells showed a decrease in the percentage of cells in S phase and a slight increase of those in G_1 phase. This study documents that ovarian cancer cells can undergo changes typical of apoptosis after exposure to fenretinide.

Clinically, the benefit of fenretinide was noted in a chemoprevention study in women with early stage breast cancer. In a randomized clinical trial supported by the National Cancer Institute performed at the Istituto Nazionale Tumori, Milan, Italy, women with T1 or T2, N0, M0 breast cancer were randomized to fenretinide (200 mg) daily for 5 years, or no treatment.[39] During the 5 years of intervention, six patients in the control group developed ovarian carcinoma, whereas no case of ovarian carcinoma occurred during the same time period in the fenretinide group. The difference in the incidence rate of ovarian carcinoma in the two groups was statistically significant ($P = 0.0162$). Of interest and as expected, the protective effect of fenretinide was lost when the drug was discontinued. Two patients subsequently developed ovarian cancer 10 and 30 months, respectively, after fenretinide was discontinued. Clearly, there is a drug effect on the ovaries and the manner by which it creates this effect is crucial to the development of preventive strategies for high-risk women.

Progestin

Pregnancy and oral contraceptive use provide considerable protection against ovarian cancer. According to the Cancer and Steroid Hormone Study of the Centers for Disease Control and Prevention, the relative risk for ovarian cancer decreased to 0.6 in women who used oral contraceptives for a minimum of 3 months and to 0.4 in women after more than 5 years of use.[40] The protective effect was still present up to 10 years after drug discontinuation.

While it is accepted that oral contraceptives protect against ovarian cancer in general, it is important to know whether they also protect against hereditary forms of ovarian cancer. Narod *et al.*[41] enrolled 270 women with hereditary ovarian cancer and 161 of their sisters as controls in a case-control study. All the patients carried a pathogenic mutation in either *BRCA1* or *BRCA2*. Lifetime histories of oral contraceptive use were obtained and compared. The adjusted odds ratio for ovarian cancer associated with any past use of oral contraceptives was 0.5. The risk decreased with prolonged duration of use. Oral contraceptive use protected against ovarian cancer both for carriers of *BRCA1* and *BRCA2*.

In the past, it was thought that pregnancy and oral contraceptives provided protection against ovarian cancer by suppressing ovulation. It is believed that chronic repeated ovulation without pregnancy-associated rest periods contributes to neoplasia of the ovarian epithelium.[42] Fathalla *et al.*[42] noted that the ovarian surface epithelium—a single cell layer encompassing the ovary and originating from the same mesodermal celomic epithelium that lines the peritoneal cavity—undergoes swift proliferation during the 24 hours after ovulation. Invaginations of the epithelium to form clefts and inclusion cysts within the ovarian stroma are most striking just after ovulation. Casagrande *et al.*[43] extended this concept to decreased cancer risk correlated with anovulation resulting from oral contraceptive use. Cramer and Welch[44] noted that the ovarian epithelium continually invaginates throughout life to form clefts and inclusion cysts. Under excessive gonadotropin (follicle stimulating hormone (FSH) or luteinizing hormone (LH)) stimulation of the ovarian stroma and resulting stimulation by estrogen or estrogen precursors, the epithelium may undergo proliferation and malignant transformation. They resolved that factors affecting systemic estrogen regulation would therefore sway gonadotropin stimulation and, indirectly, the paracrine estrogen environment of the ovarian epithelial cells. The gonadotropin model is compatible with the known protective effects of parity and oral contraceptive use, inverse associations seen in the great majority of ovarian cancer studies.[45,46]

Regarding oral contraceptive usage, it is unknown whether the synthetic progestational components in these drugs contribute directly to the decreased risk consistently seen with duration of use. Progesterone, with its increased activity during pregnancy, may have a protective role in the etiology of ovarian cancer. The maternal FSH and LH levels drop with the increase in trophoblast human chorionic gonadotropin (hCG) during the first month of pregnancy. After the seventh week, there is massive placental production of progesterone.[47] In addition, the placenta extracts maternal adrenal androgens, which remain at stable maternal serum concentrations while both production and utilization rates increase; maternal serum estrone and estradiol are made from the adrenal androgens.[47] This suggests that the protective aspect of pregnancy may not be mediated by suppression of ovulation but may be due to the 8–9 months of elevated progesterone. It is unlikely to be due to the pregnancy estrogens, since most of the evidence relating estrogens to risk of ovarian cancer points either to no effect or to increase in risk.[48]

The contraceptive progestins vary in their androgenic and estrogenic properties. However, given that the progestational potency of the synthetic 19-nortestosterone progestins is more than 100 times that of progesterone, and that serum levels of progestins absorbed form oral contraceptives are comparable to luteal-phase progesterone levels, the net progestation environment within the ovary is likely to be quite high.[49,50] Thus the decreased risk of ovarian cancer with oral contraceptive use could also be due to the cyclic progestational climate.

A study which supports the idea that combined oral contraceptives offer ovarian cancer protection beyond that from suppression of ovulation is a case-control study that enrolled subjects who used only progestin types of oral contraceptives.[51] These progestin-only formulations do not totally suppress ovulation and some ovulatory cycles typically occur.[52] Approximately 40% of women using this method can have regular ovarian function with normal estrogen and luteal-phase progesterone synthesis.[53] In this study, relative to never use of progestin-only contraceptives, the risks were 0.39 for use less than 3 years and 0.21 for use greater than 3 years ($P = 0.009$).[51] Thus, the progestin-only contraceptives create a progestational hormonal environment with a reduced risk that cannot, in total, be attributed to ovulation suppression. Given that combined oral contraceptives convey a similar degree of protection but with less ovulation, risk reduction associated with ovulation suppression cannot comprise the total protection given by the combined preparations and the net benefit is probably due to the progestational component.

Clinical trial evaluating fenretinide as a chemopreventive agent for ovarian cancer

Through access to ovaries of individuals with a strong family history of ovarian cancer, there is the unique opportunity to examine tissue where there is a very high probability that malignant transformation will occur sometime during the individual's lifetime. Histologic findings may, therefore, identify a pre-

neoplastic ovary and for the first time provide potential target lesions to determine whether any chemopreventive agent can alter the phenotype. Success in this protracted format would justify long-term treatment with an active agent and provide an alternative to oophorectomy for prophylaxis.

Preclinical and clinical studies indicate that fenretinide has an important influence on the proliferation of ovarian carcinoma, and support further research in order to understand ovarian carcinogenesis and the role of fenretinide on its inhibition in high-risk populations. By examining the ovarian tissue from both fenretinide and placebo-treated females, the mechanism by which it causes this protective effect can begin to be determined.

Individuals with increased risk for ovarian cancer who have agreed to undergo a prophylactic oophorectomy may elect immediate oophorectomy, or be placed on a randomized study of fenretinide versus placebo for 6 months prior to oophorectomy. Ovarian tissue from premenopausal females who have undergone hysterectomies for reasons other than cancer or risk for ovarian cancer comprise a fourth patient group. After 6 months of fenretinide, placebo, or observation, all patient groups will have had oophorectomies and will be compared with respect to nine cellular markers:

(1) surface epithelial papillomatosis;
(2) surface epithelial invaginations;
(3) surface epithelial pseudostratification;
(4) inclusion cysts;
(5) TUNEL—a direct marker of apoptosis;
(6) immunohistochemistry of single-stranded DNA—a direct marker of apoptosis;
(7) *bcl–2* expression—a marker of apoptosis regulation;
(8) *bax* expression—a marker of apoptosis regulation; and
(9) Mib–1 proliferation.

Comparisons between the placebo and fenretinide group may be regarded as controlled, but pair-wise comparisons will be extended to all groups (Fig. 22.1).

Study population

Females of all ethnic backgrounds who are 18 years or older and who have been recommended to undergo a prophylactic oophorectomy because of their increased risk for ovarian cancer are eligible to participate. The decision for a woman to undergo prophylactic oophorectomy must be based on one of the following criteria.

1. Increased risk for ovarian cancer secondary to evidence of a genetic defect (*BRCA1* or *BRCA2*).
2. Increased risk for ovarian cancer secondary to a family history of one or more first-degree relatives diagnosed with ovarian cancer prior to the age of 50 years.
3. Increased risk for ovarian cancer secondary to a family history of more than one first-degree relative diagnosed with ovarian cancer (any age) *and* one or more first- or second-degree relative diagnosed with breast or ovarian cancer (any age).

These high-risk subjects will be asked to schedule their surgery in approximately 6–7 months such that they may participate on

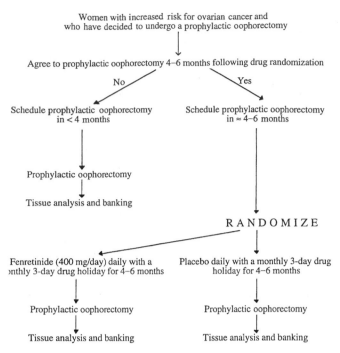

Fig. 22.1 Schema of clinical trial evaluating fenretinide as a chemopreventive agent for ovarian cancer.

Clinical trial

Seventy-one patients will be randomized to treatment with fenretinide or placebo. Assuming a 10% 'drop-out' rate, 32 subjects per arm will be evaluable. The placebo arm will provide information on the variability of the proposed biomarker assays and is ideal to assess whether there is a change in surrogate markers with fenretinide. As noted, all patients will undergo an oophorectomy and there is no known risk from a 6–12-month delay.

Fenretinide (400 mg/day) or placebo will be taken daily for 28 days every 30 days for 6 months. Each subject will have a monthly 3-day drug holiday to prevent visual toxicity (night blindness). Based upon previous clinical studies with fenretinide, it is expected that participants in this study will be able to tolerate the treatment regimens. All participants will be monitored closely for side-effects. Should there be evidence of Grade 2 or greater side-effects (Common Toxicity Criteria version 2.0), dose reduction will occur after holding the medication until resolution of symptoms.

Three techniques will be utilized to assess compliance: personal interview, pill counts, and serum drug level monitoring during the treatment period. Measurement of retinol, fenretinide, and its main metabolite, 4-MPR (*N*-(?4-methoxyphenyl) retinamide) in plasma will be analyzed by high-performance liquid chromatography (HPLC).[54]

Following the 4–6-month treatment period, participants will undergo their planned prophylactic oophorectomy. The ovarian tissue obtained during the subject's prophylactic oophorectomy will be processed routinely by the Pathology Department prior to tissue submission for research purposes.

Surrogate endpoint biomarkers

Each of the following precancerous lesions or histopathological markers (HPM) will be counted separately:

(1) surface epithelial papillomatosis;
(2) surface epithelial invaginations;
(3) surface epithelial pseudostratification; and
(4) inclusion cysts.

These lesions will be evaluated using a quantitative as well as qualitative approach in order to establish differences induced by the cancer preventive treatment.

In addition to a conventional pathological evaluation of the presence or absence of the four epithelial HPMs, including the histopathological grade of the lesions[10] by two pathologists, a quantitative analysis of the extent and number of the four epithelial HPMs will be carried out using a computerized image analyzer with morphometric software (Autocyte-Roche Pathology Work Station, Videoplan Software, Elon College, NC, USA).

Immunohistochemistry will be used to determine the percentage of proliferating cells in each sample by immunohistochemical detection of Mib–1 protein (nuclear antigen Ki–67).[55,56] The percentage of Mib–1 positive cells will be evaluated in each type of HPM as the percentage of positively stained cells per total cell population of each HPM lesion.

Two direct markers of apoptosis (TUNEL and immunohistochemistry of single-stranded DNA) as well as two apoptosis-

this study and contribute to the determination of ovarian carcinogenesis as well as the benefit of drug therapy. Prophylactic surgery is an elective procedure which can be performed safely in 6–12 months, a time frame which is very unlikely to be associated with any significant change in risk of ovarian cancer.

Should there be any subjects who are unwilling to enroll on this study because they are uncomfortable in scheduling their prophylactic oophorectomy for 6–7 months, they will be recommended to proceed with their surgery immediately. However, they will be asked to allow blood and ovarian tissue samples to be taken at the time of surgery for research purposes. This will allow additional tissue from high-risk individuals for baseline biomarker analysis to help determine the variability between individuals over time.

Since the disease is uncommon in minority subgroups and there are no strong reasons to expect different effects of therapy in different racial/ethnic subgroups, since the study sample size is small, the study will not have separate accrual targets for different subgroups. Treatment assignment in the study is not stratified on race or ethnicity. Subset analyses in this study to assess any potentially race or ethnicity treatment effects will be conducted when possible.

All participants will have a medical history and physical examination performed by a physician to ensure they are in good medical health. All subjects must have an ECOG performance status of 0–1 and a life expectancy of at least 12 months. Subjects may not be currently receiving chemotherapy, radiotherapy, or other investigational treatments. Subjects will not have major cardiac, respiratory, neurologic, or psychiatric disabilities.

related proteins that are frequently employed to evaluate apoptosis regulation (Bcl–2 and Bax) will be utilized. As before, apoptosis markers will be evaluated in each epithelial HPM separately.

Discussion

An understanding of the molecular events in gene–environmental interactions which lead to carcinogenesis in the ovary will identify specific targets for future therapy as well as for prevention strategies. Effective prevention strategies will require selection of high-risk individuals and identification of surrogate markers (precancerous lesions and biomarkers) which can serve as intermediate endpoints for prevention trials without waiting for an actual decrease in cancer incidence.

Successful completion of the fenretinide study will advance ovarian cancer prevention in several ways. The clinical trial of fenretinide as a chemopreventive agent will establish a model system in ovarian cancer, which can be used to study additional chemopreventive agents such as progestin. The premalignant phenotype in ovaries obtained from women undergoing prophylactic oophorectomies because of a perceived high risk for ovarian cancer will be validated. In addition, molecular studies on cells obtained from these women will be critical to identifying early genetic changes leading to this disease and new specific targets.

Acknowledgements

This work was supported by the United States Department of Defense and by The Ovarian Cancer Research Foundation, Inc.

References

1. Parker, S.L., Tong, T., Bolden, S. et al. (1997). Cancer Statistics, 1997. CA Cancer J. Clin., 47, 5–27.
2. Sightler, S., Boike, G., Estape, R.E. et al. (1991). Ovarian cancer in women with prior hysterectomy: a 14-year experience at the University of Miami. Obstet. Gynecol.,78, 681–4.
3. Averette, H.E., Hoskins, W., Nguyen, H.N. et al. (1993). National survey of ovarian carcinoma: I. A patient care evaluation study of the American College of Surgeons. Cancer, 71, 1629–38.
4. Boike, G., Averette, H.E., Hoskins, W. et al. (1993). National survey of ovarian carcinoma: IV. Women with prior hysterectomy: a failure of prevention. Gynecol. Oncol., 49, 112.
5. Nguyen, H.N., Averette, H.E., and Janicek, M. (1994). Ovarian carcinoma: A review of the significance of familial risk factors and the role of prophylactic oophorectomy in cancer prevention. Cancer, 74, 545–55.
6. Ravnikar, V. (1990). Physiology and treatment of hot flashes. Obstet. Gynecol., 75(Suppl.), 3–8.
7. Ettinger, B., Genant, H.K., and Cann, C.E. (1987). Postmenopausal bone loss is prevented by treatment with low-dosage estrogen with calcium. Ann. Intern. Med., 106, 40–5.
8. Bush, T.L., Barrett-Connor, E., and Cowan, L.D. (1987). Cardiovascular mortality and noncontraceptive use of estrogen: results from the Lipid Research Clinics Program Follow-up Study. Circulation, 75, 1102–9.
9. Gallion, H.H. and Park, R. (1995). Developing intervention/prevention strategies for individuals at high risk of developing hereditary ovarian cancer. J. Natl Cancer Inst., 17, 103–6.
10. Salazar, H., Godwin, A., Daly, M. et al. (1996). Microscopic benign and invasive malignant neoplasms and a preneoplastic phenotype in prophylactic oophorectomies. J. Natl Cancer Inst., 88, 1810–20.
11. Auersperg, N., Maines-Bandiera, S., Booth, J. et al. (1995). Expression of two mucin antigens in cultured human ovarium surface epithelium: Influence of a family history of ovarian cancer. Am. J. Obstet. Gynecol., 173, 558–65.
12. Fearon, E.R. and Vogelstein, B. (1990). A genetic model for colorectal tumorigenesis. Cell, 61, 759–67.
13. Bulten, J., van der Laak, J.A., Gemmink, J.H. et al. (1996). Mib–1, a promising marker for the classification of cervical intraepithelial neoplasia. J. Pathol., 178, 268–73.
14. Tamboli, P., Amin, M.B., Schultz, D.S. et al. (1996). Comparative analysis of the nuclear proliferative index (Ki–67) in benign prostate, prostatic intraepithelial neoplasia, and prostatic carcinoma. Mod. Pathol., 9, 1015–19.
15. Van Hoeven, K.H., Ramondetta, L., Kovatich, A.J. et al. (1997). Quantitative image analysis of Mib–1 reactivity in inflammatory, hyperplastic and neoplastic endocervical lesions. Int. J. Gynecol. Pathol., 16, 15–21.
16. Williams, G.T. and Smith, C.A. (1993). Molecular regulation of apoptosis: genetic controls on cell death. Cell, 74, 777–9.
17. Wright, S.C., Zhong, J., and Larrick, J.W. (1994) Inhibition of apoptosis as a mechanism of tumor promotion. FASEB J., 8, 654–60.
18. Reddy, B.S., Wang, C.X., Samaha, H. et al. (1997). Chemoprevention of colon carcinogenesis by dietary perillyl alcohol. Cancer Res., 57, 420–5.
19. Samaha, H.S., Kelloff, G.J., Steele, V. et al. (1997). Modulation of apoptosis by sulindac, curcumin, phenylethyl–3-methylcaffeate, and 6-phenylhexyl isothiocyanate: apoptotic index as a biomarker in colon cancer chemoprevention and promotion. Cancer Res., 57, 1301–5.
20. Oridate, N., Lotan, D., Mitchell, M.F. et al. (1995). Inhibition of proliferation and induction of apoptosis in cervical carcinoma cells by retinoids: implications for chemoprevention. J. Cell. Biochem., 23(Suppl.), 80–6.
21. Oridate, N., Suzuki, S., Higuchi, M. et al. (1997). Involvement of reactive oxygen species in N-(4-hydroxyphenyl) retinamide-induced apoptosis in cervical carcinoma cells. J. Natl Cancer Inst., 89, 1191–8.
22. Hsieh, T.C., Ng, C. and Wu, J.M. (1995). The synthetic retinoid N-(4-hydroxyphenyl) retinamide (4-HPR) exerts antiproliferative and apoptosis-inducing effects in the androgen-independent human prostatic JCA–1 cells. Biochem. Mol. Biol. Int., 37, 499–506.
23. Roberson, K.M., Penland, S.N., Padilla, G.M. et al. (1997.) Fenretinide: Induction of apoptosis and endogenous transforming growth factor beta in PC–3 prostate cancer cells. Cell Growth Differ., 8, 101–11.
24. Buja, L.M., Eigenbrodt, M.L., and Eigenbrodt, E.H. (1993). Apoptosis and necrosis. Basic types and mechanisms of cell death. Arch. Pathol. Lab. Med., 117, 1208–14.
25. Gavrieli, Y., Sherman, Y., and Ben-Sasson, S.A. (1992). Identification of programmed cell death in situ via specific labeling of nuclear DNA fragmentation. J. Cell. Biol., 119, 493–501.
26. Frankfurt, O.S., Robb, J.A., Sugarbaker, E.V. et al. (1996). Monoclonal antibody to single-stranded DNA is a specific and sensitive cellular marker of apoptosis. Exp. Cell Res., 226, 387–97.
27. Reed, J.C. (1994). Bcl–2 and the regulation of programmed cell death. J. Cell. Biol., 124, 1–6.
28. Hsu, S.Y., Lai, R.J., Finegold, M. et al. (1996). Targeted overexpression of Bcl–2 in ovaries of transgenic mice leads to decreased follicle apoptosis, enhanced folliculogenesis, and increased germ cell tumorigenesis. Endocrinology, 137, 4837–43.
29. Strobel, T., Swanson, L., Korsmeyer, S. et al. (1996). BAX enhances paclitaxel-induced apoptosis through a p53-independent pathway. Proc. Natl Acad. Sci. USA, 93, 14094–9.
30. Krajewska, M., Krajewski, S., Epstein, J.I. et al. (1996). Immunohistochemical analysis of bcl–2, bax, bcl-X, and mcl–1 expression in prostate cancers. Am. J. Pathol., 148, 1567–76.

31. Manetto, V., Lorenzini, R., Cordon-Cardo, C. *et al.* (1997). Bcl–2 and Bax expression in thyroid tumours. An immunohistochemical and western blot analysis. *Virchows Arch.*, **430**, 125–30.

32. Thompson, J.N., Howell, J.M., and Pitt, G.A. (1964). Vitamin A and reproduction in rats. *Proc. R. Soc. Lond. B Biol.*, **159**, 510–35.

33. Bagavandoss, P. and Midgley, A.R. (1988). Biphasic action of retinoids on gonadotropin receptor induction in rat granulosa cells *in vitro*. *Life Sci.*, **43**, 1607–14.

34. Fex, G. and Johannesson, G. (1984). Radioimmunological determination of cellular retinol-binding protein in human tissue extracts. *Cancer Res.*, **44**, 3029–32.

35. De The, H., Marchio, A., Tiollais, P. *et al.* (1989). Differential expression and ligand regulation of the retinoic acid receptor α and β genes. *EMBO J.*, **8**, 429–33.

36. Roberts, A.B. and Sporn, M.B. (1992). Mechanistic interrelationships between two super-families: the steroid/retinoid receptors and transforming growth factor -β. *Cancer Surv.*, **14**, 205–20.

37. Formelli, F. and Cleris, L. (1993). Synthetic retinoid fenretinide is effective against a human ovarian carcinoma xenograft and potentiates cisplatin activity. *Cancer Res.*, **53**, 5374–6.

38. Supino, R., Crosti, M., Clerici, M. *et al.* (1996). Induction of apoptosis by fenretinide (4HPR) in human ovarian carcinoma cells and its association with retinoic acid receptor expression. *Int. J. Cancer*, **65**, 491–7.

39. DePalo, G., Veronesi, U., Camerini, T. *et al.* (1995). Can fenretinide protect women against ovarian cancer? *J. Natl Cancer. Inst.*, **87**, 146–7.

40. The Cancer and Steroid Hormone Study of the Centers for Disease Control and Prevention (1987). The reduction in risk of ovarian cancer associated with oral contraceptive use. *N. Engl. J. Med.*, **316**, 650–5.

41. Narod, S.A., Risch, H., Moslehi, R. *et al.* (1998). Oral contraceptives and the risk of hereditary ovarian cancer. Hereditary ovarian cancer clinical study group. *N. Engl. J. Med.*, **339**, 424–8.

42. Fathalla, M. (1971). Incessant ovulation—A factor in ovarian neoplasm? *Lancet*, **2**, 163.

43. Casagrande, J.T., Louie, E.W., Pike, M.C. *et al.* (1979). Incessant ovulation and ovarian cancer. *Lancet*, **2**, 170–3.

44. Cramer, D.W. and Welch, W.R. (1983). Determinants of ovarian cancer risk. II. Inferences regarding pathologensis. *J. Natl Cancer Inst.*, **71**, 717–21.

45. Franceschi, S., Parazzini, F., Negri, E. *et al.* (1991). Pooled analysis of 3 European case-control studies of epithelial ovarian cancer: III. Oral contraceptive use. *Int. J. Cancer*, **49**, 61–5.

46. Whittemore, A., R., H., Itnyre, J. *et al.* (1992). Characteristics relating to ovarian cancer risk: Collaborative analysis of 12 U.S. case-control studies II. Invasive epithelial ovarian cancers in white women. *Am. J. Epidemiol.*, **136**, 1184–203.

47. Yen, S.S. (1994). Endocrinology of pregnancy. In *Maternal-fetal medicine: principles and practice*, Vol. 3, (ed. R.K. Creasy and R. Resnik), pp. 382–412. W.B. Saunders, Philadelphia.

48. Risch, H.A. (1998). Hormonal etiology of epithelial ovarian cancer, with a hypothesis concerning the role of androgens and progesterone. *J. Natl Cancer Inst.*, **90**, 1774–86.

49. King, R.J. and Whitehead, M.I. (1986). Assessment of the potency of orally admininstered progestins in women. *Fertil. Steril.*, **46**, 1062–6.

50. Ryder, T.A., Mobberley, M.A., and Whitehead, M.I. (1995). The endometrial nucliolar channel system as an indicator of progestin potency in HRT. *Maturitas*, **22**, 31–6.

51. Rosenberg, L., Palmer, J.R., Zauber, A.G. *et al.* (1994). A case-control study of oral contraceptive use and invasive epithelial ovarian cancer. *Am. J. Epidemiol.*, **139**, 654–61.

52. King, R.J. (1991). Biology of female sex hormone action in relation to contraceptive agents and neoplasia. *Contraception*, **43**, 527–42.

53. Stubblefield, P.G. (1993). Contraception. In *Textbook of gynecology*, (ed. L.J. Copeland, J.F. Jarrell, and J.A. McGregor), pp. 156–88. W. B. Saunders, Philadelphia.

54. Formelli, F., Clerici, M., and Campa, T. *et al.* (1993). Five-year administration of fenretinide: pharmacokinetics and effects on plasma retinol concentrations. *J. Clin. Oncol.*, **11**, 2036–42.

55. Cattoretti, G., Becker, M.H.G., Key, G. *et al.* (1992). Monoclonal antibodies against recombinant parts of the Ki–67 antigen (MIB 1 and MIB) 3 detect proliferating cells in microwave-processed formalin-fixed paraffin sections. *J. Pathol.*, **168**, 357–63.

56. Wilkinson, E.J. and Hendricks, J.B. (1994). Quality control considerations for Ki–67 and quantitation in paraffin-embedded tissue. *Abstract presented at the Workshop on Quantitative Pathology in Chemoprevention Trials, NCI. February, San Diego.*

23. Biologic effect of progestins on the ovarian epithelium: cancer prevention through apoptosis?

Gustavo C. Rodriguez, David Walmer, Mark Cline, Hannah Krigman, Regina Whitaker, Pamela D. Isner, Bruce Lessey, Connette McMahon, Jeffrey Marks, James Petitte, Donna Carver, Kenneth Anderson, Andrew Berchuck, John Barnes, and Claude Hughes

Introduction

Epithelial ovarian cancer remains a highly lethal malignancy. It is the fourth leading cause of cancer deaths among women in the United States, and causes 140 000 deaths annually in women worldwide.[1] Although there is no established pharmacological chemopreventive approach to this disease, the well-known association between oral contraceptive pill (OCP) use and lower subsequent ovarian cancer risk suggests that an effective chemopreventive approach is possible. If the mechanism underlying the protective effect of OCPs can be elucidated, then it may be possible to devise a pharmacological chemopreventive strategy that is more effective than OCPs, while possibly eliminating side-effects associated with OCPs, and not interfering with ovulation.

The reduction in the risk of ovarian cancer in women who have used combination estrogen–progestin oral contraceptives for at least 3 years is approximately 40%, and this protective effect increases with the duration of use and persists for up to two decades after discontinuation of use.[2–6] A large body of epidemiologic evidence has linked ovulation with ovarian cancer risk, leading to the widespread belief that the protective effect of OCP use is due to the ability of these agents to inhibit ovulation.[7–8] However, we questioned that presumption because routine oral contraceptive use results in a disproportionately greater protective effect than that which could be attributed solely to ovulation inhibition. For example, oral contraceptive use for 3 years, or approximately 10% of a woman's reproductive lifetime, confers a 30–50% reduction in the risk of ovarian cancer, rather than 10%. We proposed that these data are more consistent with the hypothesis that oral contraceptives exert a protective effect through some other profound biologic effect on the ovary unrelated to ovulatory inhibition.

In search of biologic effects of OCPs that have the potential to confer protective effects against ovarian cancer, we have performed a study in primates that suggests that the OCP has a potent apoptotic effect on the ovarian epithelium, mediated by the progestin component. In subsequent studies performed *in vitro*, we have induced apoptosis in transformed, immortalized cultured human ovarian epithelial cells treated with progestins, suggesting that progestins may have a direct apoptotic effect on the human ovarian epithelium.

The apoptosis molecular pathway is one of the most important mechanisms *in vivo* for the eradication of genetically damaged cells that have the potential to become malignant. In addition, there is mounting evidence that induction of apoptosis underlies the protective effect of a number of known chemopreventive agents. The finding that progestins activate this critical pathway in the ovarian epithelium raises the possibility that progestin-mediated apoptotic effects underlie the protection against ovarian cancer afforded by routine OCP use, and not ovulation inhibition as has been previously assumed. This forms the basis for an investigation of the progestin class of drugs as chemopreventive agents for epithelial ovarian cancer.

Levonorgestrel induces apoptosis of ovarian epithelial cells in cynomolgus macaques

We have recently had the opportunity to study the long-term biologic effect of the contraceptive Triphasil on the ovaries of cynomolgus macaques. The remarkable similarity of this non-human primate to humans, particularly in regard to its 28-day menstrual cycle, makes this primate model ideal for designing experiments pertinent to human ovarian and reproductive biology.[9–11] The purpose of our study was to search for biologic effects that had the potential to be responsible for the known chemopreventive effects of oral contraceptives. Given the importance of the apoptosis pathway *in vivo* for elimination of cells that have sustained DNA damage, we elected to investigate whether long-term oral contraceptive exposure induced apoptosis in the primate ovarian epithelium.

One-hundred-and-thirty young, adult female cynomolgus macaques (*Macaca fascicularis*), with an average age of 4.75 years, were randomized into a study designed to test the long-term biologic effects of the contraceptive Triphasil, including effects on the cardiovascular system, breast, and reproductive organs. Forty of the animals were sacrificed early for baseline cardiovascular and lipoprotein studies, and an additional 14 animals died during the course of the study, primarily from trauma and diarrheal diseases. One primate was excluded because ovarian tissue was not available for study. The remaining 75 animals were necropsied at the completion of the thirty-fifth month of the study. The study was performed at the Bowman Gray School of Medicine primate facility after approval by The Animal Care and Use Committee.

The macaques were prospectively randomized into four groups to receive a diet for 35 months that contained either:

(1) no hormones,
(2) the combination oral contraceptive Triphasil, which is comprised of the estrogen ethinyl estradiol and the progestin levonorgestrel,
(3) the estrogenic component of Triphasil (ethinyl estradiol) alone, or
(4) the progestin component of Triphasil (levonorgestrel) alone.

Hormones in the latter two groups were administered in the same dosage and schedule that occurs in a typical Triphasil regimen. Doses were scaled on the base of caloric intake, which takes into account species differences in metabolic rate, and this is the accepted way to achieve dosages comparable to those used by women. The human-equivalent doses were thus: 6 days of 0.030 mg ethinyl estradiol plus 0.050 mg levonorgestrel, followed by 5 days of 0.040 mg ethinyl estradiol plus 0.075 mg levonorgestrel, followed by 10 days of 0.030 mg ethinyl estradiol plus 0.125 mg levonorgestrel, followed by 7 days of no treatment. This cyclic regimen was repeated every 28 days continuously for 35 months. During the third week of the last month of the study the animals were sacrificed and the ovaries were removed and preserved.

From each animal in the study, one ovary was flash frozen and saved for future molecular studies, and the other was formalin fixed, and paraffin embedded. Five-micron sections taken from the middle of each paraffin-embedded ovary were mounted on charged slides. The ovarian epithelium was examined for morphologic and immunohistochemical evidence of apoptosis after staining with the Apoptag-plus Kit (Oncor, Gaithersburg, MD, USA). The Kit specifically labels the 3' end of DNA fragments in cells undergoing DNA fragmentation, a characteristic of apoptosis.[12]

Dark-brown nuclear staining easily identified cells undergoing apoptosis. Tonsillar and DNAase-digested tissue sections were used as positive controls.

To calculate the percentage of ovarian epithelial cells undergoing apoptosis, both the total number of ovarian epithelial cells and the number undergoing apoptosis were counted on each 5-μm section. The median proportion of cells undergoing apoptosis was calculated for each treatment group. The Kruskal–Wallis Test was used to perform multiple comparisons of all pairs of treatment,[13] and the statistical analysis was carried out using the BMDP statistical software package.[14] At each step in this study, including the histologic examinations of the ovaries, the investigators were blinded with regard to the treatment group associated with each ovary.

All animals were sacrificed during the third week of the last month of the study. Thus, control animals, which were expected to have spontaneous and regular ovulatory cycles, were sacrificed randomly at various stages of the menstrual cycle, and could be expected to vary with regard to their endogenous hormonal state. In order to determine the endogenous hormonal milieus of primates from the control group, the endometrium of control primates was dated using standard histologic morphologic criteria by one of the authors (MC), who was blinded to the apoptosis data.[9,15]

Marked morphologic differences were observed in the ovarian epithelia from the different treatment groups. In the control and ethinyl estradiol-treated monkeys, the ovarian epithelium typically had a lush appearance, with epithelial cells containing abundant cytoplasm and visible microvilli at the surface. Apoptotic cells were rarely seen (Figs 23.1 and 23.2). In contrast, in the progestin-treated monkeys, both those treated with Triphasil (ethinyl estradiol plus levonorgestrel) and those treated with levonorgestrel alone, the ovarian epithelium contained numerous brown-staining apoptotic cells (Figs 23.3 and 23.4). Additional morphologic findings in the epithelium of progestin-treated monkeys included the tendency for patches of the surface of the ovary to be devoid of epithelium, and for the epithelium to

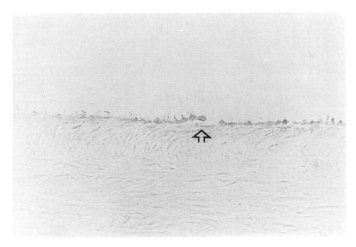

Fig. 23.1 Ovarian section from control group of macaques (20×, stained with Apoptag-plus stain). One positively staining brown cell present (arrow).

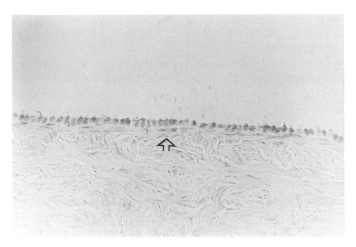

Fig. 23.2 Ovarian section from group treated with ethinyl estradiol only (20×, stained with Apoptag-plus stain). The epithelium is thick, and contains numerous microvilli (arrow).

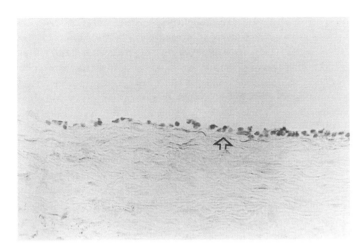

Fig. 23.3 Ovarian section from the combination (Triphasil) ethinyl estradiol and levonorgestrel-treated group (20×, stained with Apoptag-plus stain). Numerous apoptotic epithelial cells present (arrow), interspersed between non-apoptotic, non-staining cells.

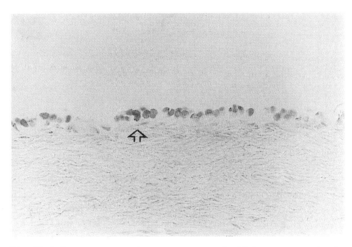

Fig. 23.4 Ovarian section from group treated with levonorgestrel only (20×, stained with Apoptag-plus stain). Numerous brown-staining epithelial cells (arrow) with abnormal morphology present.

contain many cells with sparse cytoplasm that appeared to be detaching from the ovarian surface. The most dramatic morphologic and immunohistochemical evidence of apoptotic changes was noted in the ovarian epithelium of the primates treated with levonorgestrel alone.

The median percentage of ovarian epithelial cells undergoing apoptosis for each of the treatment groups is shown in Table 23.1. The median percentage of apoptotic ovarian epithelial cells in the control group of monkeys not receiving any hormones was 3.9%. As compared to controls, there was a statistically significant four-fold increase ($P > 0.01$) in the percentage of apoptotic ovarian epithelial cells in the primates receiving Triphasil in the diet.

Comparison of the groups of primates receiving exogenous hormones revealed striking differences in the degree of ovarian epithelial apoptosis; from a very low level of 1.8% in those receiving ethinyl estradiol alone (not significantly different than controls), to a very high level of 24.9% in the primates receiving levonorgestrel alone. The apoptotic rate in this latter group was over six times greater than the level observed in the control and

Table 23.1 Apoptotic effect of hormone treatment on macaque ovarian epithelium

Study group	Number	Median percent of apoptotic cell counts	Range of percent of apoptotic cell counts
Control	20	3.9	0.1–33.0
Hormone treated			
Ethinyl estradiol	20	1.8	0.1–28.6
Combination pill	17	14.5	3.0–61.0
Levonorgestrel	18	24.9	3.5–61.8
Multiple comparisons:	Control vs levonorgestrel ($P < 0.001$)		
	Combination pill vs ethinyl estradiol ($P < 0.001$)		
	Ethinyl estradiol vs levonorgestrel ($P < 0.001$)		
	Control vs combination pill ($P < 0.01$)		

ethinyl estradiol-only treated monkeys ($P > 0.001$). Because the only difference between the combination pill group and the estrogen-only treated group is the presence of the levonorgestrel component of the combination pill, and because the degree of apoptosis in the ovarian epithelium in the estrogen-alone group was not significantly different than that of the control group, these data suggest that the increased degree of apoptosis in the ovarian epithelium in combination pill-treated monkeys is due to the effect of the progestational component (levonorgestrel) of the combination pill. Moreover, the higher rate of apoptosis measured in the ovarian epithelium of monkeys that received the progestational agent alone as compared to the monkeys that received the combination pill, although not statistically significant, suggests that progestin-only treatment may be more effective in inducing apoptosis in the ovarian epithelium than estrogen–progestin combination treatment. These data demonstrate the novel finding that oral contraceptive exposure induces apoptosis in the ovarian epithelium, and that the progestin component of the pill is responsible for this effect.

Histologic dating of the endometrium in monkeys from the control group revealed that the majority (14 of 20, or 70%) were sacrificed during the luteal phase of the menstrual cycle, indicating a bias in the control group toward an endogenous progestin milieu. It is worth noting that despite this bias in controls, significantly more apoptosis was observed in the ovarian epithelium of monkeys receiving levonorgestrel. This significant difference held up even after excluding from analysis the control monkeys who were sacrificed during the follicular (estrogenic) phase of the menstrual cycle. These data add further support to the notion that the contraceptive progestin levonorgestrel has a potent apoptotic effect on the ovarian epithelium, and suggests that this effect is more potent than that induced by endogenous progesterone. The relatively small number of control monkeys in the follicular phase of the menstrual cycle precluded a valid statistical analysis comparing the degree of apoptosis in the ovarian epithelium of control monkeys in the follicular versus luteal phases of the menstrual cycle.

Direct apoptotic effects of progestins on ovarian epithelial cells

The discovery that progestins induce apoptosis in the ovarian epithelium led us to search for potential mechanisms of action underlying these apoptotic effects. It is possible that progestins induce the expression of factors in the ovarian stroma, which then induce apoptosis via a paracrine effect in the adjacent ovarian epithelium. Conversely, it is possible that progestins exert a direct apoptotic effect on the ovarian epithelium, mediated by the progestin receptor. In order to identify target sites of action for progestin in the ovary, we first examined the normal human ovary for expression of the progesterone receptor. Immunohistochemical staining for progesterone receptor was performed on normal frozen ovarian tissue samples obtained from 40 women who underwent oophorectomy as part of a gynecologic procedure performed for benign gynecologic indications. The progesterone

receptor was consistently expressed by the ovarian epithelium in all cases, including the epithelium from ovaries from both pre- and postmenopausal women (Fig. 23.5a). In addition, progesterone receptor expression was detected in the ovarian epithelium lining inclusion cysts trapped within the ovarian stroma (Fig. 23.5b). Progesterone receptor expression was absent in all non-epithelial areas of the ovary. Not surprisingly, we found similar expression of the progesterone receptor in the ovarian epithelium in primates (cynomolgus macaque). In separate experiments, we have demonstrated expression of both the A and B isoforms of the progestin receptor *in vitro* in several ovarian cancer cell lines (OVCA 420, 429, 432, 433; OVCAR3, DOV–13), as well in cell-culture-derived non-malignant human ovarian epithelium (Fig. 23.6). Although the physiologic role of the progesterone receptor within the ovarian epithelium remains to be elucidated, localization of progesterone receptor to the ovarian epithelium suggests a functional role for progestins in ovarian epithelial cells.

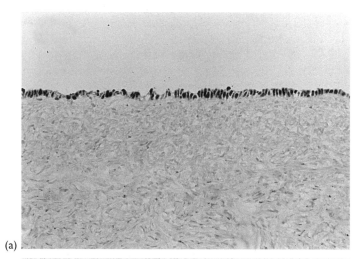

(a)

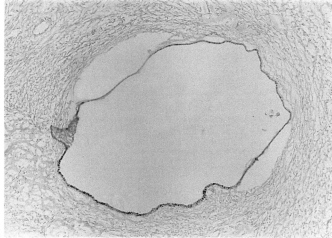

(b)

Fig. 23.5 Frozen section of normal human ovary demonstrating dark-brown nuclear immunohistochemical staining for the progesterone receptor in: (a) the surface ovarian epithelium; and (b) ovarian epithelial cells lining inclusion cysts.

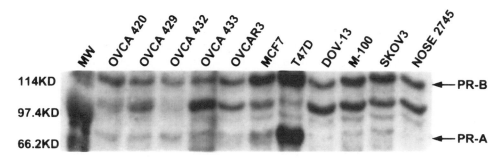

Fig. 23.6 Western blot analysis for progesterone receptor from cell lysates derived from normal ovarian epithelial cell culture (NOSE 2745), spontaneously transformed culture derived from normal ovarian epithelium (M-100), and ovarian cancer cell lines (OVCA 420, 429, 432, 433, OVCAR3, DOV-13, and SKOV3), demonstrating expression of both the A and B isoforms of the progestin receptor. MCF7 and T47D are progesterone receptor-positive breast cancer cell lines.

In addition, M–100 cells were grown to confluence in 60-mm dishes and then treated with levonorgestrel (100 µM) for 12, 24, 48, 72, and 96 hours. Then, cells were harvested, centrifuged at 6000 g for 10 minutes and the resultant pellets were resuspended in 200 µl nuclei lysis buffer (5 M guanidine thiocyanate, 25 mM sodium citrate pH 7.0, 100 mM β-mercaptoethanol). DNA was precipitated with an equal volume of isopropanol at –70 °C for 1 hour. Samples were centrifuged for 30 minutes at 12 000 g at 4 °C, and the DNA pellets were washed in 70% ethanol at room temperature. Pellets were resuspended in TE buffer and incubated overnight at 37 °C with 0.5 mg/ml RNAase A (Sigma Chemical Co., St. Louis, MO, USA). Pellets were again resuspended and an optical density reading at 260 nm wavelength was obtained on a Perkin–Elmer Lambda 3B UV/vis spectrophotometer to determine the concentration of DNA. Equal amounts of each DNA sample were then subjected to electrophoresis on a horizontal 1.5% agarose gel containing ethidium bromide, and visualized under UV illumination. DNA ladders indicative of apoptosis were observed at 48, 72, and 96 hours in M-100 cells treated with levonorgestrel, with no evidence of apoptosis observed in control cultures treated with the appropriate control vehicle solution (Fig. 23.7). Collectively, these experiments are the first to demonstrate a direct apoptotic effect of progestins on non-malignant ovarian epithelial cells.

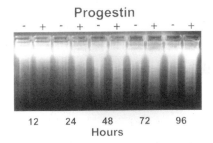

Fig. 23.7 Effect of levonorgestrel on apoptosis in the spontaneously transformed human ovarian epithelial cell line M-100. A DNA ladder consistent with apoptosis is seen at 48, 72, and 96 hours.

Chemoprevention of ovarian cancer with apoptosis-inducing agents: the case for progestins

It is widely accepted that the process of apoptosis involves a specific series of genetically directed events that eventually lead to the death and efficient disposal of the cell.[16,17] With regard to cancer prevention, the apoptosis pathway is one of the most important *in vivo* mechanisms that functions to eliminate cells that have sustained DNA damage and which are thus prone to malignant transformation.[18] Therefore it is possible that agents which selectively increase apoptosis in the ovarian epithelium may confer protection against the development of ovarian cancer.

There is mounting evidence that the apoptosis molecular pathway can be exploited for the chemoprevention of cancer. A number of known chemopreventive agents have been shown to induce apoptosis in the target tissues that they protect from malignant transformation. These agents include the retinoids,[19–27] dietary flavanoids,[28] anti-inflammatory drugs,[29] monoterpenes,[30–31] S-adenosyl-L-methionine,[32] and selenium.[33–34] Apoptosis-inducing agents have been shown to prevent development of lymphoid, colon, and mammary cancers in rodents, and are now being evaluated in human clinical trials.

The oral contraceptive may indeed represent the most significant chemopreventive agent developed to date. Routine use of the OCP reduces the subsequent risks of the two most common gynecologic malignancies—endometrial and ovarian cancer—by approximately 50%. We have demonstrated that oral contraceptives, via the progestin component, induce apoptosis in the ovarian epithelium, the target site for ovarian cancer, similar to what has been shown in the target tissues for other chemopreventive agents. Thus it is likely that induction of the apoptosis pathway in the ovarian epithelium may be a major mechanism underlying the protective effect of OCPs, rather than ovulation inhibition as has been previously presumed. An accelerated rate of apoptosis induced by progestin may facilitate the steady removal of epithelial cells from the ovarian surface, increasing the likelihood that cells containing DNA damage and possessing the potential to transform into epithelial ovarian carcinoma will undergo programmed cell death rather than survive, thereby decreasing the risk of epithelial ovarian cancer.

The concept that progestin-induced apoptosis of the ovarian epithelium is responsible for the chemopreventive effect of oral contraceptives is a complete departure from the widely accepted theory that suppression of 'incessant ovulation' is responsible for this reduced risk.[35] The 'incessant ovulation' hypothesis for ovarian cancer is based on epidemiologic evidence demonstrating that the risk of ovarian cancer correlates positively with the number of ovulatory cycles in a woman's lifetime.[7] Factors associated with decreased ovulation, such as increased parity, breast-feeding, and estrogen/progestin combination oral contraceptive use, have been shown to decrease the risk of ovarian cancer; whereas factors associated with increased ovulation, such as early menarche, late menopause, and nulliparity, increase the risk.[8,36,37] In addition, the long-term use of ovarian hyperstimulants such as clomiphene, which induces ovulation, has been shown to be associated with an increased risk of ovarian cancer in some women.[38] It is likely that years of ovarian epithelial damage, associated with ovulation, results in the accumulation of molecular aberrations in ovarian epithelial cells, which, if sufficient, can lead to neoplastic transformation. By increasing the apoptotic tendency of ovarian epithelial cells that have incurred genetic damage, oral contraceptive progestins may function to enhance the apoptotic death of dysplastic or aberrant cells that are not yet malignant, thereby decreasing the risk of epithelial ovarian cancer. Similarly, it is possible that pregnancy, which represents a high-progestin state, confers protection against ovarian cancer through a mechanism which involves apoptotic effects on the ovarian epithelium in addition to, or rather than, through ovulation inhibition.

Although not statistically significant, we found a greater degree of ovarian epithelial cell apoptosis in animals treated with levonorgestrel alone as compared to treatment with Triphasil, which contains both ethinyl estradiol and levonorgestrel. This suggests the possibility that if the apoptosis pathway is indeed the mechanism mediating the chemopreventive effects of oral contraceptives, that agents comprised solely of a progestin may confer a greater chemopreventive effect than those comprised of estrogen and progestin. More importantly, if apoptotic effects caused by progestins are primarily responsible for the chemopreventive effects of OCPs, then it may be possible to develop a chemopreventive strategy using progestins at a dose and schedule that do not inhibit ovulation in young women, or in anovulatory women such as those who are menopausal. In addition, this opens up the possibility that other agents which selectively induce apoptosis in the ovarian epithelium may confer chemopreventive effects, while sparing the undesired side-effects of progestins.

The limited epidemiologic data that are available regarding the relationship between treatment with progestin-only contraceptives and epithelial ovarian cancer have shown no significant change in ovarian cancer risk in women who have used depo-medroxy-progesterone acetate.[39,40] It is possible, however, that these studies did not demonstrate a decreased risk of ovarian cancer in medroxy-progesterone acetate users due to methodological limitations, which include insufficient numbers of study subjects, low mean age of cases studied, as well as very limited data regarding long-term effects. Alternatively, it is possible that lack of a protective effect associated with medroxy-progesterone acetate may be due to the fact that it is a different class of progestin than the 19-nortestosterone derivatives, and that the 19-nortestosterone derivatives, which are the common progestin components of combination oral contraceptives, may be more effective in conferring a chemopreventive effect than progesterone, or progesterone derivatives.

A recent and well-designed epidemiologic study suggests that long-term use of hormone replacement with estrogen alone may increase the risk of fatal ovarian carcinoma.[41] The mechanism underlying this increased risk is unclear. Whereas epithelial ovarian cancer is not known to be an estrogen-dependent disease, it is interesting to speculate that estrogens may increase the risk of ovarian cancer by lowering the apoptotic susceptibility of the ovarian epithelium. Although there was no statistical difference in the degree of apoptosis in the ovarian epithelium between monkeys treated with ethinyl estradiol alone versus controls, or between those treated with Triphasil and those receiving levonorgestrel alone, the lowest degree of apoptosis in our study was noted in the group of monkeys treated with ethinyl estradiol alone, and the addition of ethinyl estradiol to levonorgestrel (Triphasil group) resulted in a lower degree of apoptosis than treatment with levonorgestrel alone. It remains to be determined whether the addition of a progestin to an estrogen for hormone replacement in postmenopausal women would negate the potential estrogen-related increased risk of ovarian cancer and confer additional chemopreventive benefits.

It is likely that the maximal chemopreventive potential of OCPs has not been achieved. The protective effect conferred by OCP use against ovarian cancer has been presumed to be due to effects related to inhibition of ovulation, thereby limiting the potential protective benefits of these agents to women who are ovulatory and/or who desire contraception. If the mechanism(s) underlying the protective effect of OCPs can be thoroughly understood, and are found to include a potent biologic effect that is unrelated to ovulation (such as apoptosis), then it may be possible to devise a chemopreventive strategy that is more effective at prevention of ovarian cancer than routine OCP use, and that can be applied to all women, including those who are postmenopausal.

Our preliminary studies suggest that progestin activates the apoptosis pathway in the ovarian epithelium, raising the possibility that this class of hormone can be used for the chemoprevention of ovarian cancer, thereby reducing the risk of this lethal cancer in women. The ultimate goal will be to elucidate a chemopreventive strategy using the best 'apoptosis-inducing' agents in the ovarian epithelium, in the ideal pattern of administration, and that can be employed in all women, including those who are postmenopausal, in order to significantly reduce the risk of subsequent ovarian cancer. If routine use of the OCP can achieve a dramatic 50% reduction in risk of ovarian cancer, then it is possible that exploitation of the underlying mechanism responsible for the protective effect will yield a protective effect which is vastly superior. The impact on epithelial ovarian cancer, as a disease, would be dramatic.

The potential role of the domestic fowl for ovarian cancer chemoprevention research

We believe that the domestic fowl has great potential as an animal model for studying chemoprevention of ovarian cancer. The only known animal model with a high incidence of spontaneous ovarian adenocarcinoma is the domestic fowl.[42–43] Fredrickson[43] reported that in two flocks of hens with initial ages of either 2 or 3 years, followed prospectively until ages 3.9–4.2 years, there were 33 cases of ovarian adenocarcinoma in 236 chickens. This gives an incidence of 14% in the 2-year period of observation. First suggested as a model for research in ovarian cancer more than 20 years ago,[43] we know of no investigators who have taken advantage of the hen as a model to assess possible preventative approaches for ovarian cancer in women.[43–45] It is likely that the high ovulatory rate, with its associated disruption and repair of the ovarian surface epithelium, leads to the acquisition of genetic damage in ovarian epithelial cells, resulting in a high incidence of ovarian cancer.

In addition to its known high incidence of ovarian cancer, there are other features of the domestic fowl that make it attractive for studying chemoprevention of ovarian cancer, particularly with progestin agents:

(1) The ovulatory cycle in the domestic fowl has been extensively studied and previously characterized, and is highly regulated by gonadotropins, estrogens, androgens, and progestin.[46,47]
(2) Under standard conditions, the domestic fowl ovulates on almost a daily basis. However, anovulation can be induced under controlled conditions that include dietary restriction. It has been shown in a long-term (1-year) study in broiler hens, for example, that dietary restriction to maintain pullet weight (beneath the minimum required to support egg production) causes complete cessation of ovulation.[48] Thus, ovulation in the domestic fowl can be carefully controlled, allowing the design of experiments that can test the relative importance of ovulation inhibition versus molecular biologic effects of contraceptives hormones or other agents with regard to chemoprevention of ovarian cancer.
(3) Expression and regulation of known effectors of apoptosis, such as Bax, Bcl-2, and p53, have been studied extensively in the domestic fowl.[49–56]
(4) The ovarian epithelium in the domestic fowl expresses progesterone receptor in both the A and B isoforms.[57,58]
(5) We have been able to induce apoptosis with the progestin levonorgestrel in cultured normal ovarian epithelial cells from the chicken, using the same technique described above for human ovarian epithelium (Fig. 23.8).

Thus, the domestic fowl represents an animal model which spontaneously develops ovarian cancer; expresses receptor for progestin in the ovarian epithelium, our target site of interest for prevention; and our proposed intervention with progestins induces a relevant surrogate endpoint biomarker effect of apoptosis in our target site of interest.

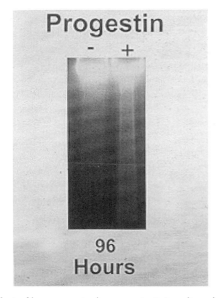

Fig. 23.8 Effect of levonorgestrel on apoptosis in cultured normal ovarian epithelial cells from the chicken. A DNA ladder consistent with apoptosis is seen at 96 hours.

We are currently performing a careful histological and molecular examination of benign and malignant chicken ovaries. The chicken ovary is comprised of an outer cortex containing ova surrounding a medulla. A single layer of germinative epithelial cells overlies the cortex (Fig. 23.9).[59] Hundreds of small follicular cysts project from the surface. The surface epithelium is highly convoluted, with extensive invaginations and folds (Fig. 23.10). Initial findings indicate that ovarian cancers form a tubular–glandular pattern, are cytokeratin positive, and stain negatively for intracellular ovalbumin (Figs 23.11 and 23.12). In contrast, oviductal tumors, which also are common in the chicken, are cytokeratin negative, contain periodic acid–Schiff (PAS)-positive eosinophilic droplets in the apical cytoplasm, and are ovalbumin positive (Figs 23.13 and 23.14).

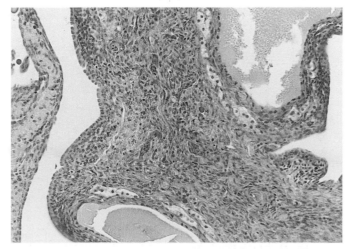

Fig. 23.9 Hematoxylin and eosin; normal chicken ovary (70×).

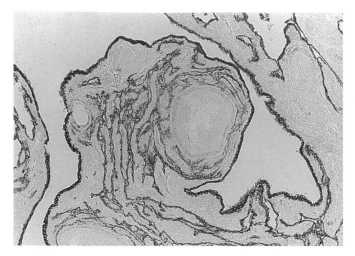

Fig. 23.10 Normal chicken ovary stained with anti-cytokeratin antibody AE1, demonstrating intense expression of cytokeratin in the surface epithelium.

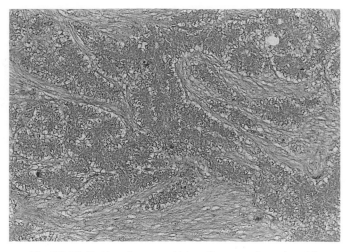

Fig. 23.13 Oviductal cancer, chicken (hematoxylin and eosin).

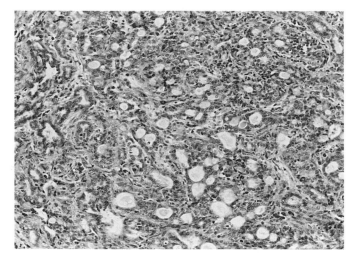

Fig. 23.11 Ovarian adenocarcinoma in the chicken, demonstrating a tubular-glandular pattern (Giemsa stain).

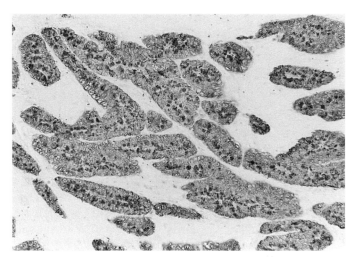

Fig. 23.14 Oviductal cancer, chicken, stained for ovalbumin.

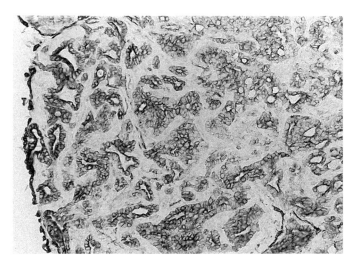

Fig. 23.12 Ovarian adenocarcinoma in chicken. Section stained with the anti-cytokeratin antibody AE1.

Additionally, we are performing a 2-year study in the domestic fowl, designed to test the hypothesis that progestin confers chemoprevention against ovarian cancer. In addition, our study will test the hypothesis that the protective effect of progestin is due to a biologic effect independent of ovulation. This project will take advantage of a long-neglected animal model to show the feasibility of prevention of ovarian cancer by progestins in women. Demonstration that progestin treatment confers chemoprevention in our avian animal model, particularly in hens who are anovulatory, would provide strong support of our hypothesis that the protective effect of contraceptive agents is due to a biologic effect caused by progestins, and not due to ovulation inhibition. More importantly, demonstration of a chemopreventive effect by progestin would then lead to other similar avian chemopreventive trials, designed to identify the optimal progestins, in the optimal doses and schedules, as a prelude to consideration of chemopreventive trials in women.

Conclusion

Given the relevance of the apoptosis pathway for the protection of normal tissues from neoplastic transformation, the finding that a progestin can activate this vital pathway in the ovarian epithelium in a relevant primate model suggests that progestins deserve further evaluation as potential ovarian cancer chemopreventive agents. In addition, the finding that progestin can induce apoptosis in normal human ovarian epithelium *in vitro* not only lends support to our primate data but also suggests that progestins have a direct apoptotic effect on the ovarian epithelium. If the mechanism underlying the protective effects of OCPs involves the apoptotic effects of progestins, and not ovulation inhibition, it may be possible:

(1) to develop a chemopreventive strategy using progestins; and
(2) to apply this strategy to a broad portion of the population, including women at high genetic risk of ovarian cancer and women who do not ovulate (i.e. postmenopausal women), who represent the age group at highest risk for the disease.

It is interesting to speculate that a preventive approach which exploits the molecular mechanism underlying the protective effect of OCPs may be markedly more effective at reducing ovarian cancer risks than routine OCP use.

References

1. American Cancer Society (1996). *Cancer facts and figures,* Yearly Publication. American Cancer Society, Atlanta, GA.
2. Rosenberg, L., Palmer, J.R., Zauber, A.G. *et al.* (1994). A case-control study of oral contraceptive use and invasive epithelial ovarian cancer. *Am. J. Epidemiol.,* **139** (7), 654–61.
3. Stanford, J.L., Thomas, D.B., Ray, R.M. *et al.* (1989). Epithelial ovarian cancer and combined oral contraceptives: The WHO collaborative study of neoplasia and steroid contraceptives. *Int. J. Epidemiol.,* **18** (3), 538–45.
4. Lee, N.C., Wingo, P.A., Gwynn, M.L. *et al.* (1987). The reduction in risk of ovarian cancer associated with oral-contraceptive use. *N. Engl. J. Med.,* **316,** 650–5.
5. Gross, T.P. and Schlesselman, J.J. (1994). The estimated effect of oral contraceptive use on the cumulative risk of epithelial ovarian cancer. *Obstet. Gynecol.,* **83** (3), 419–24.
6. Franceschi, S., Parazzini, F., Negri, E. *et al.* (1991). Pooled analysis of three European case-control studies of epithelial ovarian cancer: III, Oral contraceptive use. *Int. J. Cancer,* **49,** 61–5.
7. Wu, M.L., Whittemore, A.S., Paffenbarger, R.S. Jr *et al.* (1987). Personal and environmental characteristics related to epithelial ovarian cancer. *Am. J. Epidemiol.,* **28** (6), 1216–27.
8. Greene, M.H., Clark, J.W., and Blayney, D.W. (1984). The epidemiology of ovarian cancer. *Semin. Oncol.* **II** (3), 209–25.
9. Brenner, R.M. and Slayden, O.D. (1994). Cyclic changes in the primate oviduct and endometrium. In *The physiology of reproduction,* (ed. E. Knobil and J.D. Neill), pp. 541–69. Raven Press, New York.
10. Hotchkiss, J. and Knobil, E. (1994). The menstrual cycle and its neuroendocrine control. In *The physiology of reproduction,* (ed. E. Knobil and J.D. Neill), pp. 711–36. Raven Press, New York.
11. Kaiserman-Abramof, I. and Padykula, H. (1989). Ultrastructural epithelial zonation of the primate endometrium (rhesus monkey). *Am. J. Anat.,* 13–30.
12. Wijsman, J.H., Jonker, R.R., and Keijzer, R. (1993). A new method to detect apoptosis in paraffin sections: *In situ* end-labeling of fragmented DNA. *J. Histochem. Cytochem.,* **41,** 7–12.
13. Hollander, M. and Wolfe, D.A. (1973). *Nonparametric statistical methods.* Wiley, New York.
14. *BMDP Statistical Software Manual* (1992). University of California Press, Los Angeles, CA, pp. 459–61.
15. Ferenczy, A. (1987). Anatomy and histology of the uterine corpus. In *Blaustein's pathology of the female genital tract,* (3rd edn), pp. 257–91. Springer-Verlag, Berlin.
16. Lockshin, R.A. and Zakeri, Z. (1996). The biology of cell death and its relationship to aging. In *Cellular aging and cell death,* pp. 167–80. Wiley-Liss, Inc.,
17. Lowe, S.W. and Ruley, H.E. (1996). p53-Dependent apoptosis in tumor progression and in cancer therapy. In *Cellular aging and cell death,* pp. 209–34. Wiley-Liss, Inc.,
18. Canman, C.E., Chen, C.-Y., Lee, M.-H. *et al.* (1994). DNA damage responses: p53 induction, cell cycle perturbations, and apoptosis. *Cold Spring Harbor Symp. Quant. Biol.,* **LIX,** 277–86.
19. Chan, L.N., Zhang, S., Cloyd, M. *et al.* (1997) N-(4-hydroxyphenyl) retinamide prevents development of T-lymphomas in AKR/J mice. *Anticancer Res.,* **17,** 499–503.
20. Ponzoni, M., Bocca, P., Chiesa, V. *et al.* (1995). Differential effects of N-(4-hydroxyphenyl) retinamide and retinoic acid on neuroblastoma cells: apoptosis versus differentiation. *Cancer Res.,* **55** (4), 853–61.
21. Delia, D., Aiello, A., Lombardi, L. *et al.* (1993). N-(4-hydroxyphenyl) retinamide induces apoptosis of malignant hemopoietic cell lines including those unresponsive to retinoic acid. *Cancer Res.,* **53** (24), 36–41.
22. Seewaldt, V.L., Kim, J.H., Caldwell, L.E. *et al.* (1995). All-*trans*-retinoic acid mediates G1arrest but not apoptosis of normal human mammary epithelial cells. *Cell Growth Differ.,* **6** (7), 863–9.
23. Lotan, R. (1996). Retinoids in cancer chemoprevention. *FASEB J.,* **10** (9), 1031–9.
24. Sankaranarayanan, R. and Mathew, B. (1996). Retinoids as cancer-preventive agents. *IARC Sci. Publ.,* **139,** 47–59.
25. Toma, S., Isnardi, L., Raffo, P. *et al.* (1997). Effects of all-*trans*-retinoic acid and 13-*cis*-retinoic acid on breast-cancer cell lines: growth inhibition and apoptosis induction. *Int. J. Cancer,* **70** (5), 619–27.
26. Oridate, N., Lotan, D., Mitchell, M.F. *et al.* (1995). Inhibition of proliferation and induction of apoptosis in cervical carcinoma cells by retinoids: implications for chemoprevention. *J. Cell Biochem. Suppl.,* **23,** 80–6.
27. Dolivet, V., Ton Van, J., Sarini, J. *et al.* (1996) [Current knowledge on the action of retinoids in carcinoma of the head and neck]. *Rev. Laryngol. Otol. Rhinol. (Bord),* **117** (1), 19–26.
28. Kuo, S.M. (1996). Antiproliferative potency of structurally distinct dietary flavonoids on human colon cancer cells. *Cancer Lett.,* **110** (1–2), 41–8.
29. Thompson, H.J., Jiang, C., and Lu, J. (1997). Sulfone metabolite of sulindac inhibits mammary carcinogenesis. *Cancer Res.,* **57** (2), 267–71.
30. Reddy, B.S., Wang, C.X., Samaha, H. *et al.* (1997). Chemoprevention of colon carcinogenesis by dietary perillyl alcohol. *Cancer Res.,* **57** (3), 420–5.
31. Gould, M.N. (1997). Cancer chemoprevention and therapy by monoterpenes. *Environ. Health Perspect.,* **105** (Suppl.), 977–9.
32. Pascale, R.M., Simile, M.M., De Miglio, M.R. *et al.* (1995). Chemoprevention by S-adenosyl-L-methionine of rat liver carcinogenesis initiated by 1,2-dimethylhydrazine and promoted by orotic acid. *Carcinogenesis,* **16** (2), 427–30.
33. Thompson, H.J., Wilson, A., Lu, J. *et al.* (1994). Comparison of the effects of an organic and an inorganic form of selenium on a mammary carcinoma cell line. *Carcinogenesis,* **15** (2), 183–6.
34. el-Bayoumy, K., Upadhyaya, P., Chae, Y.H. *et al.* (1995). Chemoprevention of cancer by organoselenium compounds. *J. Cell Biochem. Suppl.,* **22,** 92–100.
35. Casagrande, J.T., Pike, M.C., Ross, R.K. *et al.* (1979). 'Incessant ovulation' and ovarian cancer. *Lancet,* 170–2.

36. Whittemore, A.S., Harris, R., Itnyre, J. *et al.* (1992). Characteristics relating to ovarian cancer risk: collaborative analysis of 12 US case-control studies. *Am. J. Epidemiol.,* **136,** 1212–20.

37. Bast, R.C. Jr and Berchuck, A. (1994). Ovarian cancer. Principles of internal medicine. In *Principles of internal medicine,* (ed. Harrison), pp. 1853–8.

38. Rossing, M.A., Daling, J.R., Weiss, N.S. *et al.* (1994). Ovarian tumors in a cohort of infertile women. *N. Engl. J. Med.,* **331** (12), 771–6.

39. Liang, A.P., Levenson, A.G., Layde, P.M. *et al.* (1983). Risk of breast, uterine corpus, and ovarian cancer in women receiving Medroxy-progesterone injections. *J. Am. Med. Assoc.,* **249,** 2909–12.

40. Stanford, J.L. and Thomas, D.B. (1991). Depot-medroxyprogesterone acetate (DMPA) and risk of epithelial ovarian cancer. *Int. J. Cancer,* **49,** 191–5.

41. Rodriguez, C., Call, E.E., Coates, R.J. *et al.* (1995). Estrogen replacement therapy and fatal ovarian cancer. *Am. J. Epidemiol.,* **41** (9), 828–35.

42. Wilson, J.E. (1958). Adeno-carcinomata in hens kept in a constant environment. *Poultry Sci.,* **37,** 1253.

43. Fredrickson, T.N. (1987). Ovarian tumors of the hen. *Environ. Hlth Perspect.,* **73,** 35–51.

44. Lingeman, C.H. (1974). Etiology of cancer of the human ovary: A review. *J. Natl Cancer Inst.,* **53,** 1603–18.

45. Mutch, D.G. and Williams, S. (1994). Biology of epithelial ovarian cancer. *Clin. Obstet. Gynecol.,* **37,** 406–22.

46. Etches, R.J. and Petitte, J.N. (1990). Reptilian and avian follicular hierarchies: Models for the study of ovarian development. *J. Exp. Zoo Suppl.,* **4,** 112–22.

47. Woolveridge, I. and Peddie, M.J. (1997). The inhibition of androstenedione production in mature thecal cells from the ovary of the domestic hen (*Gallus domesticus*): evidence for the involvement of progestins. *Steroids,* **62,** 214–20.

48. Dun, I.C. and Sharp, P.J. (1992). The effect of photoperiodic history on egg laying in dwarf broiler hens. In *Physiology and reproduction. Poultry Sci.,* **71,** 2090–8.

49. Johnson, A.J., Bridgham, J.T., Witty, J.P. *et al.* (1997). Expression of *bcl–2* and *nr–13* in hen ovarian follicles during development. *Biol. Repro.,* **57,** 1097–103.

50. Eguchi, Y., Ewert, D.L., and Tsujimoto, Y. (1992). Isolation and characterization of the chicken *bcl–2* gene: expression in a variety of tissues including lymphoid and neuronal organs in adult and embryo. *Nucleic Acids Res.,* **20** (16), 4187–92.

51. Mayr, B., Schaffner, G., Kurzbauer, R., Reiginger, M., and Schellander, K. (1995). Sequence of an exon of tumour suppressor p53 gene—a comparative study in domestic animals: mutation in a feline comparative study in domestic animals; mutation in a feline solid mammary carcinoma. *Br. Vet. J.,* **151** (3), 325–9.

52. Rampalli, A.M. and Zelenka, P.S. (1995). Insulin regulates expression of c-fos and c-jun and suppresses apoptosis of lens epithelial cells. *Cell Growth Differ.,* **6** (8), 945–53.

53. Qin, S., Inazu, T., Takata, M. *et al.* (1996). Cooperation of tyrosine kinase p72syk and p53/56lyn regulates calcium mobilization in chicken B cell oxidant stress signaling. *Eur. J. Biochem.,* **236** (2), 443–9.

54. Evans, D.L. and Mansel, R.E. (1995). Molecular evolution and secondary structural conservation in the B-cell lymphoma leukemia 2 (bcl–2) family of proto-oncogene products. *J. Mol. Evol.,* **41** (6), 775–83.

55. Takayama, S., Cazals-Hatem, D.L., Kitada, S. *et al.* (1994). Evolutionary conservation of function among mammalian, avian, and viral homologs of the bcl–2 oncoprotein. *DNA Cell Biol.,* **13** (7), 679–92.

56. Vilgrasa, X., Mezquita, C., Mezquita, J. *et al.* (1997). Differential expression of bcl–2 and bcl-x during chicken spermatogenesis. *Mol. Reprod. Dev.,* **47** (1), 26–9.

57. Bai, W., Rowan, B.G., Allgood, V.E. *et al.* (1997). Differential phosphorylation of chicken progesterone receptor in hormone-dependent and ligand-independent activation. *J. Biol. Chem.,* **272** (16), 10457–63.

58. Allgood, V.E., Zhang, Y., O'Malley, B.W. *et al.* (1997). Analysis of chicken progesterone receptor function and phosphorylation using an adenovirus-mediated procedure for high-efficiency DNA transfer. *Biochemistry,* **36** (1), 224–32.

59. Hodges, R.D. (1974). *The history of the fowl,* pp. 326–47. Academic Press, New York.

24. The current status of screening for ovarian cancer

Usha Menon and Ian J. Jacobs

Introduction

Ovarian cancer is the fourth most common malignancy in women in the UK, with nearly 6000 cases diagnosed each year. It is mainly a disease of older postmenopausal women. As the cancer is largely asymptomatic when confined to the ovaries, the majority of cases are diagnosed at an advanced stage. This leads to a high case fatality rate with over 4000 deaths each year.

Our ability to screen for this disease is hampered by deficiencies in our knowledge of the molecular and biological events involved in ovarian carcinogenesis. A true precursor lesion for ovarian cancer has not been identified, limiting the goal of screening to detection of asymptomatic, early stage disease based on the hypothesis that outcomes will improve if the cancer is diagnosed and treated in the early stages. Optimism is based on the results of a randomized control trial of ovarian cancer screening using a multimodal screening strategy incorporating serum CA125 and ultrasound.[1] Median survival (72.9 months) was significantly increased in women with ovarian cancer in the screened group when compared to the control group (41.8 months). The difference was not biased by lead time as survival was measured from the time of randomization rather than diagnosis. Analysis also revealed no bias between the two groups regarding ascertainment of cancers, treatment in specialist centres, and follow-up. However, it is important to note that there is to date no evidence that screening improves ovarian cancer mortality for women in any risk group. In addition, there are disadvantages associated with screening and new strategies need to be evaluated extensively prior to implementation.

Screening tests

Biochemical, morphological, vascular, and cytological tumour markers have all been explored, and it is now clear that ovarian cancer can be detected in asymptomatic women using a variety of screening tests.[2] Two distinct strategies have emerged: one ultrasound based, with transvaginal scanning as the primary test, and the other blood based, with measurement of the serum tumour marker CA125 as the primary test and ultrasound as the secondary test (multimodal screening).

Serum tumour markers

Serum CA125 is the tumour marker most extensively investigated in ovarian cancer screening. This is an antigen expressed by fetal amniotic and coelomic epithelium. In the adult, it is found in tissue derived from coelomic epithelium (mesothelial cells of the pleura, pericardium, and peritoneum) and Müllerian epithelium (tubal, endometrial, and endocervical). The surface epithelium of normal fetal and adult ovaries does not express the determinant, except in inclusion cysts, areas of metaplasia, and papillary excrescences.[3] Interest in CA125 as a screening test was triggered by the fact that over 83% of patients with epithelial ovarian cancer had CA125 levels greater than 35 U/ml.[4,5] Elevated levels were found in 50% of patients with stage I disease and more than 90% of women with more advanced stages.[6] In addition, it became apparent that CA125 could be elevated in the preclinical asymptomatic phase of the disease, as raised levels were found in 25% of 59 stored serum samples collected 5–12 years prior to the diagnosis of ovarian cancer.[7]

As is apparent from Table 24.1, the specificity and positive predictive value (PPV) of CA125 used on its own to screen for ovarian cancer is limited.[8] This has been improved markedly by a variety of developments:

1. The addition of pelvic ultrasound as a second-line test to assess ovarian volume and morphology (multimodal screening) (Table 24.1).
2. Limiting ovarian cancer screening in the general population to postmenopausal women, who are at increased risk of ovarian cancer but have a lower incidence of benign conditions associated with CA125 elevation (endometriosis, uterine fibroids) and do not undergo physiological changes such as pregnancy and menstruation that lead to false-positive elevation of CA125.[9] A CA125 greater than 30 U/ml in an asymptomatic postmenopausal woman is associated with a 36-fold increased risk of ovarian cancer in the subsequent year.[10]
3. The introduction of new CA125 immunoassays. It is now known that the CA125 antigen carries two major antigenic domains, classified as A, the domain-binding monoclonal antibody OC125, and B, a domain-binding monoclonal antibody M11. Heterologous assays (CA125II) using both mono-

clonal antibodies (M11, OC125), in place of the original homologous assay with monoclonal antibody OC125 alone, has improved the specificity of the marker for the detection of early ovarian cancer.[11]

4. A more sophisticated approach to interpretation of CA125 results. Detailed analysis of over 50 000 serum CA125 values, involving 22 000 volunteers followed up for a median of 8.6 years, in the study by Jacobs et al.[1,12] has revealed that CA125 levels in women without ovarian cancer were static or decreased with time, while preclinical levels associated with malignancy tended to rise. This allowed the formulation of separate complex change-point statistical models of the behaviour of serial preclinical CA125 levels for cases and controls. These models take into account a woman's age-related risk of ovarian cancer and her CA125 profile with time.[13,14] The ROC (risk of ovarian cancer) for an individual is calculated using a computerized algorithm based on the Bayes theorem, which compares each individual's serial CA125 levels to the pattern in cases, compared to controls. The closer the CA125 profile to the CA125 behaviour of known cases of ovarian cancer, the greater the risk of ovarian cancer. The final result is presented as the individual's estimated risk of having ovarian cancer, so that a ROC of 2% implies a risk of 1 in 50. This approach is part of the multimodal screening strategy used by Jacobs et al. in The Royal London/St. Bartholomew's pilot randomized control trial of ovarian cancer screening[15] and will be used in the United Kingdom Collaborative Trial of Ovarian Cancer Screening (UKCTOCS) (see Fig. 24.1).[16]

The sensitivity of CA125 using multimodal screening has been reported as 78.6–100% at 1 year.[12,17] Among the strategies introduced to increase sensitivity are:

1. Modifying the cut-off value for CA125. A serum CA125 of 35 U/ml, initially measured using the homologous assay and representing 1% of healthy female blood donors, is usually accepted as the upper limit of normal.[4] An upper limit of normal of 35 U/ml is an arbitrary cut-off and may not be ideal for certain populations. For example, in postmenopausal women or in patients after hysterectomy CA125 levels tend to be lower than in the general population and lower cut-offs may be more appropriate; 20 U/ml and 26 U/ml have been suggested.[18,19]

2. Use of the ROC algorithm. The increase in sensitivity in comparison to a single cut-off value of CA125 is achieved because women with normal but rising levels are identified as being at increased risk.

3. Use of other serum markers in addition to CA125, as certain tumours (e.g. mucinous cystadenocarcinomas) are less likely to be associated with elevated CA125 levels than serous cancers. Among the newly described tumour markers, plasma lysophosphatidic acid (LPA), a bioactive phospholipid with mitogenic and growth-factor-like activities, may have a potential role in ovarian cancer screening. Elevated LPA levels were detected in 9 of 10 patients with stage I ovarian cancer and all 24 patients with stage II, III, and IV ovarian cancer. In comparison, only 28 of 47 had elevated CA125 levels, including 2 of 9 patients with stage I disease.[20] Larger studies are required to clarify the role of LPA in primary screening.

Table 24.1 Prospective ovarian cancer screening studies using serum CA125 as the primary test in the general population

Ref. no.	Study	Main features	Screening strategy	No. screened	No. of invasive epithelial ovarian cancers detected	No. of positive screens	No. of positive screens/cancer detected
CA125 only							
8	Einhorn et al. 1992	Age ≥ 40 years	Serum CA125	5550	6,2 stage I	175[a]	29
Multimodal approach: CA125 (level 1 screen), then USS (level II screen)							
1	Jacobs et al. 1999	Age ≥ 45 years (median 56); postmenopausal	RCT; serum CA125; TAS/TVS, if CA125↑; 3 screens	10 958	6, 3 stage I	29	4.8
10, 12, 32	Jacobs et al. 1988, 1993, 1996	Age ≥ 45 years (median 56); postmenopausal	Serum CA125; TAS, if CA125↑	22 000	11, 4 stage I	41	3.7
17	Adonakis et al. 1996	Age ≥ 45 years (mean 58)	Serum CA125; TVS, if CA125↑	2000	1(1), 1 stage I	15	15
31	Grover et al. 1995	Age ≥ 40 years (median 51) or with family history (3%)	Serum CA125; TAS/TVS, if CA125↑	2550	1, 0 stage I	16	16
Total					19(1)	101	5.3

[a] Not all of these women underwent surgical investigation as the study design involved intensive surveillance rather than surgical intervention.

RCT, randomized controlled trial; TAS, transabdominal ultrasound; TVS, transvaginal ultrasound.

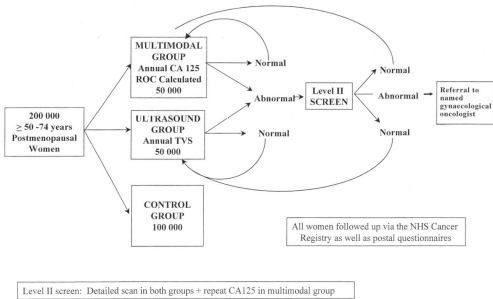

Level II screen: Detailed scan in both groups + repeat CA125 in multimodal group

Fig. 24.1 United Kingdom Collaborative Trial of Ovarian Cancer Screening (UKCTOCS).

Transvaginal ultrasound

Transvaginal ultrasonography is used in all screening strategies, either as the sole screening modality or as a secondary test in multimodal screening (Tables 24.1 and 24.2). The aim is to detect the earliest possible architectural changes in the ovary that accompany carcinogenesis. Both ovarian volume and morphology are assessed, with cut-offs for volume ranging from 10 to 20 ml, depending on menopausal status. Persistence of ultrasound features on repeat scanning 6–10 weeks following detection of abnormalities on the initial screening scan helps reduce false-positive rates. The lack of physiological changes in ovarian volume in postmenopausal women improves the specificity in this group compared to premenopausal women.

Most screening protocols use a weighted scoring system or morphological index based on ovarian volume, outline, presence of papillary projections, and cyst complexity (i.e. number of locules, wall structure, thickness of septae, and echogenicity of fluid). Based on gross anatomical changes at the time of surgery, papillary projections have the highest, and simple cysts and septal thickness the lowest, correlation with a diagnosis of ovarian malignancy.[21] As data regarding outcome accumulates with long-term follow-up of the participants of the early screening trials, it has been possible to further define the risk of ovarian cancer associated with various ultrasound findings. Postmenopausal women from the general population with an elevated serum CA125 level but normal ovarian morphology on ultrasound were found to have a cumulative risk (CR) of ovarian cancer during 6.8 years of median follow-up, of 0.15% (95% confidence interval (CI) 0.02–1.12), which was similar to that of the entire population (0.22%, 95% CI 0.18–0.30). In contrast, postmenopausal women with an elevated serum CA125 level and abnormal ovarian morphology on ultrasound had a CR of 24% (95% CI 15–37) and a significantly increased relative risk of 327 (95% CI 156–683).[22]

The use of ovarian morphology to interpret pelvic ultrasound may increase sensitivity, and use of complex ovarian morphology may increase the positive predictive value of a multimodal screening strategy.[23] Similar follow-up of participants of the largest ultrasound-based ovarian cancer screening trial has established that unilocular ovarian cysts less than 10 cm in diameter are found in 3.3% of asymptomatic postmenopausal women over 50 years of age, and are associated with a minimal risk for ovarian cancer. In contrast, complex ovarian cysts with wall abnormalities or solid areas are associated with a significant risk for malignancy.[24] Such data are invaluable in determining optimal strategies for operative intervention in screening trials.

General population screening

During the past decade, large prospective studies of screening for ovarian cancer have been performed. Tables 24.1 and 24.2 summarize the prospective ovarian cancer screening studies in the general population. It should be noted that some of the 'ovarian cancers' detected by screening in these studies are not primary invasive epithelial ovarian cancers. Mortality is unlikely to be reduced significantly by screen detection of granulosa cell or borderline epithelial tumours, which have a good prognosis regardless of screening. The data suggest that sequential multimodal screening has superior specificity and positive predictive value compared to strategies based on transvaginal ultrasound alone. For each case of ovarian cancer detected, five women underwent surgery in the multimodal studies, compared to 28 women in the studies using ultrasound alone. However, ultrasound as a first-line test may offer greater sensitivity for early stage disease, given that 20/31 (64.5%) cancers detected using ultrasound alone were stage I, compared to 8/19 (42%) cancers detected by the multimodal

Table 24.2 Prospective ovarian cancer screening studies using ultrasound as the primary test in the general population

Ref. No.	Study	Main features	Screening strategy	No. screened	No. of invasive epithelial ovarian cancers detected[a]	No. of positive screens	No. of positive screens/cancer detected
	USS only approach:						
	USS (level I screen), then repeat USS (level II screen)						
33	Pavlik et al. 2000	Age ≥ 50 years and postmenopausal or ≥ 30 years with family history	TVS; annual screens; mean 4 screens/woman	14 469	11 (6) 5 Stage I	180	16.3
34	De Priest et al. 1997						
35	van Nagell et al 1995						
36	Hayashi et al. 1999	Age ≥ 50 years	TVS	23 451	3 (3)	258	[b]
38	Tabor et al. 1994	Aged 46–65 years	TVS	435	0	9	
37	Campbell et al. 1989	Age ≥ 45 years (mean 53) or with family history (4%)	TAS; 3 screens at 18-monthly intervals	5479	2 (3); 2 stage I	326	163
39	Millo et al. 1989	Age ≥ 45 years or postmenopausal (mean 54)	USS (not specified)	500	0	11	
40	Goswamy et al. 1983	Age 39–78, postmenopausal	TAS	1084	1; 1 stage I		
	USS and CDI (level I screen)						
41	Kurjak et al. 1995	Aged 40–71 years (mean 45)	TVS and CDI	5013	4; 4 stage I	38	9.5
42	Vuento et al. 1995	Aged 56–61 years (mean 59)	TVS and CDI	1364	(1)	5	
	USS (level 1) and other test (level II screen)						
43	Parkes et al. 1994	Aged 50–64 years	TVS then CDI if TVS positive	2953	1; 1 stage I	15[c]	15
44	Holbert et al. 1994	Postmenopausal; aged 30–89 years	TVS then CA125 if TVS positive	478	1; 1 stage I	33[d]	33
45	Schingalia et al. 1994	Aged 50–69	TAS, then aspiration/biopsy	3541	2; 0 stage I	98	9.5
Total					25 (13)	873	34.9

CDI, colour Doppler imaging; RCT, randomized controlled trial; TAS, transabdominal ultrasound; TVS, transvaginal ultrasound.

[a] Primary invasive epithelial ovarian cancers. The borderline/granulosa tumours detected are shown in parentheses.

[b] Only 95 women consented to surgery and there are no follow-up details on the remaining.

[c] 86 women had abnormal USS prior to CDI.

[d] Only 11 of these women underwent surgery.

strategy. An ultrasound-based strategy may have a greater impact on ovarian cancer mortality, albeit at a higher price in terms of surgical intervention for false-positive results.

The data serve to emphasize the need for a randomized control trial that will, in addition to establishing the impact of screening on ovarian cancer mortality, also comprehensively tackle the issues of target population, compliance, health economics, and physical and psychological morbidity of screening. The UK Collaborative Trial of Ovarian Cancer Screening (UKCTOCS) jointly funded by the Medical Research Council (MRC), the Cancer Research Campaign (CRC), the Imperial Cancer Research Fund (ICRF), and the NHS Research and Development aims to achieve these objectives.[16] The three-armed randomized controlled trial due to start shortly will involve 200 000 postmenopausal women, aged 50–74 years, randomized in a 1 : 1 : 2 ratio to ultrasound screening, multimodal screening, and a control group who will not be screened. Participants will be invited from regional age/sex registers, overcoming the inherent flaws of self-referral. Screening will occur in 12 collaborating gynaecological oncology centres in the UK and participants randomized to screening will undergo six screens at annual intervals, as shown in Fig. 24.1. The small proportion of women with abnormal results will be referred for specialist surgical assessment. The primary endpoint of the study is ovarian cancer mortality at 7 years after randomization. The trial has 90% power to detect a 30% reduction in ovarian cancer mortality in the screened groups

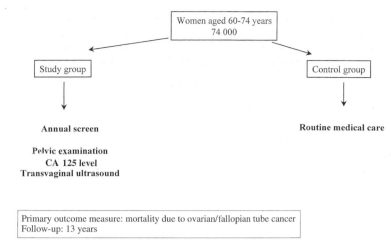

Fig. 24.2 National Cancer Institute sponsored screening trial for prostatic, lung, colorectal, and ovarian cancers (PLCO trial).

compared to the control group. Additional endpoints will include quality of life, health economics, morbidity, and compliance with screening. The performance of the two screening strategies will also be compared. The results of the trial will form the basis for an informed decision about the implementation of general population screening for ovarian cancer. The other large randomized control trial of ovarian cancer screening in the general population is the NIH PLCO study in the USA (Fig. 24.2).[25]

Screening high-risk populations

Hereditary syndromes account for approximately 5–10% of ovarian cancers. Various schemes have been suggested for stratifying women into different categories of risk for breast and ovarian by virtue of a family history, genetic predisposition, or both. A survey by Vasen *et al.*[26] of the European Familial Breast Cancer Collaborative Group found that the population designated 'high risk' for ovarian cancer by members of the group were *BRCA1* and *BRCA2* mutation carriers, members from breast/ovarian cancer families, and, in some centres, from 'breast cancer only' families with an early onset of breast cancer. These women were then offered ovarian cancer screening. Pharoah *et al.*[27] reviewed the relevance of family history in defining the target population for familial ovarian cancer screening, and has proposed the adoption of a unified management strategy in the UK. Women at significant risk of ovarian cancer defined by the eligibility criteria (Table 24.3) of the UK Familial Ovarian Cancer Screening Study,[28] should be offered screening, with central registration of all data for analysis and refinement of management protocols. Women who fall outside the proposed criteria should receive accurate and supportive information, but should not be offered screening. These women are eligible to participate in the ovarian cancer screening trials in the general population.

In 'high-risk' women, screening is frequently advocated, although the efficacy of such surveillance or other measures to reduce risk in these individuals, or even in those who carry cancer-predisposing mutations (*BRCA1* and *BRCA2* or DNA mis-

match repair gene mutations), is unknown. The results of prospective familial ovarian cancer screening trials are shown in Table 24.4. Screening can be problematic as this population often includes premenopausal women who have a higher incidence of false-positive CA125 elevations and ultrasound abnormalities. In addition, recent reports by Karlan *et al.* suggest that multifocal peritoneal serous papillary carcinoma may be a phenotypic variant of familial ovarian cancer and may be difficult to detect using current screening strategies.[29] A sample of 1261 'high-risk' women over 35 with a family history of ovarian, breast, colon, or endometrial carcinoma, or a personal history of breast cancer, underwent 6082 screens as part of a familial ovarian cancer screening programme launched in 1991. Screening with transvaginal ultrasound, colour Doppler imaging, and CA125 was initially performed biannually until 1995 and then annually. Two borderline ovarian cancers, one stage I invasive ovarian cancer and seven peritoneal serous papillary carcinoma were diagnosed. Three of the seven peritoneal cancers were undetected by screening and

Table 24.3 Eligibility criteria for UK Familial Ovarian Cancer Screening Study

An eligible woman must be over 35 years of age and a first-degree relative[a] of an affected member of an 'high-risk' family. High risk families are defined by the following criteria:

1. two or more first-degree relatives with ovarian cancer;
2. one first-degree relative with ovarian cancer, and one first-degree relative with breast cancer diagnosed under 50 years of age;
3. one first-degree relative with ovarian cancer, and two first- or second-degree[b] relatives with breast cancer diagnosed under 60 years of age;
4. an affected individual with one of the known ovarian cancer-predisposing genes;
5. three first-degree relatives with colorectal cancer, with at least one diagnosed before the age of 50 years and at least one first-degree relative with ovarian cancer.

A family history of cancer should be confirmed by histopathology report or death certification, or a documented mutation of an ovarian cancer-causing gene.

[a] A first-degree relative is mother, sister, or daughter

[b] A second-degree relative is grandmother, grand-daughter, aunt, or niece.

Table 24.4 Prospective ovarian cancer screening studies in women with a family history of ovarian or other cancer, or a personal history of breast cancer

Study	No. screened (premenopausal %)	Population	Screen positives[a] (%)	No. of invasive EOC detected (borderline tumours)	Probability of ovarian cancers at diagnostic intervention PPV (%)	Cancers in screen-negative women
TVS and CA125						
Dorum et al. 1996 (46)	180[b]	Aged >25; (mean 43);	16(8.9)	4 (3)	25	Not stated[c]
Dorum et al. 2000 (30)	803	F/H of Br/Ov cancer	Not stated	16 (4)	Not clear	Not stated
Muto et al. 1993 (47)	384 (85.4)	Aged >25; F/H of Ov cancer	15 (3.9)	0		Not stated
Menkiszak et al. 1998 (48)	124 (6 monthly)	Aged >20; F/H of Br/Ov cancer	Not available	1 (3)	Not available	Not available
TVS, CDI, and CA125						
Karlan et al. 1993, 1999 (29, 49)	1261 (75)	Aged >35; F/H of Ov, Br, Endo,	Not stated (2); 1 Stage 1 Colon cancer; P/H Br cancer	1 EOC, 3 PP		4 PP (5, 6, 15, 16 months)
Schwartz et al. 1995 (50)	247	Aged >30; F/H of Ov cancer	1 (0.4)	0		Not stated
Belinson et al. 1995 (51)	137	Aged >23 (mean 43); F/H of Ov cancer	2 (1.5)	1	50	Not stated
TVS and CDI						
Bourne et al. 1993 (52)	1000 (60)	Aged >17; (mean 47); F/H of Ov cancer	52 (5.2)	2 (1); 2 Stage 1	3.8	2 PP (2, 8 months)
	601		9 (1.5)	1 (2)	11.1	3 EOC (24–44 months)
Weiner et al. 1993 (53)	600	P/H Br cancer	12 (3)	3; 1 Stage 1	25	Not stated
Total	5157			28		

CDI, colour Doppler imaging; EOC, epithelial ovarian cancer; F/H, family history; P/H, personal history; PP, primary peritoneal cancer; PPV, positive predictive value; TVS, transvaginal ultrasound.

[a] Following positive secondary screens.

[b] Not included in total in view of a more recent update on the trial.

[c] A further 13 women underwent oophorectomy for breast cancer, two had ovarian cancer not detected by TVS.

developed as interval cancers 5, 6, and 16 months after the last screen. Annual transvaginal ultrasound and CA125 testing may also fail to detect ovarian cancer in the early stages. Sixteen ovarian cancers (15 in women > 40 years of age) including four borderline, were detected during a 5-year prospective trial (June 1992–1997) of 845 women from breast/ovarian and ovarian cancer families. Ten of the 12 invasive ovarian cancers were stage III.[30] Women in the high-risk population who request screening should be counselled about this current lack of evidence for the efficacy of both CA125 and ultrasound screening, and the associated false-positive rates. Many will still opt for screening despite understanding the risks and limitations.

Conclusion

Many aspects of ovarian cancer screening are still poorly understood, including the rate of disease progression, whether or not benign masses are a risk factor for subsequent malignant disease, and to what extent transvaginal ultrasonography and CA125 detect different cancers. New markers, such as LPA, are under development. Women in the general population should be advised to participate in large-scale ovarian cancer screening trials until definitive data on the impact of screening on ovarian cancer mortality becomes available. These include the NIH PLCO Trial in the USA and the UK Collaborative Trial of Ovarian Cancer Screening.

The latter also aims to address health economics, quality of life, and morbidity issues. Women in the high-risk population who request screening should be counselled about the current lack of evidence for the efficacy of both CA125 and ultrasound screening, and the associated false-positive rates.

Acknowledgements

U.M. was funded by a Clinical Training Fellowship Grant from the St Bartholomew's Hospital Joint Research Board.

References

1. Jacobs, I.J., Skates, S.J., Macdonald, N. *et al.* (1999). Screening for ovarian cancer: a pilot randomised controlled trial. *Lancet*, 353, 1207–10.
2. Bell, R., Petticrew, M., and Sheldon, T. (1998). The performance of screening tests for ovarian cancer: results of a systematic review. *Br. J. Obstet. Gynaecol.*, 105, 1136–47.
3. Kabawat, S.E., Bast, R.C. Jr, Bhan, A.K. *et al.* (1983). Tissue distribution of a coelomic-epithelium-related antigen recognized by the monoclonal antibody OC125. *Int. J. Gynecol. Pathol.*, 2 (3), 275–85.
4. Bast, R.C. Jr, Klug, T.L., St John, E. *et al.* (1983). A radioimmunoassay using a monoclonal antibody to monitor the course of epithelial ovarian cancer. *N. Engl. J. Med.*, 309 (15), 883–7.
5. Canney, P.A., Moore, M., Wilkinson, P.M., and James, R.D. (1984). Ovarian cancer antigen CA125: a prospective clinical assessment of its role as a tumour marker. *Br. J. Cancer*, 50 (6), 765–9.
6. Jacobs, I. and Bast, R.C. Jr (1989). The CA 125 tumour-associated antigen: a review of the literature. *Hum. Reprod.*, 4 (1), 1–12.
7. Zurawski, V.R. Jr, Orjaseter, H., Andersen, A., and Jellum, E. (1988). Elevated serum CA 125 levels prior to diagnosis of ovarian neoplasia: relevance for early detection of ovarian cancer. *Int. J. Cancer*, 42 (5), 677–80.
8. Einhorn, N., Sjovall, K., Knapp, R.C. *et al.* (1992). Prospective evaluation of serum CA 125 levels for early detection of ovarian cancer. *Obstet. Gynecol.*, 80 (1), 14–18.
9. Rosenthal, A. and Jacobs, I. (1998). Ovarian cancer screening. *Semin. Onc.*, 25 (3), 315–25.
10. Jacobs, I.J., Skates, S., Davies, A.P. *et al.* (1996). Risk of diagnosis of ovarian cancer after raised serum CA 125 concentration: a prospective cohort study. *BMJ*, 313, 1355–8.
11. Verheijen, R.H., von Mensdorff-Pouilly, S., van Kamp, G.J., and Kenemans, P. (1999). CA 125: fundamental and clinical aspects. [Review]. *Semin. Cancer Biol.*, 9, 117–24.
12. Jacobs, I., Davies, A.P., Bridges, J. *et al.* (1993). Prevalence screening for ovarian cancer in postmenopausal women by CA 125 measurement and ultrasonography. *BMJ*, 306 (6884), 1030–4.
13. Skates, S.J., Xu, F.J., Yu, Y.H. *et al.* (1995). Toward an optimal algorithm for ovarian cancer screening with longitudinal tumor markers. *Cancer*, 76, 2004–10.
14. Skates, S.J., Chang, Y., Xu, F.J. *et al.* (1996). A new statistical approach to screening for ovarian cancer. *Tumor Biol.*, 17, 45.
15. The Royal Hospitals Trust (1996). *Randomised trial of screening for ovarian cancer (protocol)*. Ovarian Cancer Screening Unit, The Royal Hospitals Trust.
16. Department of Gynaecological Oncology, St Bartholomew's and the London School of Medicine and Dentistry (2000). *UK Collaborative Trial of Ovarian Cancer Screening (protocol)*. Ovarian Cancer Screening Unit, Department of Gynaecological Oncology, St Bartholomew's and the London School of Medicine and Dentistry, London.
17. Adonakis, G.L., Paraskevaidis, E., Tsiga, S. *et al.* (1996). A combined approach for the early detection of ovarian cancer in asymptomatic women. *Eur. J. Obstet. Gynecol. Reprod. Biol.*, 65 (2), 221–5.
18. Alagoz, T., Buller, R.E., Berman, M. *et al.* (1994). What is a normal CA125 level? *Gynecol. Oncol.*, 53 (1), 93–7.
19. Bon, G.G., Kenemans, P., Verstraeten, R. *et al.* (1996). Serum tumour marker immunoassays in gynaecologic oncology: establishment of reference values. *Am. J. Obstet. Gynecol.*, 174 (1 Pt 1), 107–14.
20. Xu, Y., Shen, Z., Wiper, D.W. *et al.* (1998). Lysophosphatidic acid as a potential biomarker for ovarian and other gynecologic cancers. *JAMA*, 280, 719–23.
21. Granberg, S., Wikland, M., and Jansson, I. (1989). Macroscopic characterization of ovarian tumors and the relation to the histological diagnosis. criteria to be used for ultrasound evaluation. *Gynecol. Oncol.*, 35 (2), 139–44.
22. Menon, U., Talaat, A., Jeyarajah, A.R. *et al.* (1999). Ultrasound assessment of ovarian cancer risk in postmenopausal women with CA125 elevation. *Br. J. Cancer*, 8, 1644–7.
23. Menon, U., Talaat, A., Rosenthal, A.N. *et al.* (1999). Performance of ultrasound as a second line test to serum CA125 in ovarian cancer screening. *Br. J. Obstet. Gynaecol.*, 107 (2), 165–9.
24. Bailey, C.L., Ueland, F.R., Land, G.L. *et al.* (1998). The malignant potential of small cystic ovarian tumors in women over 50 years of age. *Gynecol. Oncol.*, 69, 3–7.
25. Kramer, B.S., Gohagan, J., Prorok, P.C., and Smart, C. (1993). A National Cancer Institute sponsored screening trial for prostatic, lung, colorectal, and ovarian cancers. *Cancer*, 71 (2 Suppl.), 589–93.
26. Vasen, H.F., Haites, N.E., Evans, D.G. *et al.* (1998). Current policies for surveillance and management in women at risk of breast and ovarian cancer: a survey among 16 European family cancer clinics. European Familial Breast Cancer Collaborative Group. *Eur. J. Cancer*, 34, 1922–6.
27. Pharoah, P.D., Stratton, J.F., and Mackay, J. (1998). Screening for breast and ovarian cancer: the relevance of family history. [Review] *Br. Med. Bull.*, 54, 823–38.
28. Department of Gynaecological Oncology, St Bartholomew's and the London School of Medicine and Dentistry (2001). *UKCCR National Familial Ovarian Cancer Screening Study (protocol)*. Ovarian Cancer Screening Unit, Department of Gynaecological Oncology, St Bartholomew's and the London School of Medicine and Dentistry, London.
29. Karlan, B.Y., Baldwin, R.L., Lopez-Luevanos, E. *et al.* (1999). Peritoneal serous papillary carcinoma, a phenotypic variant of familial ovarian cancer: implications for ovarian cancer screening. *Am. J. Obstet. Gynecol.*, 180, 917–28.
30. Dorum, A., Heimdal, K., Lovslett, K. *et al.* (1999). Prospectively detected cancer in familial breast/ovarian cancer screening. *Acta Obstet. Gynecol. Scand.*, 78 (10), 906–11.
31. Grover, S., Quinn, M.A., Weidman, P. *et al.* (1995). Screening for ovarian cancer using serum CA125 and vaginal examination: report on 2550 females. *Int. J. Gynecol. Cancer*, 5, 291–5.
32. Jacobs, I., Stabile, I., Bridges, J. *et al.* (1988). Multimodal approach to screening for ovarian cancer. *Lancet*, 1 (8580), 268–71.
33. Pavlik, E.J., Johnson II, T.L., DePriest, P.D. *et al.* (2000). Continuing participation supports ultrasound screening for ovarian cancer. *Ultrasound Obsstet. Gynecol.*, in press.
34. DePriest, P.D., Gallion, H.H., Pavlik, E.J. *et al.* (1997). Transvaginal sonography as a screening method for the detection of early ovarian cancer. *Gynecol. Oncol.*, 65 (3), 408–14.
35. Van Nagell, J.R. Jr, Gallion, H.H., Pavlik, E.J., and DePriest, P.D. (1995). Ovarian cancer screening. *Cancer (Suppl.)*, 76, 2086–91.
36. Hayashi, H., Yaginuma, Y., Kitamura, S. *et al.* (1999). Bilateral oophorectomy in asymptomatic women over 50 years old selected by ovarian cancer screening. *Gynecol. Obstet. Invest.*, 47 (1), 58–64.
37. Campbell, S., Bhan, V., Royston, P. *et al.* (1989). Transabdominal ultrasound screening for early ovarian cancer. *BMJ*, 299, 1363–7.

38. Tabor, A., Jensen, F.R., Bock, J.E., and Hogdall, C.K. (1994). Feasibility study of a randomised trial of ovarian cancer screening. *J. Med. Screen.*, 1 (4), 215–19.

39. Millo, R., Facca, M.C., and Alberico, S. (1989). Sonographic evaluation of ovarian volume in postmenopausal women: a screening test for ovarian cancer? *Clin. Exp. Obstet. Gynecol.*, 16 (2–3), 72–8.

40. Goswamy, R.K., Campbell, S., and Whitehead, M.I. (1983). Screening for ovarian cancer. *Clin. Obstet. Gynaecol.*, 10, 621–43.

41. Kurjak, A., Shalan, H., Kupesic, S. *et al.* (1994). An attempt to screen asymptomatic women for ovarian and endometrial cancer with transvaginal color and pulsed Doppler sonography. *J. Ultrasound Med.*, 13 (4), 295–301.

42. Vuento, M.H., Pirhonen, J.P., Makinen, J.I. *et al.* (1995). Evaluation of ovarian findings in asymptomatic postmenopausal women with color Doppler ultrasound. *Cancer*, 76 (7), 1214–18.

43. Parkes, C.A., Smith, D., Wald, N.J., and Bourne, T.H. (1994). Feasibility study of a randomised trial of ovarian cancer screening among the general population. *J. Med. Screen.*, 1 (4), 209–14.

44. Holbert, T.R. (1994). Screening transvaginal ultrasonography of postmenopausal women in a private office setting. *Am. J. Obstet. Gynecol.*, 170 (6), 1699–703.

45. Schingalia, P., Brondelli, L., Cicognani, A. *et al.* (1994). A feasibility study of ovarian cancer screening: does fine-needle aspiration improve ultrasound specificity? *Tumori*, 80, 181–7.

46. Dorum, A., Kristensen, G.B., Abeler, V.M. *et al.* (1996). Early detection of familial ovarian cancer. *Eur. J. Cancer*, 32A (10), 1645–51.

47. Muto, M.G., Cramer, D.W., Brown, D.L. *et al.* (1993). Screening for ovarian cancer: the preliminary experience of a familial ovarian cancer center. *Gynecol. Oncol.*, 51 (1), 12–20.

48. Menkiszak, J., Jakubowska, A., Gronwald, J., Rzepka-Gorska, I., and Lubinski, J. (1998). Hereditary ovarian cancer: summary of 5 years of experience [in Polish]. *Ginekol. Pol.*, 69 (5), 283–7.

49. Karlan, B.Y., Raffel, L.J., Crvenkovic, G. *et al.* (1993). A multidisciplinary approach to the early detection of ovarian carcinoma: rationale, protocol design, and early results. *Am. J. Obstet. Gynecol.*, 169 (3), 494–501.

50. Schwartz, P.E., Chambers, J.T., and Taylor, K.J. (1995). Early detection and screening for ovarian cancer. *J. Cell. Biochem.*, 23, 233–7.

51. Belinson, J.L., Okin, C., Casey, G. *et al.* (1995). The familial ovarian cancer registry: progress report. *Cleve. Clin. J. Med.*, 62 (2), 129–34.

52. Bourne, T.H., Campbell, S., Reynolds, K.M. *et al.* (1993). Screening for early familial ovarian cancer with transvaginal ultrasonography and colour blood flow imaging. *BMJ*, 306 (6884), 1025–9.

53. Weiner, Z., Beck, D., Shteiner, M. *et al.* (1993). Screening for ovarian cancer in women with breast cancer with transvaginal sonography and color flow imaging. *J. Ultrasound Med.*, 12 (7), 387–93.

25. Optimizing the use of ultrasonography in ovarian cancer screening

Paul DePriest

Introduction

Ovarian cancer continues to be the leading cause of gynecologic cancer death in the United States. It is estimated that 25 400 new cases of ovarian cancer were diagnosed in 1998, and that 14 500 women died of disease in that same year.[1]

Since 1960, there has been only moderate improvement in the overall survival of patients with ovarian cancer. Women continue to present with advanced disease where survival is limited despite radical surgical debulking and aggressive chemotherapy. Landis and colleagues, for example, reported in 1998 that only 25% of women with ovarian cancer presented with localized ovarian cancer.[1] Survival rates are directly related to stage at detection.[1] The 5-year survival of women with localized ovarian cancer is 93% compared to only 25% in patients with advanced-stage disease.

If ovarian cancer could be diagnosed in an early stage, it is logical that survival rates should increase. Many investigators[2–7] have studied this hypothesis. Utilizing serum markers and ultrasonography as early detection methods, physician scientists have attempted to screen populations of women for ovarian cancer. Preliminary results of these screening trials have shown that ovarian cancer can be detected at an early stage. However, there are lingering concerns regarding the costs and accuracy of such methods. The following is a review of the use of ultrasonography as an early detection method for ovarian cancer. The discussion will primarily address techniques of optimizing the accuracy of sonography in screening for ovarian carcinoma.

Ultrasound for ovarian cancer screening

Campbell, in 1989, reported the use of transabdominal ultrasound (TAS) for the early identification of ovarian cancer.[4] In this study, 5479 asymptomatic women underwent screening. Five cases of ovarian cancer were detected, and all were stage I lesions. It appeared that TAS was useful in detecting ovarian cancer; however, there were several concerns about this strategy. Women undergoing abdominal ultrasound screening had to have a full bladder. This added to the time needed to screen patients. Additionally, utilization of the abdominal probe yielded relatively low-resolution images. These lower-resolution images are less likely to differentiate benign from malignant masses.

In 1987, a transvaginal sonographic screening (TVS) program was begun at the University of Kentucky. TVS was chosen because this technique eliminated the need for a full bladder and allowed high-resolution imaging. Subsequently, over 14 000 women have been screened in the Kentucky TVS screening trial. In this project, TVS is performed using a standard ultrasound unit with a 5.0 MHz vaginal transducer. The test is usually painless and best performed with the bladder empty. A complete screening examination can be performed in 5–10 minutes. A permanent hard copy of each sonogram is generated for inclusion in the patient record. Each ovary is measured in three dimensions, and ovarian volume is calculated using the prolate ellipsoid formula:

$$\text{volume} = L \times H \times W \times 0.523.$$

An ovarian volume of 20 cm^3 or greater in premenopausal women and of 10 cm^3 or greater in postmenopausal women is considered abnormal. These values are two standard deviations (SD) above published values for normal ovarian volume in premenopausal and postmenopausal women.[8] In addition, any internal papillary projection from the tumor wall is considered abnormal. The screening algorithm used at the University of Kentucky is illustrated in Fig. 25.1. A woman with an abnormal screen is scheduled to have a repeat sonogram in 6–8 weeks. If the repeat examination is abnormal, she undergoes a pelvic examination, color Doppler assessment of tumor blood flow, a serum CA–125 determination, and morphologic indexing of the tumor. Operative removal of the tumor is then recommended. The surgery is performed by laparoscopy or laparotomy.

Using this algorithm, screening results on 8500 asymptomatic women were reported by van Nagell and colleagues.[9] One hundred and twenty-one women (1.4%) had a persisting abnormality on TVS and underwent surgical tumor removal. Eight patients had ovarian cancer, and 57 had serous cystadenomas. Six of the patients with ovarian cancer had stage I disease, one patient had stage IIC disease, and one patient had stage IIIB cancer. Only one of these patients had palpable ovarian enlargement on clini-

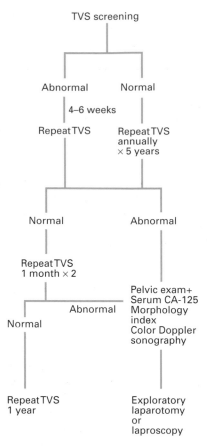

Fig. 25.1 Transvaginal sonography screening algorithm. *, Abnormal volume: ovarian volume > 10 cm³, postemenopausal; or abnormal morphology: papillary projection into a cystic ovarian tumor.

Table 25.1 Macroscopic characterization of ovarian tumors related to histopathology

Macroscopic characteristics	Malignant (number of women)	Total
Unilocular	1 (0.3%)	296
Unilocular-solid	4 (2%)	203
Multilocular	20 (8%)	229
Multilocular-solid	147 (36%)	209
Solid	31 (39%)	80
Total	203	1017

cal examination, and only one patient had an elevated serum CA125. There were 8379 women with normal screens. One patient with a family history of ovarian cancer was noted to have ovarian cancer at prophylactic oophorectomy 11 months after a normal screen (false-negative result). This patient is alive and well 3 years after surgery and chemotherapy. There were approximately 20 000 patient screening years in this trial and no deaths from primary ovarian cancer in the screened population. The authors concluded that TVS could detect early ovarian cancer. Furthermore, the authors conclude that while TVS could detect ovarian cancer, there was a low positive predictive value (PPV) (7%). This large ongoing ultrasound screening trial has provided a great deal of experience with sonographic ovarian evaluation. Ultrasound screening is most successful in postmenopausal women in which there is little functional fluctuation of ovarian size.

The difficulty with the use of TVS for ovarian cancer screening has been its lack of positive predictive value. While the sensitivity of this test is acceptable (>85%), its specificity (98.7%) and positive predictive value (7%) are too low.[10] The reason for the low positive predictive value is the utilization of rather simplistic abnormality criteria. As noted above, in the Kentucky trial, ovarian volume and the presence of a papillary projection from the wall of an ovarian tumor were the only criteria which mandated surgery. If more stringent criteria were used, a much higher positive predictive value could be obtained.

In an attempt to increase the positive predictive value of ovarian ultrasound, investigators have developed scoring systems which quantitate gray-scale sonographic characteristics. In 1989, Granberg et al. reported the ovarian macroscopic characteristics of 1017 women who underwent surgery for a pelvic mass.[11] Ovarian tumors were classified macroscopically and sonographically as unilocular (296), unilocular with a solid component (203), multilocular (229), multilocular with a solid component (209), or predominately solid (80). The corresponding rates of malignancy are shown in Table 25.1.

Small, unilocular, smooth-walled tumors were associated with a very low risk of malignancy. Granberg and coworkers, in 1990, reported on 180 women undergoing surgery for a pelvic mass who were evaluated with vaginal sonography preoperatively.[12] Vaginal sonographic findings correlated well with the macroscopic findings at the time of surgery (96%). The authors found that except in unilocular tumors, the ovarian volume correlated with the risk of malignancy. Furthermore, the presence of a papillary projection was indicative of cancer.

Sassone and colleagues subsequently published a discrete scoring index for use with vaginal sonography.[13] The scoring system was developed to aid in differentiating benign from malignant ovarian masses. The authors studied TVS images of 143 patients who underwent surgery for an ovarian mass. The morphology characteristics analyzed in this study were inner-wall characteristics, wall thickness, septation, and echogenicity. Each morphologic component could receive a score between 1 and 5. The component scores were tallied and a total ultrasound score awarded for each tumor. Using a total score of 9 or more as indicative of ovarian malignancy, the authors reported a sensitivity of 100%, a specificity of 83%, and a positive predicitive value of 37%.

In 1993 and 1994, the Kentucky Group published two reports on a morphology index used to quantitate sonographic images.[14,15] The first study evaluated a morphology indexing system which was composed of three morphologic component scores: ovarian volume, wall structure, and septal structure (Fig. 25.2).

The component scores were added to yield a total morphology index score (MI). Using a cutoff score of 5 or more, all ovarian cancers could be identified. The overall positive predictive value

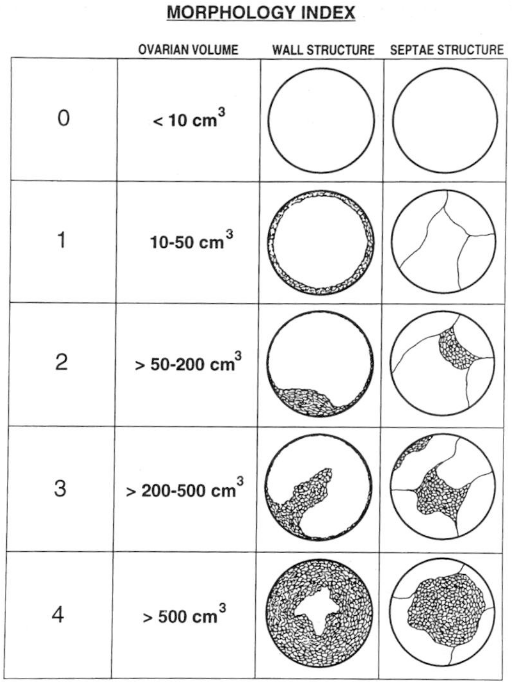

MORPHOLOGY INDEX

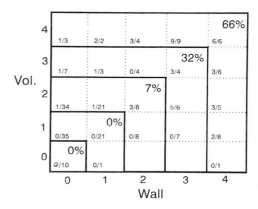

Fig. 25.2 Morphology Index to quantitate transparant ultrasound images of the ovary (14,15)

Table 25.2 Statistical performance of the morphology index scores using a value ≥ 5 indicative of malignancy

Test	
Sensitivity	0.89
Specificity	0.73
Positive predictive value	0.46
Negative predictive value	0.96

was 32%. When only postmenopausal women were analyzed, the PPV rate was 45%.

A multi-institutional trial was then performed to evaluate the performance of the morphology index.[15] Two hundred and thirteen patients who had preoperative sonograms were evaluated. Morphology index scores were assigned after thorough evaluation of each sonogram. The MI score for 169 benign ovarian tumors was 3.3 ± 1.8 as compared to a score of 7.3 ± 1.9 in ovarian malignancies. The statistical performance of the MI score may be seen in Table 25.2. A univariate analysis showed that both ovarian volume and wall structure score correlated directly to risk of malignancy. Using these two variables, a nomogram was constructed which defined four discrete risk zones for malignancy (Fig. 25.3). In this nomogram, risk of malignancy varied from 0% in zone 1 to 66% in zone 4.

In 1994, Lerner and colleagues[16] published a revised system for ovarian morphology scoring based on the original morphology index reported by Sassone et al.[13] Using a multilogistic regression analysis, the authors simplified the scoring system to include wall structure (0, 2, 3), shadowing (0, 1), septa (0, 1), and echogenicity (0, 3). Three hundred and twelve patients were evaluated. The revised system yielded a sensitivity of 96.8%, specificity 0.77%, positive predictive value 29.4%, and a negative predictive value of 99.4%. The advantages of the new system were ease of application and less interobserver variation.

Finally, Ferrazzi and colleagues[17] in 1997 presented a scoring index and compared it to those described previously.[10] This system employed component scores for wall structure, septations, vegetations, and echogenicity. The diagnostic accuracy of the five scoring systems was tested by application to sonograms performed on 330 women with ovarian neoplasms. Two hundred and seventy-one masses were benign and 69 were malignant. The statistical performance of the five scoring systems is presented in Table 25.3.

The authors concluded that the new system performed better than existing indices. However, all morphology index systems had high and similar diagnostic accuracy in differentiating benign from malignant ovarian neoplasms (50–70%).

The five morphology indexes presented above utilize one sonographic examination performed at a point in time. This method of evaluation does not exploit the fact that a predominant difference between cancer and normal tissue is the relative rate of increase of tissue mass.

Skates and colleagues were the first to employ this concept with tumor markers.[18] The authors retrospectively analyzed serial CA125 levels in a screening population. These authors found that not only was the initial serum marker value predictive of malignancy, but the relative rate of increase in serum marker concentration was also important. It is possible that the rate of change of

Fig. 25.3 Nomogram of risk of malignancy based upon ovarian volume and cyst wall structure on trans????? Ultrasound (15)

Table 25.3 Statistical performance of morphology scoring systems in tumors ≤ 5 cm

Authors	Sensitivity	Specificity	PPV	Accuracy (tumor ≤ 5 cm)
DePriest	88	40	28	52
Ferrazzi	87	67	41	69
Lerner	87	59	36	63
Granberg	87	49	31	53
Sassone	74	65	36	63

tissue mass (volume, wall structure) may help differentiate benign from malignant lesions sonographically.

Using this concept, Ueland and colleagues evaluated the change of sonographic morphology scores over time in early ovarian cancer versus benign lesions.[19] Ovarian masses were identified sonographically in the Kentucky screening program. Masses were evaluated for ovarian volume, wall structure, and septal structure at least twice at 6-week intervals. The slopes of ovarian volume measurements were calculated. The rate of increase in volume in ovarian cancer was 1.42 versus 1.00 in benign ovarian lesions ($P = 0.06$). While this difference did not reach statistical significance, this trend is even more hopeful since most of the cancers were stage I. Future analysis of the morphology index will focus on this dynamic characteristic of ovarian tumors.

While sonographic morphology indexing can increase the positive predictive value of ultrasound, several caveats must be considered. First, vaginal and abdominal ovarian sonography are more accurate in postmenopausal women. In this group of patients, there is less functional ovarian enlargement. Also, in postmenopausal women, there is a lower rate of teratomas, endometriomas, and inflammatory lesions, which are difficult to sonographically differentiate from malignant lesions. Secondly, most of the ultrasound morphology studies evaluated patients who presented with symptoms which led to the diagnosis of a mass. In screening studies, the ovarian lesions are usually smaller and ovarian cancers more likely to be early stage.[4-7] Therefore, the performance of the morphology scoring systems could be negatively affected, particularly if the sensitivity is low. Thirdly, ovarian cancer prevalence is highest in women over 50 years of age. Therefore, each of the indices should perform optimally when the population screened has a higher prevalence of disease.

Considering these caveats, ultrasound screening should be limited to postmenopausal women, or to women at a significantly higher risk than the background population (i.e. family history). Also, sensitive morphologic scoring systems which accurately differentiate benign from malignant lesions should be employed.

Changing technology will help optimize sonographic screening for ovarian cancer. For example, three-dimensional imaging will aid in a more accurate evaluation of ovarian architecture. However, this technology must be inexpensive and portable, and results must be reproducible, if it is to positively impact screening. The use of serum marker determinations and color Doppler evaluations as second-line studies could aid in ultrasound screening.[20,21] However, any second-line study must be highly sensitive so that ovarian cancers will not be overlooked.

In conclusion, optimization of ultrasound for ovarian cancer screening can be achieved by focusing on higher-risk populations (postmenopausal, positive family history), utilizing morphology scoring systems and recognition of the dynamic nature of ovarian lesions. Further improvement in ultrasound screening accuracy may be realized with advances in technology (three-dimensional, color Doppler) and the addition of tumor marker analysis.

References

1. Landis, S.H., Murray, T., Bolden, S. *et al.* (1998). Cancer statistics, 1998. *CA*, **48**, 6–29.
2. Jacobs, I., Davies, A.P., Bridges, J. *et al.* (1993). Prevalence screening for ovarian cancer in postmenopausal women by CA 125 measurement and ultrasonography. *Br. Med. J.*, **306**, 1030–4.
3. Einhorn, N., Sjovall, K., Knapp, R.C. *et al.* (1992). Prospective evaluation of serum CA 125 levels for early detection of ovarian cancer. *Obstet. Gynecol.*, **80**, 14–18.
4. Campbell, S., Bhan, V., Royston, P. *et al.* (1989). Transabdominal ultrasound screening for early ovarian cancer. *Br. Med. J.*, **299**, 1363–7.
5. DePriest, P.D., van Nagell, J.R., Gallion, H.H. *et al.* (1993). Ovarian cancer screening in asymptomatic postmenopausal women. *Gynecol. Oncol.*, **51**, 205–9.
6. Bourne, T.H., Campbell, S., Reynolds, K.M. *et al.* (1993). Screening for early familial ovarian cancer with transvaginal ultrasonography and colour blood flow imaging. *Br. Med. J.*, **306**, 1025–9.
7. van Nagell, J.R. and DePriest, P.D. (1998). Screening for epithelial ovarian cancer. In *Controversies in the management of ovarian cancer*, (ed. D.M. Gershenson and W.P. McGuire). Churchill Livingstone, New York.
8. Goswamy, R.K., Campbell, S., and Whitehead, M.I. (1983). Screening for ovarian cancer. *Clin. Obstet. Gynecol.*, **10**, 621–43.
9. van Nagell, J.R., Gallion, H.H., Pavlik, E.J. *et al.* (1995). Ovarian cancer screening. *Cancer*, **76**, 2086–91.
10. DePriest, P.D., Gallion, H.H., Pavlik, E.J. *et al.* (1997). Transvaginal sonography as a screening method for the detection of early ovarian cancer. *Gynecol. Oncol.*, **65**, 408–14.
11. Granberg, S., Wikland, M., and Jansson, I. (1989). Macroscopic characterization of ovarian tumors and the relation to the histological diagnosis: criteria to be used for ultrasound evaluation. *Gynecol. Oncol.*, **35**, 139–44.
12. Granberg, S., Norstrom, A., and Wikland, M. (1990). Tumors in the lower pelvis as imaged by vaginal sonography. *Gynecol. Oncol.*, **37**, 224–9.
13. Sassone, A.M., Timor-Tritsch, I., Artner, A. *et al.* (1991). Transvaginal sonographic characterization of ovarian disease: evaluation of a new scoring system to predict ovarian malignancy. *Obstet. Gynecol.*, **78**, 70–6.
14. DePriest, P.D., Shenson, D., Fried, A. *et al.* (1993). A morphology index based on sonographic findings in ovarian cancer. *Gynecol. Oncol.*, **51**, 7–11.
15. DePriest, P.D., Varner, E., Powell, J. *et al.* (1994). The efficacy of a sonographic morphology index in identifying ovarian cancer: a multi-institutional investigation. *Gynecol. Oncol.*, **55**, 174–8.
16. Lerner, J.P., Timor-Tritsch, I.E., Federman, A. *et al.* (1994). Transvaginal ultrasonographic characterization of ovarian masses with an improved, weighted scoring system. *Am. J. Obstet. Gynecol.*, **170**, 81–5.
17. Ferrazi, E., Zanetta, G., Dordoni, D. *et al.* (1997). Transvaginal ultrasonographic characterization of ovarian masses: comparison of five scoring systems in a multicenter study. *Ultrasound Obstet. Gynecol.*, **10**, 192–7.
18. Skates, S.J., Feng-Ji X., Yin-Hua, Y. *et al.* (1995). Towards an optimal algorithm for ovarian cancer screening with longitudinal tumour markers. *Cancer*, **76**, 2004–10.
19. Ueland, F., DePriest, P.D., DeSimone, C.P. *et al.* (1999). An analysis of a morphology index in predicting ovarian cancer with transvaginal sonography. *Gynecol. Oncol.*, **72**, 514.
20. Fleischer, A.C., Rodgers, W.H., Kepple, D.M. *et al.* (1993). Color Doppler sonography of ovarian masses: a multiparameter analysis. *J. Ultrasound Med.*, **12**, 41–8.
21. Davies, A.P., Jacobs, I., Woolas, R. *et al.* (1993). The adnexal mass: benign or malignant? Evaluation of a risk of malignancy index. *Br. J. Obstet. Gynecol.*, **100**, 927–31.

26. Doppler ultrasound derived indices in screening and diagnosis of ovarian cancer

Kenneth J. W. Taylor and Andrea Lundell

Introduction

An occasional conference such as the Helene Harris Memorial Trust Fora allows a timely opportunity to gauge the progress in the fight against ovarian cancer. In the past decade remarkable advances have been made. The availability of CA125 as a tumor marker for epithelial ovarian cancer has allowed the earlier detection of recurrence and has also helped to increase or decrease suspicion of malignancy when a pelvic mass is discovered on physical examination.[1]

Unfortunately, there remain some limitations for CA125 in large-scale screening studies since, when applied to a large population of apparently normal women in whom the prevalence of ovarian cancer is low, many false positives are found. Einhorn *et al.*[2] tested 5550 healthy Swedish women for CA125 levels above 30 μg/ml. One hundred and seventy-five women tested positive, of whom only six proved to have ovarian cancer (false-positive rate 96.6%). Three other women proved to have ovarian cancer despite normal CA125 levels. False positives are most commonly due to common gynecological disorders, including fibroids, endometriosis, or ovarian cysts, as well as liver disease and pregnancy.

A major limitation for the use of CA125 is the fact that it may remain at normal levels in 23–50% of patients with early ovarian cancer, so that sensitivity as well as specificity is limited for large-scale screening.[3] Nevertheless, it has been used successfully by Jacobs *et al.*,[4] and has indeed resulted in the detection of early ovarian cancers.

In clinical practice, it is found that the pattern of elevation of CA125 levels may be more important than the absolute level. In chronic conditions such as endometriosis or fibroids, levels commonly oscillate between 40 and 80 μg/ml, whereas a rapidly escalating level is strongly indicative of a progressive malignancy.

The other remarkable advance is the development of endovaginal transducers utilizing high-frequency ultrasound (EVUS), typically in the range of 5–9 MHz. Such broad-band transducers are important for producing the superb resolution that has become the general standard in practice. Not only do these devices produce first-rate gray-scale images of the ovaries but, in addition, they provide dramatic scans of pelvic vascularity, together with the ability to sample the waveform from any blood vessel in any organ within the imaged field. By the mid–1980s, we had documented the cyclic flow associated with ovulation and described luteal flow as having a resistive index (RI) of 0.52 + 0.1.[5] In later work, we defined the flow associated with the developing placenta. This flow was important since it allowed us to recognize the gestational process, even if it were sonographically abnormal and even if it were extrauterine. The methodology therefore became important in the diagnosis of ectopic pregnancy.[6]

It was the recognition of neovascularity that allowed definition of functional ovarian flow and that of placentation. The importance of neovascularity was first recognized by Judah Folkman in 1971.[7] Realizing the limitations of diffusion, Folkman proposed that the neovascularity that supplied tumors was produced by the host in response to angiogenic factors secreted by the tumor. The definition and delineation of this vascularity, as an aid in the diagnosis of tumors, has been used widely in angiography, and similar attempts have been made using color flow ultrasound with pulse Doppler. We have described neovascularity in a variety of tumors, including liver, kidney, breast, and ovary.[8–10]

In an analysis of tumor flow in a variety of tumors, we found that 80% of tumors showed very high velocities, with or without high diastolic velocities. Such high velocities correlated well with the presence of arteriovenous fistulae, which are well recognized angiographic features of many tumors.[8] In approximately 20% of tumors, tumor flow was characterized by very low resistance. This correlated histologically with the presence of sinusoidal tumor spaces with little or no media to the tumor blood vessels and, on angiography, contrast medium became trapped in these areas, giving rise to prolonged staining.[8]

It was shortly after the publication of these papers that Kurjak *et al.*[11] published a startling finding that an RI of 0.4 provided an almost complete separation between benign and malignant in a very large group of ovarian tumors.[11] Of 56 malignant ovarian masses, they reported that 54 had an RI of 0.4 or less. Of 624 benign masses, 623 had an RI greater than 0.4. This provided a positive predictive value of 98.2%, a negative predictive value of

99.7%, a sensitivity of 96.4%, a specificity of 99.8%, and an accuracy of 99.5%. Clearly, such dramatic results required further investigation and confirmation. An account of our investigations into the efficacy of RIs and velocity criteria, both for differentiating the nature of a known ovarian mass and in screening for early ovarian cancer, is reported here.

Screening at Yale

The Yale screening clinic for the early detection of ovarian cancer commenced in 1990 and it has continually recruited women who have at least one first-degree relative with a history of ovarian cancer.[12] To date, 252 women have been screened, with follow-up by repeat ultrasound scanning, a mail survey to the participants, and by reference to the Connecticut Tumor Registry. The protocol was approved by the Human Investigation Committee at Yale University.

After recruitment, patients are interviewed by a medical social worker, who takes their personal history, their family history, and their medical history. They are then seen by an oncologic gynecologist. The patient then undergoes bimanual and rectal examination and if this is normal, ultrasound examination is deferred for 3 months. If a mass is found on this initial examination, immediate referral for an endovaginal ultrasound is made. At this stage, blood is taken for CA125 and a number of other experimental tumor markers, including lipid-associated sialic acid (LSA), NB/70K, and urinary gonatropin fragment (UGF).

During the first year, physical examination is performed twice, and alternating with these examinations two endovaginal ultrasound exams are performed. In the second and subsequent years, there is one pelvic examination, which is alternated with an endovaginal ultrasound examination.

The endovaginal examinations are performed in the Department of Diagnostic Imaging and utilize the ATL (Advanced Technology Laboratory, Bothell, Washington, USA) HDI, the 3000 and 5000 using a 9–5 MHz endovaginal transducer. This not only produces high-quality gray-scale ultrasound but also provides color-flow imaging and pulse Doppler. The woman is invited to insert the probe herself.

The examination consists of viewing the uterus, noting the size, the thickness of the endometrium, and the presence of any fibroid, Nabothian cysts, or other pathology such as adenomyosis. The adnexa are then examined and the size of the ovaries measured. An ovarian volume is calculated assuming that the ovary is a prolate ellipse, and the upper volume for a normal premenopausal ovary is taken to be 18 ml. The upper limit for the volume of a postmenopausal ovary has been quoted as 10 ml, but in our observations 6 ml is the upper limit and this was used in these studies.

The presence of any cysts is noted and the cysts are measured. Any enlargement of the ovaries is noted and any mass described in terms of size and consistency. Color flow is then utilized to look for vascularity within the ovary. Every attempt is made to examine women within the first 8 days of their menstrual cycle to decrease the possibility of luteal flow, but residual luteal flow is not unusual.

Ovarian flow must be carefully differentiated from uterine flow, which is seen medial to the ovary from the region of the cornuum. Uterine flow demonstrates a diastolic notch, whereas ovarian flow does not. In the past literature, uterine arterial flow from the region of the cornuum has frequently been stated to be 'normal ovarian' flow. In the areas of displayed color flow, pulse Doppler is then utilized to calculate the maximum peak systolic velocity and the minimum resistive index (RI) is calculated. These two values are noted for subsequent analysis. The same procedure is repeated in the other adnexus.

We have data on 201 premenopausal women, with a mean age of 42 + 5.4 years and a range of 27–56 years. Of all ovaries present, 97% were imaged. Thirty-three cysts larger than 3 cm were present. Of these 33 cysts, 19 resolved spontaneously (56.7%). The size of these cysts ranged up to 10.9 cm and the mean diameter was 4.75 ± 2 cm. Doppler-detected flow was found in 77.5% of these ovaries and peak systolic velocities ranged from 0.4 to 98 cm/s, with a mean of 12 ± 8.36 cm/s. The resistive indices showed a mean of 0.61 ± 0.16 and demonstrated a range of 0.26–1.

Gynecological surgery was carried out on 13 of these premenopausal patients, two of which were prompted by our results. One of these was a solid adnexal mass with high velocities, which proved to be a pedunculated fibroid. This false positive occurred earlier in our experience and subsequently we have diagnosed many other similar cases successfully. It is important to compare the texture of the mass with the texture of the myometrium and, in addition, to look for the vascular pedicle connecting the pedunculated fibroid to the body of the uterus. If there is still uncertainty, patients should undergo magnetic resonance imaging (MRI) before surgery is considered.

A further false-positive result was due to a misinterpretation by a junior attending physician. A partially solid and cystic mass was seen with peak systolic velocities of 28 cm/s and an RI of 0.4, and was assumed to be cancer. On hearing of this finding, the patient went to a New York cancer institution to have it removed, where it proved to be a hemorrhagic corpus luteal cyst. Such hemorrhagic cysts may persist for weeks, or even months, and be seen in the succeeding cycle.

Fifty-six postmenopausal women, with an age range of 45–88 years and a mean age of 61 ± 8.2 years, were studied. The visualization rate of their ovaries was 85.4%.

Detectable flow was noted in 62% of the ovaries visualized. Peak systolic velocities of 1.4–33 cm/s, with a mean value of 7.9 ± 4.8 cm/s, were detected. The mean resistive index was 0.76 ± 0.2 with a range of 0.3–1. These low RIs were associated with peak systolic velocities of less than 10 cm/s.

There were 12 cysts larger than 1.5 cm, with a range from 1. 9 to 10.9 cm. Four of these cysts resolved spontaneously and three were removed surgically. In total, there were eight cases involving gynecological surgery, of which only one was stimulated by our study. A thickened endometrium was seen by EVUS and at surgery; this proved to be a carcinoma of the endometrium. These data are limited since no ovarian cancers were detected but one colon cancer and one renal cell cancer were detected.

For the purpose of this chapter, it is important to note that the value of Doppler was very limited in this screening study.

Diagnosis of the normality of an ovary was based on its size and sonographic appearance. If any vascularity were demonstrated, this did not contribute to our diagnosis. Indeed, in the presence of a sonographically normal ovary, the Doppler findings were ignored, since they were at the best, superfluous, and at the worst, misleading. In the two false positives, the presence of high velocities and low impedance as determined by Doppler encouraged us to make a false-positive diagnosis. In the diagnosis that was made of an endometrial cancer, the abnormality was a sonographic finding of a thickened endometrium, and the presence of any Doppler signals did not influence that diagnosis. Although low impedance signals have been documented in carcinoma of the endometrium, we have also seen them in endometrial hyperplasia and endometritis.[13]

It may therefore be concluded that color flow and Doppler are of little or no proven value in screening for ovarian cancer.

The value of Doppler indices in the evaluation of adnexal masses in premenopausal women

The population of premenopausal patients in this study was scanned at Yale for a 3.7-year period and comprised 114 premenopausal and perimenopausal women, with a mean age of 40 ± 9 years and a range of 9–55 years. The peak systolic velocity (PSV) for benign masses in this population was 20.37 ± 13.93 cm/s, with a range of 4.3–71.2 cm/s (Fig. 26.1). The mean PSV for malignant ovarian masses was 23.24 ± 17.11 cm/s, with a range of 5–60 cm/s. These PSVs are not statistically significantly different ($P < 0.40$). Thus, in the premenopausal population PSV cannot be used to distinguish between benign and malignant ovarian pathology.

Examination of the RI values demonstrated a similar trend. In the premenopausal group of women, the average RI of benign

masses was 0.59 ± 0.16, with a range of 0.21–1. For malignant ovarian masses, the mean RI was 0.54 ± 0.1 with a range of 0.4–0.71. These two populations are not statistically different ($P < 0.1$). Receiver operator characteristic (ROC) curves were generated to provide cutoff values in the premenopausal population. The optimum PSV was 25 cm/s, which only had a 55.6% sensitivity and a 72% specificity. ROC evaluation also provided an RI value of 0.5, which gave a sensitivity of 55.6% and a specificity of 69%. Both these performances are too poor to be used for diagnostic purposes.

The value of Doppler indices in the evaluation of adnexal masses in postmenopausal women

The similarity between tumor blood flow and that found in the functioning corpus luteum suggests that there will be much more overlap between hemorrhagic corpus luteal cysts and tumors seen in the premenopausal population than will occur in the postmenopausal population. One might therefore predict that color flow and pulse Doppler will be of greater value in postmenopausal women than in premenopausal women.

To test this hypothesis, we can use available data on a cohort of women seen by one of the authors (K.T.) between 1992 and 1998, for each of which there is a tissue diagnosis. This cohort of women was chosen because the author included prospectively the highest peak systolic velocity and the lowest resistance within any mass visualized in the report, the results of which are now available for review and analysis.

The cohort of women with proven malignant masses consisted of 25 women, with the tumor histology shown in Table 26.1. Of these 25 women with malignant masses, all but four demonstrated flow (84%) (Fig. 26.2). The mean PSV in the 21 tumors that demonstrated vascularity was 29 cm/s, with a standard deviation of 16.2 cm/s and a range of 0–78 cm/s. The mean RI was 0.50 ± 0.1, with a range of 0.33–0.67. Only four of the 21 showing vascularity demonstrated RIs below 0.4.

The poorly differentiated carcinomas tended to have the highest velocities, at 28, 41, 78, 37 and 17 cm/s, with one showing no flow (Figs 26.3, 26.4).

There were 62 proven benign masses with 18 demonstrating no evidence of flow (Fig. 26.5). Thus, 71% demonstrated flow. The histology of the postmenopausal benign masses is given in Table 26.2. Of the 44 benign tumors that demonstrated flow, the mean PSV was 12.9 cm/s, with a standard deviation of 11.0 cm/s (Fig. 26.6). The range of velocities in the benign tumors was from

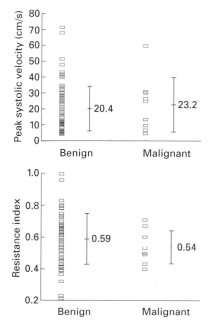

Fig. 26.1 Peak systolic velocity in benign and malignant masses in premenopausal women. Values are means ± SD.

Table 26.1 Postmenopausal women: histology of malignant tumors

Mucinous adenocarcinoma	1
Serous adenocarcinoma	7
Poorly differentiated carcinoma	6
Cyst adenofibroma (LMP[a])	4
Mixed Müllerian	2
Carcinoid	1
Endometrioid	4
Total:	25

[a] LMP, low malignant potential.

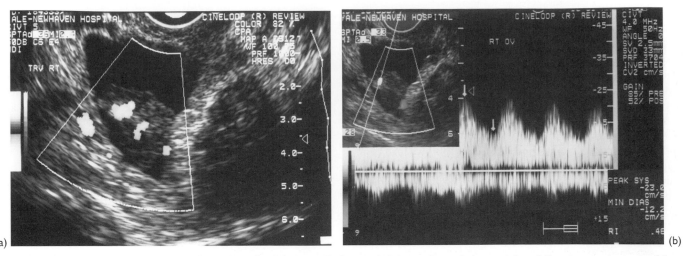

Fig. 26.2 A 78-year-old patient presented with an irregular right ovary. Endovaginal ultrasound revealed a partially solid/cystic mass measuring 26 × 20 × 22 mm. (b) Peak velocities were 23 cm/s and the RI was 0.46. A diagnosis of ovarian cancer was made and pathology revealed a cyst adenocarcinoma.

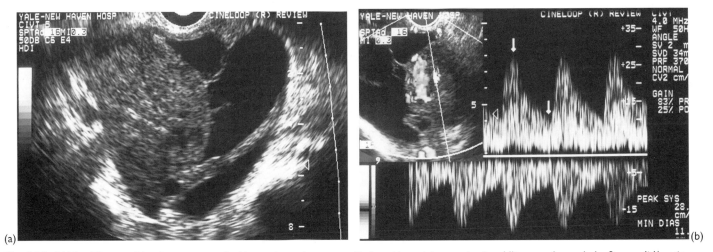

Fig. 26.3 (a) This 72-year-old patient presented with ovarian enlargement disclosed by pelvic examination. Ultrasound revealed a 8 cm solid/cystic mass with thick septations. (b) The solid portion was vascularized and demonstrated a peak systolic velocity of 28 cm/s and an RI of 0.6. Surgery disclosed a poorly differentiated carcinoma.

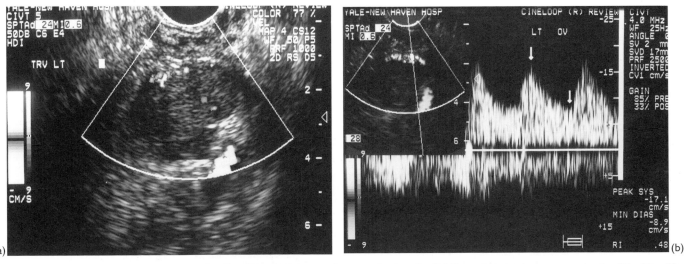

Fig. 26.4 (a) An 80-year-old woman presented with enlarged ovary on pelvic examination. On EVUS a solid mass was seen, measuring 27 × 37 × 32 mm and giving a volume of 16 ml, which is too large for a postmenopausal ovary. The CA125 was over 2000 U/ml. (b) Doppler revealed a peak systolic velocity of 70 cm/s and an RI of 0.48. Surgery revealed a poorly differentiated carcinoma.

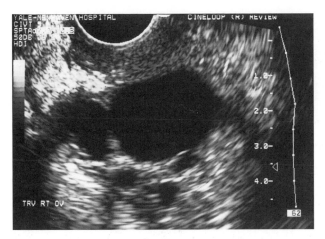

Fig. 26.5 A 60-year-old woman presented with enlarged ovary detected by pelvic examination. EVUS revealed two cysts separated by a strand of normal-appearing ovary. Overall, it measured 57 × 39 × 44 mm. No vascular signals were detected. Surgery revealed a cyst adenofibroma.

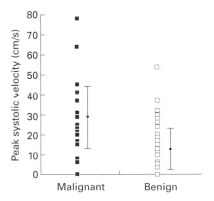

Fig. 26.6 Peak systolic velocity in postmenopausal masses. Means ± SD are shown.

0 to 54 cm/s, the latter seen in a teratoma. The mean RI in the benign tumors that demonstrated flow was 0.58 ± 0.15, and 6 of the 44 demonstrated an RI of less than 0.4.

In further statistical analysis, we used the unpaired Student's t-test to compare the parameters of the benign and malignant tumors that demonstrated detectable flow. The velocities were statistically different with $P = 0.01$. The RIs were not significantly different ($P > 0.08$).

Conclusion

These results, and those reported by other authors, effectively disprove the claim that RIs can be used to discriminate between benign and malignant ovarian masses.[14–16] The finding that PSVs in malignant tumors are statistically significantly higher than in benign tumors in postmenopausal women is in accord with our clinical observations, but of little clinical value, as ovarian cancers may have no detectable vascularity. It is of little value to observe that in a large population, the PSV is significantly higher. We therefore must regress to managing our patients as having ovarian

Table 26.2 Postmenopausal women: histology of benign tumors

Paratubal cyst	7
Serous cyst	10
Benign cystic teratoma	6
Cystadenofibroma	10
Brenner tumor	1
Inflammatory mass	1
Mucinous cystadenoma	4
Serous cystadenoma	13
Endometrioma	4
Fibroma	5
Fibrothecoma	1
Total	62

cancer when there is a solid, or solid and cystic, enlargement of the ovary. The demonstration of high velocities under these conditions only adds confidence to the diagnosis made on sonographic morphology. Enhancement of masses by contrast media aids in the diagnosis of malignancy by CT, and it would be expected that a similar improvement in diagnosis may occur by the use of an ultrasonic contrast agent, as these become clinically available.[17] At present, they are being applied to improve diagnosis of liver metastasis and in the diagnosis of renal artery stenosis. Their application to the diagnosis of ovarian tumors is likely to follow in the near future.

References

1. Niloff, J.M., Klug, T.L., Schaetzl, E. *et al.* (1984). Elevation of serum CA125 in carcinomas of the fallopian tube, endometrium, and endocervix. *Am. J. Obstet. Gynecol.*, 148 (8), 1057–8.
2. Einhorn, N., Sjoval, K., Knapp, R.C. *et al.* (1992). Prospective evaluation of serum CA125 levels for early detection of ovarian cancer. *Obstet. Gynecol.*, 80, 14–18.
3. Mann, W.J., Patsner, B., Cohen, H., and Loesch, M. (1988). Preoperative serum CA125 levels in patients with surgical stage I invasive ovarian cancer. *J. Natl Cancer Inst.*, 80, 208–9.
4. Jacobs, I.J., Skates, S., Davies, A.P. *et al.* (1996). Risk of ovarian cancer after raised serum CA125 concentration: A prospective cohort study. *BMJ*, 313, 1355–8.
5. Taylor, K.J.W., Burns, P.N., Wells, P.N.T. *et al.* (1985). Ultrasound Doppler flow studies of the ovarian and uterine arteries. *Br. J. Obstet. Gynecol.*, 92, 240–6.
6. Taylor, K.J.W., Ramos, I.M., Feyock, A.L. *et al.* (1989). Ectopic pregnancy: duplex Doppler evaluation. *Radiology*, 73, 93–7.
7. Folkman, J., Merler, E., Abernathy, C., and Williams, G. (1971). Isolation of a tumor factor responsible for angiogenesis. *J. Exp. Med.*, 133, 275–88.
8. Taylor, K.J.W., Ramos, I.M., Carter, D., *et al.* (1988). Correlation of Doppler US tumor signals with neovascular morphologic features. *Radiology*, 166, 57–62.
9. Ramos, I.M., Taylor, K.J.W., Kier, R. *et al.* (1988). Tumor vascular signals in renal masses: Detection with Doppler US. *Radiology*, 168, 633–7.
10. Taylor, K.J., Ramos, I., Morse, S.S. *et al.* (1987). Focal liver masses: differential diagnosis with pulsed Doppler US. *Radiology*, 164, 643–7.
11. Kurjak, A. and Zalud, I. (1992). Transvaginal colour Doppler in the differentiation between benign and malignant ovarian masses. In *Ovarian cancer 2 Biology, diagnosis and management*, (ed. F. Sharp, W.P. Mason, and W. Creasman), p. 261. Chapman & Hall Medical, London.
12. Schwartz, P.E., Chambers, J.T., Taylor, K.J.W. *et al.* (1991). Early detection of ovarian cancer: background, rationale, and structure of the Yale early detection program. *Yale J. Biol. Med.*, 64, 557–71.

13. Campbell, S., Bourne, T., Crayford, T., and Pittrof, R. (1993). The early detection and assessment of endometrial cancer by transvaginal colour Doppler ultrasonography. *Europ. J. Obstet. Gynecol. Reprod. Biol.*, **49** (1–2), 44–5.

14. Jain, K.A. (1994). Prospective evaluation of adnexal masses with endovaginal gray-scale and duplex and color Doppler US. Correlation with pathologic findings. *Radiology*, **191** (1), 63–37.

15. Levine, D., Feldstein, V.A., Babcook, C.J., and Filly, R.A. (1994). Sonography of ovarian masses: poor sensitiviity of resistive index for identifying malignant lesions. *Am. J. Rad.*, **162** (6), 1355–9.

16. Salem, S., White, L.M., and Lai, J. (1994). Doppler sonography of adnexal masses: the predictive value of the pulsatility index in benign and malignant disease. *Am. J. Rad.*, **163** (5), 1147–50.

17. Goldberg, B.B., Liu, J.B., and Forsberg, F. (1994). Ultrasound contrast agents: a review. *UMB*, **20** (4), 319–33.

27. Differentiating the risk of ovarian cancer calculation from CA125 velocity: a new concept for optimizing CA125 screening for ovarian cancer

Steven J. Skates

Introduction

CA125 is a blood test[1] that has been approved by the US Food and Drug Administration (FDA) for detection of recurrence of ovarian cancer following primary therapy. Since it is simple and inexpensive, regular CA125 measurement as the primary test may be an acceptable and economically feasible method of screening for ovarian cancer. Screening is an appealing approach to reducing mortality from ovarian cancer, since most cases are detected at a late stage with very poor prognosis, while the few cases detected at an early stage have excellent prognosis.[2] The missing information required to determine the value of CA125 screening is its impact on ovarian cancer mortality through identifying disease at an early stage and the rate of screen-induced surgery on women without ovarian cancer from false-positive screening results. Only preliminary clinical trials have addressed these issues so far, with encouraging but inconclusive results,[3,4] although planning for a definitive trial is under way.

The standard interpretation of a CA125 test is to declare the result positive if the value exceeds 35 U/ml.[1] In prospective clinical pilot trials, annual CA125 testing using this interpretation (or a 30 U/ml cutoff) for referral to pelvic ultrasound detected ovarian cancer prior to the occurrence of clinical symptoms in the majority of cases.[3,4] The standard CA125 interpretation in a pilot randomized screening trial found a significant increase in ovarian cancer survival time, avoiding lead-time bias by measuring survival time from the date of randomization.[5] Ovarian cancer mortality dropped by 50% in the screened arm compared to the control arm, although this difference did not reach statistical significance. The results of these trials provided the basis for the funding of a definitive three-arm screening trial of ovarian cancer, with the first arm using the CA125 test as a primary screen, the second arm using ultrasound as the primary screen, and the third arm being the control group.

Screening for ovarian cancer is a delicate balance between identifying as many cases as possible at an early stage while achieving the lowest rate possible of screen-induced surgeries on women without ovarian cancer per screen-detected case. Jacobs and Bast[6] suggest that the rate of 10 surgeries from false-positive screening results per true case of screen-detected ovarian cancer is the maximum rate that should be considered acceptable. To give the CA125 test the greatest chance of maximum impact while achieving the required balance, we felt that a systematic approach to the optimization of CA125 screening was essential.

It was noted previously that the behavior over time of CA125 values provided additional information on the presence of ovarian cancer.[7] In most ovarian cancer cases where serial CA125 values were available prior to detection of the disease, CA125 values rose exponentially. The exponential behavior likely reflects doubling of tumor volume over fixed time-intervals, which is mathematically equivalent to an exponential rise. In contrast, in most women without ovarian cancer CA125 values were relatively stable over time. However, such insight has only led to *ad hoc* rules for incorporating the longitudinal CA125 information in a screening strategy. One example of an *ad hoc* rule based on serial CA125 values is to use estimates of doubling time or, equivalently, the slope (on the logarithmic scale)—or CA125 velocity—to make screening decisions.

This article discusses a new concept that was developed systematically to extract the additional information in longitudinal CA125 values, and apply it in a screening strategy. The additional information is extracted using the 'risk of ovarian cancer calculation' (ROCC), and the new screening strategy is termed the 'risk of ovarian cancer algorithm' (ROCA).[8] We differentiate the ROCC from the concept of CA125 'velocity' or slope, and ROCA from *ad hoc* rules based on the velocity. The next section outlines the behavior of CA125 in cases and controls. Then a qualitative assessment of risk is discussed, and examples which differentiate the two concepts are provided. An introduction, with only a few elementary mathematical formulae, to a quantitative method for calculating the risk is given, and the final section suggests briefly how the risk may be utilized in a strategy termed ROCA.

CA125 trajectories in cases and controls

Expected CA125 profiles in cases and controls

The first step in developing systematic methods for extracting the information in longitudinal CA125 values is to model the expected CA125 levels over time in subjects that are known cases through long-term follow-up, and to develop a separate model for controls. Graphs of longitudinal CA125 values from many control subjects confirm that each subject has a stable baseline expected CA125 value around which the observed CA125 values fluctuate.[8] In subjects subsequently confirmed as cases (usually by histological examination of resected ovaries), expected CA125 levels are initially stable but at a time point prior to clinical detection begin to rise exponentially. Figure 27.1 illustrates the expected CA125 behavior for a case, with the left-hand graph displaying CA125 values on the original scale, and the right-hand graph displaying CA125 values on the logarithmic scale. On the original scale, an exponential rise follows a flat profile until clinical detection occurs, at which point treatment intervention typically alters the CA125 behavior. On the logarithmic scale, the exponential CA125 rise becomes a linear rise, and the prior flat profile behaves in the same way as the profile of women without ovarian cancer (controls). It is likely that tumor inception (if indeed such a concept can be well defined biologically) occurs on or before the change-point, and unlikely that it occurs after the change-point. Therefore in subsequent graphs we label the time after the change-point as 'tumor present', and refer to this pattern as an 'elbow' profile.

Sources of CA125 variability

If CA125 behaved exactly like the expected graphs of Fig. 27.1, then differentiating cases from controls would be straightforward, because any change (increase) in CA125 levels would indicate the presence of disease. However, unexplained CA125 variability exists both within a subject over time, and between subjects, due to assay and biological variability. These multiple sources of CA125 variability are the reason that serial CA125 levels are not straightforward to interpret. The next step in systematically extracting information about the presence of ovarian cancer ('tumor present') is to describe quantitatively the sources of CA125 variability for both cases and controls. The top-left graph of Fig. 27.2 displays the sources of variability arising from CA125 differences between women. We quantified these sources of variability by using advanced statistical analyses, termed Markov chain Monte-Carlo techniques, applied to data from the largest CA125 screening reported to date.[5]

Two main sources of CA125 variability are due to: (1) variation in the baseline level, and (2) variation in the slope after the change-point. Arrows cover approximately 95% of the distribution across the population of subjects for each source of between-

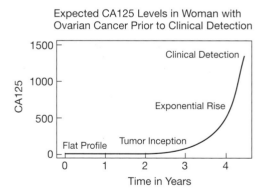

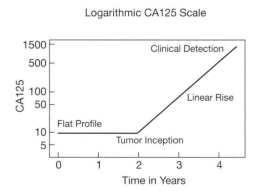

Fig. 27.1 The expected CA125 trajectory over time prior to clinical detection of ovarian cancer. Expected levels assume no variation due to biological or assay variability, and only steadily rising values due to the presence of undetected ovarian cancer. An exponential rise is expected on the original CA125 scale, as displayed in the left-hand graph, which transforms to a linear rise when the vertical axis is logarithmic, as displayed in the right-hand graph.

subject variability. The top-right graph of Fig. 27.2 displays the CA125 variability within a woman due to changes over time and to assay variability. Notice that the scales of both axes have been eliminated, since effectively the expected graph can be moved around—horizontally in time, since tumor inception occurs at different time points for each case, and vertically, since each woman has her own baseline. The baseline will most likely lie within the arrows indicated in the previous graph. Also notice that the within-person variability is substantially smaller than the between-person variability. If the two were equal, or the within variability exceeded the between variability, then longitudinal values would only provide a small increase in information over a single absolute level. The bottom-left graph of Fig. 27.2 displays the corresponding variation in CA125 values over time within a control subject. Given the level of within-subject variation, it is possible that serial CA125 levels from a control subject will appear with an 'elbow', especially if the duration after an apparent change-point is short. Assessing the relative likelihood that a given CA125 sequence is due to the presence of ovarian cancer rather than within-control-subject variation is the next step in developing a systematic approach to the interpretation of serial CA125 values.

The qualitative risk of ovarian cancer

Qualitative assessment

To qualitatively assess the risk of having ovarian cancer, we examine the relative likelihood that a particular CA125 trajectory can be explained by a flat profile, compared to being explained by an 'elbow' profile. This assessment needs to account for the systematic components as well as the between-subject and within-subject sources of variability. The more likely the observed sequence of CA125 values can be explained by a flat profile together with within-person variability, compared to an 'elbow' profile, the lower the risk of having ovarian cancer. Essentially, this approach is a pattern-matching comparison, where the pattern is any part of the expected profile. By 'part' we imply that the pattern does not have to be the full 'elbow' profile, but, for example, could be a part following the change-point, which would match steadily increasing CA125 values with no evidence of an 'elbow'. We explain later how this qualitative comparison is quantified through the systematic application of Bayes' theorem.

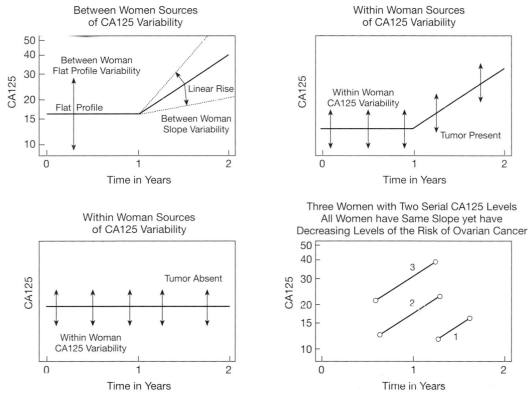

Fig. 27.2 The top-left graph displays the between-women sources of CA125 variability, both in the flat profile and the linear rise on the logarithmic scale. The extent of the arrows indicate 95% population variation. The top-right graph displays the extent of within-subject CA125 source of variability due to assay and biological variability within a woman when ovarian cancer develops. The tumor is believed to be present while the expected CA125 levels are rising, and possibly present before the change-point. The bottom-left graph displays the extent of variability within a woman who does not develop ovarian cancer during the screening process. In both these graphs labels for the time axis (horizontal) and the CA125 axis (vertical) have been deliberately omitted to indicate that the pattern of the profile can move both in time and CA125 value, although the latter is constrained for most women by the first set of arrows in the top-left graph. The bottom-right graph displays pairs of CA125 values from three women. All CA125 sequences have the same slope, but it is argued in the text that the risks of having ovarian cancer differ substantially between these women.

Differentiating CA125 velocity and the risk of ovarian cancer

Consider the bottom-right graph of Fig. 27.2, which displays longitudinal CA125 values at two time points for three subjects. All three women are subjects in a CA125 screening program, are asymptomatic at the time points for which CA125 is measured, and we do not know whether ovarian cancer is present or not. It is clear that all three women have the same slope—or CA125 'velocity'—yet consideration of the expected CA125 trajectories and the sources of variability provides convincing support for the conclusion that the three women have very different risks of ovarian cancer being present. This consideration is further supported by the intuitive interpretations of clinical researchers in the field of ovarian cancer screening with CA125, who interpret the three example CA125 paths with very different qualitative assessments of the risk of ovarian cancer. The first woman's CA125 trajectory (1) is readily explained by the within-subject CA125 variability in a flat profile, even though the slope is close to the expected slope of a case. In one sense, this is partly because the time between the two CA125 values is relatively short, and small variations over short duration can lead to high values of the slope.

The second woman's CA125 trajectory (2) starts at the same level, increases at the same rate, but ends at a considerably higher CA125 value than for the first woman because the duration between measurements is greater. It is more difficult to explain this trajectory by a flat profile and the within-subject variability, although the change in CA125 is not too far outside the 95% range. The trajectory is more readily explained by the increasing part of an 'elbow' profile. Consideration of these two examples have led to the suggestion that slopes should only be acted upon when measured over a minimum duration, such as 6 months or 1 year. However, the next example illustrates that such an *ad hoc* approach still does not differentiate between two subjects with clearly differing chances of having ovarian cancer.

The third trajectory (3) has the same slope and the same duration between measurements as the second trajectory. Yet since the initial (and final) CA125 values are substantially greater than for the second woman, the third woman is at even higher risk of having ovarian cancer than the second (and first) woman. This elevated risk is due to the final CA125 value not being readily explained by the combination of within- and between-woman CA125 flat profile sources of variability. It is for this reason that the CA125 scale is indicated in this fourth figure. In contrast, a profile consonant with the presence of ovarian cancer, with a component increasing due to the presence of ovarian cancer, readily explains the observed CA125 trajectory. Therefore the risk of having ovarian cancer is significantly higher for the third woman than for the second woman, even though their slopes are identical and their durations between the measurements are identical.

In summary, by comparing the observed CA125 trajectories with patterns of expected CA125 profiles and knowledge of between- and within-subject sources of variation, we can qualitatively rank the risks of having ovarian cancer in certain situations which are not differentiated by CA125 'velocity'. *Ad hoc* rules which attempt to ameliorate problems of the velocity concept create further problems. We have described a systematic approach which does not suffer these problems. However, it does require a quantitative method for comparing CA125 trajectories when intuition is not sufficiently accurate, and which can accommodate a varying number of CA125 measurements, and variable durations between the measurements.

Quantifying the risk of ovarian cancer

To achieve the full benefit of a systematic approach based on the risk of having ovarian cancer, it is necessary to go beyond the qualitative stage and develop methods to quantify the risk. Given a method to calculate the risk, efficient strategies for screening based on longitudinal CA125 values can be devised and implemented.

As motivation, consider Fig. 27.3, which displays hypothetical CA125 trajectories measured 3-monthly for one woman with ovarian cancer prior to clinical detection and six women without ovarian cancer (controls) over the same time period. The trajectories are deliberately chosen to be (almost) identical for the first 9 months. By the end of 18 months, the exponential CA125 rise due to the presence of undetected ovarian cancer, which appears linear on the logarithmically scaled vertical axis, clearly differentiates the case from all controls, whose CA125 profiles are generally stable over time. However, the earlier in time the case is detected, the greater the chance of detecting the disease at an early stage. By the end of 12 months, two controls still have the same profile as the case, one-third the number of controls that had the same profile at 9 months. Thus, the risk for the two controls and one case (at that point in time we do not know the status of either the case or the controls) has increased by a factor of three. If this risk could be calculated, then a screening decision might be made on the basis of the risk level. For example, for a sufficiently high level of risk, immediate transvaginal ultrasound might be indicated, as may occur for the three women with continuing rising CA125 values at 12 months. While it is clear which women are at greater risk in this contrived example, more general CA125 patterns may not be easily comparable in terms of the risk of disease.

Two concepts of risk

The risk of eventually *developing* ovarian cancer and the risk of having ovarian cancer are two distinct, although related, concepts. While epidemiologists most often use the term 'risk' in the first sense, in this article the term risk refers to the 'risk of *having* ovarian cancer' unless explicitly noted otherwise. Epidemiological studies of the first concept have identified use of oral contraceptives, especially for longer than 5 years, and increasing parity as protective risk factors, and vaginal talc use, increasing age, Caucasian race, and presence of a *BRCA1* or *BRCA2* mutation as factors that increase the risk of developing ovarian cancer. The definitive trial mentioned in the introduction excludes women with a relevant genetic mutation or a family history suggestive of a mutation, since it would be unethical to randomize such women to a control arm. Aside from the genetic risk factors, age is the next strongest risk factor, so proposed ovarian cancer screening

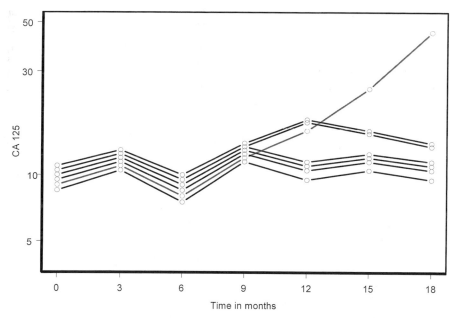

Fig. 27.3 This graph displays hypothetical CA125 values in six women without ovarian cancer, and one women with ovarian cancer prior to clinical detection. While all CA125 values from control subjects track the CA125 values from the case for the first 9 months, fewer track after 12 months, and none after 15 months. By 18 months the differentiation between the case and the controls is obvious. We aim to quantify the risk based on serial CA125 values, so that cases are detected as early as possible by efficiently separating higher-risk women from lower-risk women.

trials focus on postmenopausal women. Three-quarters of ovarian cancer cases occur in the corresponding age group. Additional reasons to focus on this population are that the two candidate testing modalities, CA125 measurements and transvaginal sonography (TVS), are far less likely to give false-positive results in this population compared with premenopausal women.

Quantification begins with the baseline risk of *having* ovarian cancer, prior to any CA125 measurements. This is the prevalence of disease, and it is related to the incidence of ovarian cancer and the duration of preclinical disease. Incidence is the number of new cases developing within a given time period in a cohort of women apparently disease free at the beginning of the time period. Typically, incidence is age related and specified in 1- or 5-year age intervals, the time period is 1 year, and the size of the cohort is 100 000. In northern Europe and the US, annual incidence in postmenopausal women ranges from 40–50 cases per 100 000 apparently disease-free women, or approximately 1 in 2000 per year. Preliminary evidence from ultrasound screening trials suggests that the preclinical duration is approximately 2 years. The prevalence, or risk of having ovarian cancer, is the product of the incidence and the preclinical duration, that is, approximately 1 in 1000. This baseline risk could then be modified by measurement of the other risk factors for developing ovarian cancer, such as oral contraceptive use and parity.

In developing an efficient screening strategy, it is (almost) axiomatic that more resources should be devoted to subjects with higher risk of *having* ovarian cancer. For example, if in one subgroup there were 10 women with (asymptomatic) ovarian cancer, and in another same-sized subgroup only 1 woman with (asymptomatic) ovarian cancer, then more screening resources should be devoted to the first subgroup, where the risk is tenfold greater

than the second subgroup. Any approach that does not use the risk to direct screening resources could easily allocate more resources to a lower risk group than a higher risk group, and such an approach would be inefficient. Therefore, quantitatively assessing the risk of *having* ovarian cancer is a crucial step in designing an efficient screening program.

Risk from one biomarker measurement

Measuring a biomarker further modifies the risk of having a target disease. A perfect biomarker would separate all (asymptomatic) cases from all other subjects. No such biomarker exists for ovarian cancer (nor for any other disease as far as I am aware). To calculate the risk, given a single biomarker measurement in a new subject, requires a study of biomarker levels in disease-free subjects and subjects with the disease. Rigorous implementation of such a study necessitates a gold standard procedure to classify subjects into the two classes. For ovarian cancer the gold standard is surgery followed by pathological examination of the resected ovaries. Since it is impossible to apply this gold standard to every subject in a large study, the biomarker study employs surrogate endpoints instead. Two approaches are used to address this problem. The first uses a case-control design with clinically detected ovarian cancer cases as surrogates for asymptomatic cases and apparently healthy women as surrogates for disease-free women. The second utilizes a cohort design and classifies the subjects by target disease status through follow-up of all subjects after a fixed time interval, such as 1 or 2 years for ovarian cancer. Neither approach is perfect. The first gives biomarker data on clinically detected cases which are usually more advanced than asymptomatic cases, introducing a bias; while the second usually has far fewer cases, leading to greater imprecision for the distribution of the biomarker in cases. We will ignore these issues in the following discussion.

The distribution of the biomarker in the two groups is graphed by two histograms, one for the cases and the other for the disease-free subjects, a hypothetical 1 : 1 case-control example is given in Fig. 27.4. Often the distributions are summarized by fitting a density to the histograms, especially when there are few cases. The continuous lines in Fig. 27.4 illustrate the fitting of densities to both cases and controls. In this hypothetical example, higher values of the biomarker give a greater chance of being a case, that is, having the disease. For any given biomarker value, the relative odds of having the target disease is given by the relative heights of the histograms at the measured value. For example, for a new subject with a biomarker value of 34, which is between values 32 and 36 on the histogram, there were 195 cases and 114 controls, as indicated by the first vertical line. The relative odds (or odds ratio) of being a case are then 195 : 114 or 1.7 : 1. To account for the case-control approach of the study, the relative odds are multiplied by the prior odds, which is simply the prevalence (as a probability) transformed to odds. With a baseline risk prior to measuring the biomarker of 1 in 1000, or baseline odds of 1 : 999, the odds change to 1 in 580 with the new biomarker measurement of 34. At a biomarker value of 53, as indicated by the second vertical line, the case to control ratio is 302 : 43 or 7 : 1, which modifies the baseline odds from 1 : 999 to 1 : 140, or a risk of 1/(140 + 1) = 0.7%.

Summarizing the histogram with a statistical density

Instead of retaining all the counts within each histogram bin for the cases and controls, a statistical density often adequately summarizes the two distributions. In the example given in Fig. 27.4, bell-shaped curves closely follow the histogram bin heights. A convenient bell-shaped density is the normal (or Gaussian) distribution, which is determined by the mean and the standard deviation. For a new biomarker value, the distance from the mean in terms of standard deviations is the z-score. The normal density for the z-score is proportional to $\exp(-1/2\ z^2)$ which is the formula for the bell-shaped curve. The relative odds are then estimated by the ratio of the controls' normal density to the cases' normal density at a new subject's biomarker value, or $\exp(-1/2\ z^2)/\exp(-1/2\ z^{*2})$. The variable z is the distance in standard deviations of the marker value from the mean of the cases, and z^* is the distance from the mean of the controls (assuming the standard deviation is the same for cases and controls). As the marker level moves further away from the mean of the controls and closer to the mean of the cases, z^* increases and the density for the controls, $\exp(-1/2\ z^{*2})$, diminishes, while z decreases and the density for the cases, $\exp(-1/2\ z^2)$, increases. Thus the relative odds of being a case increases as the biomarker value moves away from the mean of the controls and towards the mean of the cases, as expected.

In the hypothetical distributions of Fig. 27.4, which are plotted on the logarithmic marker value scale, the mean for the cases is

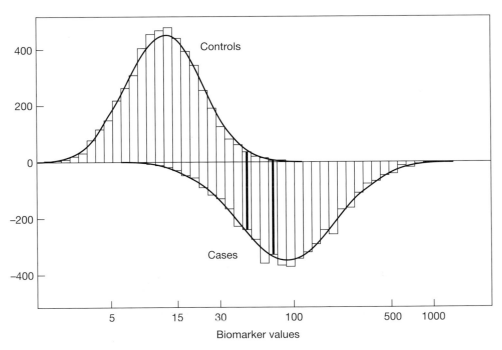

Fig. 27.4 Hypothetical distributions of a biomarker from a case-control study are displayed in two histograms. The top histogram displays the distribution of marker values in controls, while the bottom histogram gives the distribution for cases. The first vertical line compares the number of cases to number of controls for a marker level between 32 and 36, while the second vertical line compares the same quantities for a marker level of 53. The ratio of cases to controls gives the relative odds of being a case for a particular small range of marker levels. By smoothing the histograms with density estimates, the relative odds can be estimated for a specific value of the biomarker.

$\log(90) = 4.5$, for the controls it is $\log(10) = 2.3$, and the common standard deviation is 0.7. Thus for a new marker value of 34 (3.53 on the logarithmic scale), $z_1 = (3.53 - 4.5)/0.7 = -1.39$, while $z_2 = (3.53 - 2.3)/0.7 = 1.76$. The normal density corresponding to cases is proportional to $\exp(-1/2 \ z^2) = 0.38$, and for the controls is $\exp(-1/2 \ z^{*2}) = 0.21$, so the estimate of the relative odds is $0.38/0.21 = 1.8 : 1$. This estimate is close to the relative odds of $1.7 : 1$ obtained above from the relative heights of the two histograms at the marker value of 34.

If the sample sizes are large, as in the example displayed in Fig. 27.4, the means and standard deviations are estimated with great accuracy. However, when the sample sizes are moderate the means and standard deviations are not estimated precisely, and in fact have standard errors. This imprecision is an additional source of (statistical) variability which needs to be accounted for; since we do not know their true value, we average over the distribution of their possible values. Statistical methods exist which provide many values representing the possible ranges of the means and standard deviations. In this situation, the densities for the cases and controls are calculated for each possible value of the means and standard deviations, and then averaged. The ratio of the two averaged densities (one for cases and one for controls) is the final estimate of the relative odds.

Quantifying the risk from multiple biomarker measurements

When multiple biomarker measurements taken over time are available, a generalization of the above procedure is used to calculate the relative odds. Suppose we know the expected baseline

CA125 level for a subject, and measure CA125 values at multiple points in time, as depicted in the top-left graph of Fig. 27.5. Given the within-subject CA125 variability, the z^* score is calculated for each CA125 value, giving $z^{1*}, z^{2*}, \dots, z^{5*}$. Since CA125 measurements fluctuate about the mean level independently of each other, the combined density for all the measurements is the product of the densities for each individual measurement (probabilities for independent events multiply). Thus the combined density is the product $\exp(-1/2 \ z^*_1{}^2) \exp(-1/2 \ z^*_2{}^2)\dots \exp(-1/2 \ z^*_5{}^2) = \exp(-1/2 \ (z^*_1{}^2 + z^*_2{}^2 + z^*_5{}^2))$. Effectively the sum of squared z^* values for multiple CA125 measurements replaces the squared z^* value for a single measurement.

Since we do not know the true baseline level for a subject, we average the density over the possible values of the baseline level. The possible values are obtained from the distribution across women specified by the first arrows in Fig. 27.2. The average density is the final estimate of the density under the assumption that the woman is a control subject.

A similar calculation is performed to calculate the density under the assumption that the woman is a case, that is, has undetected ovarian cancer. In this situation, the expected behavior of the CA125 values is part of an 'elbow' profile. Suppose we know the expected trajectory over time. Then for each point in time, we calculate the z score as the number of within standard deviations the value is from the expected trajectory as shown in the top-right graph of Fig. 27.5. With this sequence of CA125 values, $z_1 = z^*_1, z_2 = z^*_2, z_3 = z^*_3$, but z_4 and z_5 are much larger than the corresponding z scores assuming a control subject as in the top-left graph of Fig. 27.5, namely z^*_4 and z^*_5. Therefore the sum of squared z values for the cases is much larger than the sum of squared z^* values for

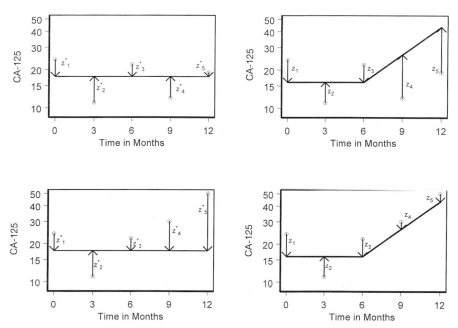

Fig. 27.5 The top two graphs display CA125 values from a control subject that does not develop ovarian cancer during the observed time period. The top-left graph displays the z scores for a flat profile, giving a better fit than an elbow profile as displayed in the top-right graph. The text explains how a sequence of z scores is converted to a density. The bottom two graphs display a sequence of CA125 values from a case, and illustrate the better fit an elbow profile provides compared to a flat profile. These four graphs demonstrate that our approach to calculating the relative odds, and hence the risk, on the basis of the ratio of two densities, provides a systematic approach to interpreting single and multiple CA125 values.

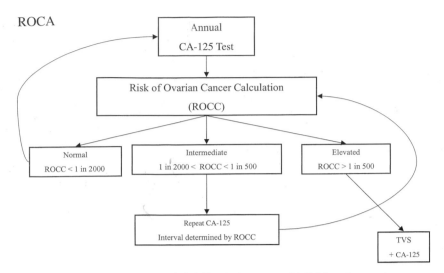

Fig. 27.6 A schema for implementing the risk of ovarian cancer (ROCC) calculation in a CA125-based screening strategy, referred to as the risk of ovarian cancer algorithm (ROCA).

the controls, and consequently the density for cases is much less than the density for controls. We average the density for cases over all the possible values of the elbow profile, as indicated by the two sets of arrows in Fig. 27.2. We find that the average density for cases is much less than the average density for controls. Hence the relative odds for the sequence of CA125 values given in the top row of Fig. 27.5 is much less than one, indicating very little chance that the subject has ovarian cancer.

In contrast, with the sequence of CA125 values displayed in the bottom row of Fig. 27.5, a much smaller set of z scores is obtained for the cases (bottom-right graph) than z^* scores for the controls (bottom-left graph). Hence for this particular elbow profile, the density for cases is much larger than the density for controls. When averaged over all the possible elbow profiles for the cases, and all possible flat profiles for the controls, the density of the cases is much greater than the density for the controls. The relative odds are then much greater than one, and the final odds of having ovarian cancer can be significantly raised from baseline odds.

When this approach is applied to the three sequences of CA125 values displayed in the bottom-right graph of Fig. 27.2, it is clear that an elbow profile will fit the first sequence (line 3) much better than a flat profile. This is due both to the initial value, the slope, and the duration of the rise, and not just to the slope alone. A better way of stating the same point is that the best-fitting elbow profile fits much better than the best-fitting flat profile within the likely ranges of flat and elbow profiles. This systematic approach of calculating the final odds of having ovarian cancer (or risk) summarizes all the information about the presence of ovarian cancer contained in the sequence of CA125 values within one number. The slope does not summarize all the information. It can be similarly verified that the final odds is smaller for the second sequence (line 2), and even smaller for the third sequence (line 1) in the bottom-right graph of Fig. 27.2.

The risk of ovarian cancer algorithm

Having determined the optimal method to summarize the information about the presence of ovarian cancer in the CA125 values, much research remains to be done to determine the optimal method of using the ROCC. We briefly mention one method of implementing the ROCC in a CA125-based screening strategy for ovarian cancer.

We suppose that the context of the CA125 screening program is a regular (e.g. annual) CA125 measurement on all subjects. Also, a screening program will have limited resources, and more expensive tests such as transvaginal ultrasound will be limited to women at elevated risk. After each CA125 test, the risk will be evaluated on all CA125 measurements to date, and a screening decision will be made based on the level of the risk. For most women, the risk will be sufficiently low, such as lower than the baseline risk, to recommend returning for the next CA125 test at the regularly scheduled time (in 1 year). For women at greater than normal risk, but still not considered elevated enough for referral to ultrasound, a possible screening decision is to provide another CA125 test before their next annual test. In this intermediate-risk group, women whose risk is above but close to normal, this extra CA125 test might be performed in 6 months time. For women below but close to elevated risk, this extra CA125 test might be performed within the next 1 or 2 months. Thus a suggested strategy based on the ROCC, termed the risk of ovarian cancer algorithm (ROCA), could be implemented following the schema displayed in Fig. 27.6. Optimizing the cutoff points of risk which determine intermediate and elevated risk, while maintaining high sensitivity and positive predictive value, while constraining the resources expended is the topic of ongoing research.

References

1. Bast, R.C. Jr, Klug, T.L., St John, E. *et al.* (1983). A radioimmunoassay using a monoclonal antibody to monitor the course of epithelial ovarian cancer. *N. Engl. J. Med.*, **309**, 883–7.

2. Young, R.C., Walton, L.A., Ellenberg, S.S. *et al.* (1990). Adjuvant therapy in stage I and stage II epithelial ovarian cancer. Results of two prospective randomized trials [see comments]. *N. Engl. J. Med.*, **322**, 1021–7.

3. Einhorn, N., Sjovall, K., Knapp, R.C. *et al.* (1992). Prospective evaluation of serum CA 125 levels for early detection of ovarian cancer. *Obstet. Gynecol.*, **80**, 14–18.

4. Jacobs, I., Davies, A.P., Bridges, J. *et al.* (1993). Prevalence screening for ovarian cancer in postmenopausal women by CA 125 measurement and ultrasonography [see comments]. *BMJ*, **306**, 1030–4.

5. Jacobs, I.J., Skates, S.J., MacDonald, N. *et al.* (1999). Screening for ovarian cancer: a pilot randomised controlled trial. *Lancet*, **353**, 1207–10.

6. Jacobs, I. and Bast, R.C. Jr (1989). The CA 125 tumour-associated antigen: a review of the literature. *Hum. Reprod.*, **4**, 1–12.

7. Zurawski, V.R. Jr, Sjovall, K., Schoenfeld, D.A. *et al.* (1990). Prospective evaluation of serum CA 125 levels in a normal population, phase I: the specificities of single and serial determinations in testing for ovarian cancer. *Gynecol. Oncol.*, **36**, 299–305.

8. Skates, S.J., Xu, F.J., Yu, Y.H. *et al.* (1995). Toward an optimal algorithm for ovarian cancer screening with longitudinal tumor markers. *Cancer*, **76**, 2004–10.

28. Socio-economics of ovarian cancer screening

Nicole Urban, Martin McIntosh, Lauren Clarke, Ian Jacobs, Beth Karlan, Garnet Anderson, and Charles Drescher

Introduction

There is growing support for an ovarian cancer screening randomized controlled trial (RCT), but there is debate regarding choice of a protocol to be tested. To have an important public-health impact, the protocol should be suitable for use in average-risk post-menopausal women. Because the protocol is likely to become the standard of care if a suitable level of efficacy is demonstrated in a trial, it should be cost-effective when applied in the population of women to whom results will be generalized. Because the trial must have sufficient power, and power depends in part on the expected mortality reduction, it should yield high mortality reduction. The strategy should be efficient in the sense that it yields years of life saved (YLS) at minimum cost, and cost-effective in the sense that cost per YLS does not exceed what society is willing to pay.

To identify promising screening strategies, we estimated the mortality reduction and cost-effectiveness of three candidate ovarian cancer screening protocols applied at varying intervals in two alternative populations of women. The candidate protocols were transvaginal sonography (TVS) as a first-line screen,[1,2] a multimodal strategy using CA125 as a first-line screen followed by TVS if CA125 exceeds 30 U/ml,[3,4] and an approximation of the risk of cancer (ROC) algorithm proposed by Skates *et al.*[5] The screening intervals were 6, 12, 18, and 24 months. The populations were women aged 50–64 and 50–80 years.

Performance characteristics of the strategies were estimated using a microsimulation model as described previously.[6] Methods for estimating mortality reduction, YLS, and costs are described, and results regarding mortality reduction, efficiency, and cost-effectiveness are reported. In addition, methods and results of validation and sensitivity analyses are reported. We hope that this work will be useful in the design of an ovarian cancer screening trial. It is not intended to encourage ovarian cancer screening outside the context of a RCT, or to replace a RCT as a means of demonstrating screening efficacy.

Methods

Estimation methods

A stochastic microsimulation (computer) model was used to estimate the mortality reduction, years of life saved (YLS), and costs attributable to ovarian cancer screening. In this model, screening strategies are evaluated when applied to a hypothetical cohort of 1 million women aged 50 in 1998. Screening begins at age 50 and continues until age 64 or 80. In both cases, the perspective is societal and screening outcomes are measured over the entire lifetimes of the women. The 12 screening strategies vary in frequency of the screen (6, 12, 18, or 24 months), the algorithm for using CA125 (single threshold rule or change over time), and use of TVS (as primary or second-line screen).

The model is *stochastic* in the sense that randomness is introduced to simulate the 'luck' of an individual woman. The model has four components: natural history, disease detection, survival, and outcomes reporting. A surrogate measure of disease aggressiveness is used to link the natural history, detection, and survival components. Women with aggressive tumors are assumed to experience worse survival regardless of the stage of their disease at diagnosis. Conversely, women with slower growing tumors will experience better survival regardless of their mode of detection.

Each component requires input parameters that are based on analysis of public-use data or reports in the literature. A *base-case* is defined using assumptions that are plausible given current knowledge of ovarian cancer disease progression and detection. The model predicts (rather than assumes) the outcomes of screening such as mortality reduction, stage shifts, lead time, and survival gains for different screening protocols. These outcomes are not fixed by the model inputs, allowing a high degree of validation for these important model outputs.

Table 28.1 Distribution of ovarian cancer by age and stage

	Age (years)											
	30–34	35–39	40–44	45–49	50–54	55–59	60–64	65–69	70–74	75–79	80–84	85+
Percent of ovarian cancer at each ages	2.2%	3.9%	5.3%	7.3%	8.5%	11.2%	14.3%	14.6%	12.7%	9.3%	6.5%	4.0%
Stage distribution within an age range												
Local	54.0%	39.7%	35.5%	28.5%	26.1%	22.2%	18.3%	15.9%	14.9%	15.4%	13.8%	11.6%
Regional	11.0%	14.4%	12.1%	14.4%	14.4%	12.5%	13.3%	13.2%	11.9%	11.6%	12.9%	10.9%
Distant	35.0%	45.9%	52.4%	57.0%	59.5%	65.3%	68.4%	70.9%	73.2%	73.0%	73.3%	77.5%

Natural history component

The natural history component represents four types of women: healthy women, women who develop benign ovarian disease but do not develop ovarian cancer (benigns), women who develop cancer but die of other causes before the cancer is diagnosed (latents), and women who develop symptomatic cancer (cases). Competing risks of dying cancer free or developing cancer are derived on an age-specific basis from US Census Bureau life tables[7] and SEER (surveillance, epidemiology, and end results)[8] public use data from the National Cancer Institute (NCI). Age-specific and lifetime risks are generated using the method described in SEER publications.[9] Rates of incidence of cancer, ages at onset, and stage at diagnosis in the absence of screening are chosen to match national data from the United States, as shown in Table 28.1.

The age at cancer onset is determined by measuring backwards from the age of the woman and stage at diagnosis of the cancer at clinical detection and diagnosis. Cancer is assumed to progress from local through regional to distant disease. Disease *duration* is defined as the total time it takes the cancer to progress from its smallest detectable size to death in the absence of treatment. The total duration of untreated disease is approximated to be 28.5 months on average. Women are assumed to have localized disease for an average of 9 months, regional disease for an average of 4.5 months, and advanced disease for an average of 15 months, 12 months with abdominal spread and 3 months with metastases to distant sites. These assumptions are not empirically based, but reflect the beliefs of clinicians.[10] Women are randomly assigned a disease duration so that some have rapidly progressing tumors while others have relatively slow-growing tumors.

Detection component

The detection component describes the behavior of the screening tests as a function of the characteristics of the tumor at the time of the screen. The probability that the screen will detect the tumor increases with tumor age. Benign conditions and natural variability in healthy women affect the probability that the screen will be falsely positive. The model accommodates two general tests, TVS and tumor markers such as CA125, that can be combined in various ways. Additionally, the model supports results-based

scheduling, which allows for the simulation of callbacks for indeterminate results. The model generates true- and false-positive tests based on the characteristics of the woman and the tumor at the time of the screen.

Assumptions about TVS

TVS is assumed to be 100% sensitive x months after tumor inception (the beginning of disease stage I). If the woman's disease aggressiveness is above the median for all women, then $x = 0$; otherwise, x is uniformly distributed from 0 to 6 months, proportional to disease aggressiveness. These assumptions imply that half of cancers are immediately detectable by TVS while the rest become detectable within 6 months of inception, and that rapidly progressing cancers are detectable sooner.

Specificity of TVS is determined by the presence of benign ovarian conditions that generate false positives. A secondary imaging screen is used to distinguish benign from malignant conditions. Because inception rates for benign conditions are unknown, the model was calibrated to observed rates of false positives at the first and subsequent screens among postmenopausal women reported by Campbell *et al.*[11] Conditions observed in the Campbell series were reproduced, including the age distribution of the population screened, the time between screens and compliance with screening schedules. To reflect the use of TVS[1] rather than transabdominal ultrasound (TAU),[12] rates of false positives were adjusted by a factor of 0.58, based on TVS results for a prevalence screen reported by Van Nagell.[1]

Reports suggest that the use of systematic morphology rating systems[13] can improve TVS sensitivity and that the rate of false positives per woman screened can be reduced to between 0.3% and 0.7%.[2,14] Resulting rates of false positives generated by the simulation model are shown in Table 28.2. To yield these results, the inception of benign conditions that would generate false positives was modeled as 102 and 58 per 100 000 women annually in women younger and older than 50, respectively. Reports suggest that color Doppler imaging (CDI)[15] can be useful in distinguishing benign from malignant ovarian masses prior to surgery. In the model its specificity for malignancy was assumed to be 0.55 among masses identified by TVS.

Table 28.2 False-positive rates of transvaginal sonography (TVS) by screen reported by Campbell et al.[11] and generated by the model

	Reported by Campbell	Generated by model	
		Using TAU	Using TVS
1st screen	3.1%	3.1%	1.8%
2nd screen	1.8%	1.8%	1.1%
3rd screen	1.0%	1.1%	0.6%
Overall	1.9%	2.1%	1.2%

Representation of CA125

Each woman is assigned a level of CA125 for each test performed during the screening period, based on its level at the time of the test. Her mean CA125 level is randomly generated from an exponential distribution. Among healthy women, CA125 is highly variable because the natural levels of CA125 vary among women. In addition, each woman's CA125 varies around its own natural level, and there is laboratory measurement error. Following Skates and Singer, among 95% of cases the level of CA125 is assumed to increase exponentially over time as the tumor grows.[10] CA125 increases exponentially from its baseline with time since tumor inception, at a rate that depends inversely on disease duration. In addition, we assume that in 10% of women with benign ovarian conditions, CA125 behaves as if the condition were malignant (as described below). These assumptions are consistent with reported rates of positivity of CA125 among women with benign pelvic masses.[3]

Data from the Karlan series (1250 women screened periodically for up to 7 years at the Gilda Radner Ovarian Cancer Screening Program in Los Angeles) were analyzed to estimate the between- and within-woman variance of CA125 in healthy women. These data suggest that about 58% of the variance in CA125 is attributable to variance over time within women, while the remaining 42% is attributable to variance in the mean levels among women. Data from Jacobs' prevalence screen suggest that the overall mean of CA125 in healthy postmenopausal women is 10 U/ml and that about 1.5% of women have CA125 above 30 U/ml. These data are consistent with experience in the PLCO trial that 0.5% of women have CA125 above 35 U/ml.[16]

Survival component

The survival component describes the survival experience of women diagnosed at localized, regional, and distant disease, relative to other-cause mortality. Ten-year relative survival curves were estimated from cross-sectional SEER data for the years 1985–1989, within 5-year age categories and stage at diagnosis. Relative survival is the observed survival probability for the specified time interval adjusted for the expected survival, in this case a ratio of observed survival among cases divided by expected survival generated from the US population matched by race, sex, age, and date.[9] Women with aggressive tumors (short disease durations) are assumed to experience worse survival regardless of their stage at diagnosis.

Outcomes reporting component

The performance of screening is measured as the difference between the experience of the women when screened versus not screened. Mortality reduction is measured as the decrement in deaths due to ovarian cancer divided by the ovarian cancer deaths occurring in the absence of screening, among cases with disease present during the screening period. Death is assumed to be attributable to ovarian cancer if it occurs at a younger age than death in the absence of ovarian cancer. Age at death from cancer is selected from the relevant age- and stage-specific relative survival curve based on the randomly selected aggressiveness of the tumor. If screening results in diagnosis of cancer at a different age or stage, the age at death from cancer will usually change as a result of screening. Age at death from other causes is independently randomly selected from the all-cause mortality distribution curve, adjusted for ovarian cancer mortality. If the age at death from cancer exceeds the randomly selected life expectancy of the woman, her death is attributed to other causes rather than to her cancer.

For cost-effectiveness analysis, the health benefits of the screening program are measured in years of life saved (YLS). For each woman, YLS is the difference between the age at death with and without the screen. For each woman, the YLS from a screening strategy is defined as the difference in age at death with and without screening, regardless of the cause of death. The monetary benefit (cost) of the strategy is similarly the difference in costs with and without the screen, including treatment, screening, and diagnosis costs.

All costs are measured in 1998 US dollars and all costs and benefits are discounted by 3% to 1998, the time at which the investment decision is made. Discounting has the effect of weighting costs and benefits that occur in the future less heavily than those that occur immediately; it is appropriate in the context of trial design when considering the costs and benefits of intervening in the population after the protocol tested in the trial is adopted.[17,18] The model simulates a large number of women, calculating discounted YLS and costs for each, then sums over all women.

The costs of screening and diagnosis are assumed for the base case to be $25 for CA125, $50 for TVS, and $4500 for laparoscopy, including both physician and facility fees. Although charges for TVS are usually much higher than this (over $100), it has been reported that when high volumes of women are screened the costs per screen could be as low as $25.[19]

The costs of initial and ongoing treatment for ovarian cancer over the 15 years following diagnosis, within stage of diagnosis, were estimated from SEER-Medicare data.[20] Costs for the first 5 years are shown in Table 28.3. Savings in treatment costs, the monetary benefits of screening, are calculated for each case with a shift from distant to local or regional stage, or from regional to

Table 28.3 Costs (in 1998 US dollars) of initial and ongoing treatment for ovarian cancer

Year post-diagnosis	Stage I	Stage II	Stage III	Stage IV
Year 1	$21,345	$34,148	$37,531	$37,531
Year 2	$2,970	$10,567	$14,050	$14,050
Year 3	$3,127	$7,442	$11,861	$11,861
Year 4	$3,555	$4,741	$9,023	$9,023
Year 5	$2,120	$5,194	$7,810	$7,810

local stage, as the difference in the net present value of the costs over her remaining lifetime with and without the screen. It is possible for treatment costs to be higher with than without the screen.

Validation methods

We have validated our model by assessing its ability to reproduce or predict the results of published screening studies. Specifically, we have demonstrated that the results of the screening pilot study conducted by Jacobs *et al.*[3,4] are consistent with the predictions of the natural history and detection components of our model. To the extent that we cannot validate our model with external information, sensitivity analyses have been performed using revised model parameters that indicate plausible ranges that these parameters may take yet still be consistent with the outcomes of the trials. The sensitivity analyses and validation results are presented in the results section.

Source of data for validation

Jacobs *et al.* reported the results of two studies that we have used for model validation: a prevalence screen study that screened 22 000 women, and a RCT that randomized the same 22 000 women to a screened group and a no-screening control group. Both studies screened subjects using the multimodal strategy involving CA125 above 30 U/ml as a first-line screen to select women for TVS.[3] The prevalence screen was a one-time only screen, but the RCT had three annual screens. There was a substantial delay between the prevalence screen and the RCT, with women not being randomized for the RCT for up to 3 years after the prevalence screen.

The microsimulation natural history and screening components mimic the experience of these 22 000 women. We have evaluated the microsimulation model by determining the degree to which it may predict the findings of Jacobs' trial. We were particularly interested in the ability of the model to reproduce certain important outcomes that are not fixed by the model inputs. With the prevalence screen we evaluated the total number of cancers, the rate of screen detection versus interval cancers, and the stage distribution at detection for cases by their detection mode (i.e. stage distribution for screen detected, screened but clinically detected, and interval cancer cases). With the RCT, we evaluated the stage distribution at detection by treatment arm and detection mode and the mean lead time.

Hypothesis testing

We evaluated the trial formally in a manner similar in spirit to Fisher's randomization test. We configured the simulation model independently from the study results, and treated its validity as a null hypothesis, *H0: model is valid*. We then used the model to replicate the Jacobs studies 1000 times. These 1000 simulated trials described a predictive distribution under the null hypothesis, and the fraction of values as extreme or more extreme than found by Jacobs approximated a one-sided *P* value that evaluated the null hypothesis; low *P* values suggested that our model is invalid. To be conservative, we used a one-sided *P* value with a cutoff at 0.025.

Estimation of lead time

We will discuss briefly how we defined lead time and estimated it in the Jacobs trial because it is such an important summary of screening performance. An individual's lead time is the number of days between her screen detection and the time when her clinical detection *would have occurred* had she not been screened. The average lead time, a summary of screening performance, is the average of the individual lead times for all screen-detected subjects. Within the microsimulation model we can identify the individual lead times and so can compute the mean from them directly, but this is not possible in screening trials. However, we can still estimate the mean lead time as follows.

An intention to treat evaluation of lead time, one that ignores screen detection status, would compute the difference of average duration from randomization to detection for the screened and unscreened groups. Because the screened group includes both screen-detected and clinically detected subjects, this intention to treat estimate is biased too small for estimating the lead-time effect of screen detection. We can adjust for the bias with the following formula (here *TDx* is the time from randomization to cancer diagnosis):

$$\text{Mean Lead Time} = \frac{\textit{Average}\,(\textit{TDx}\text{ Screened Group}) - \textit{Average}\,(\textit{TDx}\text{ Control Group})}{\text{Percent of screen group detected by screening}}$$

The numerator of the above expression is the intention to treat estimate. The assumptions needed for this estimator to be valid are quite general, and are found in McIntosh.[21] The mean lead time calculation above, when applied to screening trial data having appropriate follow-up past the final screen, estimates the mean of the individual lead times. By 'appropriate follow-up' we mean that the follow-up past the final screen exceeds the preclinical period of the disease, so that the number of cancers in the control group catches up with the number of cancers in the screened group.

Analyses performed using the model

To provide a benchmark against which to evaluate candidate strategies, we defined a hypothetical 'perfect' screening test with sensitivity and specificity of 100% and a cost of $25. We analyzed mortality reduction first for the perfect screen, to define the limits of screening at various intervals under different assumptions about the overall duration of the disease. We then identified *efficient* strategies from among the 12 candidate screening strategies for each age group of women, comparing them to the perfect screen as a benchmark. Efficient strategies are defined as those that achieve a given level of YLS at minimum cost. Efficient and other strategies of interest were ranked by YLS so that *incremental cost per YLS* (CPYLS) could be estimated.

Screening strategies analyzed

Table 28.4 describes the three screening protocols. In all protocols, if TVS cannot be performed or is inadequate, transabdominal ultrasound is employed. All employ immediate laparoscopy for

Table 28.4 Ovarian cancer screening strategies

TVS: TVS (transvaginal sonography) is performed as a first-line screen. If TVS is positive, the woman is referred for laparoscopy

CA125 elevation: CA125 is performed as a first-line screen. If CA125 exceeds 30 U/ml the woman is referred for TVS. If TVS is positive, she is referred for laparoscopy

ROC algorithm: CA125 is performed as a first-line screen. If CA125 is rising, the woman is referred for TVS, or recalled for repeat CA125 to confirm an exponential rise. If TVS is positive, she is referred for laparoscopy

definitive diagnosis. If malignancy is confirmed, laparotomy and oophorectomy are performed. If a significant benign condition is found by laparoscopy, it is surgically explored, prophylactic oophorectomy is performed, and periodic screening is discontinued. Each of the three protocols is evaluated in a periodic screening program with screening intervals of 6, 12, 18, and 24 months, applied either to women aged 50–64 or 50–80.

Approximation of the ROC algorithm

One of the screening strategies we evaluated was the ROC algorithm, which relies on analysis of CA125 change over time to detect an exponential rise in the marker. Designed by Skates, this elegant approach uses all of the available data from prior screens in a multimodal strategy. It results in 2% of women screened by CA125 being referred *directly* from the first CA125 screen to TVS each year, and 13% being recalled for repeat CA125 in 6 weeks to 6 months, depending on their CA125 levels and changes. Following the recall, a woman can be referred for TVS, recalled again for CA125, or returned to annual screening. Up to five recall CA125 tests can be performed before a woman is scheduled for her next annual screen 12 months from the last recall. At recall, another 2% of women are referred for TVS, for a total of 2.26% at each annual screen.

The ROC algorithm uses a model of how the markers behave both before and after the onset of cancer in a computationally intensive manner to substantially increase the efficiency of CA125 compared to the more traditional single-threshold use. For simplicity and computational efficiency, we approximated the ROC algorithm in the simulation model using parametric empirical Bayes (PEB) methods.[22,23] The ROC algorithm assumes that markers increase at an exponential growth rate after the onset of cancer and uses this assumption to maximize the efficiency of screening with CA125. The PEB approximation, like the ROC algorithm, uses a woman's individual screening history to determine her screening status, and assumes the same underlying pre-cancer marker behavior as the ROC algorithm. However, the PEB does not specifically represent the post-cancer marker behavior, instead assuming only a general elevation in CA125. Although the PEB approximation captures much of the efficiency gain of the ROC algorithm, it cannot achieve all of it. Thus, the ROC algorithm may achieve greater performance than we present here.

Results

Mortality reduction

Mortality reduction, the percent reduction in deaths due to ovarian cancer, was estimated for a hypothetical 'perfect' screening test under various assumptions about the duration of the disease, the frequency of screening, and the characteristics of the women screened. The results of the simulation suggest that frequent screening is needed if the disease duration is short. As can be seen in Fig. 28.1a, screening women aged 50–64 could reduce their mortality from ovarian cancer by as much as 50% if screening were performed every 6 months. Less frequent screening could achieve the same mortality reduction only if the disease progresses more slowly than we have assumed. For any given duration of disease, mortality reduction falls as the frequency of screening decreases. Similarly, for any given screening frequency, mortality

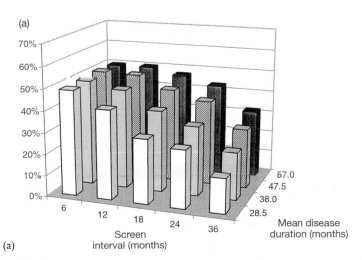

(a)

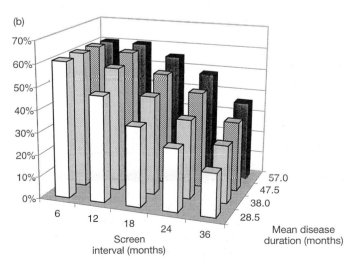

(b)

Fig. 28.1 Mortality reduction using the hypothetical screen with sensitivity and specificity of 100%, screening women aged (a) 50–64 years and (b) 50–80 years.

reduction falls as the duration of the disease decreases. The pattern is the same if women aged 50–80 are screened but the mortality reduction is about 10 percentage points higher.

Identification of efficient strategies

The microsimulation model was used to identify efficient screening strategies for each age group. For each of the 12 candidate protocols, total costs and years of life saved (YLS) attributable to each of the strategies were estimated. Efficient strategies are identified by plotting each strategy where Y = costs per 1 000 000 women screened and X = YLS per 1 000 000 women screened, as shown in Fig. 28.2. The strategies are identified by a prefix denoting the protocol and a suffix indicating the number of months between screens. Candidate protocols are transvaginal sonography (TVS) as a first-line screen, a multimodal strategy (E30) using CA125 as a first-line screen followed by TVS if CA125 exceeds 30 U/ml, and an approximation of the risk of cancer (ROC) algorithm. The efficient strategies are those for which no other strategy exists which yields the same (or more) YLS at a lower cost. The perfect screen is also included in these figures as a point of reference to depict the room for improvement with improved screening technology. It is based on a hypothetical first-line screen that is 100% sensitive and specific and costs $25.

As shown in the figures, the ROC approximation is efficient relative to TVS and E30. The ROC algorithm used annually performs

as well at lower cost than TVS used as a first-line screen every 18 months. Similarly, the ROC algorithm used every 6 months outperforms TVS used as a first-line screen annually. However, it does not perform as well as the 'perfect' screen.

Cost-effectiveness of efficient strategies

Cost-effectiveness is reported only for selected strategies, based on the results of the efficiency analysis. The single threshold rule (E30) is not competitive, so it is dropped from the analyses. The ROC algorithm is more efficient than TVS but the differences are small, so the ROC and TVS are considered for both age groups of women at screening intervals that yield mortality reduction and costs per YLS saved in a desirable range. As can be seen from Fig. 28.3, screening the older women using these strategies is more efficient than restricting screening to women aged 50–64.

The cost-effectiveness and related performance characteristics of selected strategies are shown in Table 28.5. To show the limits of a screening program given base-case assumptions regarding the natural history of the disease, the performance characteristics of a hypothetical 'perfect screen' used annually are also shown. The efficient strategies are shown in bold. The estimates suggest that if screening is confined to women aged 50–64, the ROC algorithm used at a 6-month interval might reduce mortality by 36%, saving 7 years of life per case at a cost of $32 000 per YLS. If women aged 50–80 are screened, the ROC algorithm used annually might

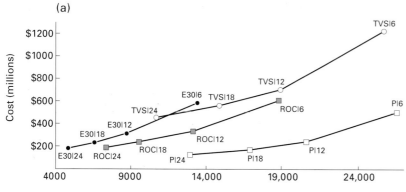

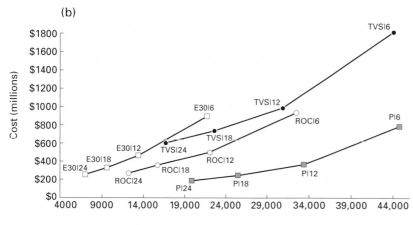

Fig. 28.2 Efficiency of various ovarian cancer screening strategies in women aged (a) 50–64 years and (b) 50–80 years. Costs and benefits discounted at 3%.

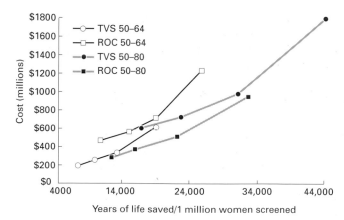

Fig. 28.3 Efficiency of screening women aged 50–64 versus 50–80 years, using TVS or the ROC algorithm. Costs and benefits discounted at 3%.

reduce mortality by 31%, saving an average of 4 years of life per case at a cost of $23 000 per YLS.

Validation and sensitivity analyses

The validation results are demonstrated visually by Fig. 28.4, which uses the screening trial lead time (top row) and number of cancers found at the prevalence screen (bottom row) to assess the model fit. The middle column of each row shows the validation when using the base-case configuration discussed throughout the chapter. The columns to the left and right are used for sensitivity analysis, and are discussed below. The middle, top-row histogram represents the 1000 mean lead times found by the simulation model, and the solid vertical line through the histogram represents the mean lead time found by Jacobs (see discussion of lead time calculation that follows). Because the line falls well within the range of the histogram, we conclude that the model's lead time finding is consistent with Jacobs' RCT lead time. Put another way, the Jacobs result is well within the range of the stochastic noise of the simulation model. The area more extreme than the Jacobs' lead time, the area to the right of the solid line, represents the P

value; here $P = 0.493$. The bottom row, middle histogram represents the number of cancer cases found at the prevalence screen, and the vertical line represents the number found by Jacobs. The P value equals 0.031, is greater than the 0.025 cutoff, and so is consistent with Jacobs' results to the customary levels, but is low enough that we will evaluate it in a sensitivity analysis below.

Table 28.6 summarizes all quantitative measures used in the validity tests performed using the Jacobs results. The table has size columns, which are: name of measure (see below), the value observed in the Jacobs studies, the median value of the 1000 simulations, the low and high values for a 95% prediction interval, and a P value to assess the test. The prediction interval describes the range in which 95% of the 1000 simulated values fall. If the Jacobs results fall in this range then we cannot reject the null hypothesis of a valid model. The P value represents the percentage of observations that are more or as extreme as the Jacobs value. These are one-sided P values and so should be compared to a 0.025 level for rejection. The rows are divided into three categories by their measures. The 'control group' section gives the total number of cases found in the control group during the entire 7-year period of screening and follow-up, and gives the percentage of the cancers found in stage I. The 'screen group' section gives the percentage of the screen group cancers found in stage I, and the 'screen detected' section evaluates the subset of subjects whose cancer was detected by screening, giving their number and the fraction of early stage cancers. The 'prevalence screen' section includes measures in the last three rows, including the number of positive screens (i.e. elevated CA125 and positive sonography), the total number of cancers found at the prevalence screen, and the fraction of cancers found in stage I.

Validation sensitivity test

The base-case simulations represented in Table 28.6 and in Fig. 28.4 suggest that overall our microsimulation is consistent with Jacobs' results. However, one important measure, the number of diagnosed cancers at the prevalence screen, may be too low. One possible reason for this underdiagnosis is an inaccurate approximation to the disease duration. The standard configura-

Table 28.5 Cost-effectiveness of alternative strategies for women aged 50–64 and 50–80 years

Strategy	% Cases detected by screen	% Cases detected in Stage I	Sensitivity (based on 1 yr of follow-up)	YLS/case	Surgeries/ detected cancer	Cost/YLS (discounted)	% Mortality reduction
Women aged 50–64 years							
Perfect (12)	82.8%	75.0%	81.7%	7.69	1.00	$11 748	41.5%
ROC (6)	**72.9%**	**67.3%**	**75.2%**	**6.96**	**4.35**	**$32 591**	**36.4%**
TVS (12)	79.3%	68.2%	79.1%	7.00	11.68	$37 316	37.0%
TVS (18)	75.3%	52.0%	82.9%	5.57	12.28	$37 862	27.0%
ROC (12)	**65.4%**	**48.8%**	**68.3%**	**4.89**	**3.63**	**$25 419**	**26.7%**
Woman aged 50–80 years							
Perfect (12)	84.0%	73.9%	83.7%	6.21	1.01	$11 109	47.0%
ROC (6)	**78.2%**	**70.5%**	**78.9%**	**6.03**	**3.23**	**$29 323**	**45.1%**
TVS (12)	81.6%	67.5%	81.6%	5.71	6.35	$32 286	42.3%
TVS (18)	70.9%	52.3%	84.9%	4.20	7.09	$32 843	31.8%
ROC (12)	**70.9%**	**50.5%**	**71.9%**	**4.10**	**2.72**	**$23 133**	**31.0%**

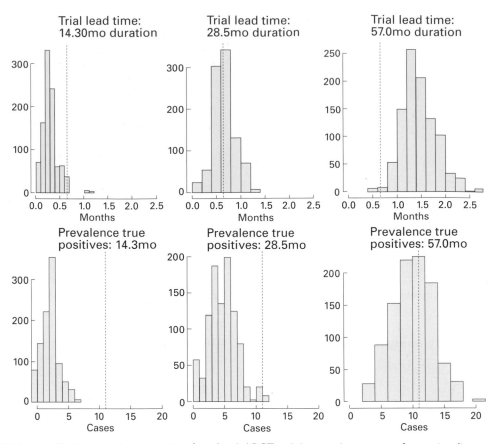

Fig. 28.4 Validation of lead time and true positives from Jacobs' RCT and the prevalence screen for varying disease duration.

Table 28.6 Summary of validation study hypothesis tests (*P* value), upper (high) and lower (low) 95% intervals, and median, for comparison to values found by Jacobs for selected outcome measures. *P* values are one sided, so the traditional cutoff should be 0.025

Validation measure	Observed in Jacobs study	Median of 1000 simulations	Low	High	P value
Lead time	0.650	0.651	0.198	1.143	0.493
Control group					
Total cases in control	20.000	28.000	19.000	36.000	0.061
Percent Stage I	0.050	0.182	0.045	0.326	0.046
Screen group					
Percent stage I	0.250	0.219	0.053	0.378	0.375
Screen detected cancers					
Total screens detected	6.000	7.000	3.000	13.275	0.472
Percent stage I	0.500	0.300	0.000	0.714	0.185
Prevalence screen cancers					
Predictive positive	41.000	52.000	33.000	67.000	0.101
Total cancers	11.000	5.000	1.000	11.000	0.031
Percent stage I	0.273	0.250	0.000	0.667	0.384

tion uses the stage lengths reported by Skates and Singer,[10] giving stage I a mean duration of 9 months. These values are used in the base-case (center column) simulations used in the validation. The histograms in the left and right columns of Fig. 28.4 represent the model's predictions when the stage durations are halved or doubled. The left column of Fig. 28.4 shows that halving the stage lengths makes the model inconsistent with both the prevalence

screen and the RCT. The right column of figures, representing the results of doubling the stage lengths, gives the prevalence screen a good fit, but now makes the RCT lead time too large to be consistent with Jacobs' results. From this we can conclude that the value of stage length that gives the best overall validity lies between the 9-month stage I length used in the base case and the 18-month stage I duration. To be conservative, we used the 9-month stage I duration as our base case. This avoids overfitting the model to the relatively small Jacobs cohort, and also gives conservative estimates of screening performance.

Discussion

Conclusions

An algorithm to detect exponential rise in CA125 compares favorably with TVS as a first-line screen, but requires more frequent screening to achieve the same mortality reduction and YLS. Based on the assumption that TVS and CA125 cost $50 and $25 respectively, our estimates suggest that use of the CA125 change over time (ROC approximation) algorithm at a 6-month interval in women aged 50–64 might reduce ovarian cancer mortality by over 30% for a cost per YLS of under $35 000. TVS used annually as a first-line screen in the same age group performs comparably, at a cost per YLS of just over $35 000. An RCT is needed to test the efficacy of TVS and/or the ROC algorithm in reducing ovarian cancer mortality.

Mortality reduction and cost-effectiveness are improved if women aged 50–80 are screened: the ROC algorithm used annually achieves 30% mortality reduction in this age group for under $30 000 per YLS. This is because older women experience poorer survival when they are diagnosed at a late stage, but similar survival when diagnosed at an early stage. In addition, older women are more likely than younger women to be diagnosed with advanced cancer in the absence of screening, as shown in Table 28.1.

Limitations

The predictions of a microsimulation model are only as good as the assumptions it is based on. In particular, predictions regarding mortality reduction must be interpreted with caution. They are based on assumptions regarding improvement in survival resulting from stage shifts; such improvements have not been demonstrated in an RCT. In addition, measurement of mortality reduction is based on the presence of disease during the screening period, an unobservable phenomenon. Mortality is measured over the entire screening period, with follow-up for the lifetime of the woman. For all these reasons, the mortality reduction reported here should not be expected in an RCT.

Many aspects of ovarian cancer screening are still poorly understood, including the rate of disease progression, whether or not benign masses are a risk factor for subsequent malignant disease, and to what extent TVS and CA125 detect different cancers.[24] Although color Doppler imaging (CDI) offers an opportunity to improve significantly the positive predictive value (PPV) of imaging, the sensitivity of imaging is largely determined by assumptions about the average duration of the disease and the periodicity of the screen. As reported in Table 28.5, if the average duration of stage I disease is 9 months, the model predicts that in an annual screening program the sensitivity cannot be higher than 84%, even if it is assumed that all tumors are immediately detectable by imaging.

Quality of life effects of screening should also be considered, including long-term effects of false positives and oophorectomy. New markers are under development, such as lysophosphatidic acid (LPA),[25] and molecular discoveries may lead to the identification of many more. It is possible that eventually a panel of markers will be identified that, used together as a first-line screen in a multimodel strategy involving imaging, will yield higher sensitivity and therefore greater mortality reduction than currently available strategies. Our understanding of ovarian cancer disease progression and detection will be improved by analysis of data from a large, well-designed RCT. It is time to plan an international trial or set of trials to test the hypothesis that screening and early detection prevent mortality from ovarian cancer.

References

1. van Nagell, J.R. Jr, Depriest, P., Puls, L. *et al.* (1991). Ovarian cancer screening in asymptomatic postmenopausal women by transvaginal sonography. *Cancer*, **68**, 458–62.
2. Parkes, C.A., Smith, D., Wald, N.F., and Bourne, T.H. (1994). Feasibility study of a randomised trial of ovarian cancer screening among the general population. *J. Med. Screen.*, **1**, 209–14.
3. Jacobs, I., Davies, A.P., Bridges, J. *et al.* (1993). Prevalence screening for ovarian cancer in post-menopausal women by CA 125 measurement and ultrasonography. *BMJ*, **306**, 1030–4.
4. Jacobs, I., Skates, S.J., MacDonald, N. *et al.* (1999). Screening for ovarian cancer: a pilot randomized controlled trial. *Lancet*, **353** (9160), 1207–10.
5. Skates, S., Jacobs, I., and Knapp, R. (1998). Quantifying risk of ovarian cancer using longitudinal CA125 levels. In *Ovarian Cancer 5*, (ed. F. Sharp), pp. 187–97. Isis Medical Media, Oxford.
6. Urban, N., Drescher, C., Etzioni, R., and Colby, C. (1997). Use of a stochastic simulation model to identify an efficient strategy for ovarian cancer screening. *Control Clin. Trials*, **18**, 251–70.
7. US Department of Health and Human Services (1985). *US Decennial Life Tables for 1979–81*. United States Life Tables, vol. 1, number 1.
8. Kosary, C.L., Ries, L.A.G., Miller, B.A. *et al.* (1995). *SEER Cancer Statistics Review 1973–1992*. NIH Publication No. 96–2789, National Cancer Institute.
9. Wun *et al.* (1998). Estimating lifetime and age-conditional probabilities of developing cancer. *Lifetime Data Analysis*, **4**, 169–86.
10. Skates, S.J. and Singer, D.E. (1991). Quantifying the potential benefit of CA125 screening for ovarian cancer. *J. Clin. Epidemiology*, **44**, 365–80.
11. Campbell, S., Bhan, V., Royston, P. *et al.* (1989). Transabdominal ultrasound screening for early ovarian cancer. *BMJ*, **299**, 1363–7.
12. Campbell, S., Royston, P., Bhan, V *et al.* (1990). Novel screening strategies for early ovarian cancer by transabdominal ultrasonography. *Br. J. Obstet. Gynaecol.*, **97**, 304–11.
13. DePriest, P.D., Varner, E., Powell, J. *et al.* (1994). The efficacy of a sonographic morphology index in identifying ovarian cancer by transabdominal ultrasonography. *Br. J. Obstet. Gynaecol.*, **97**, 302–11.
14. Bell, R., Petticrew, M., and Sheldon, T. (1998). The performance of screening tests for ovarian cancer: results of a systematic review. *Br. J. Obstet. Gynaecol.*, **105**, 1136–47.
15. Bourne, T., Campbell, S., Steer, C. *et al.* (1989). Transvaginal color flow imaging; a possible new screening technique for ovarian cancer. *BMJ*, **299**, 1367–70.
16. Prorok, presented in London, April 1997.
17. Detsky, A.S. (1990). Using cost-effectiveness analysis to improve the efficiency of allocating funds to clinical trials. *Stat. Med.*, **9**, 173–84.
18. Urban, N. and Baker, M. (1989). The Women's Health Trial as an investment. *Medical Decision Making*, **9**, 59–64.

19. Pavlik, E.J., van Nagell, J.R. Jr, DePreist, P.D. *et al.* (1995). Participation in transvaginal ovarian cancer screening: Compliance, correlation factors and cost. *Gynecol. Oncol.*, **57**, 395–400.

20. Etzioni, R., Urban, N., and Baker, M. (1995). Estimating the costs attributable to a disease with application to ovarian cancer. *J. Clin. Epidemiol*, **49**, 95–103.

21. McIntosh, M.W. (1999). Instrumental variables for evaluating screening trials: estimating the benefit of detecting cancer by screening. *Stat. Med.*, **30**; 18(20), 2775–94.

22. Morris, C.N. (1983). Parametric empirical Baye inference: theory and applications. *JASA*, **78**, 47–65.

23. Efron, B. and Morris, R. (1977). Stein's paradox in statistics. *Sci. Am.*, **236**, 119–27.

24. Karlan, B., Baldwin, R., Lopez-Luevanos, E. *et al.* (1999). Peritoneal serous papillary carcinoma, a phenotypic variant of familial ovarian cancer: indications for ovarian cancer screening. *Am. J. Obstet. Gynecol.*, **180**, 917–28.

25. Xu, Y., Shen, Z., Wiper, D. *et al.* (1998). Lysophosphatidic acid as a potential biomarker for ovarian and other gynecologic cancers. *JAMA*, **280**(8), 719–23.

29. The management of familial ovarian cancer

Paul D. Pharoah and James Mackay

Introduction

Knowledge about the epidemiology and genetics of cancer has accrued rapidly over the past two decades, partly as a result of prodigious advances that have been made in molecular genetics. However, there is a substantial hiatus between this knowledge and its application to clinical practice, with ovarian cancer providing a notable example.

In the 1950s, families in which transmission of ovarian cancer occurs according to the rules of Mendelian inheritance were first described. Subsequently, in the 1960s and 1970s, a variety of hereditary cancer syndromes were defined, including the Lynch syndrome and hereditary breast–ovarian cancer syndrome, which include ovarian cancer as part of the characteristic phenotype. The genes that cause these syndromes were then mapped and isolated during the 1980s and 1990s.

When an individual presents to a family cancer specialist because she has concerns about ovarian cancer, there are three fundamental questions that need to be addressed before that specialist can confidently advise and manage the individual:

1. Is the aggregation of cancer in this family due to a fault in one of the known cancer susceptibility genes?
2. What are the cancer risks in this individual and other members of her family?
3. Can anything be done to reduce or eliminate the cancer risk?

Although we are particularly concerned with the management of familial ovarian cancer, the risks of other cancers may also be substantial and possible interventions to reduce these additional risks have to be considered. It should also be noted that, in general, the answers to these questions are related. For example the ovarian cancer risk will depend on whether or not there is a mutation in the *BRCA1* or *BRCA2* susceptibility genes.

In this chapter we will review the science that addresses each of these questions in turn, and also highlights many areas of uncertainty. We then discuss how this scientific background can be applied to provide a framework for the management of the individual who presents with a family history of ovarian cancer.

Inherited ovarian cancer

We will address the first question (Is the aggregation of cancer in this family due to a fault in one of the known cancer susceptibility genes?), by first describing the known susceptibility genes. We will then consider the evidence that one of these genes accounts for the aggregation of cancer seen in any given family.

The aggregation of ovarian cancer in families usually occurs in three forms. Site-specific familial ovarian cancer is the familial clustering of ovarian cancer in the absence of other cancer phenotypes in the family. In this context a familial cluster is usually considered to be the presence of two or more ovarian cancers occurring in first-degree relatives. Ovarian cancer in families is more commonly associated with early onset breast cancer as part of the hereditary breast–ovarian cancer syndrome (HBOC).[1] Finally, ovarian cancer may also occur in families with hereditary non-polyposis colorectal carcinoma (HNPCC or the Lynch syndrome). The management of these families is mainly concerned with the management of the risk of colorectal carcinoma, and will not be considered further here.

Site-specific familial ovarian cancer and the hereditary breast–ovarian cancer syndrome

No gene that confers increased susceptibility to ovarian cancer alone has yet been isolated, and so site-specific familial ovarian cancer and the hereditary breast–ovarian cancer syndrome are part of the same spectrum.

BRCA1 on chromosome 17q12–21 was the first major breast–ovarian cancer susceptibility gene locus to be identified. Convincing evidence for the locus was first published in 1990, and came from a linkage study of 23 families with multiple cases of breast cancer among relatives.[2] *BRCA1* was subsequently cloned in 1994.[3,4] Prior to its identification, other linkage studies had indicated that *BRCA1* was responsible for a large proportion of families with cases of breast cancer only (45%) and virtually all families with cases of breast cancer in association with epithelial ovarian cancer, and site-specific ovarian cancer families.

A second major breast ovarian cancer locus (*BRCA2*) was mapped to chromosome 13q12–13 in 1995[5] and the gene isolated 1 year later.[6] Initial studies indicated that the majority of families with evidence against linkage to the *BRCA1* locus were linked to *BRCA2*.

Proportion of ovarian cancer families due to BRCA1 and BRCA2

There have been many studies of the contribution of *BRCA1* and *BRCA2* to hereditary breast and ovarian cancer families.[7] Most of these studies have been based on families that have been ascertained because of the aggregation of breast cancer. An analysis of 237 families with at least four cases of breast cancer has been performed by the Breast Cancer Linkage Consortium to estimate the proportion of families that are due to *BRCA1* and *BRCA2*.[8] Families were selected without regard to the occurrence of ovarian or other cancers. Using a combination of mutation data and linkage data, it was estimated that 52% of families were due to *BRCA1*, 32% of families were due to *BRCA2*, and 16% of families were not due to either gene. As predicted from previous studies using linkage data alone, almost all families with breast and ovarian cancer were due either to *BRCA1* (81% of families) or *BRCA2* (14% of families). However, these results may not apply to families ascertained because of the clustering of ovarian cancer.

There have been two studies of families ascertained because of ovarian cancer clustering. The largest study was based on 112 families registered with the UKCCCR Familial Ovarian Cancer Register, that have been tested for mutations in *BRCA1* and *BRCA2*.[9] The proportion of these families that were found to have a mutation varied according to the extent of the family history (Table 29.1).

The majority of families with an extensive family history (at least four members affected with ovarian or breast cancer) can be accounted for by *BRCA1*, with a handful due to *BRCA2*. Nevertheless, even in these families, no mutation was found in nearly a third of families. In the 'two cases of ovarian cancer only' families, *BRCA1* and *BRCA2* accounted for only one-fifth of families.

A segregation analysis of these families suggested that a combination of chance clustering of sporadic cases and insensitivity of the methods may account for the *BRCA1/2*-negative families. However, the possibility that other susceptibility genes exist (as yet unidentified) could not be excluded.

Cancer risks associated with BRCA1 and BRCA2 mutations

A variety of methods have been used to estimate the breast and ovarian cancer penetrance for *BRCA1* and *BRCA2*. Several of these have used data derived from multiple-case breast and breast/ovarian cancer families. Others have used data from population breast and ovarian cancer case series. Ford *et al.* obtained a direct estimate of breast and ovarian cancer risks by examining the risks of second cancers in individuals with breast cancer from 33 families linked to *BRCA1*[10] and Easton *et al.* used the same families to estimate cancer-specific penetrance of *BRCA1* by maximizing the LOD score over different penetrance functions.[11] The maximum LOD score method has also been used to estimate *BRCA2* penetrance using *BRCA2* mutation families from the Breast Cancer Linkage Consortium.[8] Hopper *et al.* estimated penetrance using pedigree data from 18 *BRCA1* and *BRCA2* mutation carriers ascertained through a population-based series of breast cancer cases diagnosed under the age of 40.[12] Similarly, Antoniou *et al.* used family history data from 12 *BRCA1* mutation carriers identified from an unselected series of 374 ovarian cancer cases.[13] Thorlacius *et al.* identified 69 carriers and 506 non-carriers of the *BRCA2* mutation 999del5 in a population-based series of breast cancer cases, and compared the history of cancer in first-degree relatives of carriers and non-carriers.[14] Whittemore *et al.* derived penetrance estimates for *BRCA1* from a segregation analysis of breast–ovarian cancer families ascertained via three population-based case-control studies of ovarian cancer.[15] In another study, estimates of the penetrance of *BRCA1* and *BRCA2* mutations were based on the family histories of 120 Ashkenazi Jews in whom one of three different founder mutations common to this population had been identified.[16] The breast and ovarian cancer risks estimated by these studies are shown in Figs 29.1–29.4.

Breast cancer risks for *BRCA1* and *BRCA2* appear to be similar, but those derived from population-based studies of breast cancer,[12,14] ovarian cancer,[13,17] and the Ashkenazi Jewish population[16] are lower than those derived from the multiple-case families.[10,11] Ovarian cancer risks derived from high-risk families are higher for *BRCA1*[10,11] than for *BRCA2*.[8] Of the population-based studies, the ovarian cancer risk for *BRCA1* reported by Antoniou *et al.*[13] was similar to that for high-risk families, whereas Whittemore *et al.* reported a risk that was somewhat lower,[15] and close to the ovarian cancer risk estimated by Struewing for *BRCA1* and *BRCA2* combined.[16] A low ovarian cancer penetrance for

Table 29.1 UKCCR Familial Ovarian Cancer Register study of ovarian cancer associated with *BRCA1* and *BRCA2*

Family history of cancer[a]	No. of families	BRCA1 (%)	BRCA2 (%)
At least two cases of ovarian cancer and at least two cases breast cancer	18	56	5
At least three cases ovarian cancer and no more than one case breast cancer	27	63	7
Two cases of ovarian cancer and one case breast cancer	17	29	18
Two cases of ovarian cancer and no cases of breast cancer	50	16	4
Total	112	36	7

[a]Confirmed cases of ovarian cancer diagnosed at any age, breast cancer diagnosed at age < 60 years.

THE MANAGEMENT OF FAMILIAL OVARIAN CANCER

211

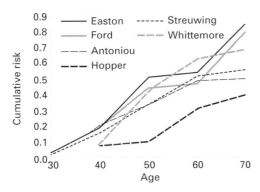

Fig. 29.1 Cumulative breast cancer risk in *BRCA1* mutation carriers. Population-based studies are indicated by a dotted line. Studies reported by Hopper *et al.* and Struewing *et al.* report penetrance estimates for *BRCA1* and *BRCA2* combined. References: Antoniou *et al.* (1999),[13] Easton *et al.* (1995),[11] Ford *et al.* (1994),[10] Hopper *et al.* (1999),[12] Struewing *et al.* (1997),[16] and Whittemore *et al.* (1997).[15]

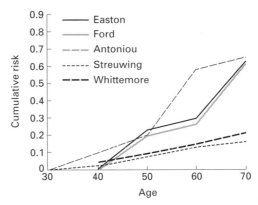

Fig. 29.2 Cumulative ovarian cancer risk in *BRCA1* mutation carriers. References: Antoniou (1999),[13] Easton (1995),[11] Ford (1994),[10] Struewing (1997),[16] and Whittemore (1997).[15]

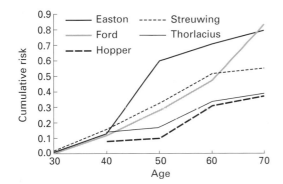

Fig. 29.3 Cumulative breast cancer risk in *BRCA2* mutation carriers. Studies reported by Hopper *et al.* and Struewing *et al.* report penetrance estimates for *BRCA1* and *BRCA2* combined. References: Easton *et al.* (1995),[11] Ford *et al.*, (1998),[8] Hopper *et al.* (1999),[12] Struewing *et al.* (1997),[16] and Thorlacius *et al.* (1998).[14]

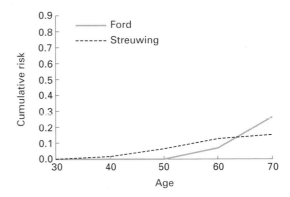

Fig. 29.4 Cumulative ovarian cancer risk in *BRCA2* mutation carriers. References: Ford (1998)[8] and Struewing *et al.* (1997).[16]

BRCA1 and *BRCA2* combined was also reported by Hopper *et al.*[12] In this study a specific ovarian cancer risks estimate was not reported, as no first- or second-degree relatives of the 18 mutation carriers were affected with ovarian cancer.

In addition to breast and ovarian cancer, *BRCA1* appears to confer slightly increased risks of prostate and colon cancer.[10] Likewise, mutations in *BRCA2* confer, in addition to risk of female breast cancer, male breast cancer and ovarian cancer, increased risks of prostate cancer, pancreatic cancer, gall bladder and bile duct cancer, stomach cancer, and malignant melanoma.[18]

The breast and ovarian cancer risk estimates described above are based on the assumption that the risks associated with all mutations are the same. There are, however, good data to support the hypothesis of allelic risk heterogeneity, that is that different mutations confer different risks. First, data from the BCLC suggest that the risk of ovarian cancer in a family varies between different families linked to the *BRCA1* locus. In the majority of these families there appears to be a high risk of breast cancer but a relatively low risk of ovarian cancer, while in a minority of families there appears to be an equally high risk of both breast and ovarian

cancer. Easton *et al.*[11] have shown that the observed patterns of disease risk are much better explained by a model with two different *BRCA1* susceptibility alleles; one conferring a cumulative breast cancer risk of 91% by age 70 and an ovarian cancer risk of 32%, the other conferring a breast cancer risk of 70% and an ovarian cancer risk of 84%. Furthermore, analysis of these and additional BCLC data suggested that when mutations occur in the first two-thirds of the *BRCA1* gene, the risk of ovarian cancer relative to breast cancer in the family is significantly higher than when truncating mutations occur in the last third of the gene.[19] A similar genotype–phenotype correlation with respect to risks of breast and ovarian cancer is seen in *BRCA2*. However, in *BRCA2*, mutations that occur in families with a high risk of ovarian cancer are clustered in a central portion of the gene, which has been termed the 'ovarian cancer cluster region'.[20]

The cause of the observed difference in the breast cancer penetrance estimated from the population-based studies and the high-risk families is not clear. Assuming that the difference is not simply due to chance, there must be some variation in penetrance between carriers. In principle, this could be due to allelic heterogeneity in risk, but the allelic heterogeneity described above is insufficient to account for the difference observed. A more important potential explanation is that there may be other factors that modify risk. These could be modifier genes or non-genetic factors, some of which may be related to lifestyle.

Gene–gene and gene–environment interactions

There is mounting evidence to support the assertion that the risks of cancer in *BRCA1* and *BRCA2* families are modified both by genetic background and environmental factors.

Low parity is a well-established risk factor for sporadic breast cancer and has also been shown to be associated with an increased breast cancer risk in women found by haplotype analysis to carry *BRCA1* mutations.[21] In contrast, the risk of ovarian cancer in *BRCA1* carriers was found to increase significantly with increasing parity, which is the opposite effect to that seen for sporadic ovarian cancer.[21] Cigarette smoking is thought to have minimal effect on sporadic breast cancer risk, but in one study, subjects with *BRCA1* or *BRCA2* gene mutations and breast cancer were significantly more likely to have been non-smokers than control (unaffected) subjects with mutations.[22] As with sporadic cancer, oral-contraceptive use may reduce the risk of ovarian cancer in women with pathogenic mutations in the *BRCA1* or *BRCA2* gene.[23]

Genes that have been shown to alter cancer risks in mutation carriers include *HRAS1* and the androgen receptor gene (*AR*). Rare alleles of a variable number tandem repeat (VNTR) polymorphism located about 1 kb downstream of the *HRAS1* proto-oncogene on chromosome 11p15.5 confer an increased risk of breast cancer.[24] These alleles do not seem to be associated with an increased risk of breast cancer in *BRCA1* carriers, but they may be associated with an increased risk of ovarian cancer.[25] Breast cancer risk does appear to be altered by a polymorphism in the *AR* gene; age at breast cancer diagnosis is earlier among *BRCA1* mutation carriers with very long *AR* CAG repeats.[26] A preliminary report from the same group has also suggested that the steroid hormone metabolism gene, *AIB1*, may alter breast cancer risk in *BRCA1* mutation carriers.[27]

Cancer risks in ovarian cancer families

However, in the case of women for whom a genetic cause has not been found, the risks of developing breast and ovarian cancer are less clear. In these cases, family cancer specialists must rely on the results of epidemiological studies performed on families with similar strong histories of ovarian cancer in order to estimate their patients' risks.

The majority of women with a family history of ovarian cancer have a single first-degree relative affected with ovarian cancer. For them, the risk of developing ovarian cancer is small. Meta-analysis of data from 15 case-control studies has shown that for women with a single first-degree relative affected with ovarian cancer, the relative risk of developing ovarian cancer is 3.1 (95% CI = 2.6–3.7),[28] which equates to a cumulative risk of 4% by age 70.

Only two studies have estimated this risk in women with two or more affected relatives, and these estimates have had wide confidence limits.[29,30] Easton *et al.* (1996) found the relative risk of death from ovarian cancer to be 24.15 (95% CI = 6.58–61.85) in a population-based cohort study of women with two first-degree relatives with confirmed ovarian cancer.[29] By contrast, in a population-based case-control study, Schildkraut *et al.* (1988) found the relative risk of developing ovarian cancer to be 2.10 (0.20–12.9) for women with two affected relatives.[30] A combined analysis of data from these studies estimated the relative risk of developing ovarian cancer to be 11.7 (5.3–25.9) for these women.[28]

Three studies have published estimates of the risk of developing breast cancer for women with two or more relatives with ovarian cancer. In the same study as described above, Easton *et al.* (1996) observed three breast cancer deaths compared to 0.68 expected deaths based on population death rates (relative risk (RR) = 4.41, 0.89–12.89).[29] In a retrospective cohort study of women with two or more relatives with reported ovarian cancer, Jishi *et al.* (1995) found the relative risk of developing breast cancer to be 2.52 (1.68 3.65).[31] Finally, Claus *et al.* (1993) calculated the lifetime risk of developing breast cancer to be 31% in a population-based case-control study of women with two first-degree relatives with ovarian cancer.[32] This approximates to a relative risk of 3.5. All these studies have wide confidence limits.

Data from the UKCCCR Familial Ovarian Cancer Register have been used to obtain more precise estimates of ovarian and breast cancer risks to women in ovarian cancer families. A cohort of unaffected women in these families has been followed for up to 8 years, and the number of observed incident cancers compared with the number expected based on national-, age-, sex-, and period-specific incidence rates for England and Wales. A total of 10 893 person years of follow-up data from 316 families were used for the ovarian cancer risk analysis and 11 936 person years of follow-up data from 319 families for the breast cancer risk analysis. The relative risk of ovarian cancer was found to be 7.18 (95% CI 3.82–12.3), declining from 16.0 (6.40–32.9) in women under 50 to 4.38 (1.60–9.52) in women aged 50 years and older. For breast cancer, the relative risk for women under 50 was 3.74 (2.04–6.28) and 1.79 (1.02–2.90) for women 50 years of age and older (average RR = 2.36, 1.59–3.37). These correspond to absolute risks by age 70 of 11% for ovarian cancer and 15% for breast cancer. When the analyses were restricted to families that had tested negative for mutations in the breast/ovarian cancer susceptibility genes, *BRCA1* and *BRCA2*, the ovarian cancer risk was 11.59 (3.12–29.7) and that of breast cancer 3.32 (1.52–6.31). The cumulative ovarian and breast cancer risks corresponding to these relative risk estimates are shown in Figs 29.5 and 29.6. For the purposes of counselling women in these families about their cancer risks, an important finding is that even in families where no mutation has been found, a substantial risk of both breast and ovarian cancer remains. This may suggest that other breast/ovarian cancer genes are segregating in these families, although the possibility of undetected *BRCA1/2* mutations must also be considered.

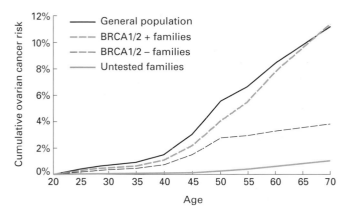

Fig. 29.5 Cumulative risk ovarian cancer in women with a strong family history of ovarian cancer. The cancer risk in the *BRCA1/2* families is less than cumulative risks associated with *BRCA1/2* mutations, because some women from these families will not be carriers of the mutation, and are therefore at population risk.

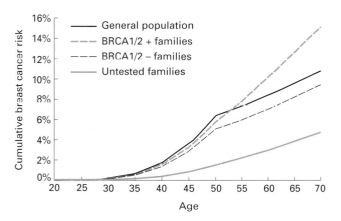

Fig. 29.6 Cumulative risk of breast cancer in women with strong family history of ovarian cancer.

Management of risk

There are three fundamental approaches to minimizing disease morbidity: the prevention of incident disease (primary prevention), the early detection of prevalent disease (secondary prevention), and the improved treatment of established disease (tertiary prevention). In the context of ovarian and breast cancer, primary prevention includes both interventions such as hormonal manipulation/chemoprophylaxis and prophylactic surgery. Early detection of ovarian cancer may be carried out using serum markers and/or ultrasound examination of the ovaries, which has been extensively reviewed in Chapters 00 and 00. For breast cancer, the mainstay of early detection is regular mammography, while the role of magnetic resonance imaging as a screening tool is being evaluated.

Ovarian cancer

Chemoprophylaxis

Ovarian cancer incidence in women at risk may be reduced by hormonal manipulation with the oral contraceptive pill. The use of combined oestrogen–progestin oral contraceptive type medication has been associated with decreased risk of ovarian cancer, not only in the general population, but also in women with a family history of ovarian cancer[33] and women with a mutation in *BRCA1* or *BRCA2*.[23] However, the benefit may be outweighed by the enhancement of breast cancer risk associated with exogenous oestrogens.[34]

Prophylactic surgery

Two studies have estimated the effect of bilateral prophylactic oophorectomy (BPO) on reducing ovarian cancer risk in women who may be at elevated ovarian cancer risk because of family history. Struewing *et al.*[35] studied 346 non-oophorectomized and 44 oophorectomized women in 'high-risk' families. Two post-BPO cases of intra-abdominal carcinomatosis and eight ovarian cancers in the non-BO group were observed. After adjusting for age and duration of follow-up, these results suggested a 50% risk reduction, but the study was too small to achieve statistical significance. Piver *et al.*[36] studied 324 women from the Gilda Radner Familial Ovarian Cancer Registry who underwent BPO, and reported six cases of intra-abdominal carcinomatosis 1–27 years following surgery. These suggest that BPO may reduce risk in women with *BRCA1* or *BRCA2* mutations, although no studies of BPO in women who carry a mutation in *BRCA1* or *BRCA2* have been reported.

Early detection

Currently available screening strategies for ovarian cancer consist of transvaginal ultrasound (TVS) and measurement of serum levels of CA125. The efficacy of these in the general population has been discussed previously. The data available on screening high-risk women is scanty. In a study of both transabdominal and transvaginal ultrasonography in self-referred women with a first- or second-degree relative with ovarian cancer, abnormalities requiring surgical exploration were found in 3.8% of screened women, of whom only 10% were found to have ovarian cancer (5 of 6 had stage I disease).[43] Five additional cases of cancer not detected by screening (three ovarian and two peritoneal) were reported 2–44 months after the last ultrasound.

In another study of 386 women with a first-degree relative or multiple second-degree relatives with ovarian cancer, using ultrasound and CA125, 15 women underwent exploratory laparotomies, 10 as a result of abnormal ultrasound findings alone, three as a result of abnormal CA125 levels and ultrasound findings, and two women because of rising CA125 levels. No cancer was identified in any of these women, one of whom sustained unrecognized small bowel damage requiring further surgery.[48] In a more recent study, 1261 women with a significant family history were followed up with transvaginal ultrasound with colour Doppler imaging and tumour marker estimation, including

CA125, initially every 2 years and then annually from 1995, giving a total of 6082 screening visits.[49] Three stage I ovarian cancers and seven cases of peritoneal serous papillary carcinoma were identified. All three cases of ovarian cancer were identified because of an abnormal ultrasound, and four of the seven peritoneal carcinoma cases were identified because of abnormal ultrasound (two cases) or elevated CA125 levels (two cases). The other three cases of peritoneal cancer were identified because of the development of abdominal or pelvic pain at 5, 6, and 15 months after their last normal screening visit. One of the Ashkenazi *BRCA1* mutations (185delAG) was identified in three of the seven patients with peritoneal cancer. Preliminary molecular data suggest that the primary peritoneal carcinomata were multifocal.

The authors do not clarify details of the family history inclusion criteria needed before volunteers were offered a place on this screening programme and it is unclear how many truly high-risk women were involved. These results do suggest that even if screening strategies involving serial CA125 measurement and regular ultrasound imaging are cost-effective in the postmenopausal normal-risk population, this may not be the case in the high- and moderate-risk population. Large, robust prospective clinical trials examining different screening strategies in the high- and moderate-risk groups are required urgently.

Breast cancer

Chemoprophylaxis

Possibilities for primary prevention of breast cancer have been restricted by our limited understanding of the aetiology of the disease. Although epidemiological studies in humans have consistently demonstrated that early menarche, late menopause, nulliparity, late age at first full-term pregnancy, and postmenopausal obesity are associated with significantly increased risk of breast cancer,[50] the potential to modify these risk factors in either the individual or the population is minimal. These factors are all thought to operate by increasing oestrogen exposure, which raises the possibility of primary prevention by hormonal manipulation. The potential for such chemoprevention was first confirmed by the observation that adjuvant therapy of primary breast cancer with tamoxifen reduced the incidence of contralateral breast cancer. Tamoxifen, however, has potentially serious side-effects and its use in a primary prevention setting could only be justified in women at high risk. Subsequently, several randomized controlled trials have been set up to test the hypothesis that tamoxifen reduces breast cancer risk in women at high risk of breast cancer. The first of these to report found a significantly reduced incidence of breast cancer in the women treated with tamoxifen,[51] although there were concerns that non-breast cancer morbidity and mortality was elevated. Two studies have been published since, and neither of these found a significant reduction in breast cancer incidence.[52,53] However, newer selective oestrogen receptor modulators, such as raloxifene, have a much more favourable side-effect profile, and may therefore prove more suitable as an agent for primary prevention. In a small study evaluating the effect of raloxifene on fractures in postmenopausal women, breast cancer incidence was assessed as a secondary endpoint and was found to be reduced by 76%.[54] Large

clinical trials are now in progress and should provide definitive results within a few years.

Prophylactic bilateral mastectomy

Prophylactic mastectomy is the only intervention for which there are good data on effectiveness. In women at moderate to high risk of breast cancer, the risk reduction is 90%.[55] Prophylactic oophorectomy may also reduce breast cancer risk by 50%.[56] However, surgical approaches are likely to be rejected by many women.

Early detection

The mainstay for secondary prevention of breast cancer is regular mammographic examination of the breast, which has been shown to reduce breast cancer mortality in women over the age of 50 in several clinical trials. Meta-analyses of these trials have shown that mammography will produce a relative reduction in breast cancer mortality of around 30% in these women.[57] The effectiveness of mammographic screening in younger women is controversial. A US National Cancer Institute workshop concluded that there was no proof of benefit for women under the age of 50,[58] although evidence of benefit in women aged 40–49 is mounting.[59] Even if the relative risk reduction were the same as in older women, the absolute benefit would be considerably reduced because breast cancer is less common in this age group. As a consequence the cost effectiveness of mammography in younger women is reduced and is likely to limit its application in the general population. However, the absolute benefit could potentially be improved by limiting mammography in young women to those at increased risk of breast cancer because of some other factor.

Unresolved issues

It is clear that there remain several unresolved issues that limit our ability to counsel women from ovarian cancer families:

1. Do the breast and ovarian cancer risks associated with mutations in *BRCA1* and *BRCA2* differ in site specific ovarian cancer families?
2. Are there genetic or environmental modifiers of risk?
3. What is the effectiveness of the various interventions to reduce cancer risks in women with a mutation in *BRCA1* or *BRCA2*?
4. What is the effectiveness of the various interventions to reduce cancer risks in women at increased risk because of family history in the absence of an identifiable inherited cause?

Nevertheless, a framework for managing these women, based on what is already known about familial and inherited ovarian (and breast) cancer, is essential for the delivery of clinical care.

Management framework

This framework is based on the strategy of stratifying women presenting with a family history of ovarian cancer into three risk categories based on the strength of that history: high risk, moderate risk, and low risk.

High risk

Inclusion criteria

- Four or more relatives affected at any age by breast or ovarian cancer.
- Three relatives affected with breast or ovarian cancer, with an average age of diagnosis of the breast cancer of less than 60 years.
- Two relatives affected by breast cancer, with an average age at diagnosis of less than 40 years.
- One relative with both breast and ovarian cancer at any age.

Management

If there is an alive, affected individual in the family, we offer to start searching for *BRCA1/2* mutations. If a mutation is identified in the family, then we offer direct genetic testing to unaffected family members if they wish it. Unaffected individuals who have been identified as carriers have a variety of options to choose from in the management of their breast and ovarian cancer risk. These have been described above.

Moderate risk

Inclusion criteria
- The family contains two or more individuals with ovarian cancer who are first-degree relatives.
- The family contains one individual with ovarian cancer and one individual with breast cancer diagnosed under 50 years who are first-degree relatives.
- The family contains one individual with ovarian cancer and two individuals with breast cancer diagnosed under 60 years who are connected by first-degree relationships.
- The family contains an affected individual with a mutation of one of the known ovarian cancer predisposing genes.
- The family contains three individuals with colorectal cancer, with at least one case diagnosed before 50 years, as well as one case of ovarian cancer, and all of these individuals are connected by first-degree relationships
- One first-degree female relative aged less than 40 years with breast cancer.

Families in which affected individuals are connected by second-degree relationships through an unaffected male are also eligible.

Management
Women from moderate-risk families who are over 35 and who have an affected first-degree relative are offered entry into the UKCCCR familial ovarian screening study, a single-arm prospective study of annual CA125 estimation and annual ultrasonography, after a full discussion of the potential false-negative and false-positive results.[60]

The advantages and disadvantages of prophylactic bilateral salpingo-oophorectomy are discussed, emphasizing particularly the important age-related issues; that the risk of developing ovarian cancer below the age of 40 is low, and the incidence of short- and long-term side-effects is higher in women undergoing oophorectomy at a younger age. The implications of the results outlined in the paper of Karlan *et al.*[49] discussed under the section on screening for the practice of prophylactic oophorectomy remain unclear, but should be mentioned.

Low risk

Inclusion criteria
Individuals with a family history of ovarian cancer which does not fit the moderate-risk criteria.

Management
These individuals should be informed that their risk of developing ovarian cancer is higher than that of an individual of the same age without a family history, and at present this increased risk is not considered significant. This slightly begs the question of how high the risk has to be before it is considered significant. Women in the moderate-risk group have a 15% or higher lifetime risk of developing ovarian cancer, but the choice of where to set the level of significance is purely arbitrary.

Consistent information-giving through primary care, secondary care in breast and gynaecology units, and tertiary care in cancer genetics centres is particularly important in gaining and retaining public confidence. Different strategies for achieving this remain high on the research agenda.

Conclusions

- Our knowledge of the genetic epidemiology of ovarian cancer is increasing.
- There are several crucial gaps in the present body of knowledge.
- Optimal clinical care demands that we use the available knowledge despite the shortcomings to plan, explain, and deliver the available management options within a coherent and understandable framework.

Acknowledgements

Dr Paul D. Pharoah and Dr James Mackay are funded by the Cancer Research Campaign.

References

1. Lynch, H.T., Guirgis, H.A., and Albert, S. (1974). Familial association of carcinoma of the breast and ovary. *Surg. Gynecol. Obstet.*, **138**, 717.
2. Hall, J.M., Lee, M.K., Newman, B. *et al.* (1990). Linkage of early onset familial breast cancer to chromosome 17q21. *Science*, **266**, 120–2.
3. Miki, Y., Swensen, J., Shattuck-Eidens, D. *et al.* (1994). A strong candidate for the 17 linked breast and ovarian cancer susceptibility gene *BRCA1*. *Science*, **266**, 66–71.
4. Futreal, P.A., Liu, Q., Shattuck-Eidens, D. *et al.* (1994). *BRCA1* mutations in primary breast and ovarian carcinomas. *Science*, **266**, 120–2.

5. Wooster, R., Neuhausen, S.L., Mangion, J. *et al.* (1995). Localization of a breast cancer susceptibility gene, *BRCA2*, to chromosome 13q12–13. *Science*, **265** (5181), 2088–90.

6. Wooster, R., Bignell, G., Lancaster, J. *et al.* (1995). Identification of the breast cancer susceptibility gene *BRCA2*. *Nature*, **378**, 789–92.

7. Gayther, S.A., Pharoah, P.D.P., and Ponder, B.A.J. (1998). The genetics of inherited breast cancer. *J. Mamm. Gland Biol. Neoplasia*, **3** (4), 365–76.

8. Ford, D., Easton, D.F., Stratton, M. *et al.* (1998). Genetic heterogeneity and penetrance analysis of the *BRCA1* and *BRCA2* genes in breast cancer families. *Am. J. Hum. Genet.*, **62** (3), 676–89.

9. Gayther, S.A., Russell, P., Harrington, P. *et al.* (1999). The contribution of germline *BRCA1* and *BRCA2* mutations to familial ovarian cancer: No evidence for other ovarian cancer-susceptibility genes. *Am. J. Hum. Genet.*, **65**, 1021–9.

10. Ford, D., Easton, D.F., Bishop, D.T. *et al.* (1994). Risks of cancer in *BRCA1* mutation carriers. *Lancet*, **343**, 692–5.

11. Easton, D.F., Ford, D., Bishop, D.T., Breast Cancer Linkage Consortium. (1995). Breast and ovarian cancer incidence in *BRCA1*-mutation carriers. *Am. J. Hum. Genet.*, **56** (1), 265–71.

12. Hopper, J.L., Southey, M.C., Dite, G.S. *et al.* (1999). Population-based estimate of the average age-specific cumulative risk of breast cancer for a defined set of protein-truncating mutations in *BRCA1* and *BRCA2*. *Cancer Epidemiol. Biomarkers Prev.*, **8** (9), 741–7.

13. Antoniou, A.C., Gayther, S.A., Stratton, J.F. (1999). Risk models for familial breast and ovarian cancer. *Genet. Epidemiol.*

14. Thorlacius, S., Struewing, J.P., Hartge, P. *et al.* (1998). Population-based study of risk of breast cancer in carriers of *BRCA2* mutation. *Lancet*, **352** (9137), 1337–9.

15. Whittemore, A.S., Gong, G., and Itnyre, J. (1997). Prevalence and contribution of *BRCA1* mutations in breast cancer and ovarian cancer: results from three U.S. population-based case-control studies of ovarian cancer. *Am. J. Hum. Genet.*, **60** (3), 496–504.

16. Struewing, J.P., Hartge, P., Wacholder, S. *et al.* (1997). The risk of cancer associated with specific mutations of *BRCA1* and *BRCA2* among Ashkenazi Jews. *N. Engl. J. Med.*, **336**, 1401–8.

17. Whittemore, A.S. (1997). Risk of breast cancer in carriers of *BRCA* gene mutations. *N. Engl. J. Med*, **337** (11), 788–9.

18. Breast Cancer Linkage Consortium (1999). Cancer risks in *BRCA2* mutation carriers. *J. Natl Cancer Inst.*, **91** (15), 1310–16.

19. Gayther, S.A., Warren, W., Mazoyer, S. *et al.* (1995). Germline mutations of the *BRCA1* gene in breast and ovarian cancer families provide evidence for a genotype–phenotype correlation. *Nature Genet.*, **11** (4), 428–33.

20. Gayther, S.A., Mangion, J., Russell, P. *et al.* (1997). Variation of risks of breast and ovarian cancer associated with different germline mutations of the *BRCA2* gene. *Nature Genet.*, **15** (1), 103–5.

21. Narod, S.A., Goldgar, D., Cannon Albright, L. *et al.* (1995). Risk modifiers in carriers of BRCA1 mutations. *Int. J. Cancer*, **64** (6), 394–8.

22. Brunet, J.S., Ghadirian, P., Rebbeck, T.R. *et al.* (1998). Effect of smoking on breast cancer in carriers of mutant *BRCA1* or *BRCA2* genes. *J. Natl Cancer Inst.*, **90** (10), 761–6.

23. Narod, S.A., Risch, H., Moslehi, R. *et al.* (1998). Oral contraceptives and the risk of hereditary ovarian cancer. *N. Engl. J. Med.*, **339** (7), 424–8.

24. Krontiris, T.G., Devlin, B., Karp, D.D. *et al.* (1993). An association between the risk of cancer and mutations in the HRAS1 minisatellite locus. *N. Engl. J. Med.*, **329** (8), 517–23.

25. Phelan, C.M., Rebbeck, T.R., Weber, B.L. *et al.* (1996). Ovarian cancer risk in *BRCA1* carriers is modified by the *HRAS1* variable number of tandem repeat (VNTR) locus. *Nature Genet.*, **12** (3), 309–11.

26. Rebbeck, T.R., Kantoff, P.W., Krithivas, K. *et al.* (1999). Modification of *BRCA1*-associated breast cancer risk by the polymorphic androgen-receptor CAG repeat. *Am. J. Hum. Genet.*, **64** (5), 1371–7.

27. Rebbeck, T.R., Kantoff, P.W., Krithivas, K. *et al.* (1999). *Modification of breast cancer risk in* BRCA1 *mutation carriers by the* AIB1 *gene*. American Association for Cancer Research Annual Meeting, March, Philadelphia.

28. Stratton, J.F., Pharoah, P.D.P., Smith, S.K. *et al.* (1998). A systematic review and meta-analysis of family history and risk of ovarian cancer. *Br. J. Obstet. Gynecol.*, **105**, 493–9.

29. Easton, D.F., Matthews, F.E., Ford, D. *et al.* (1996). Cancer mortality in relatives of women with ovarian cancer: the OPCS study. *Int. J. Cancer*, **65**, 284–94.

30. Schildkraut, J.M. and Thompson, W.D. (1988). Familial ovarian cancer: a population-based case-control study. *Am. J. Epidemiol.*, **128** (3), 456–66.

31. Jishi, M.F., Itnyre, J.H., Oakley-Girvan, I.A. *et al.* (1995). Risks of cancer among members of families in the Gilda Radner Familial Ovarian Cancer Registry. *Cancer*, **76** (8), 1416–21.

32. Claus, E.B., Risch, N., and Thompson, W.D. (1993). The calculation of breast cancer risk for women with a first degree family history of ovarian cancer. *Breast Cancer Res. Treat.*, **28** (2), 115–20.

33. Piver, M.S., Baker, T.R., Jishi, M.F. *et al.* (1993). Familial ovarian cancer. A report of 658 families from the Gilda Radner Familial Ovarian Cancer Registry 1981–1991. *Cancer*, **71** (2 Suppl), 582–8.

34. Collaborative group on hormonal factors in breast cancer. (1996). Breast cancer and hormonal contraceptives: collaborative reanalysis of individual data on 53297 women with breast cancer and 100239 women without breast cancer from 54 epidemiological studies. *Lancet*, **347**, 1713–27.

35. Struewing, J.P., Watson, P., Easton, D.F. *et al.* (1995). Prophylactic oophorectomy in inherited breast/ovarian cancer families. *J. Natl Cancer Inst. Monogr.*, **17**, 33–5.

36. Piver, M.S., Jishi, M.F., Tsukada, Y., and Nava, G. (1993). Primary peritoneal carcinoma after prophylactic oophorectomy in women with a family history of ovarian cancer. A report of the Gilda Radner Familial Ovarian Cancer Registry. *Cancer (Philadelphia)*, **71** (9), 2751–5.

37. Bell, D.A. and Scully, R.E. (1994). Early *de novo* ovarian carcinoma. A study of fourteen cases. *Cancer (Philadelphia)*, **73** (7), 1859–64.

38. Scully, R.E., Mark, E.J., and McNeely, B.U. (1986). Case records of the Massachusetts General Hospital—Case 40–1986. *N. Engl J. Med.*, 952–956.

39. Tobacman, J.K., Tucker, M.A., Kase, R. *et al.* (1982). Intra-abdominal carcinomatosis after prophylactic oophorectomies in ovarian-cancer-prone families. *Lancet*, (Oct. 9), 795–7.

40. Pecorelli, S., Odicino, F., and Tessadrelli, A. (1996). Primary and interval debulking surgery for advanced disease. In *Ovarian cancer*, (1st edn), (ed. F. Sharp, T. Blackett, R. Leake, and J. Berek), pp. 105–9. Chapman & Hall Medical, London.

41. Campbell, S., Bhan, V., and Royston, P. (1989). Transabdominal ultrasound screening for early ovarian cancer. *BMJ*, **299**, 1363–7.

42. DePriest, P.D., van Nagell, J.R., Gallion, H.H. *et al.* (1993). Ovarian cancer screening in asymptomatic postmenopausal women. *Gynecol. Oncol.*, **51** (2), 205–9.

43. Bourne, T.H., Campbell, S., Reynolds, K.M. *et al.* (1993). Screening for early familial ovarian cancer with transvaginal ultrasonography and colour blood flow imaging. *BMJ*, **306**, 1025–9.

44. Zurawski, V.R., Orjaseter, H., Andersen, A. *et al.* (1988). Elevated serum CA 125 levels prior to diagnosis of ovarian neoplasia: relevance for early detection of ovarian cancer. *Int. J. Cancer*, **42**, 677–80.

45. Helzlsouer, K., Bush, T.L., Alberg, A.J. *et al.* (1993). Prospective study of serum CA125 levels as markers of ovarian cancer. *JAMA*, **269** (9), 1123–6.

46. Jacobs, I.J., Skates, S., Davies, A.P. *et al.* (1996). Risk of diagnosis of ovarian cancer after raised serum CA 125 concentration: a prospective cohort study. *BMJ*, **313**, 1355–8.

47. Jacobs, I., Davies, A.P., Bridges, J. *et al.* (1993). Prevalence screening for ovarian cancer in postmenopausal women by CA 125 measurement and ultrasonography. *BMJ*, **306**, 1030–4.

48. Einhorn, N., Sjovall, K., Knapp, R.C. (1992). Prospective evaluation of serum CA 125 levels for early detection of ovarian cancer. *Obstet.Gynecol.*, **80** (1), 14–18.

49. Karlan, B.Y., Baldwin, R.L., Lopez-Luevanos, E. *et al.* (1999). Peritoneal serous papillary carcinoma, a phenotypic varian of familial ovarian cancer: Implications for ovarian cancer screening. *Am. J. Obstet. Gynecol.*, **180** (4), 917–28.

50. Kelsey, J.L., Gammon, M.D., and John, E.M. (1993). Reproductive factors and breast cancer. *Epidemiol. Rev.*, **15**, 36–47.

51. Fisher, B., Costantino, J.P., Wickerham, D.L. *et al.* (1998). Tamoxifen for prevention of breast cancer: report of the National Surgical Adjuvant Breast and Bowel Project P–1 Study. *J. Natl Cancer Inst.*, **90** (18), 1371–88.

52. Powles, T., Eeles, R., Ashley, S. *et al.* (1998). Interim analysis of the incidence of breast cancer in the Royal Marsden Hospital tamoxifen randomised chemoprevention trial. *Lancet*, **352** (9122), 98–101.

53. Veronesi, U., Maisonneuve, P., Costa, A. *et al.* (1998). Prevention of breast cancer with tamoxifen: preliminary findings from the Italian randomised trial among hysterectomised women. Italian Tamoxifen Prevention Study. *Lancet*, **352** (9122), 93–7.

54. Cummings, S.R., Eckert, S., Krueger, K.A. *et al.* (1999). The effect of raloxifene on risk of breast cancer in postmenopausal women: results from the MORE randomized trial. *J. Am. Med. Assoc.*, **281** (23), 2189–97.

55. Hartmann, L.C., Schaid, D.J., Woods, J.E. *et al.* (1999). Efficacy of bilateral prophylactic mastectomy in women with a family history of breast cancer. *N. Engl J. Med.*, **340** (2), 77–84.

56. Rebbeck, T.R., Levin, A.M., Eisen, A. *et al.* (1999). Breast cancer risk after bilateral prophylactic oophorectomy in *BRCA1* mutation carriers. *J. Natl Cancer Inst.*, **91** (17), 1475–9.

57. Kerlikowske, K., Grady, D., Rubin, S.M. *et al.* (1995). Efficacy of screening mammography: a meta-analysis. *J. Am. Med. Assoc.*, **273**, 149–54.

58. Fletcher, S.W., Black, W., Harris, R. *et al.* (1993). Report of the international workshop of screening for breast cancer. *J. Natl Cancer Inst.*, **85**, 1644–56.

59. Feig, S.A. (1997). Increased benefit from shorter screening mammography intervals for women ages 40–49 years. *Cancer*, **80**, 2035–9.

60. Mackay, J. and Jacobs, I.J. The UKCCCR Familial Ovarian Cancer Screening Study.

Part 5

Diagnostic and prognostic techniques

30. Clinical diagnosis including paraneoplastic syndromes

Chris N. Hudson, Thomas J. Ind, and O. Marigold Curling

Introduction: presentation and diagnosis

The ovary is the site of origin for a greater variety of primary neoplasms than any other organ in the body (Table 30.1).[1] Ovarian cancer arises in an inaccessible intrapelvic situation and, because the majority of metastases are transcoelomic and remain intraperitoneal, it is not surprising that the clinical manifestations of this malignancy are non-specific and show great variability. Moreover, the natural history of ovarian cancer embraces a range of activity, from the rapid and relentless aggression of highly anaplastic tumours on the one hand, to the other end of a spectrum of malignancy, where a group of tumours of such low-grade activity exists[2] that in any individual case the pathologist may be in doubt about the actual malignant potential (see Chapter 10). The manifestations of ovarian malignant disease are thus so protean that it has been questioned whether the clinical disease should be classed as a gynaecological disorder.[3]

There is a general lack of awareness of the potential for diagnostic confusion in the allied subspecialties of internal medicine, colo-proctology, and urology; specialists in these disciplines, even those who treat cancer arising in other organs, may not appreciate that modern concepts of the management of ovarian cancer differ fundamentally in some respects from principles applied to the management of malignant disease in other sites.

In this chapter the range of clinical manifestations of ovarian malignancy and some of the problems of diagnosis are reviewed. Special diagnostic techniques are discussed in following chapters. Many of the data on which this review is based have been derived from a prospective clinicopathological study of 966 cases of primary ovarian malignancy entered into an ovarian tumour registry run in the North-East Thames Region of London and the Home Counties of the UK.[4]

General presentation: analysis of symptoms

Pain and abdominal swelling provide the most obvious complaints. The latter may be ascribed to the primary ovarian mass, epigastric omental plaque or ascites, or a combination of these. Pain and swelling were noted in the authors' series at presentation in 47% and 57%, respectively, often, of course, together.

The *gastroenterological manifestations* of ovarian malignancy deserve much wider recognition. In the authors' series, dyspepsia was recorded in 10%. Vomiting also occurred in 10%, and alteration of bowel habit in 16%. Concentration of symptoms in the upper abdomen may be misleading and ultrasonic examination, including the pelvis, and tumour marker screening should at least be offered, even if more expensive imaging is not considered to be indicated. With increasing sophistication of diagnostic measures, the importance of clinical pelvic examination, even just rectal examination, should not be overlooked as providing a clue to the origin of vague abdominal, even upper abdominal, symptoms.

Urinary symptoms are somewhat less common (13%). Pressure on the bladder provoking urinary frequency occurred more commonly than retention due to impaction on the pelvis. Retroperitoneal extension can produce ureteric obstruction with understandable sequelae.

The fact that 3% of ovarian cancer cases were recorded as '*incidental findings*', hitherto unsuspected and noted only during an examination or operation for some unrelated cause, emphasizes the need for, and likely rewards from, improving screening and diagnostic facilities (see Chapter 24).

Presentation with extra-abdominal disease

Manifestations of extra-abdominal disease can include nodal metastases (especially inguinal or supraclavicular), pleural effusion, and uncommon deposits in breast, lung, bone, or skin, including the umbilicus ('Sister Joseph's nodule').

Pleural effusion alone does not allocate a patient to stage IV unless malignancy is confirmed by exfoliative cytology. Rarely, respiratory symptoms may dominate the clinical scene and an ovarian primary source may be occult or even undetectable. The authors found radiological evidence of pleural effusion noted at presentation in 5%, of which barely half were clinically detectable.

Table 30.1 Histological classification of ovarian tumours

I. Common 'epithelial' tumours

A. Serous tumours
  1. Benign
    (a) cystadenoma and papillary cystadenoma
    (b) surface papilloma
    (c) adenofibroma and cystadenofibroma
  2. Of borderline malignancy (carcinomas of low malignant potential)
    (a) cystadenoma and papillary cystadenoma
    (b) surface papilloma
    (c) adenofibroma and cystadenofibroma
  3. Malignant
    (a) adenocarcinoma, papillary adenocarcinoma, and papillary cystadenocarcinoma
    (b) surface papillary carcinoma
    (c) malignant adenofibroma and cystadenofibroma

B. Mucinous tumours
  1. Benign
    (a) cystadenoma
    (b) adenofibroma and cystadenofibroma
  2. Of borderline malignancy (carcinoma of low malignant potential)
    (a) cystadenoma
    (b) adenofibroma and cystadenofibroma
  3. Malignant
    (a) adenocarcinoma and cystadenocarcinoma
    (b) malignant adenofibroma and cystadenofibroma

C. Endometrioid tumours
  1. Benign
    (a) adenoma and cystadenoma
    (b) adenofibroma and cystadenofibroma
  2. Of borderline malignancy (carcinomas of low malignant potential)
    (a) adenoma and cystadenoma
    (b) adenofibroma and cystadenofibroma
  3. Malignant
    (a) carcinoma
      (i) adenocarcinoma
      (ii) adenoacanthoma
      (iii) malignant adenofibroma and cystadenofibroma
    (b) endometrioid stromal sarcomas
    (c) mesodermal (Müllerian) mixed tumours, homologous and heterologous

D. Clear cell (mesonephroid) tumours
  1. Benign: adenofibroma
  2. Of borderline malignancy (carcinomas of low malignant potential)
  3. Malignant: carcinoma and adenocarcinoma

E. Brenner tumours
  1. Benign
  2. Of borderline malignancy (proliferating)
  3. Malignant

F. Mixed epithelial tumours
  1. Benign
  2. Of borderline malignancy
  3. Malignant

G. Undifferentiated carcinoma

H. Unclassified epithelial tumours

II. Sex cord stromal tumours

A. Granulosa-stromal cell tumours
  1. Granulosa cell tumours

  2. Tumours in the thecoma—fibroma group
    (a) thecoma
    (b) fibroma
    (c) unclassified
B. Androblastomas: Sertoli–Leydig cell tumours
  1. Well differentiated
    (a) tubular androblastoma; Sertoli cell tumour (tubular adenoma of Pick)
    (b) tubular androblastoma with lipid storage; Sertoli cell tumour with lipid storage (folliculome lipidique of Lecène)
    (c) Sertoli–Leydig cell tumour (tubular adenoma with Leydig cells)
    (d) Leydig cell tumour; hilus cell tumour
  2. Of intermediate differentiation
  3. Poorly differentiated (sarcomatoid)
  4. With heterologous elements

C. Gynandroblastoma

D. Unclassified

III. Lipid (lipoid) cell tumours

IV. Germ cell tumours

A. Dysgerminoma

B. Endodermal sinus tumour

C. Embryonal carcinoma

D. Polyembryoma

E. Choriocarcinoma

F. Teratomas
  1. Immature
  2. Mature
    (a) solid
    (b) cystic
      (i) dermoid cyst (mature cystic teratoma)
      (ii) dermoid cyst with malignant transformation
  3. Monodermal and highly specialised
    (a) struma ovarii
    (b) carcinoid
    (c) struma ovarii and carcinoid
    (d) others

G. Mixed forms

V. Gonadoblastoma

A. Pure

B. Mixed with dysgerminoma or other form of germ cell tumour

VI. Soft tissue tumours not specific to ovary

VII. Unclassified tumours

VIII. Secondary (metastatic) tumours

IX. Tumour like conditions

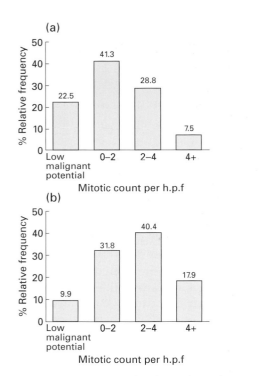

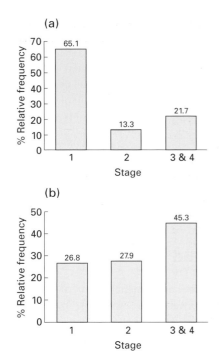

Fig. 30.1 Primary ovarian cancer patients, distribution by grade, (a) 84 cases aged under 40 years; (b) 882 cases aged 40 years and over (cases from North-East Thames Region, UK).

Fig. 30.2 Primary ovarian cancer, common epithelial tumours; distribution by stage for (a) 59 patients aged less than 40 years; (b) 705 patients aged 40 years and over (cases from North-East Thames Region, UK).

Nodal metastases may be amenable to local as well as, or instead of, systemic therapy. However, in younger patients (especially male) it has been found that some who present with the finding of apparently anaplastic carcinoma in lymph nodes appear to have occult germ cell tumour of genital or extragenital origin.[5] A search for the appropriate tumour marker should therefore always be carried out because these tumours may be amenable to radical chemotherapy.

Age

No age is exempt from ovarian neoplasia, although it is very rare in prepubertal girls. A small cell ovarian carcinoma in a 14-month-old girl was reported by Florell *et al.* (1999).[6] The peak incidence of ovarian malignancy is around 54 years of age[7] and there is a broad distribution in the decades either side of this peak, which is some 15 years after the peak incidence of benign ovarian cysts (Figs 30.1, 30.2).[8] There are variations due to age distribution according to histopathology, the most obvious being the tendency for most tumours of germ cell origin to arise in the under–30 age group (Fig. 30.3). Although these tumours are uncommon, they are of such importance that the possibility of their presence should always be suspected when a questionably sinister gonadal tumour is discovered in a young person (of either sex). Early investigation for the appropriate tumour markers can elucidate the problem before inappropriate treatment is undertaken (see Chapters 11 and 31). The dysgerminoma, however, has

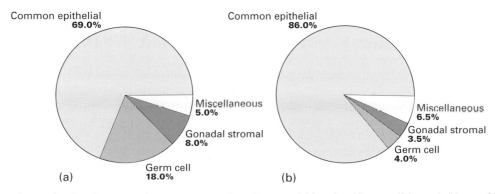

Fig. 30.3 Relative prevalence of main primary ovarian cancer groups in patients aged (a) under 40 years (84 cases); (b) over 39 years (882 cases). (North-East Thames Ovarian Cancer Study.)

a much broader distribution into later adult life, and those tumours which arise by secondary malignant transformation in a pre-existing benign cystic teratoma have a peak incidence in an older age group.[9] Tumours of gonadal stromal and some of surface epithelial origin, especially small cell carcinoma, may nevertheless also arise in the younger group of patients.

Although some epithelial tumours are anaplastic and run an aggressive course in all age groups, in general when these tumours arise in patients below the age of 40 they tend to be better differentiated and less malignant than those in the over–40 age group, and also less advanced (Figs 30.1, 30.2). In all stages, the prognosis for those under the age of 35 is better[10] and worse over the age of 65.[11]

Genetic and constitutional factors

Although a familial and genetically determined predisposition to epithelial ovarian cancer is responsible for only a small proportion of the clinical cases of this disorder, they are of considerable importance and these syndromes are discussed in detail in Chapter 4. Certain other associations, such as the Peutz–Jeghers syndrome,[12] are recognized. Aberrations of germ cell biology are important. Patients with gonadal dysgenesis are at increased risk from germ cell neoplasia, particularly if a Y chromosome is present, even in a mosaic. These patients may be of short stature with primary amenorrhoea and may show other features of Turner's syndrome, but this is not universal. Such a constitutional diathesis should raise the level of suspicion. If these genetic configurations are confirmed, then in an individual with the external characteristics of a female, the question of prophylactic gonadal ablation at an appropriate time may be a consideration.[13] Optimum timing is important, because if castration is carried out too early, skeletal development may be interrupted. Ovarian cancer has been described in identical twins.[14]

Parity

Low parity has long been recognized as a risk factor for ovarian cancer.[15] There has been much debate about the complex nature of this apparent association (Chapter 2).[16] The greatest risk is associated with nulliparity in a woman who has never taken oral contraception (Fig. 30.4). A single pregnancy may offer some independent protective effect,[17] but the principal feature would appear to be the suppression of ovulation by pregnancy, lactation, or oral contraception.[18] The protective effect of oral contraception is now well documented (see Chapter 22).

It is not clear whether the circumstances surrounding involuntary infertility may themselves predispose to ovarian malignancy or whether the association is secondary to the consequent nulliparity. In the authors' series, 33% of 394 nulliparous patients reported 10 years' involuntary infertility and the occurrence of this symptom in the whole group was in the order of 10%. Venn *et al.* (1995)[19] calculated that there was an increased incidence of ovarian cancer amongst a cohort of women attending for assisted

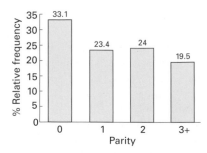

Fig. 30.4 Parity distribution for 764 patients with common epithelial ovarian cancer (from North-East Thames Region, UK).

reproduction, but no significant differences among those receiving ovulation induction therapy and hence increased folliculogenesis, although Whittemore *et al.* (1992)[20] concluded that there was likely to be a small increase in risk from the use of fertility drugs.

An apparent association with social class may reflect no more than demographic variations in reproductive behaviour; this may also confound reports of ethnic variation in prognosis. Whatever the apparent cause, the occurrence of vague or non-specific symptoms in a nulliparous female in the perimenopausal years should enhance the index of suspicion for occult ovarian malignancy.

Fibroids

As uterine fibroids are also more common in nulliparous women of this age group, they constitute a potential cause of diagnostic confusion. They may also coexist in 10–15% of cases.[21] The embarrassment of making a confident preoperative diagnosis of fibroids, only to be faced at laparotomy with ovarian malignancy adherent to the uterus, may usually be avoided by the use of diagnostic ultrasound.[22] Although ultrasound cannot indicate malignancy in an ovarian cyst with confidence, the value of the study in a case considered to be fibroids lies in the potential to show either that the clinically detectable pelvic mass is not entirely uterine, or that at least in part the consistency may be cystic or otherwise not characteristic of a benign leiomyoma. Under such circumstances, the need for more advanced imaging and tumour marker investigation would become apparent (see Chapters 32, 33, and 34), adding greatly to the precision of preoperative diagnosis.[23]

Concurrent pregnancy

Ovarian malignancy in association with pregnancy is very rare (1 : 18 000 deliveries).[24] Half the patients known to the authors with concurrent pregnancy had tumours of germ cell origin, which is not surprising as the age distribution of these coincides with the younger reproductive years, as opposed to the older peak incidence of common epithelial tumours. Mechanical obstetric obstruction and torsion are recognized manifestations of ovarian tumours in pregnancy. The diagnosis of ovarian tumour may be made coincidentally at Caesarean section. Vaginal examination and ultrasound scanning in the first trimester of pregnancy may reveal adnexal pathology. However, a cyst deep in the pouch of Douglas may not impinge sufficiently on the scanned field to ensure that it is not overlooked. Once the fundus of the pregnant uterus has risen from the pelvis, any ovarian tumour, unless trapped in the pouch of Douglas, will be displaced into the upper abdomen and no longer accessible to examining fingers in the vagina. If an ovarian cyst in pregnancy is flaccid and adjacent to an equally soft uterus, distinction by abdominal palpation may also be almost impossible. Asymmetry of the uterus may be suspected or the condition mistaken for a degenerating leiomyoma. Diagnostic ultrasound will have a crucial role in the elucidation of suspicious adnexal swellings in pregnancy, because unnecessary intervention for a corpus luteum cyst is to be deprecated. Accurate observations on the consistency and loculation of an adnexal swelling are necessary before a decision on the need for intervention is made. If a decision for conservatism is made, then serial observations are mandatory. Although the most common malignant ovarian tumour associated with pregnancy is the dysgerminoma, the authors have seen both solid teratoma and yolk sac tumour. One corollary of the association of pregnancy with the latter tumours is that elevated levels of pregnancy-associated plasma proteins and carcino-placental antigens, such as α-fetaprotein, lose their specificity as tumour markers.

Prior hysterectomy

A debate continues on the desirability of prophylactic oophorectomy performed at the time of hysterectomy.[25] The principal risks of postmenopausal hormonal replacement therapy appear to be those of imbalanced endometrial stimulation, and this factor is, of course, absent in those patients treated by hysterectomy. Nevertheless, other more subtle side-effects of long-term replacement therapy may be present, but they are not such as to prevent the use of hormone replacement therapy in patients after ovarian and uterine ablation. However, the balance between the benefits and unwelcome consequences of prophylactic ovarian ablation cannot be entirely achieved using endocrinological and oncological data alone. The psychological and emotional sequelae of castration should not be lightly overlooked by clinicians. It is absolutely clear that removal of normal ovaries should not be regarded as a trivial encore to hysterectomy, and there is case law to the effect that unconsented ovarian ablation is a breach of professional conduct.

All this may be small consolation to a patient who develops ovarian malignancy, having previously undergone hysterectomy, particularly if the interval is short. It is undoubtedly true that the surgical treatment of ovarian malignancy arising in a patient who has already undergone hysterectomy is technically more difficult. There appears, however, to be little evidence that the genital pathology that provided the indication for surgical hysterectomy is also associated with a higher incidence of subsequent ovarian cancer, and there is a suggestion that the risk of ovarian cancer after hysterectomy is actually reduced.[15] The incidence of prior hysterectomy in the authors' series was 4%.

Ovarian conservation after, or even at, the menopause may be considered altruistic, but most hysterectomy operations are carried out for menstrual disturbance and thus, by definition, are carried out before the menopause. It is prudent therefore that consent should encompass the possibility of oophorectomy. It may well be that the woman will be prepared to leave the decision to the surgeon if the normality of the ovary is in doubt, but this agreement should be prospectively clear.

Menopausal status

There is a steep rise in the occurrence of ovarian malignancy after the menopause,[26] which raises the question of whether the increase in circulating gonadotrophins at that time could be relevant. Age at menopause and the history of prior menstrual disturbance have not been reported consistently in carcinoma of the ovary, in contrast to such a relationship with malignancy of the endometrium. In a multiple logistic regression of the authors' data, age at menopause was not shown to be independently related to outcome.

Abnormal vaginal bleeding

In spite of the above, abnormal uterine bleeding is sometimes associated with malignant ovarian disease, and this may not always be a coincidence.

Hormonal stimulation of the endometrium and coincidental endometrial carcinoma

Postmenopausal bleeding is a dramatic demonstration of abnormal uterine stimulation. This symptom may occasionally be the presenting symptom of a small ovarian tumour of gonadal stromal origin and paradoxically is more likely when the causative tumour is benign, particularly a thecoma. Rather more commonly, endometrial stimulation may be the result of stromal luteinization, which can occur in surface epithelial tumours and also even in secondary deposits arising within the ovary from a primary tumour elsewhere. In the authors' series, postmenopausal bleeding was present as an initial symptom in 20% of those women with common epithelial cancers who presented after the menopause. The endometrium in such cases may show hyperplasia or even carcinoma. In the authors' series, in the 293 cases of ovarian malignancy, in which endometrium was also available for examination, hyperplasia was found in 63 and carcinoma in 39.

Endometrial malignancy

Postmenopausal bleeding will, in any event, commonly cause a patient to seek medical advice. Even if a large abdominopelvic mass is discovered, the possibility of endometrial involvement or associated neoplasia will not normally be overlooked. Aspiration endometrial biopsy and transvaginal ultrasound may clinch the diagnosis. The occasional association between ovarian cancer and concomitant endometrial malignancy was clearly the basis for the traditional teaching that hysterectomy should be regarded as an essential part of the basic treatment of malignant ovarian disease. It is now recognized that this association is largely with those surface epithelial tumours with endometrioid elements, either pure or mixed.[27] Thus a selective approach to hysterectomy may sometimes be practised in cases of unilateral disease entirely confined to the ovary when conservation of reproductive function is desired. If such a management plan is determined after the negative preliminary screen, it would be prudent to carry out concurrent hysteroscopy with a full endometrial sample by curettage for histological examination. Although endometrial carcinoma is most commonly a disease of the postmenopausal age group, some 20% of such patients present before the menopause, and it seems likely that these patients have a somewhat greater association with endometrioid ovarian malignancy. Clinicians should be aware that endometrial carcinoma in such cases may have produced no abnormal uterine bleeding and the possibility of its presence should not be overlooked. The authors found that 16 out of the 39 patients with concomitant endometrial and ovarian cancer had reported no abnormal uterine bleeding.

The specific linkage between endometrial carcinoma and endometrioid ovarian carcinoma suggests that hysterectomy is not *per se* invariably necessary for the optimum treatment of disease of other histological types, even when more advanced. The uterus and the broad ligaments are, however, an important part of the tumour bed which therefore require removal as part of *optimal* cytoreduction for locally extensive disease. However, hysterectomy could not be said to add to the therapeutic effect of *palliative* cytoreduction in advanced intra-abdominal malignancy, only adding to the magnitude of the surgical intervention.

Endocrine syndromes associated with ovarian malignancy

In addition to the uterine effects of hormones produced by some gonadal stromal tumours referred to above, there are also some germ cell tumours which may rarely produce evidence of virilization due to androgen production (see Chapter 11). Such hormonal activity may be considered appropriate to the tissue of origin, even though this has undergone malignant transformation. Furthermore, a germ cell tumour of one ovary contains tissue which produces chorionic gonadotrophin, which may achieve levels sufficient to promote the formation of theca lutein cysts in the contralateral ovary. This phenomenon should not be mistaken for bilateral neoplastic involvement, as the cyst formation is exactly comparable to that which is known to occur in gestational trophoblastic disease. Other onco-fetal products (α-fetoprotein, α_1-antitrypsin) do not provoke recognizable clinical syndromes. They are found in some cases of germ cell tumour[28] and rarely in androblastoma (Chapter 31).[29]

Paraneoplastic syndromes

Paraneoplastic syndromes are systemic manifestations of cancer that cannot readily be explained by the local metastatic effects of a tumour or of hormones indigenous to the tissue in which the tumour arises. Endocrine manifestations, as a consequence of oversecretion of normal ovarian hormones by ovarian tumours as illustrated above, should not, by definition, be classed as paraneoplastic or para-endocrine syndromes.[30] Paraneoplastic syndromes may be divided into five broad groups, between which there may well be some overlap. These may be classed as endocrine, neurological, haematological/vascular, dermatological, or osteo-articular. The presentation and occurrence of paraneoplastic syndromes among the patients with primary ovarian cancer in the authors' series were reported by Hudson *et al.* (1993).[31] There were single examples of probable paraneoplastic syndromes in the series, suggesting that the prevalence of any individual syndrome is probably of the order of 1 : 1000.

There is unlikely to be a single explanation for these rare and interesting clinical syndromes—indeed, their very rarity is one of the most puzzling features. The fact remains that ovarian cancer, with a greater diversity probably than any other human site of primary malignancy, has a well-recorded association with a full range of paraneoplastic syndromes. Within this range is a number of 'collagen' disorders, for which there may be an established or theoretical immunological basis.[32] It is pertinent, therefore, that ovarian cancer is clearly among the more immunogenic tumours,[33] and that antibodies to a number of tissue antigens not normally present have been found in patients with ovarian cancer.[34,35] Furthermore, circulating immune complexes have also been demonstrated in the sera of patients with metastatic epithelial ovarian cancer.[36] Circumstantial evidence of a direct effect may be adduced from the paraneoplastic nephrotic syndrome, in which the cause has been suggested to be glomerular deposition of immune complexes.[37] Another most striking demonstration of an autoimmune basis for a paraneoplastic syndrome is the expression of a particular type of Purkinje cell antibody in some patients with ovarian carcinoma, the antibody being associated with subacute cerebellar degeneration (see below). These antibodies have not been found in the serum of patients with small cell carcinoma of the lung, who also developed cerebellar degeneration. A mechanism of peripheral activation of specific cytoreduction T lymphocytes has been proposed.[38]

Subgroups

Endocrine/metabolic

Hormone production not appropriate to tissue normally found in the ovary can derive from endocrine tissue in a teratoma. This is out of context here unless the teratoma is malignant. In clinical practice, this is confined to the monophyletic variants. Although struma ovarii (thyroid) is the most important, a clinical syndrome may also be found with primary ovarian argentaffinoma, some cases of which may behave in a malignant fashion.[39] Such tumours, benign or malignant, will release serotonin directly into the systemic circulation to produce the carcinoid syndrome with episodic flushing. Under other circumstances, the 'flushing' syndrome normally denotes hepatic metastatic disease because the serotonin output from a primary tumour draining into the hepatic portal system will be inactivated in the liver. It is necessary to realize that the ovary is an important site for metastasis from any primary tumour within the GI tract and that malignant carci-

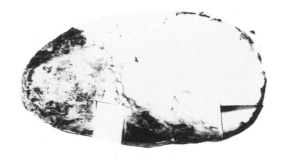

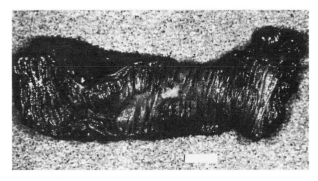

Fig. 30.5 Intestinal carcinoid presenting with ovarian metastasis (Department of Medical Illustration, Westmead Hospital, New South Wales, Australia).

noid is no exception (Fig. 30.5). If ovarian carcinoid syndrome is diagnosed, it is imperative that a thorough search for an occult intestinal primary should be made.[40]

An 'inappropriate antidiuretic hormone secretion' syndrome has occasionally been described in gynaecological (and other) cancers. Persistent hyponatraemia is a feature and the syndrome has been described in immature teratomas of the ovary.[41]

An 'ectopic ACTH' syndrome has also been described in a number of sites for malignancy, notably the bronchus. Cases have been described with ovarian tumours in which the production of ectopic ACTH or cortisol has been sufficient to produce Cushing's syndrome.[42,43]

Hypercalcaemia in advanced malignant disease is recognized in the presence of osseous metastases. However, it may arise as a result of paraneoplastic endocrinopathy. A role for prostaglandins has been suggested.[44] Within the female genital tract this has been described with carcinoma of the endometrium and ovary. The ovarian association seems particularly to be with mesonephroid 'clear cell' tumours, which some would regard as an endometrioid variant.[45] In addition, hypercalcaemia has been described in association with small cell carcinoma, a rare ovarian tumour occurring in a younger age group.[46,47] Isolated examples of hypercalcaemia have been reported with mucinous cystadenocarcinoma,[48] serous cystadenocarcinoma,[49] and with squamous cell carcinoma arising in a pre-existing benign cystic teratoma.[50] Clinical presentation may represent 'the tip of the iceberg' and more cases may come to light from biochemical screening.

Clinical syndromes have been described in cases of ectopic production of gastrointestinal hormones. Gastrin from a mucinous cystadenocarcinoma has been responsible for the Zollinger–Ellison syndrome.[51] Likewise, hypoglycaemia with the secretion of an insulin-like substance[52] and hyperamylasaemia have been reported.[53]

Vascular/haematological

Although erythrocytosis (polycythaemia) and ectopic erythropoetin production may be true paraneoplastic phenomena, perhaps correctly classified under the endocrine heading,[54] within gynaecological practice there is found a curious 'mechanical' association of polycythaemia with certain tumours between the leaves of the broad ligament, most commonly benign leiomyoma.[55] One such case of secondary polycythaemia associated with an intraligamentary malignant ovarian tumour was reported in the authors' series. This intraligamentary tumour was a mucinous cystadenocarcinoma. The reason for this curious anatomical association is unclear.

Haemolytic anaemia is a recognized paraneoplastic phenomenon and has also been described in association with benign cystic teratoma.

Coagulation and venous disorders are important in malignant disease of the ovary, but the issue of a paraneoplastic effect is clouded by venous circulatory embarrassment from pressure effects within the pelvis and abdomen. Nevertheless, there is an observed increased incidence over that expected of ovarian (and pancreatic) cancer in patients presenting with thromboembolism.[56] There is, moreover, an accepted association with thrombophlebitis migrans, in which the primary tumour may be occult.[57] In one case in the authors' series, the diagnosis of ovarian malignancy was only achieved after a search for a possible occult primary in such a situation. Even with a serious complication such as venous gangrene, the ovarian tumour may not hitherto have been apparent.[58]

A case of polyarteritis nodosa in the authors' series was considered to be probably paraneoplastic.

Osteo-articular disease

There is overlap between this clinical subgroup and that of dermatological manifestations. The 'collagen' disorders of systemic sclerosis (scleroderma)[59] and dermatomyositis have a well-recognized association with visceral malignancy, including ovarian cancer.[60,61]

Rheumatoid arthritis is a collagen disorder with an autoimmune basis. It would be difficult to establish a paraneoplastic connection in any particular case, although this has been suggested.

Reflex sympathetic dystrophy ('shoulder–hand' syndrome), of which palmar fasciitis (Dupuytren's contracture) is a feature, has a described association with endometrioid ovarian cancer. This is another example of a paraneoplastic syndrome which may antedate the discovery of the underlying neoplasm.[62]

Dermatological conditions

The dermatological manifestations of occult visceral malignancy are well known, and of great interest to dermatologists. Apart from the two collagen disorders mentioned above, acanthosis nigricans is a dermatological condition which may be related to gynaecological malignancy, including ovarian cancer.[63] Patchy hyperkeratosis and pigmentation may occur, including odd sites such as the axilla.[64]

A patchy purpuric rash on the extremities has shown leucocyto-clastic vasculitis as a paraneoplastic presentation of a malignant ovarian tumour.[65]

Neurological conditions

Several neurological conditions have been reported in a para-neoplastic relation to ovarian cancer, namely neuromyopathy,[66] necrotizing myelopathy,[67] lower motor neuron paralysis,[68] and limbic-encephalitis.[69] One particular condition has aroused very considerable interest. This is the occurrence of subacute cerebellar degeneration.[70] In such patients with ovarian cancer, there is expression of a particular type of Purkinje cell antibody.[71] In such cases, it has been suggested that these antibodies might have a role as a tumour marker,[72] even though the paraneoplastic neuropathy does not always appear.[73] Therapeutic plasmapheresis has been attempted.[74]

Other associations

Thyroid adenoma has been associated with malignant ovarian androblastoma,[29] but the basis of any relationship is unclear.

An association between Hashimoto's disease, clinical dermato-myositis, and ovarian carcinoma has been reported.[75]

Retroperitoneal fibrosis Although often idiopathic, there is a recognized association of this condition with malignant disease.[76] Rarely, ovarian cancer, particularly when recurrent, may spread in retroperitoneal lymphatics with the evocation of a very fibrous response, so that the clinical features of retroperitoneal fibrosis dominate or mask other evidence of active ovarian malignancy. A similar mechanism can produce the radiological appearance of lymphangitis carcinosa as opposed to pulmonary or pleural metastases.

Length of history

Not unnaturally, the presenting symptoms of patients with advanced-stage disease (IIb, III, and IV) differ somewhat from

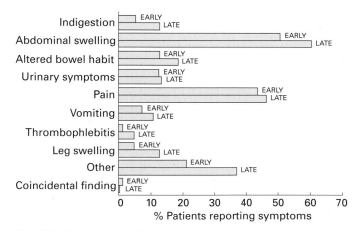

Fig. 30.6 Non-gynaecological presentation symptoms of patients with primary ovarian cancer; variation between early disease (stages I, IIa) and late disease (stages IIb, III, and IV) (966 cases from the North-East Thames Region, UK).

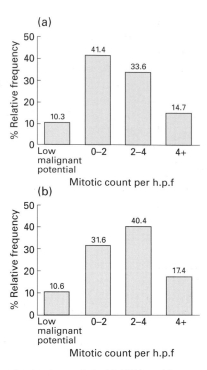

Fig. 30.7 Distribution by grade in (a) 125 long-history cases (greater than 12 months); (b) 739 short-history cases (less than 6 months) (1.7% ungraded).

those with disease confined to the ovaries (Fig. 30.6). Owing to the silent nature of the initial stages of ovarian malignancy, there is little correlation between the duration of symptoms and the stage of disease. All symptoms represent either an accident to, or extension of, a primary ovarian tumour. Thus the longer duration of premonitory symptoms may actually be a reflection of lower biological activity. In the authors' series, 52% of patients with a presenting history longer than 12 months were recorded as having well-differentiated tumours of low grade, as opposed to 42% of those presenting within 6 months of the onset of symptoms (Fig. 30.7). Early diagnosis based solely upon the correct interpretation of symptoms is unlikely to be rewarded by significant improvement in therapeutic results.

The relevance of biological behaviour to presentation and management plan

The biological behaviour of tumours of low potential malignancy is currently of great interest. The histological recognition is discussed in detail in Chapter 10. The majority of patients with borderline tumours present in stage I (83% in the authors' series). For these, the term 'of low malignant potential' is entirely apposite. There is, however, a continuous spectrum of malignant activity of ovarian neoplasia. The line drawn between borderline and 'invasive' ovarian tumours is somewhat arbitrary, being based on a rather subjective definition of 'destructive stromal invasion'. This phenomenon is more easily diagnosed within the stromal stalks of serous papillary tumours than in mucinous tumours, where it may be difficult to tell whether small glandular inclusions within stromal septa represent an invasive process or small 'daughter' cysts in a multicystic lesion,[77] and is extremely difficult in clear cell tumours. The grade of serous papillary tumours tends to be much more uniform and thus less subject to sampling errors than that of mucinous tumours, which often show a complete spectrum of activity from obviously totally benign loculi to those with clearly invasive characteristics.

Borderline tumours tend to occur in the younger age group in which well-differentiated invasive tumours may also be treated relatively conservatively. For younger patients with stage I tumours, no great therapeutic decision hangs on the histopathological semantics at the less aggressive end of the spectrum. However, this is not the case in those low-grade tumours which have already metastasized at presentation and which have therefore demonstrated an actual, rather than a potential, malignant propensity. To describe such a metastasizing tumour as 'proliferative without evidence of invasion', although in a purest sense technically correct, may mislead clinicians by inappropriate analogy with the terms 'pre-invasive' and 'invasive' when applied to carcinoma of the cervix. Some women will die of proliferative (albeit non-invasive) cancer of the ovary, which is not true of pre-invasive carcinoma of the cervix unless and until it becomes invasive. However, it is true that the natural history of many of these low-grade lesions of the ovary is such that, even when metastatic, the prognosis is significantly better than that of anaplastic 'invasive' lesions. It is generally agreed that better prognosis is associated with a good response to conventional therapy, although anecdotal reports exist of prolonged survival in the face of treatment which would be regarded as inadequate under any other circumstances. Sampling errors and differences between primary tumours and metastases further compound the issue.

Late recurrences of ovarian cancer may present occasionally after a very protracted interval, particularly with tumours of gonadal stromal origin. A lapse of 20 years has been seen by the authors and has also been reported elsewhere.[78] The diagnosis of granulosa cell ovarian carcinoma in metastases may actually be quite difficult, particularly after a long time interval when the nature of the original ovarian pathology may have been forgotten or never available. The natural history, and thus management plans, for gonadal stromal tumours are different.[79]

Extragenital carcinoma metastatic to the ovary

Patients who present with symptoms attributable to a malignant ovarian mass may, in fact, have a secondary deposit arising from an unsuspected extragenital primary. The classical Krukenberg tumour is fairly easily recognized. These tumours are pink, bossellated, glistening, and rarely adherent to other structures. However, many secondary deposits do not show the classical appearance which usually implies a mucus-secreting tumour. On closer inspection, such secondary deposits may be indistinguishable from a primary ovarian malignancy and it is the histopathologist

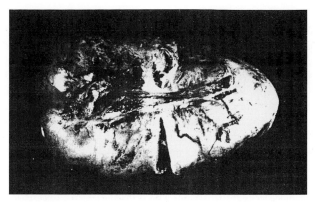

Fig. 30.8 Burkitt's lymphoma of the ovary (Photographic Unit, University College Hospital, Ibadan, Nigeria).

who first raises the possibility that the ovarian tumour may be a secondary deposit. The value and propriety of pursuing investigations to identify an unknown primary in the presence of widespread metastatic disease should be determined on an individual basis, in the light of the prognosis, quality of life, and availability of useful therapeutic intervention. With some types of tumour, the latter may be dramatic and worthwhile, for instance in appropriate parts of the world the diagnosis of Burkitt's lymphoma (Fig. 30.8) needs to be considered, particularly in younger patients.[80]

Summary of diagnosis and assessment

The natural history of malignant disease depends on five variables:

(1) age;
(2) general medical condition of the patient (Karnovsky performance score):
    (a) coincidental conditions,
    (b) those secondary to the cancerous process (e.g. cachexia, paraneoplastic syndromes);
(3) pathology:
    (a) site (primary or secondary),
    (b) tumour type,
    (c) grade (cytological, architectural);
(4) stage;
(5) treatment.

Of these factors, the first four have already been determined by the time the patient seeks medical advice and the only variable still potentially able to influence the natural history of the disease is treatment. If a treatment plan is not tailored carefully to fit in with the multivaried implications of the preceding four factors, then the chances of a successful outcome may be significantly reduced. Di Selvestro et al. (1997)[81] reported that there was no significant association between coexisting chronic medical conditions and early death.

Evidence of extra-abdominal (stage IV) disease is very important in formulating appropriate treatment and should be obtained before surgical intervention.. Full radical surgery is of little benefit, but palliative bulk reduction can be worthwhile to improve quality of life during a temporary remission, if this is achievable by chemotherapy. Because of the undoubted benefits of chemotherapy in advanced ovarian disease, and because individual tailoring of the regimen should suit both the patient and the particular tumour, it is always worthwhile establishing whether the ovary is the likely primary and this information may be obtained in the course of palliative oophorectomy. In other cases, the diagnosis may be achieved by minimally invasive means.

In malignant disease of the ovary, much of the information necessary for correct treatment planning becomes available only at or after operation. Preliminary diagnostic measures may aid, but not replace, this information. The possibilities and opportunities for asymptomatic screening are explored in Chapter 24, but the general impact of such programmes and their availability will not be apparent for decades.[82]

In the meantime, if the diagnosis is not suspected on clinical grounds, opportunities for the use even of currently available diagnostic aids may be overlooked. An operating surgeon may still be taken unawares by the finding of unexpected ovarian malignancy and may also be unacquainted with the need for, and niceties of, accurate staging (see Chapter 37), unfamiliar with the vagaries and therapeutic implications of the pathology (see Chapters 9, 10, and 11), and, finally, unprepared for the range of surgical procedures which may be appropriate for adequate primary treatment (see Chapter 37). A locally incomplete operation (perhaps rationalized as 'debulking') may compromise subsequent optimal surgical intervention.

In conclusion, therefore, an improvement in clinical awareness of this disorder must be looked for, not only amongst the general public, but, more importantly, amongst the many strands of the medical profession, including those generalist and specialist surgical practitioners of other disciplines who may encounter ovarian malignancy. Without this, there will be little hope of deriving any general benefit from the limited, but undeniable, advances being made in the management of this hitherto depressing disease.

Acknowledgements

The authors acknowledge the collaborative study of the Association of Obstetricians and Gynaecologists of North-East Thames (Metropolitan) Region and the Regional Histopathologists Group, and the related work, respectively, of the Williamson Laboratory and the Computing Unit at St Bartholomew's Hospital, London, with support from Regional funds for Locally Organised Clinical Research, the Charities Aid Foundation, and the Peel Medical Trust.

References

1. Serov, S.F., Scully, R.E., and Sobin, L.H. (1973). Histological typing of ovarian tumors. *International histological classification of tumors*, No. 9. WHO, Geneva.
2. Prendeville, J., Taylor, A.E., Carter, P.G. *et al.* (1995). A retrospective analysis of survival and natural history in 64 patients with borderline ovarian tumours. *Br. J. Obstet. Gynaec.*, **102**, 345.
3. Hudson, C.N. (1981). Ovarian cancer: a gynaecological disorder? *Ann. Roy. Coll. Surg. Engl.*, **63**, 118–25.
4. Hudson, C.N., Potsides, P., and Curling, O.M. (1991). An audit of surgical treatment of ovarian cancer in a metropolitan health region. *J. Roy. Soc. Med.*, **84**, 206.
5. Fox, R.M., Woods, R.L., Tattersall, M.H.N., and McGovern, V.J. (1979). Undifferentiated carcinoma in young men: the atypical teratoma syndrome. *Lancet*, **1**, 1316–18.
6. Florell, S.R., Bruggers, C.S., Matlak, M., Young, R.H., and Lowichik, A. (1999). Ovarian small cell carcinoma of the hypercalcemic type in a 14 month old. *Med. Ped. Oncol.*, **32**, 304–7.
7. Neijt, J.P. (1990). *Advanced ovarian cancer. Consultant series*: The role of haemopoietic growth factors, **4**, 5.
8. Bernstein, P. (1936). Tumors of the ovary: a study of 1101 cases of operations for ovarian tumor. *Am. J. Obstet. Gynec.*, **32**, 1023–39.
9. Curling, O.M., Potsides, P.N., and Hudson, C.N. (1979). Malignant change in benign cystic teratoma of the ovary. *Br. J. Obstet. Gynaec.*, **86**, 399–402.
10. Marchetti, M., Chiavelli, S., Silvestri, P., and Peron, M.L. (1995). Epithelial ovarian tumours in young women under 35 years. *Eur. J. Gynaecol. Oncol.*, **16**, 488–93.
11. T, Ind and R. Iles (1998). Prognostic markers for epithelial ovarian cancer. *Contemp. Rev. Obstet. Gynecol.*, **3**, 536–60.
12. Christian, C.D. (1971). Ovarian tumours: an extension of the Peutz–Jeghers syndrome. *Am. J. Obstet. Gynec.*, **111**, 529–34.
13. Shearman, R.P. (1981). The intersexes. In *Integrated obstetrics and gynaecology for postgraduates*, (3rd edn), (ed. C.J.Dewhurst), pp. 37–8. Blackwell Scientific Publications, Oxford.
14. Tucker, M.H.M., Fryer. J.A., and Saunders, D.M. (1982). Ovarian carcinoma in identical twins. *Aust. N.Z. J. Obstet. Gynaec.*, **22**, 113–15.
15. Booth, M., Beral, V., and Smith, P. (1989). Risk factors for ovarian cancer: a case-control study. *Br. J. Cancer*, **60**, 592–8.
16. Cramer, D.W., Hutchison, G.B., Welch, W.R., Scully, R.E., and Knapp, R.C. (1982). Factors affecting the association of oral contraceptives and ovarian cancer. *N. Engl. J. Med.*, **302**(17), 1047–51.
17. Crowther, M.E., Poulton, T.A., and Hudson, C.N. (1981). Relationship between cellular responses of parous women and ovarian cancer patients to tumour extracts. *J. Obstet.Gynaec.*, **11**, 263–7.
18. Casagrande, J.T., Louie, E.W., Pike, M.C., Roy, S., Ross, R.K., and Henderson, B.E. (1979). 'Incessant ovulation' and ovarian cancer. *Lancet*, **8135**, 170–2.
19. Venn, A., Watson, L., Lumley, J., Giles, G., King, C., and Healy, D. (1995). Breast and ovarian cancer incidence after infertility and *in vitro* fertilisation. *Lancet*, **346**, 995–1000.
20. Whittemore, A.S., Harris, R., and Itnyre, J. (1992). Characteristics relating to ovarian cancer risk: collaborative analysis of 12 US case-control studies II. *Am. J. Epidemiol.*, **136**, 1184.
21. Vara, P. and Pankamaa, P. (1946). A clinical–statistical investigation of ovarian tumors operated at the Helsinki University Clinic of Gynecology during the years 1900–1944. *Acta Obstet. Gynecol. Scand.*,**26**, (Suppl.4), 49.
22. Bourne, T. (1993). Can ovarian masses be characterized using ultrasound? [editorial;comment]. *Gynecol. Oncol.*, **51**, 4–6.
23. Jacobs, I., Stabile, I., Bridges, J., Kemsley, P., Reynolds, C., Grudzinskas, J., and Oram, D. (1988). Multimodal approach to screening for ovarian cancer. *Lancet*, **8580**, 268–71.
24. Barr, W. (1980). Current problems in diagnosis and management. In *Ovarian cancer*, (ed. C.E. Newman, C.H.J. Ford, and J.A. Jordan), pp. 1–8. Pergamon, Oxford.
25. Oram, D.H. and John, J. (1999). Should ovaries be removed at hysterectomy? In *Menorrhagia* (ed. Sheth, S. and Sutton, C.J.), pp. 265–7. Isis, Oxford.
26. Koonues, P.P., Campbell, K, Mishell, D.R. Jr, Grimes, D.A. (1989). Relative frequency of primary ovarian neoplasms: a 10 year review. *Obstet Gynecol*, **74**, 921–6.
27. Curling, O.M. and Hudson, C.N. (1975). Endometrioid tumours of the ovary. *Br. J. Obstet. Gynaecol.*, **82**, 405–11.

28. Beilby, J.O.W., Horne, C.H.W., Milne, G.D., and Parkinson, C. (1979). Alpha-fetoprotein, alpha–1-antitrypsin, and transferrin in gonadal yolk-sac tumours. *J. Clin. Path.*, **32**, 455–61.

29. Benfield, G.F.A., Tapper-Jones, L., and Stout, T.V. (1982). Androblastoma and raised serum alpha-feto protein with familial multinodular goitre. *Br. J. Obstet. Gynaecol.*, **89**, 323–6.

30. Hudson, C.N. (1979). A review of immunological aspects of gynaecological malignancy. *Br. J. Obstet. Gynaecol.*, **86**, 154–8.

31. Hudson, C.N., Curling, O.M., Potsides, P., and Lowe, D.G. (1993). Paraneoplastic syndromes in patients with ovarian neoplasia. *J. Roy. Soc. Med.*, **86**, 202–4.

32. Bennett, R.M., Ginsberg, M.H., and Thomsen, S. (1976). Carcinomatous polyarthritis. *Arthritis Rheum.*, **19**, 953–9.

33. Levin, L., McHardy, J.E., Curling, O.M., and Hudson, C.N. (1975). Tumour antigenicity in ovarian cancer. *Br. J. Cancer*, **32**, 152–9.

34. Whitehouse, J.M.A. (1973). Circulating antibodies in human malignant disease. *Br. J. Cancer*, **28** (Suppl.1), 170.

35. Gerber, M.A., Koffler, D., and Cohen, C.J. (1977). Circulating antibodies in patients with ovarian carcinoma. *Gynecol. Oncol.*, **5**, 228–32.

36. Poulton, T.A., Crowther, M.E., Hay, F.C., and Nineham, L.T. (1978). Immune complexes in ovarian cancer. *Lancet*, **2**, 72–3.

37. Hoyt, R.E. and Hamilton, J.F. (1987). Ovarian cancer associated with the nephrotic syndrome. *Obstet. Gynecol.* **70**, 513–14.

38. Albert, M.L., Darnell, J.C., Barder, A. *et al.* (1998). Tumour specific killer cells in paraneoplastic cerebellar degeneration. *Nature Med.*, **4**, 1321–4.

39. Ausell, J.K. and Stebbings, W.S.L. (1993). Carcinoid syndrome due to primary ovarian carcinoid tumour. *J. Roy. Soc. Med.*, **86**, 668.

40. Robboy, S.J., Scully, R.E., and Norris, H.J. (1974). Carcinoid metastatic to the ovary. *Cancer*, **33**, 798–811.

41. Lam, S.K. and Cheung, L.P. (1996). Inappropriate ADH secretion due to immature ovarian teratoma. *Aust. N.Z. J. Obstet. Gynaecol.*, **36**, 104–5.

42. Parsons, V. and Rigby, B. (1958). Cushing's syndrome associated with adenocarcinoma of the ovary. *Lancet*, **2**, 992–4.

43. Marieb, N.J., Spangler, S., Kashgarian, M. *et al.* (1983). Cushing's syndrome secondary to ectopic cortisol production by an ovarian carcinoma. *J. Clin. Endoc. Metab.*, **57**, 737–40.

44. Fosse R.G., Wilson, D.R., Heersche, J.N., Mills, J.R., and Murray, T.M. (1981). Hypercalcemia with ovarian carcinoma: evidence of a pathogenetic role for prostaglandins. *Cancer*, **48**, 1233–41.

45. Ross, L. and Shelley, E. (1968). Mesonephric carcinoma of the ovary producing hypercalcemia. *Am. J. Obstet. Gynec.*, **100**, 418–21.

46. Dickersin, G.R., Kline, I.W., and Scully, R.E. (1982). Small cell carcinoma of the ovary with hypercalcemia. *Cancer*, **49**, 188–97.

47. Taraszewski, R., Rosman, P.M., Knight, C.A., and Cloney, D.J. (1991). Small cell carcinoma of the ovary. *Gynecol. Oncol.*, **41**, 149–51.

48. Boyer, M., Friedlander, M., Bannatyne, P., and Atkinson, K. (1989). Hypercalcemia in association with mucinous cystadenocarcinoma of the ovary: a case report. *Gynecol. Oncol.*, **35**, 387–90.

49. Allan, S.G., Lockhart, S.P., Leonard, R.C., and Smyth, J.F. (1984). Paraneoplastic hyper-calcaemia in ovarian carcinoma. *Br. J. Med.*, **228**, 1714–15.

50. Kim, W., Bockman, R., Lemos, L., and Lewis, J.L. Jr (1981). Hypercalcemia associated with epidermal carcinoma in ovarian cystic teratoma. *Obstet. Gynecol.*, **57**, 81S–5S.

51. Connell, W.R., Newell-Price, J.D., Lowe, D.G. *et al.* (1993). Zollinger–Ellison syndrome caused by mucinous cystadenocarcinoma of the ovary. *Aust. N.Z. J. Med.*, **23**, 520–1.

52. O'Neill, R.T. and Mikuta, J.J. (1970). Hypoglycemia associated with serous cystadenocarcinoma of the ovary. *Obstet. Gynecol.*, **35**, 287–9.

53. Hayakawa, T., Kameya, A., Mizuno, R., Noda, A., Kondo, T., and Hirabayashi, N. (1984). Hyperamylasemia with papillary serous cystadenocarcinoma of the ovary. *Cancer*, **54**, 1662–5.

54. Hammond, D. and Winnick, S. (1974). Paraneoplastic erythrocytosis and ectopic erythropoietins. *Ann. N.Y. Acad. Sci.*, **230**, 219–27.

55. Menzies, D.N. (1965). Two further cases of erythrocytosis secondary to fibromyomata. *Proc. Roy. Soc. Med.*, **58**, 239.

56. Sorenson, H.T., Mellemkjaer L., Steffensen, F.H., Olsen, J.H., and Nielsen, G.L. (1998). The risk of diagnosis of cancer after primary deep venous thrombosis or pulmonary embolism. *N. Engl. J. Med.*, **338**, 1169–73.

57. Henderson, P.H. (1955). Multiple migratory thrombophlebitis associated with ovarian carcinoma. *Am. J. Obstet. Gynecol.*, **70**, 452–3.

58. Adamson, A.S., Littlewood, T.J., Poston, G.J. *et al.* (1988). Malignancy presenting as peripheral venous gangrene. *J. Roy. Soc. Med.*, **81**, 609–10.

59. Duncan, S.C. and Winkelmann, R.K. (1979). Cancer and scleroderma. *Arch. Dermatol.*, **115**, 950–5.

60. Barnes, B.E. (1976). Dermatomyositis and malignancy. *Ann. Int. Med.*, **84**, 68–76.

61. Peters, W.A., Anderson, W.A., and Thornton, W.N. Jr (1983). Dermatomyositis and co-existent ovarian cancer. A review of the compounding clinical problems. *Gynecol. Oncol* **15**, 444–6.

62. Medsger, T.A., Dixon, J.A., and Garwood, V.F. (1982). Palmar fasciitis and polyarthritis associated with ovarian carcinoma. *Ann. Int. Med.*, **96**, 424–31.

63. Haynes, H.A. and Curth, H.O. (1979). Acanthosis nigricans. In *Dermatology in general medicine*, (2nd edn), (ed. T.B. Fitzpatrick *et al.*), p. 1348. McGraw Hill, New York.

64. Dingley, E.R. and Marten, R.H. (1957). Adenocarcinoma of the ovary presenting as acanthosis nigricans. *J. Obstet. Gynaecol. Br. Cwlth*, **64**, 898–900.

65. Stashower, M.E., Rennie, T.A., Turiansky, G.W., and Gilliland, W.R. (1999). Ovarian cancer presenting as leukocytoclastic vasculitis. *J. Am. Acad. Dermat.*, **40**, 287–9.

66. Croft, P.B. and Wilkinson, M. (1964). The incidence of carcinomatous neuromyopathy with special reference to lung and breast carcinoma. In *The remote effects of cancer on the nervous system*, (eds W.R. Brain and F. Norris), pp. 44–54. Grune and Stratton, New York.

67. Young, R.R. and Richardson, E.P. (1976). Case records of the Massachusetts General Hospital. Case 26. *New Engl. J. Med.*, **294**, 1447–54.

68. Wilkins, D.J.W. (1953). Malignant Brenner tumour presenting with lower motor neurone paralysis. *J. Obstet. Gynaecol.*, **4**, 64.

69. Aydimer, A., Gurvit, H., and Baral, I. (1998). Paraneoplastic limbic encephalitis with immature ovarian teratoma. *J. Neurol. Oncol.*, **37**, 63–6.

70. Hall, D.J., Dyer, M.L., and Parker, J.C. Jr (1985). Ovarian cancer complicated by cerebellar degeneration: a paraneoplastic syndrome. *Gynecol. Oncol.*, **21**, 240–6.

71. Hetzel, D.J., Stanhope, C.R., O'Neill, B.P., and Lennon, V.A. (1990). Gynecologic cancer in patients with subacute cerebellar degeneration predicted by anti-Purkinje cell antibodies and limited in metastatic volume. *Mayo Clin. Proc.*, **65**, 1558–63.

72. Lowe, D.G. and Shepherd, J.H. (1991). Enough evidence to operate? [editorial]. *Lancet*, **337**, 1066–7.

73. Drlicek, M., Bianchi, G., Boglium, G. *et al.* (1997). Antibodies of the anti-Y0 and anti-R1 type in the absence of paraneoplastic neurological syndromes. *J. Neurol.*, **244**, 85–9.

74. Cocconi, G., Ceci, G., Juvarra, G. (1985). Successful treatment of subacute cerebellar degeneration in ovarian carcinoma with plasmapheresis. A case report. *Cancer*, **56**, 2318–20.

75. Chamberlain, M.J. and Whitaker, S.R.F. (1963). Hashimoto's disease, dermatomyositis and ovarian carcinoma. *Lancet*, **1**, 1398–400.

76. Kinder, C.H. (1979). Retroperitoneal fibrosis. *J. Roy. Soc. Med.*, **72**, 485–7.

77. Colgan, T.J. and Norris, H.J. (1983). Ovarian epithelial tumours of low malignant potential. *Int. J. Gynecol. Pathol.*, **1**, 367.

78. Lamout, C.A.R and Ashton, P.W. (1975). Observations on granulosa cell tumours, in *Diagnosis and first treatments of ovarian neoplastic cerebrations* (ed. H. DeWattesville and P. Burch), pp. 241–8. Excerpta Medica, Amsterdam.

79. Savage, P., Constenla, D., Fisher, C. *et al.* (1998). Granulosa cell tumours of the ovary. Demographics, survival and management of advanced disease. *Clin. Oncol.*, **10**, 242–5.

80. Junaid, T.A. (1981). Ovarian neoplasms in children and adolescents in Ibadan, Nigeria. *Cancer*, **47**, 610–14.

81. Di Selvestro, P., Peipert, J.S., Hogan, J.W. *et al.* (1997). Prognostic values of clinical variable in ovarian cancer. *J. Clin. Epidemiol.*, **50**, 501–5.

82. Oram, D.H., Jacobs, I.J., Brady, K., and Prys, D.A. (1990). Early diagnosis of ovarian cancer. *Br. J. Hosp. Med.* **44**, 5.

31. Serum tumour markers in the clinical management of ovarian cancer

Robert P. Woolas

Introduction

A substantial research effort has resulted in a large number of substances being proposed and recognized as serum markers for ovarian cancer. In clinical practice none has proved more useful than the measurement of CA125 levels in the evaluation of malignant epithelial tumours. Hormones such as oestrogen, inhibin, and Müllerian inhibitory substance are helpful serum markers for the detection of granulosa cell and other sex cord–stromal tumours. Among germ cell tumours differentiation along trophoblastic lines results in human chorionic gonadotrophin (hCG) expression, which is also expressed by undifferentiated embryonal carcinoma and non-gestational choriocarcinoma. Differentiation along yolk-sac pathways results in α-fetoprotein secretion. Malignant transformation in a teratoma can result in neuron-specific enolase and squamous cell carcinoma antigen expression. These latter lesions are comparatively rare, thus this chapter focuses primarily on marker expression by epithelial ovarian cancer.

CA125

Assay of CA125 levels is the most widely requested serological investigation for ovarian cancer, as 95% of malignant ovarian tumours are epithelial in origin.[1] The compound was first identified by Bast in 1981[2] through the monoclonal antibody OC125. It is expressed by most non-mucinous epithelial ovarian tumours as well as other tissues of Müllerian origin.[3] Prior to histological diagnosis, the measurement of serum CA125 levels has been shown to be useful in the discrimination of the benign from malignant adnexal mass. Very high absolute values at presentation confer information on the likely extent and possible prognosis of malignant disease.[4] Failure of CA125 levels to return to normal following primary surgery and initial chemotherapy has been associated with the degree of residual disease remaining after surgery and the likely disease course. The response to therapy may be monitored, and rising levels may be detected in advance of clinical or radiological evidence of recurrence.[5] Furthermore, among postmenopausal women the specificity of the assay is such

that a role as the first-line test in a multimodal screening programme for ovarian cancer has been proposed.[6] (See Chapter 24.)

The CA125 antigen is expressed by fetal coelomic structures.[7] In healthy women it is a secretory product found in uterine and tubal fluids, breast milk, and amniotic fluid.[8] However, normal ovarian epithelium does not express CA125, except for micro-inclusion cysts and papillary excrescences. The endometrium secretes CA125 during menses, or when involved in benign disease.[9,10] The disruption of endometrial tissue architecture at menstruation appears to allow the release of CA125 into the circulation, leading to elevated serum levels. Coelomic-derived structures such as the peritoneum, pleura, or pericardium are immunocytochemically negative for CA125 in adults. They can, however, re-express CA125 when involved in benign diseases (Table 31.1), such as pelvic infection,[11] endometriosis,[12] and conditions with benign causes of ascites, such as tuberculosis and pericarditis, or when these structures are infiltrated by malignant processes arising from any primary site.

CA125 is an antigenic determinant on a high molecular weight glycoprotein which is larger than 200 kDa. The antigen is still poorly characterized and the CA125 gene has not been identified. Attempts to obtain the sequence of the CA125 peptide backbone by expression cloning have resulted in the isolation of a zinc-finger protein that maps to a site on chromosome 17q near *BRCA1*.[13] However, this protein lacks the ability to bind OC125, suggesting that it does not express the CA125 epitope. The biological function of the glycoprotein expressing CA125 remains unknown.[14]

The OC125 monoclonal antibody was produced in BALB/c mice immunized with ovarian cancer cells derived from a serous

Table 31.1 Benign conditions known to be associated with an elevated CA125

Gynaecological	Non-gynaecological
Pregnancy	Peritonitis
Menstruation	Acute pancreatitis
Endometriosis	Peritoneal dialysis
Adenomyosis	Chronic liver disease
Pelvic inflammatory disease	Pericarditis
Ovarian cysts	Pleurisy

papillary cystadenocarcinoma cell line. Subsequent application of the OC125 antibody in an immunoradiometric assay made quantification of CA125 possible.[15] Serum levels up to 35 U/ml are considered normal, as this cutoff represents the 97.5 percentile in healthy female blood donors. In the original CA125 assay, OC125 was applied as both a capture and tracer antibody. An increasing number of CA125 levels are now analysed with the second-generation CA125 II assays.[16] These utilize the M11 as a capture antibody and the original OC125 as a tracer. This results in superior analytical performance and an assay that is more sensitive for the diagnosis of malignancy. The results of our own comparison of these two assays when tested on 429 preoperative serum samples from women presenting with a pelvic mass are shown in Table 31.2. Although the 35 U/ml cutoff threshold has generally been retained, it should be noted that alternative thresholds at a lower level 26 U/ml or 20 U/ml, particularly amongst postmenopausal women, have been proposed.[17–19]

In the initial report[15] of the use of CA125 measurement in monitoring the course of patients with ovarian cancer, serum CA125 levels were elevated above 35 U/ml in 83 of 101 patients (82%) with surgically demonstrated disease, in contrast to 1% of healthy blood donors. Rising or falling levels correlated with progression and regression of disease in 42 of 45 cases. Following these observations, over 2000 investigations have been published, both confirming these findings and also documenting the following useful applications of CA125 measurement.

Preoperative diagnosis of the adnexal mass

The advanced knowledge of the benign or malignant nature of an adnexal mass has considerable relevance to the planning, timing, and operative approach, either open or laparoscopic, that may be used for such patients. Furthermore, in the UK recent recommendations supporting the tertiary referral of all women with ovarian cancer to gynaecological cancer centres and fast track access to secondary services of all patients with suspected cancer have focused attention on the accurate assessment of women diagnosed as having a pelvic mass.[20]

Elevated levels of CA125 are found in the serum of over 85% of women presenting with ovarian cancer, but this sensitivity is reduced to approximately 50% when only those with stage I disease are considered.[21] Normal serum levels are more frequently found in association with the mucinous histological subtype of epithelial cancer and among patients with borderline ovarian tumours.[22–24] The specificity of CA125 levels, using the 35 U/ml cutoff, among women with benign adnexal lesions is in the order of 75%.[25,26] This specificity is higher among postmenopausal women, as diseases such as endometriosis or pelvic infection are less prevalent. Malkasian et al. (1988)[27] reported that a preoperative value greater than 65 U/ml had a positive predictive value of malignancy of 98% in postmenopausal patients. However, among premenopausal patients the predictive value of malignancy using the 65 U/ml cutoff was only 49%.

In the context of a diagnostic test, several strategies might be used to increase the predictive accuracy of serum assays. These include altering the cutoff threshold and use of a panel of multiple complementary markers. Decreasing the threshold for an individual assay inevitably results in a decrease in specificity. Likewise, raising the cutoff reduces sensitivity. Use of multiple markers should increase sensitivity and may or may not decrease specificity, depending on the degree of coordinate expression in both benign and malignant disease. A reduction of specificity incurred by the measurement of a panel of markers might be refined through the identification of multiple elevations,[28] or possibly through observations over time.[29] The ideal requirement is complementary and coordinate expression[30] of different markers. Numerous studies have investigated potential coordinate or complementary markers to CA125.[31–33] In a simple combination analysis, none have shown consistent improvement in discrimination among large numbers of patients, as the characteristics of the markers measured results in a trade-off between sensitivity and specificity. An electronic decision tree, classification, and regression analysis (CART)[34–36] or artificial neural network is required to improve the overall result.[37] In addition, such a programme can also integrate demographic or clinical information; for example, age or menopausal status or the results of imaging investigations.[38–40] Although these automated analytical programmes could be developed for universal application in practice,[41] the straightforward simple analysis of currently available information

Table 31.2 Comparison of original CA125 assay with CA125 II assay among 429 women with a pelvic mass

Marker	Cutoff threshold	Sensitivity (%)		Specificity (%)			
		Invasive EOC	Invasive and borderline EOC	All ovarian cancer	All gynaecological cancer	All cancer	Benign pelvic mass
Number		127	136	157	180	192	237
CA125	30 U/ml	90%	87%	85%	81%	79%	71%
CA125 II	30 U/ml	94%	91%	90%	88%	85%	67%
CA125	35 U/ml	88%	85%	84%	80%	78%	77%
CA125 II	35 U/ml	91%	88%	87%	85%	82%	71%

EOC, epithelial ovarian cancer.

remains important at the clinical interface. Thus at present the most commonly used approach to triage of these patients is that described by Jacobs et al. 1990,[42] who developed the risk of malignancy index (RMI) score. A logistic regression formula was derived from the characteristics of a consecutive series of patients presenting with an adnexal lesion. Three readily available features were combined: the patient's menopausal status, an ultrasound score based on simple morphological features of the preoperative report, and the serum CA125 level. In this equation (RMI 1) the patient's menopausal status is weighted as either 1 or 3 for pre- or postmenopausal women, and the ultrasound score is calculated as 0, 1, or 2, dependent upon the presence of none or more of the following features of an adnexal lesion: a septum, solid areas, bilaterality of the cysts, ascites, or obvious metastatic disease. These two scores are then multiplied together with the actual CA125 level to provide an objective assessment of the risk of malignancy. This result provided greater discriminatory value than any single test alone and was confirmed by Prys-Davies et al. (1993)[43] in a further prospective study. The clinical application was tested in Norway by Tinglustad et al. (1996).[44] Setting a threshold of the RMI at a level of 200 provides a sensitivity for identification of ovarian cancer in the order of 80% and excludes over 90% of benign adnexal tumours (Table 31.3). Such a threshold provides appropriate tertiary referral of almost all cases of advanced disease for cytoreductive surgery by a gynaecological oncologist but is less discriminatory for early stage cancers.[44] These authors also described modifications (RMI 2) to the original weighting in the equation of the menopausal status (4 for postmenopausal) and an ultrasound score of either 1 instead of 0, or 4 if 2 or more features of malignancy were present. This equation (RMI 2), was then prospectively evaluated in a further large series of patients[45] and two other reports using these calculations have subsequently been published.[46,47] These data relating to RMI calculations are summarized in Table 31.3. There appears to be no discriminatory difference between the RMI 1 and 2 in this pooled analysis. Using the 200 cutoff, over three-quarters of ovarian malignancies can be identified by this technique, and 9 out of 10 benign lesions excluded.

Table 31.3 Risk of malignancy index (RMI) versions 1 and 2, calculated as score >200; compiled data from five centres

Study	Year	N	% Malignant	% Sensitivity	% Specificity
RMI 1					
Jacobs	1990	143	29	86	97
Prys-Davies	1993	132	31	87	91
Tingulstadt	1996	173	32	71	96
Morgante	1999	124	25	58	95
Timmerman	2000	173	28	84	82
Timmerman	2000	230	34	76	79
Woolas	2001	246	42	80	93
Total		**1221**	**33**	**78**	**90**
RMI 2					
Tingulstadt	1996	173	32	80	92
Tingulstadt	1999	365	21	71	92
Morgante	1999	124	25	74	93
Total		**662**	**24**	**75**	**92**

This approach would not have sufficient sensitivity to ensure appropriate fast tracking, as has recently been suggested in the UK, of primary-care referrals of suspected malignancy to the cancer assessment unit. However, using a lower threshold of the RMI, or perhaps, more simply, a CA125 level of 20 U/ml or greater, would ensure the prompt treatment of 98% of women with invasive epithelial ovarian cancer in our catchment area.[48] Furthermore the proportion of patients referred to our service who have cancer appears higher and the specificity of the later reports is lower than in the earlier data (Table 31.3). No population-based data exist to inform us of the exact ratio of benign to malignant adnexal lesions in the community. However, an explanation for this shift in proportions is that the publication and dissemination of knowledge relating to CA125 levels and the risk of malignancy has already led to a more accurate primary and secondary referral practice to tertiary gynaecological oncology services.

Information available from absolute perioperative levels

In 1988 Di-Xia et al.[49] defined a new positivity criterion for CA125 of 194 U/ml as representing the 95th centile among 153 women presenting with a benign pelvic mass. The corresponding sensitivity for the identification of malignancy was 80%. It is extremely rare for postmenopausal women who have levels in excess of 300 U/ml not to have malignant disease. This is less so among premenopausal women, as endometriosis is a relatively common condition, but it should also be noted that this disease can also occur in older women taking hormone replacement therapy.[12] Conversely, patients with a serum CA125 below 20 U/ml are extremely unlikely to have advanced ovarian cancer. The negative predictive value for any stage of invasive epithelial ovarian cancer is very high at this threshold.

Although initial reports did not determine a relationship between the absolute value of CA125 and prognosis, a recent large study of prognostic factors in 201 stage I patients has been performed.[50] In a multivariate analysis the preoperative CA125 level was found to be the most powerful prognostic factor for survival ($P < 0.0001$). The risk of dying of ovarian cancer was six times higher among those women with a CA125 level above 65 U/ml. In addition, failure of CA125 levels to return to normal after apparent complete resection of a stage I tumour has also been recognized as an adverse prognostic finding and is generally regarded as an indication for consideration of adjuvant chemotherapy.

Monitoring of the disease course

Measurements of CA125 are widely applied to follow treatment response, as early information about a response could contribute to therapy being continued despite serious complications. Alternatively, in patients with progressive disease, ineffective drugs can be stopped and another treatment instituted. It has been shown that combination chemotherapy has little effect on CA125 antigen expression by ovarian cancer cells,[51] and many reports have confirmed that changes in CA125 levels reflect progression or regression in approximately 90% of instances.[14]

The rate of decline of the serum CA125 level during primary chemotherapy has proven to be a good predictor of the response.[52–55] Calculations of half-life time are a sensitive predictor of the likelihood of achieving complete remission and prolonged survival.[53, 56–58] Furthermore, an absolute level of 70 U/ml before the third course of chemotherapy has been shown to predict progression or death within 12 months better than any other prognostic indicator.[59]

Generally the course of the CA125 level confers greater information than single values and is now included in the response criteria for evaluating the results of chemotherapy trials. A serial rise of CA125 levels of 25% has been shown to predict disease progression with almost 100% specificity.[60–62] Many clinicians now withhold or change chemotherapy if there is a serial increase in CA125 levels. Definitions followed range from a serial increase of 50% for three samples, a persistent increase over 100 U/ml for more than 2 months, or a 25% increase over two samples confirmed by a fourth sample. Measurement of additional markers may be used to increase the sensitivity of this approach.[5]

Following cytoreductive surgery and/or chemotherapy, most women with advanced ovarian cancer have residual disease which is difficult to evaluate by clinical examination or imaging techniques. Niloff et al. (1986)[63] studied serial CA125 assays in 55 patients who, following treatment, were clinically and radiographically free of disease. The CA125 levels became elevated above 35 U/ml before clinical recurrence in 33 (94%), with a median lead time of 3 months.

The ability to detect clinically occult recurrence demands consideration of the advantages of further immediate treatment. Whether earlier intervention based on rising CA125 levels is associated with survival benefits when compared to treatment of symptomatic recurrence requires a randomized controlled trial, and the outcome of the Medical Research Council investigation OVO5 is awaited.[64]

Among women undergoing second-look surgery following chemotherapy, an elevated CA125 level invariably (96%) predicts the presence of residual tumour. The sensitivity of the test is less valuable, as approximately 50% of patients with persistent disease will have levels less than 35 U/ml.[65] In a review of 15 such series,[21] an elevated CA125 level was associated with residual disease in 156 of 165 patients, having a positive predictive value of 94.5%. However, a serum CA125 level below 35 U/ml was still associated with persistent tumour in 180 of 414 patients.

To determine whether decreasing CA125 levels can accurately indicate tumour response requires clear definition. Several definitions have been proposed, but only one has been appropriately validated. To be reliable, such criteria need to take into account natural variations in CA125 levels, upper limits of normal, lower limits of assay accuracy, and missing samples. An analysis of 620 patients demonstrated reliable prediction if either of the following definitions were satisfied. A 50% response has occurred if after two samples there has been a 50% decrease in serum CA125 levels confirmed by a fourth sample. Alternatively, a 75% response has occurred if there has been a serial decrease in serum CA125 level of more than 75% for three samples. In all

cases, the final sample has to be analysed at least 28 days after the previous sample.[66] The specificity of these requirements is very high. Only two patients (0.3%) had a mathematical response at the time of clinical disease progression. These definitions have predicted accurately the response to altretamine[67] and taxol,[68] but it should be noted that removal of ascites and administration of mouse antibodies can invalidate CA125 measurements.

Other serum tumour markers expressed by epithelial ovarian cancer

Many alterations in serum constituents, both quantitative and qualitative, have been documented in association with epithelial ovarian cancer. These observations of marker expression have been made primarily in relation to diagnosis and prognosis, but may also have direct relevance to prevention and treatment. The levels may reflect an influence of ovarian function, alterations of surface molecular structure[69] or a general response to malignancy.[70] Changes in circulating enzymes,[71–74] hormones,[75,76] non-specific inflammatory proteins,[77] and placental and fetal antigens[78–83] have all been identified in women with ovarian cancer.

Advances in monoclonal technology have resulted in the improved definition of antigens expressed on the malignant cell surface. Like CA125, these antigens may pass directly into the venous drainage of the ovary, or are shed from the ovarian surface into the peritoneal cavity and drain via lymphatics into the thoracic duct and hence access the venous circulation. Many of these antibodies are directed against epitopes on mucins, a family of highly glycosylated, high molecular weight (>200 kDa) glycoproteins which are distinct from the CA125 antigen.[84,85] More recently the discovery of peptide growth factors, their receptors, oncogenes, cytokines, and also tumour suppressor genes has raised the possibility that abnormal expression of these substances or gene products may provide interesting novel markers.[86,87] To date, little clinical application of this theory or knowledge has been confirmed, but autoantibodies to the p53 gene have been associated with advanced-stage tumours,[88] and high serum levels of the c-erbB2 gene product associated with a poor prognosis.[89] However, this latter assay was not helpful in discriminating benign from malignant adnexal masses.[90] Several markers have been shown to have independent expression to CA125 for detection of ovarian cancer, including NB/70K,[91,92] HMFG2,[93] lipid-associated sialic acid (LASA),[94–96] OSA,[97] CASA,[98] macrophage- colony stimulating factor (M-CSF),[99–104] OVX 1,[105,106] and monocyte chemoattractant protein–1.[107] A large number of studies have been performed using assays for markers such as CA15–3,[32,108,109] CA19–9,[32,110–113] CA72–4,[30,32,114–116] tissue polypeptide antigen (TPA),[113,117] CA54/61,[118–121] sialyl-Tn,[113,122] tumour-associated trypsin inhibitor (TATI),[32,123,124] MMMP–2,[125] soluble interleukin–2 receptor alpha,[126] soluble tumour necrosis factor (TNF),[127] and vascular endothelial growth factor (VEGF).[128,129] In some cases, such as LASA, CASA, and M-CSF, a degree of complementary activity of these markers has been demonstrated, but sufficient data confirming the benefits to patients are not available to justify recommending their use outside of further prospective clinical investigations.

Most markers studied to date have been either proteins or carbohydrates. Lipid molecules may also have application as tumour markers. Recently an ovarian cancer activating factor present in ascites, which stimulates proliferation, promotes invasion, and increases drug resistance, has been shown to be composed of a number of forms of lipophosphatidic acid (LPA). Elevated levels of LPA and the related derivative, lysophosphatidyl choline (LPC), have been found in most patients with ovarian cancer.[130] It is possible that these lipids may represent an entirely new family of ovarian tumour markers currently awaiting evaluation.

In the majority of investigations to date the measurement of additional markers has been found to reflect, rather than add to, the information provided by CA125 alone. A considerable problem is that the performance of CA125 as a tumour marker, although not perfectly specific, is quite robust. An additional issue is that, having accepted that some inconsistency of approach to investigation is inevitable with studies of this nature, the interpretation of these data is made more difficult by the problems associated with using stored sera, the diversity of assay techniques available,[131] variable reference ranges, and intra-individual differences,[132] including those between pre- and postmenopausal women.[17]

Serum markers in non-epithelial ovarian cancer

Serial measurements of human chorionic gonadotrophin (hCG), α-fetoprotein (AFP), and CA125 are essential in the monitoring of patients with ovarian germ cell tumours. These markers should also be assayed prior to surgery for complex ovarian masses in teenagers and young women. Raised levels in the absence of pregnancy are virtually diagnostic of a germ cell tumour and should prompt conservative surgery.[133] It is likely that hCG, AFP, and lactate dehydrogenase (LDH), a marker for pure dysgerminoma,[134] levels are prognostic indicators which are as important for females as they are for male germ cell tumours, where they play a major role in deciding which therapy patients receive.[135]

Elevated levels of squamous cell carcinoma antigen have been reported among 13 of 20 patients with a squamous cell carcinoma developing in a dermoid cyst.[136] However, increased serum levels of this marker have also been found in 17% of benign teratomas.[137] When a malignant neural element is present within a teratoma, neuron-specific enolase (NSE) has been documented as being expressed in 4 of 8 preoperative serum specimens, in contrast to only 2 of 30 benign cystic teratomas.[138] In addition, these authors reported NSE to be at an elevated level among 83% of six women prior to resection of a dysgerminoma.[138]

Granulosa cell tumours secrete inhibin, but such measurements are only of value preoperatively in postmenopausal women, due to the physiological secretion of this marker during the menstrual cycle.[139,140] Similarly oestrogen secretion by these tumours is less obvious when the disease presents in younger women. Follicle regulatory protein[141] and anti-Müllerian hormone[142] or Müllerian inhibitory substance (MIS) has been proposed as a marker for these lesions and other sex cord tumours.[143] The utility of the MIS assay is not confined to postmenopausal patients as this hormone is not produced by the normal postpubertal ovary.[144]

Conclusions

The measurement of serum CA125 levels can confer important clinical information on the nature and course of ovarian tumours. Numerous other substances have been documented in the serum of women with ovarian cancer. Determining whether this knowledge can be translated into improved survival prospects perhaps awaits the development of a better range of primary and salvage therapies for epithelial lesions. Young women presenting with complex ovarian masses should have levels of germ cell markers measured. The course of malignant non-epithelial lesions may often be monitored by a range of specific serum marker measurements.

References

1. Wiltshaw, E. (1990). Chemotherapy of ovarian cancer. In *Clinical gynaecological oncology*, (ed. J.H. Shepherd and J.M. Monaghan), pp. 254–78. Blackwell Scientific, Oxford.
2. Bast, R.C., Feeney, M., Lazarus, H. *et al.* (1981). Reactivity of a monoclonal antibody with human ovarian carcinoma. *J. Clin. Oncol.*, **68**, 1331–7.
3. Zurawski, V.R., Davis, H.M., Finkler, N.J. *et al.* (1988). Tissue distribution and characteristics of the CA125 antigen. *Cancer Rev.*, **11–12**, 102–18.
4. Parker, D., Bradley, C., Bogle, S.M. *et al.* (1994). Serum albumin and CA125 are powerful predictors of survival in epithelial ovarian cancer. *Br. J. Obstet. Gynaecol.*, **101**, 888–93.
5. Tuxen, M., Soletormos, G., and Dombernowsky, P. (1995). Tumor markers in the management of patients with ovarian cancer. *Cancer Treat. Rev.*, **21**, 215–45.
6. Jacobs, I.J., Skates, S.J., MacDonald, N. *et al.* (1999). Screening for ovarian cancer. A pilot randomised control trial. *Lancet*, **353**,
7. Kabawat, S.E., Bast, R.C., Bhan, A.K. *et al.* (1983). Tissue distribution of a coelomic-epithelium related antigen recognised by the monoclonal antibody OC 125. *Int. J. Gynecol. Pathol.*, **2**, 275–85.
8. Hardardottir, H., Parmely, T.H., Quirk, J.G. *et al.* (1990). Distribution of CA125 in embryonic tissue and adult derivatives of the fetal periderm. *Am. J. Obstet. Gynecol.*, **163**, 1925–31.
9. Grover, S., Koh, H., Weideman, P., and Quinn, M.A. (1992). The effect of the menstrual cycle on serum CA125 levels: a population study. *Am. J. Obstet. Gynecol.*, **167**, 1379–81.
10. Kan, Y.Y., Yeh, S.H., Ng, H.T., and Lou, C.M. (1992). Effect of menstruation on serum CA125 levels. *Asia Oceania J. Obstet. Gynaecol.*, **18**, 339–43.
11. Branagan, G., Woolas, R.P., Senapati, A., and Cripps, N.P.J. (1999). *Streptococcus milleri* infection mimicking ovarian carcinoma. *Br. J. Obstet. Gynaecol.*, **106**, 745–6.
12. Woolas, R.P., Prys-Davies, A., and Oram, D.H. (1994). Post menopausal endometriosis inadvertently detected by screening for ovarian cancer. *Obstet. Gynaecol. Today*, **5**, 20.
13. Campbell, I.G., Nicolai, H.M., Foulkes, W.D. *et al.* (1994). A novel gene encoding a B-box protein within the BRCA1 region at 17q21.1. *Hum. Mol. Genet.*, **3**, 589–94.

14. Bast, R.C., Xu, F., Yu, Y. *et al.* (1998). CA125 the past and the future. *Int. J. Biol. Markers*, **13**, 179–87.
15. Bast, R.C., Klug, T.L., St John, E. *et al.* (1983). A radioimmunoassay using a monoclonal antibody to monitor the course of epithelial ovarian cancer. *N. Engl. J. Med.*, **309**, 169–71.
16. O'Brien, T.J., Raymond, L.M., Bannon, G.A. *et al.* (1991). New monoclonal antibodies identify the glycoprotein carrying the CA 125 epitope. *Am. J. Obstet. Gynecol.*, **165**, 1857–64.
17. Bon, G.G., Kenemans, P., Verstraeten, R. *et al.* (1996). Serum tumor marker immunoassays in gynecologic oncology: establishment of reference values. *Am. J. Obstet. Gynecol.*, **174**, 107–14.
18. Alagoz, T., Buller, R.E., Berman, M. *et al.* (1994). What is a normal CA125 level? *Gynecol. Oncol.*, **53**, 93–7.
19. Woolas, R.P., Jacobs, I.J., Zu, F. *et al.* (1997). Multiple tumour marker measurements to differentiate Stage I ovarian cancer from the benign ovarian cyst. *J. Gynecol. Tech.*, **3**, 123–6.
20. NHS Executive (1999). *Guidance on commissioning cancer services. Improving outcomes in gynaecological cancers.* 16150. Department of Health.
21. Jacobs, I.J. and Bast, R.C. (1989). The CA 125 antigen a review of the literature. *Hum. Reprod.*, **4**, 1–12.
22. Bell, D.A. and Scully, R.E. (1990). Ovarian serous borderline tumours with stromal microinvasion: A report of 21 cases. *Hum. Path.*, **21**, 397–403.
23. Rice, L.W., Lasge, J.M., Berkowitz, R.S. (1992). Pre-operative serum CA125 levels in borderline tumours of the ovary. *Gynecol. Oncol.*, **46**, 226–9.
24. Tamakoshi, K., Kikkawa, F., Shibata, K. *et al.* (1996). Clinical value of CA125, CA19–9, CEA, CA72–4, and TPA in borderline ovarian tumour. *Gynecol. Oncol.*, **62**, 67–72.
25. Niloff, J.M., Klug, T.L., Schaetzl, E. *et al.* (1984). Elevation of CA 125 in carcinomas of the fallopian tube, endometrium and endocervix. *Am. J. Obstet. Gynecol.*, **148**, 1057–8.
26. Einhorn, N., Bast, R.C., Knapp, R.C. *et al.* (1986). Preoperative evaluation of serum CA 125 levels in patients with primary epithelial ovarian cancer. *Obstet. Gynecol.*, **67**, 414–16.
27. Malkasian, G.D., Knapp, R.C., Lavin, P.T. *et al.* (1988). Preoperative evaluation of serum CA 125 levels in premenopausal and postmenopausal patients with pelvic masses: Discrimination of benign from malignant disease. *Am. J. Obstet. Gynecol.*, **159**, 341–6.
28. Soper, J.T., Hunter, V.J., Daly, L. *et al.* (1990). Preoperative serum tumor associated antigen levels in women with pelvic masses. *Obstet. Gynecol.*, **75**, 249–54.
29. Jacobs, I.J., Oram, D.H., and Bast, R.C. (1992). Strategies for improving the specificity of screening for ovarian cancer with tumour associated antigens CA 125, CA15–3 and TAG–72.3. *Obstet. Gynecol.*, **80**, 396–9.
30. Bast, R.C., Knauf, S., Epenetos, A. *et al.* (1991). Coordinate elevation of serum markers in ovarian cancer but not in benign disease. *Cancer*, **68**, 1758–63.
31. Yedema, C., Massuger, L., Hilgers, J. *et al.* (1989). Preoperative discrimination between benign and malignant ovarian tumours using a combination of CA 125 and CA 15–3 serum assays. *Br. J. Cancer*, **59**, 307.
32. Gadducci, A., Ferdeghini, M., Prontera, C. *et al.* (1992). The concomitant determination of different tumor markers in patients with epithelial ovarian cancer and benign ovarian masses: Relevance for differential diagnosis. *Gynecol. Oncol.*, **44**, 147–54.
33. Jacobs, I.J., Rivera, H., Oram, D.H., and Bast, R.C. (1993). Differential diagnosis of ovarian cancer with tumour markers CA 125, CA15–3, and TAG 72.3. *Br. J. Obstet. Gynaecol.*, **100**, 1120–4.
34. Brieman, L., Friedman, J.H., Olshen, R., and Stone, C.J. (1984). *Classification and regression trees.* Wadsworth International Group, Belmont, California.
35. Clarke, L. and Pregibon, D. (1992). Tree-based models. In *Statistical models* (ed. J. Chambers and T. Hastie). Wadsworth International Group, South Pacific Grove, California.
36. Woolas, R.P., Conaway, M.R., Feng, J.X. *et al.* (1995). Combinations of multiple serum markers are superior to individual assays for discriminating malignant from benign pelvic masses. *Gynecol. Oncol.*, **59**, 111–16.
37. Zhang, Z., Barnhill, S.D., Zhang, H. *et al.* (1999). Combination of multiple serum markers using an artificial neural network to improve specificity in discriminating malignant from benign pelvic masses. *Gynecol. Oncol.*, **73**, 56–61.
38. Finkler, N.J., Benacerraf, B., Lavin, P.T. *et al.* (1988). Comparison of serum CA 125, clinical impression and ultrasound in the preoperative evaluation of ovarian masses. *Obstet. Gynecol.*, **72**, 659–64.
39. Clayton, R.D., Snowden, S., Weston, M.J. *et al.* (1999). Neural networks in the diagnosis of malignant ovarian tumours. *Br. J. Obstet. Gynaecol.*, **106**, 1078–82.
40. Tailor, A., Jurkovic, D., Bourne, T.H. *et al.* (1999). Sonographic prediction of malignancy in adnexal masses using an artificial neural network. *Br. J. Obstet. Gynaecol.*, **106**, 21–30.
41. Leaning, M.S., Gallivan, S., Newlands, E.S. *et al.* (1992). Computer system for assisting with clinical interpretation of tumour marker data. *BMJ*, **305**, 804–7.
42. Jacobs, I.J., Oram, D.H., Fairbanks, J. *et al.* (1990). A risk of malignancy index incorporating CA 125, ultrasound and menopausal status for the accurate preoperative diagnosis of ovarian cancer. *Br. J. Obstet. Gynaecol.*, **97**, 922–9.
43. Prys-Davies, A., Jacobs, I.J., Woolas, R.P. *et al.* (1993). The adnexal mass—benign or malignant? Evaluating a risk of malignancy index. *Br. J. Obstet. Gynaecol.*, **100**, 927–31.
44. Tingulstad, S., Hagen, B., Skjeldestad, F.E. *et al.* (1996). Evaluation of a risk of malignancy index bases on serum CA125, ultrasound findings and menopausal status in the pre-operative diagnosis of pelvic masses. *Br. J. Obstet. Gynaecol.*, **103**, 826–31.
45. Tingulstad, S., Hagen, B., Skjeldestad, F.E. *et al.* (1999). The risk of malignancy index to evaluate potential ovarian cancers in local hospitals. *Obstet. Gynecol.*, **93**, 448–52.
46. Morgante, G., la Marca, A., Ditto, A., De Leo, V. (1999). Comparison of two malignancy risk indices bases on serum CA125, ultrasound score and menopausal status in the diagnosis of ovarian masses. *Br. J. Obstet. Gynaecol.*, **106**, 524–7.
47. Timmerman, D., Verrelst, H., Van Holsbeke, C. *et al.* (2000). Prospective evaluation of a new risk of malignancy index. *Gynecol. Oncol.*, **76**, 255.
48. Woolas, R.P., Walter, E.J., Gornall, R. *et al.* (2001). Triage of the adnexal mass and the two week wait for suspected cancer, in press.
49. Di-Xia, C., Schwartz, P.E., and Xinguo, L. (1988). Evaluation of CA 125 levels in differentiating malignant from benign tumours in patients with pelvic masses. *Obstet. Gynecol.*, **72**, 23–7.
50. Nagile, F., Petrue, E., Medl, M. *et al.* (1995). Pre-operative CA125: an independent prognostic factor in patients with Stage I epithelial ovarian cancer. *Obstet. Gynecol.*, **60**, 197–202.
51. van Ravenswaay, Claasen, H.H., and Fleuren, G.J. (1995). The influence of combination chemotherapy on antigen expression in ovarian cancer. *Gynecol. Oncol.*, **58**, 16–23.
52. Lavin, P.T., Knapp, R.C., and Malkasian, G. (1987). CA 125 for the monitoring of ovarian carcinoma during primary therapy. *Obstet. Gynecol.*, **69**, 223–7.
53. van der Burg, M.E.L., Lammes, F.B., van Putten, W.L.J., and Stoter, G. (1988). Ovarian cancer: The prognostic value of the serum half-life of CA 125 during induction chemotherapy. *Gynecol. Oncol.*, **30**, 307–12.
54. Rustin, G.J.S., Gennings, J.N., and Nelstrop, A.E. (1989). Use of CA 125 to predict survival of patients with ovarian carcinoma. *J. Clin. Oncol.*, **7**, 1667–71.
55. Mogensen, O. (1992). Prognostic value of CA 125 in advanced ovarian cancer. *Gynecol. Oncol.*, **44**, 207–12.
56. Hawkins, R.E., Roberts, K., Wiltshaw, E. *et al.* (1989). The prognostic significance of the half life of serum CA125 in patients responding to chemotherapy for epithelial ovarian carcinoma. *Br. J. Obstet. Gynaecol.*, **96**, 1395–9.

57. Willemse, P.H.B., Aalders, J.G., De Bruign, H.W.A. *et al.* (1991). CA 125 in ovarian cancer relation between halflife, doubling time, and survival. *Eur. J. Cancer*, **27**, 993–5.

58. Gadducci, A., Zola, O., Landoni, F. *et al.* (1995). Serum half life of CA125 during early chemotherapy as an independent prognostic variable for patients with advanced epithelial ovarian cancer: results of a multicentric Italian study. *Gynecol. Oncol.*, **58**, 42–7.

59. Fayers, P.M., Rustin, G., Wood, R. *et al.* (1993). The prognostic value of serum CA125 in patients with advanced ovarian carcinoma: an analysis of 573 patients by the Medical Research Council Working Party of gynaecological cancer. *Int. J. Gynecol. Cancer*, **3**, 285–92.

60. Vergote, I.B., Bormer, O.P., and Abeler, V.M. (1987). Evaluation of serum CA 125 levels in the monitoring of ovarian cancer. *Am. J. Obstet. Gynecol.*, **157**, 88–92.

61. van der Burg, M.E.L., Lammes, F.B., and Verweij, J. (1990). The role of CA 125 in the early diagnosis of progressive disease in ovarian cancer. *Ann. Oncol.*, **1**, 301–2.

62. Rustin, G.J.S., Nelstrop, A., and Stilwell, M.A. (1992). Savings obtained by CA 125 measurements during therapy for ovarian carcinoma. *Eur. J. Cancer*, **28**, 79–82.

63. Niloff, J.M., Knapp, R.C., Lavin, P.T. *et al.* (1986). The CA 125 assay as a predictor of clinical recurrence in epithelial ovarian cancer. *Am. J. Obstet. Gynecol.*, **155**, 56–60.

64. Rustin, G. and Tuxen, M. (1996). Use of CA125 in follow up of ovarian cancer. *Lancet*, **348**, 191–2.

65. Gallion, H.H., Hunter, J.E., Van Nagel, J.R. *et al.* (1992). The prognostic implications of low serum CA125 levels prior to the second look operation for Stage II and IV epithelial ovarian cancer. *Gynecol. Oncol.*, **46**, 29–33.

66. Rustin, G.J.S., Nelstrop, A.E., McClean, P. *et al.* (1996). Defining response of ovarian carcinoma to initial chemotherapy according to CA125. *J. Clin. Oncol.*, **14**, 1545–51.

67. Rustin, G.J., Nelstrop, A.E., Crawford, M. *et al.* (1997). Phase II trial of oral altretamine for relapsed ovarian carcinoma: evaluation of defining response by serum CA125. *J. Clin. Oncol.*, **15**, 172–6.

68. Davelaar, E.M., Bonfrer, J.M.G., Verstraeten, R.A. *et al.* (1996). CA125 a valid marker in ovarian carcinoma patients treated with Paclitaxel. *Cancer*, **78**, 118–27.

69. van Niekerk, C.C., Boerman, O.C., Ramaekers, F.C.S., and Poels, L.G. (1991). Marker profile of different phases in the transition of normal human ovarian epithelium to ovarian carcinomas. *Am. J. Pathol.*, **138**, 455–63.

70. Katupodis, N., Hirshauti, Y., Geller, N., and Stock, C.C. (1982). Lipid-associated sialic test for detection of human cancer. *Cancer Res.*, **42**, 5270–5.

71. Awais, G.M. (1978). Carcinoma of the ovary and serum lactate dehydrogenase levels. *Surg. Gynecol. Obstet.*, **146**, 893–5.

72. van Kley, H., Cramer, S., and Burns, D.E. (1981). Serous ovarian neoplastic amylase (SONA). *Cancer*, **48**, 1444–9.

73. Gauduchon, C., Tilher, C., Guyonnet, C. *et al.* (1983). Clinical value serum galactosyltransferase levels in different histological types of ovarian carcinoma. *Cancer Res.*, **3**, 4491–6.

74. Ward, B.G., Cruikshank, D.J., Tucker, D.F., and Love, S. (1987). Independent expression in serum of three tumour associated antigens: CA 125, placental alkaline phosphatase and HMFG2 in ovarian carcinoma. *Br. J. Obstet. Gynaecol.*, **94**, 696–8.

75. Heinonen, P.K., Tuimala, K., Pyykko, K., and Pystynen, P. (1982). Peripheral venous concentrations of oestrogens in post menopausal women with ovarian cancer. *Br. J. Obstet. Gynaecol.*, **89**, 84–6.

76. Backstrom, T., Mahlck, C.G., and Kjellgren, O. (1983). Progesterone as a possible tumour marker for non endocrine ovarian malignant tumours. *Gynecol. Oncol.*, **16**, 129–38.

77. Lukomska, B., Olszewski, W.L., and Engeset, A. (1981). Acute phase reactive proteins and complement components and inhibitors in patients with ovarian cancer. *Gynecol. Oncol.*, **11**, 288–98.

78. Donaldson, E.S., van Nagell, J.R., Pursell, S. *et al.* (1980). Multiple biochemical markers in patients with gynaecological malignances. *Cancer*, **45**, 948–53.

79. Stall, K.E. and Martin, E.W. (1981). Plasma CEA levels in ovarian cancer patients: A chart review and survey of published data. *J. Reprod. Med.*, **26**, 73–9.

80. Kikuchi, Y., Hirose, J., Uekita, Y. *et al.* (1983). Clinical evaluation of serum CEA levels in ovarian cancer. *Gan No Rinsho*, **29**, 330–5.

81. Boot, R.C., Klug, T.L., Schaetzl, E. *et al.* (1984). Monitoring human ovarian carcinoma with a combination of CA 125, CA19–9 and carcinoembryonic antigen. *Am. J. Obstet. Gynecol.*, **149**, 533–59.

82. Nouwen, W.J., Pollet, D.E., Schelstraete, J.B. *et al.* (1985). Human placental alkaline phosphatase in benign and malignant ovarian neoplasia. *Cancer Res.*, **45**, 892–902.

83. Breitenecker, G., Neunteufel, W., Bieglmayer, C. *et al.* (1989). Comparison between tissue and serum content of CA 125, CA 19–9 and carcinoembryonic antigen in ovarian tumours. *Int. J. Gynecol. Pathol.*, **8**, 97–102.

84. Lan, M.S., Bast, R.C., Colnaghi, M.I. *et al.* (1987). Co-expression of human cancer-associated epitopes on mucin molecules. *Int. J. Cancer*, **39**, 68–72.

85. Devine, P.L., McGuckin, M.A., and Ward, B.G. (1992). Circulating tumour markers in ovarian cancer. *Anticancer Res.*, **12**, 709–18.

86. Berchuck, A., Kohler, M.F., Boente, M.P. *et al.* (1993). Growth regulation and transformation of ovarian epithelium. *Cancer*, **71**, 545–51.

87. Campbell, I.G., Foulkes, W.D., Jones, T.A., Poels, L.G., and Trowsdale, J. (1995). Cloning and molecular characterisation of monoclonal-antibody defined ovarian tumour antigens. In *Ovarian cancer 3*, (ed. F. Sharp, W.P. Mason, T. Blackett, and J. Berek), pp. 53–9. Chapman and Hall, London.

88. Vogl, F.D., Stickeler, E., Weyermann, K. *et al.* (1999). P53 autoantibodies in patients with primary ovarian cancer are associated with higher age, advanced stage and a higher proportion of p53-positive tumour cells. *Oncology*, **57**, 324–9.

89. Meden, H., Marx, D., Schauer, A. *et al.* (1997). Prognostic significance of p105 (c-erbB–2 HER2/neu) serum levels in patients with ovarian cancer. *Anticancer Res.*, **17**, 757–60.

90. Cheung, T.H., Wong, Y.F., Chung, T.K. *et al.* (1999). Clinical use of serum c-erbB–2 in patients with ovarian masses. *Gynecol. Obstet. Invest.*, **48**, 133–7.

91. Knauf, S., Anderson, D.J., Knapp, R.L., and Bast, R.C. (1985). A study of the NB/70K and CA125 monoclonal antibody radioimmunossays for measuring serum antigen levels in ovarian cancer patients. *Am. J. Obstet. Gynecol.*, **152**, 911–13.

92. Petru, E., Sevin, B.U., Averette, H.E. *et al.* (1990). Comparison of three tumor markers—CA125, lipid-associated sialic acid (LSA), and NB/70K—in monitoring ovarian cancer. *Gynecol. Oncol.*, **38**, 181–6.

93. Dhokia, B., Canney, P.A., Pectasides, D. *et al.* (1986). A new immunoassay using monoclonal antibodies HMFG1 and HMFG2 together with an existing marker CA 125 for the serological detection and management of epithelial ovarian cancer. *Br. J. Cancer*, **54**, 891–5.

94. Schwartz, P.E., Chambers, S.K., Chambers, J.T. *et al.* (1987). Circulating tumour markers in the monitoring of gynecologic malignancies. *Cancer*, **60**, 353–61.

95. Stratton, J.A., Rettenmaier, M.A., Phillips, H.B. *et al.* (1988). Relationship of serum CA 125 and lipid associated sialic acid tumour associated antigen levels to the disease status of patients with gynecologic malignancies. *Obstet. Gynecol.*, **71**, 20–6.

96. Patsner, B., Mann, W.J., Vissicchio, M., and Loesch, M. (1988). Comparison of serum CA125 and lipid-associated sialic acid (LASA-P) in monitoring patients with invasive ovarian adenocarcinoma. *Gynecol. Oncol.*, **30**, 98–103.

97. McGuckin, M.A., Layton, G.T., Bailey, M.J. *et al.* (1990). Evaluation of two new assays for tumour associated antigens, CASA and OSA, found in the serum of patients with epithelial ovarian carcinoma: comparison with CA 125. *Gynecol. Oncol.*, **37**, 165–71.

98. Ward, B.G., McGuckin, M.A., Ramm, L.E. *et al.* (1993). The management of ovarian cancer is improved by the use of cancer associated serum antigen and CA 125 assays. *Cancer*, **71**, 430–8.

99. Kacinski, B.M., Stanley, E.R., Carter, D. *et al.* (1989a). Circulating levels of CSF–1 (M-CSF) a lymphohematopoietic cytokine may be a useful marker of disease status in patients with malignant ovarian neoplasms. *Int. J. Radiat. Oncol. Biol. Phys.*, **17**, 159–64.

100. Kacinski, B.M., Bloodgood, R.S., Schwartz, P.E. *et al.* (1989b). Macrophage colony-stimulating factor is produced by human ovarian and endometrial adenocarcinoma-derived cell lines and is present at abnormally high levels in the plasma of ovarian carcinoma patients with active disease. *Cancer Cells*, **7**, 333–7.

101. Ramakrishnan, S., Xu, F.J., Brandt, S.J. *et al.* (1989). Constitutive production of macrophage colony-stimulating factor by human ovarian and breast cancer cell lines. *J. Clin. Invest.*, **83**, 921–6.

102. Olt, G.J., Berchuck, A., and Bast, R.C. Jr. (1990). Gynecologic tumor markers. *Semin. Surg. Oncol.*, **6**, 305–13.

103. Xu, F.J., Ramakrishnan, S., Daly, L. *et al.* (1991). Increased serum levels of macrophage colony stimulating factor in ovarian cancer. *Am. J. Obstet. Gynecol.*, **165**, 1356–62.

104. Gadducci, A., Ferdeghini, M., Castellanic (1998). Serum macrophage colony-stimulating factor (M-CSF) levels in patients with epithelial ovarian cancer. *Gynecol Oncol*, **70**, 111–4.

105. Xu, F.J., Yu, Y.H., Li, B.Y. *et al.* (1993). OVX1 radioimmunoassay complements CA 125 for predicting the presence of residual ovarian carcinoma at second look surgical surveillance procedures. *J. Clin. Oncol.*, **11**, 1506–10.

106. Woolas, R.P., Xu, F.J., Jacobs, I.J. *et al.* (1993). Elevation of multiple serum markers in patients with Stage I ovarian cancer. *J. Natl Cancer Inst.*, **85**, 1748–51.

107. Hefler, L., Tempfer, C., Heinze, G., *et al.* (1999) Monocyte chemoattractant protein serum levels in ovarian cancer patients. *Br. J. Cancer*, **81**, 855–9.

108. Scambia, G., Benedetti Panici, P., Biaoccchi, G. *et al.* (1988). CA 15–3 as a tumour marker in gynecological malignancies. *Gynecol. Oncol.*, **30**, 265–73.

109. Colomer, R., Ruibal, A., Genolla, J., and Salvador, L. (1989). Circulating CA15–3 antigen levels in non mammary malignancies. *Br. J. Cancer*, **59**, 283–6.

110. Magnani, J.L., Steplewski, Z., Koprowski, H., and Ginsberg, V. (1983). Identification of gastrointestinal and pancreatic cancer-associated antigen detected by monoclonal antibody 19–9 in the sera of patients as a mucin. *Cancer Res.*, **43**, 5489–92.

111. Dietel, M., Arps, H., Klapdor, R. *et al.* (1986). Antigen detection by the monoclonal antibodies CA 19–9 and CA 125 in normal and tumor tissue and patients' sera. *J. Cancer Res. Clin. Oncol.*, **111**, 257–65.

112. Motoyama, T., Watanabe, H., Takeuchi, S. *et al.* (1990). Cancer antigen 125, carcinoembryonic antigen and carbohydrate determinant 19–9 in ovarian tumors. *Cancer*, **66**, 2628–35.

113. Inoue, M., Fujita, M., Nakazawa, A. *et al.* (1992). Sialyl-Tn, Sialyl-Lewis Xi, CA19–9, CA 125, Carcinoembryonic antigen and tissue polypeptide antigen in differentiating ovarian cancer from benign tumors. *Obstet. Gynecol.*, **79**, 343–40.

114. Nuti, M., Teramoto, Y.A., Marini-Costantini, R. *et al.* (1982). A monoclonal antibody (B72.3) defines patterns of distribution of a novel tumor associated antigen in human mammary carcinoma cell populations. *Int. J. Cancer*, **29**, 539–45.

115. Jibiki, K., Takeda, M., Abe, H. *et al.* (1990). A clinical evaluation of the CA72–4 serum level as a possible tumour marker. *Gan No Rinsho*, **36**, 2146–52.

116. Negishi, Y., Iwabuchi, H., Sakunaga, H. *et al.* (1993). Serum and tissue measurements of CA72–4 in ovarian cancer patients. *Gynecol. Oncol.*, **48**, 148–54.

117. Fukazawa, I., Inaba, N., Ota, Y. *et al.* (1988). Serum levels of six tumor markers in patients with benign and malignant gynecological disease. *Arch. Gynecol. Obstet.*, **243**, 61–8.

118. Nozawa, S., Yajima, M., Udagawa, Y. *et al.* (1989). The elevation of CA 54/61 in the diagnosis of ovarian cancer—with special reference to the cooperative results of 5 institutes. *Nippon Sanka Fujinka Gakkai Zasshi*, **41**, 1823–1929.

119. Suzuki, M., Sekiguchi, I., and Tamada, T. (1990). Clinical evaluation of tumor associated mucin type glycoprotein CA 54/61 in ovarian cancers: Comparison with CA 125. *Obstet. Gynecol.*, **76**, 422–7.

120. Nozawa, S., Aoki, D., Yajima, M. *et al.* (1992). CA54/61 as a marker for epithelial ovarian cancer. *Cancer Res.*, **52**, 1205–9.

121. Kobayashi, H., Ohi, H., Sugimura, M. *et al.* (1992). Characterisation and clinical evaluation of tumor associated antigen CA54/61 identified by monoclonal antibodies MA54 and MA61 in epithelial ovarian cancer. *Gynecol. Oncol.*, **47**, 328–36.

122. Kobayashi, H., Terao, T., and Kawashima, Y. (1991). Clinical evaluation of circulating serum sialyl Tn antigen levels in patients with epithelial ovarian cancer. *J. Clin. Oncol.*, **9**, 983–7.

123. Halila, H., Lehtovirta, P., and Stenman, U.H. (1988). Tumour associated trypsin inhibitor (TATI) in ovarian cancer. *Br. J. Cancer*, **57**, 304–7.

124. Mogensen, O., Mogensen, B., and Jacobsen, A. (1990). Tumour associated trypsin inhibitor (TATI) and CA 125 in mucinous ovarian tumours. *Br. J. Cancer*, **61**, 327–9.

125. Garzetti, G.G., Ciavattini, A., Lucarini, G. *et al.* (1996). Increased serum 72 KDa metalloproteinase in serous ovarian tumors: comparison with CA125. *Anticancer Res.*, **16** (4A), 2123–7.

126. Hurteau, A.J., Woolas, R.P., Jacobs, I.J. *et al.* (1995). Soluble interleukin–2 receptor alpha is elevated in sera of patients with benign ovarian neoplasms and epithelial ovarian cancer. *Cancer*, **76**, 1615–20.

127. Onsrud, M., Shabana, A. and Austgulen, R. (1996). Soluble tumour necrosis factor receptors and CA125 in serum as markers for epithelial ovarian cancer. *Tumour Biol.*, **17**, 90–6.

128. Koehler, M.K. and Caffier, H. (1999). Diagnostic value of VEGF in women with ovarian tumours. *Anticancer Res.*, **19**, 2519–22.

129. Gornall, R., Anthony, F.W., Coombes, E. *et al.* (2001). Serum vascular endothelial growth factor (VEGF) measurements in women presenting with an adnexal mass. *Int. J. Gynecol. Cancer*, **11**, 164–6.

130. Ohita, M., Gaudette, D., Mills, G. and Holub, B. (1997). Elevated levels and altered fatty acid composition of plasma lysophosphatidylcholine (LYSOPC) in ovarian cancer patients. *Int. J. Cancer*, **71**, 31–4.

131. Milford Ward, A. and White, P.A.E. (1997). External quality assessment of commercial assays for CA125. *Contemp. Rev. Obstet. Gynaecol.*, 319–23.

132. Tuxen, M.K., Soletormos, G., Peterson, P.H.G. *et al.* (1999). Assessment of bioligical variation and analytical imprecision of CA125, CEA and TPA in relation to monitoring of ovarian cancer. *Gynecol. Oncol.*, **74**, 12–22.

133. Zalel, Y., Piura, B., Elchalal, U. *et al.* (1996). Diagnosis and management of malignant germ cell ovarian tumors in young females. *Int. J. Gynecol. Obstet.*, **55**, 1–10.

134. Kawai, M., Kano, T., Kikkawa, F. *et al.* (1992). Seven tumor markers in benign and malignant germ cell tumors of the ovary. *Gynecol. Oncol.*, **45**, 248–53.

135. Mead, G.M. on behalf of the IGCCCG (1995). International consensus prognostic classification for metastatic germ cell tumours treated with platinum based chemotherapy: final report of the International Germ Cell Cancer Collaborative Group. *Proc. Am. Soc. Clin. Oncol.*, **14**, 235.

136. De Bruijn, H.W.A., Hollema, H., Willemse, P.H.B. *et al.* (1996). Raised serum squamous cell carcinoma antigen levels in malignant transformation of mature cystic ovarian teratoma. *Int. J. Gynecol. Cancer*, **6**, 76–9.

137. Suzuki, M., Kobayashi, H., Sekiguchi, I. *et al.* (1995). Clinical evaluation of squamous cell carcinoma antigen in squamous cell carcinoma arising in cystic teratoma of the ovary. *Gynecol. Oncol.*, **52**, 287–90.

138. Kawata, M., Sekiya, S., Hatakeyama, R. and Takamizawa, H. (1989). Neurone-specific enolase as a serurm marker for immature teratoma and dysgerminoma. *Gynecol. Oncol.*, **32**, 191–7.

139. Jobling, T., Makers, P., Healy, D.L. *et al.* (1994). A prospective study on inhibin in granulosa cell tumours of the ovary. *Gynecol. Oncol.*, **55**, 285–9.

140. Cooke, I., O'Brien, M., Charnock, F.M. *et al.* (1995). Inhibin as a marker for ovarian cancer. *Br. J. Cancer*, **71**, 1046–50.

141. Rodgers, K.E., Marks, J.F., Ellefson, D.D. *et al.* (1990). Follicle regulatory protein: A novel marker for granulosa cell cancer patients. *Gynecol. Oncol.*, **37**, 381–7.

142. Rey, R.A., Lhomme, C., Marcillak, I. *et al.* (1996). Antimullaerian hormone as a serum marker of granulosa cell tumors of the ovary: comparative study with serum alpha inhibin and estradiol. *Am. J. Obstet. Gynecol.*, **174**, 958–65.

143. Gustafson, M.L., Lee, M.M., Scully, R.E. *et al.* (1992). Mullerian inhibiting substance as a marker for ovarian sex-cord tumor. *N. Engl. J. Med.*, **326**, 466–71.

144. Lane, A.H., Lee, M.M., Fuller, A.F. *et al.* (1999). Diagnostic utility of mullerian inhibiting substance determination in patients with primary and recurrent granulosa cell tumors. *Gynecol. Oncol.*, **73**, 51–5.

32. Three-dimensional ultrasound and color-flow studies

A. Kurjak and S. Kupesic

It has been known for over 25 years that the development of new blood vessels is necessary to sustain the growth, invasion, and metastasis of tumors.[1–3] Angiogenesis is crucial for sustaining tumor growth as it allows oxygenation and nutrient perfusion of the tumor as well as removal of waste products. Moreover, increased angiogenesis coincides with increased tumor cell entry into circulation and thus facilitates metastasis.[4,5] Cancer cells activate the quiescent vasculature to produce new blood vessels via an 'angiogenetic switch', often during the premalignant stages of tumor development. Data suggesting that control of angiogenesis is separate from control of cancer cell proliferation raise the possibility that drugs inhibiting angiogenesis could offer a treatment that is complementary to traditional chemotherapy, which targets tumor cells directly.[1–3,6] This exciting possibility has made research on tumor angiogenesis topical.[7–11]

Contribution of transvaginal color Doppler

Angiogenesis is a common phenomenon in malignant ovarian neoplasms, but the intensity of neovascularization may depend on the characteristics of the individual tumor.[12] Therefore, an incremental decrease of the impedance indices in the vessels of adnexal tumors may reflect the increase in angiogenesis and be an indication of the tumor's malignant potential.[13] Animal models have shown that angiogenesis can be detected by Doppler ultrasound even in a small volume of malignant tumor (25 mg).[14] These findings suggested that angiogenesis could be detected with current color Doppler ultrasound equipment even when the carcinoma is well-confined within the ovarian capsule or when it exhibits a low malignant potential. Indeed, several series showed that color and pulsed Doppler sonography can depict ovarian carcinoma at stage I.[15–17] One series detected 2 out of 18 stage I ovarian carcinomas solely by the presence of an abnormal blood flow pattern in normal-sized ovaries,[16] whereas another study found 3 out of 17 stage I cancers on the basis of abnormal blood flow (Plate 2).[17] However, in the latter study, two stage I tumors did not demonstrate flow and both were larger than 15 mm in size. It could be argued that these undiscovered malignant tumors

had a low potential to induce an angiogenic response, or that the blood vessels were so small that they were impossible to depict with current color and pulsed Doppler equipment.

The newly developed power or energy modes of color Doppler imaging afford depiction of even smaller vessels but, paradoxically, small intraparenchymal arterioles in benign and normal tissues may show a low impedance and a low-velocity blood-flow pattern, giving rise to false-positive results. Nevertheless, the tendency towards a progressive decrease in the vascular impedance from benign lesions, to borderline malignancy and early malignancy, to advanced malignancies has been reported.[13] This observation is supported circumstantially by an *in vivo* study which showed that there is a rise in vascularity with tumor progression in the melanocytic system, demonstrated by histopathology.[18] This *in vivo* information is in agreement with the notion that an increased vascular supply may facilitate tumorigenesis and aggressive biological behavior in a neoplastic system.

Since the vascular impedance measured by color Doppler in the parenchymal vessels of an adnexal tumor will not always represent the microangiogenesis itself,[19] it is possible that the signal obtained by color and pulsed Doppler demonstrates the main neovascularized channel representing the summation of downstream resistance of the vascular bed in a certain tissue block. Additionally, blood-flow parameters are not only a result of numerous blood vessels and their wall structure, but also of increased permeability of the vascular network. Because of increased permeability, stasis of blood flow and short shunts with low impedance can occur, not necessarily being the same in all parts of the tumor (Plates 3 and 4).[20] Increased interstitial pressure is another parameter that could elevate vascular impedance despite the high malignant potential.

Since the introduction of transvaginal color Doppler sonography (TVCD) in the assessment of ovarian vascularity,[21,15] attitudes concerning its usefulness in the detection of adnexal malignancies have been equally divided. The majority of the published studies on this subject agree that malignant ovarian tumors, in comparison with benign ones, have characteristic blood-flow features. However, overlap in blood-flow parameters between malignant and benign ovarian tumors is a main element of the current debate regarding attempts to achieve accurate differentiation of ovarian tumors on the basis of their vascular characteristics. A review of the literature from 1989 to the present[9,22–69] shows a clear difference between malignant and benign adnexal masses. However, over succeeding years, an increasing number of publications have demonstrated a significant overlap in the results and the fact that a large number of benign masses have blood-flow features equal to those of malignant lesions, and vice versa. The previous belief that TVCD is valuable and gives strong support in clinical decision making and management has been challenged.[58]

For the purpose of this review, we analyzed 47 articles from different institutions in countries worldwide, published since 1989.[9,22–69] Table 32.1 presents the chosen publications. Departments of obstetrics and gynecology published 38 articles on the assessment of adnexal vascularity, and the evaluation of the usefulness of transvaginal color Doppler in the clinical setting; the other nine publications were from departments of radiology. The final conclusion of the articles was evaluated as 'in favor', 'limited use,' or 'against' the usefulness of color Doppler in the assessment of the adnexal vascularity and discrimination of malignant versus benign adnexal lesions. We can see that 48.9% of the studies were in favor and 14.9% against the usefulness of the transvaginal color

Table 32.1 General attitude towards transvaginal color Doppler sonography since 1989

Author	Ref. no.	Year	Department	No. of cases	Attitude towards Doppler
Hata et al.	22	1989	Gynecology	21	In favor
Fleischer et al.	25	1991	Radiology	43	In favor
Kurjak et al.	26	1991	Gynecology	680	In favor
Weiner et al.	27	1992	Gynecology	53	In favor
Kawai et al.	28	1992	Gynecology	24	In favor
Tekay and Jouppila	29	1992	Gynecology	72	Against
Hata et al.	30	1992	Gynecology	64	Against
Kurjak et al.	31	1992	Gynecology	83	In favor
Hamper et al.	32	1993	Radiology	31	Limited
Schneider et al.	33	1993	Gynecology	55	In favor
Timor-Tritsch et al.	34	1993	Gynecology	115	In favor
Jain	35	1994	Radiology	50	Limited
Weiner et al.	36	1994	Gynecology	18	In favor
Levine et al.	37	1994	Radiology	35	Against
Brown et al.	38	1994	Radiology	44	Limited
Valentin et al.	39	1994	Gynecology	149	Against
Bromley et al.	40	1994	Gynecology	33	Limited
Carter et al.	41	1994	Gynecology	30	Limited
Prompeler et al.	42	1994	Gynecology	83	Limited
Chou et al.	43	1994	Gynecology	108	In favor
Wu et al.	44	1994	Gynecology	410	In favor
Zaneta et al.	45	1994	Gynecology	76	In favor
Salem et al.	46	1994	Radiology	102	Against
Sengoku et al.	47	1994	Gynecology	28	In favor
Sawicki et al.	48	1994	Gynecology	65	In favor
Franchi et al.	49	1995	Gynecology	129	Limited
Maly et al.	50	1995	Gynecology	102	In favor
Stein et al.	51	1995	Radiology	169	Against
Carter et al.	52	1995	Gynecology	89	Limited
Fleischer et al.	53	1995	Radiology	126	In favor
Buy et al.	54	1996	Gynecology	132	Limited
Rehn et al.	55	1996	Gynecology	259	Limited
Predanic et al.	56	1996	Gynecology	106	In favor
Tailor et al.	57	1996	Gynecology	79	Limited
Alcazar et al.	58	1996	Gynecology	51	Limited
Wheeler et al.	59	1997	Gynecology	34	Limited
Reles et al.	60	1997	Gynecology	98	In favor
Emoto et al.	9	1997	Gynecology	106	In favor
Valentin	61	1997	Gynecology	151	In favor
Takac	62	1998	Gynecology	120	Limited
Guerriero et al.	63	1998	Gynecology	192	Limited
Leeners et al.	64	1998	Gynecology	265	In favor
Angeid-Beckman et al.	65	1998	Radiology	189	Against
Brown et al.	66	1998	Gynecology	211	Limited
Buckshee et al.	67	1998	Gynecology	34	In favor
Alcazar et al.	68	1999	Gynecology	94	In favor
Valentin	69	1999	Gynecology	173	Limited

Doppler, whereas 36.2% of the studies evaluated color and pulsed Doppler ultrasound as of limited usefulness in the assessment of adnexal lesions.

Table 32.2 shows the observed results in terms of the screening parameters—sensitivity, specificity, positive predictive value, and negative predictive value—from some of the aforementioned studies. When the same results are displayed as scattergrams, demonstrating the relationship between screening parameters and the year of the publications, it is obvious that the sensitivity and specificity of the method significantly decreased following its introduction. The significant reduction of the method's sensitivity and specificity could be explained by several facts. First, transvaginal color Doppler sonography has been accepted at a large number of institutions for trials and evaluation, but different protocols were used. Secondly, different ultrasound machines were in use with different set-ups, as well as differences in the quality of the resolution and color/pulsed Doppler sensitivity. Additionally, the experience of the ultrasonographers probably also played one

Table 32.2 Screening parameters reported in the reviewed literature

Authors	Ref. no.	Sensitivity	Specificity	PPV	NPV
Hata et al.	22	100	100	100	100
Fleischer et al.	25	100	83	73	100
Kurjak et al.	26	96	99	98	99
Weiner et al.	27	94	97	94	94
Kawai et al.	28	88	100		
Tekay and Jouppila	29	82	72	35	96
Hata et al.	30	92	53	59	90
Kurjak et al.	31	96	95	96	95
Hamper et al.	32	66	76	40	90
Schneider et al.	33	94	56	47	96
Timor-Tritsch et al.	34	94	99	94	99
Jain	35	70	82		
Weiner et al.	36	86	100	92	100
Levine et al.	37	25	89		
Brown et al.	38	100	79		
Valentin et al.	39	100	53		
Bromley et al.	40	66	81		
Carter et al.	41	57	78	68	69
Prompeler et al.	42	95	86		
Chou et al.	43	88	92	85	94
Wu et al.	44	68	97		
Zaneta et al.	45	91	85		
Salem et al.	46	79	77	31	96
Sengoku et al.	47	82	92	93	79
Sawicki et al.	48	100	94	95	100
Franchi et al.	49	76	72	68	93
Maly et al.	50	100			
Stein et al.	51	43	56	56	
Fleischer et al.	53	92	86	86	98
Buy et al	54	71	67	43	87
Rehn et al.	55	67	53	22	89
Predanic et al.	56	86	83	32	98
Tailor et al.	57	88.9	81.0		
Alcazar et al.	58	100	88.6		
Takac	62	82	97	94	92
Guerriero et al.	63	58	87	48	91
Leeners et al.	64	79.6	58.2		

PPV, positive predictive value; NPV, negative predictive value.

Table 32.3 A comparison between the attitude of radiology and gynecology departments towards transvaginal color Doppler sonography

Attitude towards TVCD	Radiology departments	Gynecology departments	Total
In favor	2	21	23 (48.9%)
Limited use	3	14	17 (36.2%)
Against its usefulness	4	3	7 (14.9%)

of the major roles, as did the general attitude and belief of the facility in the capability of the new ultrasound modality. For example, only two radiology departments assessed transvaginal color Doppler as a valuable diagnostic tool, whereas seven radiology departments had divided attitudes: three described transvaginal color Doppler as a limited improvement to already used diagnostic tools, whereas the other four radiology facilities found the method completely inferior to conventional ultrasound (Table 32.3). In contrast, 21 departments of obstetrics and gynecology found transvaginal color Doppler to be very helpful, 14 found it to be of limited use, and only three of them found it to be of no use at all. This discrepancy can be explained by the general approach towards the use of color Doppler as an adjunct to conventional ultrasound. While departments of obstetrics and gynecology use this new diagnostic tool as an additional element in the clinical assessment of the patient with adnexal disease, radiologists assess adnexal lesions solely as an 'object' extracted from the whole picture of the patient with an adnexal disease. They treat the adnexal lesion as a structure that can be visualized, described, and reported without much clinical information and without any further involvement in decision making or management.

During analysis of the conflicting data, it became obvious that three groups of investigators could be distinguished. The first group reported high sensitivity and specificity of color Doppler; their opinion was that color Doppler significantly improved the accuracy of B-mode ultrasonography, but that the value of this technique in screening procedures should continue to be evaluated. The second group was less optimistic in the interpretation of their results. They found that color Doppler had some potential but did not significantly facilitate the decision-making process in their routine clinical work. The third group believed that color Doppler brought nothing new to current diagnostic procedures. They did not discuss the possibility that human skill in performing the procedure may be the problem, and put the blame on the technique itself.

The first group began using the technique in its early stage of development (mostly around 1988) and it could be claimed that a non-critical enthusiasm might have contributed to their optimistic results. Against this, it could be argued that the most powerful tool of this group is their experience with the method. The other investigators did not bring anything essentially new to the technique. For the most part, they began to use the technique after 1991 and focused their studies on the false-positive results and the overlapping of the pulsed Doppler values (particularly benign versus. malignant lesions).

There are some causes known for these incompatible results. For example, the difference in the detection and quantification of flow velocities by different machines and overall system sensitivity may well account for some variability in the results of the various reported series. Because there is no test phantom to replicate the flow velocity of the smaller vessels within the ovarian masses, it is difficult to achieve objective assessment of each machine's sensitivity and accuracy in flow determination. It is known that some systems may display a waveform from areas that do not demonstrate a color signal, while others may not detect a waveform in areas of color.

The manufacturers of ultrasound equipment, being aware of the complexity of the Doppler technique, sometimes provide present configurations for certain clinical uses that make the technique easily applicable. Because the pelvic circulation includes numerous vessels with different blood-flow characteristics, it should be recognized that preset defaults for Doppler measurements might lead to misinterpretation of results.

In such a situation, when there is no standardization in the Doppler measurement, the operator's responsibility becomes highly significant. A good basic knowledge of Doppler physics is mandatory, as is a personal sensitivity for the Doppler instrumentation. The Doppler pitfalls and artifacts must be known before it is even considered to apply the Doppler technique to patients in the clinical situation.

An interesting dispute on Doppler physics developed between Kurjak and Kupesic on one side and Levine on the other.[70] Levine commented that a reduction in ultrasound frequency of the examining transducer might decrease the number of vessels detected but did not affect the measured resistance. Kurjak and Kupesic explained that operating frequency did influence the measured resistance. The reason for that was that a higher-frequency probe yielded a small minimum sample volume. This applied particularly to the lateral (to US beam) dimension of the sample volume, since the lateral resolution is always worse than the axial and both depend on the wavelength. For a constant number of cycles per measurement pulse the axial resolution was better with higher frequency as well. This meant that for lower frequencies the detection and measurement of resistance was biased towards larger vessels. Such larger vessels branched out into smaller vessels, e.g. into two or three branches of a smaller diameter draining blood from a larger vessel. In the simplest case those would have been in a parallel combination of vessels. If there had been two such vessels they would be equivalent to one vessel (the resistance of one small vessel). In parallel combinations the more vessels, the lower the resistance. The law of combination is complicated for parallel combinations of unequal vessels, but if the vessels were equal, it would boil down to half the single resistance for parallel combination of two, one-third single resistance for a combination of three, and so forth. These resistances combine differently if they are in a series combination (i.e. one after the other—in fact a tube of varying diameter). In the series combination the resistances simply add, so that more tubes in series yield a higher overall resistance. However, in case of adnexal malignancies, there were situations where a large blood vessel branched out into a few normal vessels and one vessel of pathologically low resistance. In such a case it was very important that one could discriminate between measuring the single, low-resistance vessel and

the bulk effect of this vessel combined with a few normal vessels running parallel with it. If the sampling volume were put on the branching point, one would measure a parallel combination of normal and low-resistance vessels. In this case the overall combined resistance would have been even lower than that of the single low-resistance vessel because the other parallel branches drain from the same pool and thus reduce the overall resistance to flow. The multiple paths could both be seen, due to the lower image definition at lower frequencies. This led to overestimation of the number of low-resistance vessels, increasing the false positive rate compared to operation at higher frequencies.

Part of the controversy is engendered by differences in patient population. Clearly, the best results in terms of differentiation between benign and malignant adnexal masses are obtained in postmenopausal patients and premenopausal patients analyzed during the early proliferative phase of the menstrual cycle.

To prove our hypothesis, we tried to correlate reports on the menstrual phase when patients were examined between published articles by radiology and gynecology departments, assuming that menstrual phase can alter blood flow features of the adnexal masses, creating overlaps in results between benign and malignant lesions.[71] However, we found no correlation between the reports of the menstrual phase and the final results. From eight studies published by radiologists, five did not report on the menstrual phase (62%), whereas from 25 articles published by gynecologists, 11 studies reported the menstrual phase (44%) but still gynecologists evaluated TVCD as an inventive and useful new diagnostic tool. Therefore, no significant difference in the material and method approach, based on the report of menstrual cycle, in the assessment of adnexal vascularity was found. This observation brings us back to reality—the general attitude towards the usefulness of color Doppler is not built up on the final results, however good or bad they are, but on how the new knowledge, even sometimes minimal or insignificant in terms of statistics, can be used and applied in the clinical setting. It seems that gynecologists use this new diagnostic modality more enthusiastically and with more optimism than radiologists. Keeping in mind that the major criticism of the opponents of color flow Doppler imaging is that it adds little to the overall management of patients with pelvic masses, we will attempt to discuss and evaluate the capabilities, advantages, and benefits, as well as the disadvantages and overestimated results, produced by the use of transvaginal color and pulsed Doppler sonography in the assessment of adnexal disease. By the end of the chapter, we hope that our data and experience will support the counter-argument to that of our opponents, and prove that color Doppler flow imaging gives the clinician additional useful clinical information for determining those patients in whom early intervention is necessary, versus those in whom expectant management can be undertaken safely.

Color Doppler and malignant adnexal tumors

Use of color Doppler sonography was based on the well-established hypothesis that unrestricted growth of tumors is dependent upon angiogenesis.[72,73] The growth of new vessels and development of already existing ones are influenced by specific factors which regulate angiogenic activity.[74] Angiogenesis as a physiological phenomenon can be seen in the endometrium during the process of implantation[75] or in the ovary during folliculogenesis (plate 5).[76] However, it occurs as pathological process during oncogenesis as well.[72] Most tumors larger than 2–3 mm cannot grow further without the support of vascularization.[77] The development of an adequate vascular network and blood nourishment is crucial to the growth and development of a cancer, as well as its to metastasis.[78] Based on angiogenesis studies, tumor vasculature consists of the vessel recruited from the existing vascular network and vessels that have developed as an angiogenic response of the host vasculature to angiogenesis factors synthesized by cancer cells. Tumor vascularity tends to rise from venous rather than arterial host vasculature. Therefore, compared to the normal vessel architecture, blood vessels located at the advancing cancer front lack muscular coating and they consist mostly of endothelial lining and may contain tumor cells. Because of this characteristic architecture of the tumor blood vessels, tumor vascularization can be analyzed in terms of vessel location, vessel arrangement, and pulsed Doppler waveform signal features—shape and resistance to blood flow.

The advantages of the color Doppler technique were demonstrated and used in gynecology for the first time by groups in Zagreb and London.[21,23] The Zagreb group has studied pelvic masses, and observed low impedance intratumoral blood flow (RI < 0.41) in malignant ovarian lesions. Both groups agreed that this technique can detect ovarian cancer as early as FIGO (International Federation of Gynaecology and Obstetrics) stage Ia, and can be used as a screening technique for the disease. From those days on, nothing has essentially changed. A lot of research has been done to prove or dispute the use of color Doppler, but a final verdict has never been reached.

Schneider and co-workers[33] compared the results obtained by color Doppler, two-dimensional ultrasonography, and CA125 serum levels in 22 premenopausal and 33 postmenopausal patients with adnexal masses previously diagnosed by sonography and/or computed tomography. Although they presented RI values for each tumor, they did not report on morphological descriptions of the tumors (e.g. cystic, cystic solid, or solid) and mean size of the lesions. It is possible that, for example, the majority of malignant tumors with false-negative RI values were cystic and large. If this is true, then it is possible that neovascular signals could be easily missed or that normal pericystically located vessels with high RI values would be erroneously classified as malignant.

Weiner and colleagues[36] followed 18 patients, who had completed their treatment for pelvic tumors, by sonography, computed tomography, and measurement of serum CA125. These techniques were compared with transvaginal color Doppler and the results demonstrated a high sensitivity and specificity (86% and 100%, respectively). Color Doppler demonstrated intratumoral blood flow in all cases, but in one case the pulsatility index (PI) was high.

Data presented in the study of Schulman and colleagues[79] proved color Doppler to be useful. This study clearly showed that the morphology of adnexal masses depicted by conventional transvaginal sonography could be used in the majority of cases to determine histopathology. However, in non-specific complex lesions containing solid and cystic areas, color Doppler sonography serves as an adjunctive test for clarifying the etiology. The same method has proved to be mandatory in detection of the area of cancer in normal-sized ovaries. As we have found, an abnormal flow velocity in the ovary used in this study was defined by a resistance index of less than 0.41. Using this cutoff point, 15 cysts were predicted to be benign and histology was confirmatory, and one stage Ib ovarian cancer was detected successfully.

Predanic and co-workers[56] correlated morphological score, CA125 measurement, RI values, and peak systolic velocity values in order to evaluate which parameter works best in the detection of malignant adnexal masses. They concluded that color and pulsed Doppler sonography are as good as gray-scale sonography or serum CA125 in the assessment of adnexal disease. Applied by an experienced operator in a disciplined fashion and in correlation with other clinical findings, it will provide valuable information about adnexal masses in terms of angiogenic or growth activity.

Alcazar and co-workers[58,68] reported the overlapping of PI lowest values among benign and malignant tumors, and that this is an obstacle to establishing a clear cutoff value. These results are similar to those reported by other groups, which found a false-positive rate ranging from 24 to 76% with the use of a cutoff value of $PI_{lowest} < 1.0$. However, the use of a cutoff value of $RI_{lowest} \leq 0.45$ had a sensitivity of 100%, with an acceptable specificity of 88.6% Therefore, the lowest RI seems to be better than the lowest PI to differentiate benign from malignant adnexal masses.

In the authors' series, the mean peak systolic velocity (PSV) in malignant tumors was significantly higher than in benign masses. However, there was a considerable overlap in values, making it difficult to establish clear cutoff value. These results agreed with those reported by Valentin and colleagues[39,69] and Prompeler and colleagues.[42] Alcazar and co-workers[68] concluded that RI is the best predictor, but should not be used alone, but in conjunction with other parameters, such as tumor vessel location and peak systolic velocity.

Presence of blood vessels and vessel location

Macroscopically, the tumor vasculature can be categorized as peripheral and central vascularization.[25] Although this classification is not appropriate and anatomically correct, it may help in the assessment of ultrasonically detectable vascular position within tumor tissue. It is believed that peripherally located vessels originate from pre-existing host vasculature, while centrally located vessels develop in response to angiogenic tumor cell activity and/or due to necrotic processes. Vessels displayed within septa or papillae represent specific intratumoral branches (Plate 6). The vascular network could be used as an indicator of peripheral blood perfusion of the tumor and its growth, especially in cases of papillary projections (Plate 7). When vasculature of benign adnexal lesions is correlated with that of malignant ones, it is found that benign adnexal masses are mostly vascularized pericystically and peripherally (Plate 8), while in malignant tumors centrally located vascularization is present most frequently.[80] Although the position of the neovascularization area within tumor tissue is unpredictable, the largest number of blood vessels can be seen in the center of the malignant tumor, while peripheral neovascularization is found less often.[50] Additionally, the presence of color flow in the regular wall or septa does not indicate malignancy, although it can be seen randomly.[54]

Color Doppler sonography has the potential to discriminate malignant from benign masses in cases with 'doubtful' morphology. The usefulness of this method was reported specifically for semi-solid or solid-cystic tumors.[26,39] For example, when malignancy is suggested by morphologic features, color Doppler may help to demonstrate vascularization in malignant vegetations of volume 1 cm^3 or more. It was also shown that within malignant tumors that had small vegetations without color flow, solid irregular portions with color flow were found, allowing the diagnosis of malignancy. Therefore, high vascular resistance and absence of color flow has been considered to suggest a benign lesion.[51] Indeed, color flow can be seen in virtually all malignant adnexal lesions in most series,[15,25,26,33,35,44,46,47,64,65,81] although occasionally no flow is detected in malignant tumors.[25,28,29,35,38,80] The explanation for this difference may be sought in the actual diameter of blood vessels which can be depicted with color Doppler sonography. It was found that in benign adnexal lesions the diameter of vessels ranges from 0.01 to 0.03 mm and the number of vessels per field at magnification 10 was between 9 and 12. In borderline tumors, the diameter of vessels ranges from 0.01 to 0.1 mm and the number of vessels per field at magnification 10 was between 10 and 20, whereas in malignant tumors, the diameter of vessels ranges from 0.01 to 0.1 but the number of vessels per field at the same magnification was between 20 and 30.[54]

Vessel arrangement

Very few studies have tried to evaluate or quantify the amount of vascularity within the tumor. In one of the early series we described vessel arrangement as a diffuse or isolated vascular pattern[31] Diffuse vessel arrangement was categorized as more than one color spot displayed, whereas an isolated vessel was described when only one color spot was displayed over tumor tissue. We found that, compared to isolated vessels, diffuse vessels located within the central solid parts of tumors were almost three times more common in malignant tumors (80%) than in benign lesions (33%), suggesting that the area demonstrating diffuse vessel pattern contains high angiogenic activity.[71] These findings can be related to the previously described study where the authors found significantly larger number of blood vessels per field at magnification 10 in malignant tumors than in benign ones, 20–30 versus 8–12 blood vessels, respectively.[54] Therefore, we believe that an objective method, such as a computerized method of quantification, is needed to analyze the likelihood of malignancy on the basis of vessel density. Such a system has been described for predicting the 'vessel density' in nine cases of transplanted murine tumors and has shown excellent correlation to histopathologic

quantification.[82] The system used seems to provide an accurate depiction of vascularity while time–activity curves show greater flow in the experimental group injected with exotoxine than in the group injected with saline solution. Vascular density quantification with amplitude color Doppler sonography was shown to be more accurate when an intravascular agent was used. One of the proposed hypotheses for tumor resistance is poor delivery of chemotherapeutic agents to areas of tumors that are poorly perfused. It is therefore accepted that chemotherapy given simultaneously with an agent that increases blood flow may reach deeper areas of tumor (that are potentially hypoxic and ischemic) and give better results. The quantification scheme published by Meyerowitz et al.[82] may allow the development of a system to assess the malignant potential of the tumor and to monitor tumor response to chemotherapy on the basis of vascularity of the mass. This technique may be used to assess whether vascular density is a parameter that correlates with the likelihood of a tumor's spread and its metastatic potential. It is expected that three-dimensional imaging conjoined with color Doppler evaluation will depict overall blood flow to the tumor more accurately.

Alcazar et al[58] also used the position of tumor vessel location to predict the malignancy of a tumor. They suggested that RI_{lowest} should be used in conjunction with a vessel location parameter in order to achieve maximal accuracy. Takac[62] reported that the presence or absence of vascularization, as a parameter, did not have any predictive value, while vessel arrangement, as well as an RI of less than 0.40 allowed the prediction of malignancy with limited reliability.

Brown and co-workers[65] reported on the use of a combined morphological and Doppler scoring system. In their opinion, a solid component is the most statistically significant predictor of a malignant ovarian mass.

Valentin is cautious with the use of color Doppler for the assessment of malignancy. In her latest works,[61,69] she concludes that the degree to which Doppler examination can contribute to the differential diagnosis of pelvic tumors will depend on the proportion of multilocular cysts with solid parts in the population studied: the greater this proportion, the greater the potential of the Doppler examination to improve diagnostic accuracy.

Guerriero and co-workers[63] investigated the use of power Doppler as an additional aid in differentiating between benign and malignant tumors. By CDE (color Doppler energy) imaging (evaluation of vessel distribution), malignancy was suspected when arterial flow was visualized in an echogenic portion of a mass defined as malignant by B-mode ultrasonography (in agreement with Buy and colleagues,[54] using conventional color Doppler imaging). A mass was considered benign by transvaginal CDE imaging when no arterial flow was visualized in an echogenic portion, or when flow was seen only in the wall of a mass defined as malignant by B-mode. The authors reported that from a clinical point of view, the use of transvaginal ultrasonography associated with CDE imaging evaluation of vessel distribution seems to increase the specificity and positive predictive value of the use of transvaginal ultrasonography alone, reducing the number of false-positive results. Our own group has learned an important lesson from pathologists specializing in tumor vascularity.[8] In about 50% of malignant ovarian tumors, there is more than one area of vascularization. This is an important finding for all of us, particularly for those who are entering the field. If we are not sufficiently careful, we can easily misinterpret the high resistance of a vessel as being a neovascular signal when it is probably a pre-existing vessel with a normal wall structure.

Pulsed Doppler waveform shape

In addition to the localization of blood vessels in adnexal tumors, it was emphasized that shape of the flow curve is one of the important descriptive features of blood hemodynamics. Appearance of the early diastolic notch or indentation of the early diastolic part of the pulsed Doppler waveform signal slope has been found more often in blood vessels of benign rather than malignant lesions.[50,83] Experimental work with tumors inoculated into rabbit flanks shows that the vessels within areas of active tumor growth have a paucity of muscular tunica media and simulate sinusoids rather than well-formed arterioles. These sinusoid-like vascular spaces have been observed in liver and ovarian tumors in areas of active tumor growth. The low-velocity and impedance waveforms obtained from tumors can be explained on the basis of this type of tumor vessel.[84] In blood vessels with normally developed tunica muscularis, after systole there is a short period of relaxation of the muscle vessel wall and orthograde flow.[84] This kind of blood-flow pattern with an early diastolic notch was demonstrated in the flow curve for ovarian blood vessels during the proliferative phase of the menstrual cycle.[85] Therefore, the lack of a diastolic notch on the waveform is probably related to a lack, or relative paucity, of smooth muscle in the tunica media, which would account for the initial resistance to flow during the first

part of diastole, followed by a relaxation of the muscular wall and forward flow.[86] One must be aware that a diastolic notch can also be observed at a branch point of vessels. It has also been observed that new vessels found in the wall of a corpus luteum demonstrate the lack of a diastolic notch, perhaps due to a relative lack of a muscular coat in these newly formed vessels.[25] It seems that an early diastolic notch, although a common finding in benign cystic lesions, can be also observed in 7% of malignant multilocular-solid tumors.[39] Furthermore, Parsons has pointed out that a few larger vessels feed the vascular wreath within the wall of a corpus luteum. Interestingly enough, the flow in the 'feeding' vessel has higher impedance and velocity than that of the more distal branches.[87]

Vascular resistance to blood flow

It is clear that conflicting attitudes towards Doppler ultrasound in the evaluation of the vascular characteristics of malignant adnexal masses arise from largely different results obtained from the number of studies published in the past several years. It is also important to stress that pulsed Doppler analysis and vascular resistance to blood flow have been, and still are, one of the major features in the assessment of tumor vascular characteristics. Therefore, both the first and the latest studies concentrate on differences in terms of vascular resistance to blood flow between benign and malignant adnexal masses.[21,25,27,31,32,34,38,40–42,44,45,46,48,51,58,63–66,69]

Table 32.4 depicts how Kurjak and co-workers improved on their knowledge on vascular parameters for malignancy. Later studies found less difference in blood-flow data with larger

Table 32.4 Review of color Doppler research done by Kurjak and co-workers as their knowledge and understanding of Doppler increased. At first, only Doppler parameters were used, and nowadays various scores together with Doppler parameters achieve best clinical results

Authors	Criteria for malignancy	Sensitivity	Specificity	PPV	NPV	Accuracy
Kurjak et al. (1989)[21]	Color flow +	100	93.3	83.3	100	95
Kurjak et al. (1990)[90]	Color flow +	100	100	100	100	100
Kurjak et al. (1990)[91]	RI < 0.50	100	100	100	100	100
Kurjak and Zalud (1990)[89]	RI < 0.40	100	99.2	95.9	100	99.3
Kurjak et al. (1992)[31]	RI < 0.41	96.6	94.7	96.6	94.7	95.8
	TVS	48.3	98.1	93.3	77.9	80.7
	Color flow +	93.1	64.8	58.7	94.6	74.7
	Doppler score	89.7	98.1	96.3	96.4	95.2
	TVS + Doppler score	89.7	96.3	89.7	96.3	94
Kurjak and Predanic (1992)[88]	Multiparameter scoring system	97.3	100	100	99.2	99.4
	TVS	92.1	94.8	79.5	97.7	94.2
	Both combined	97.3	100	100	99.2	99.4
Kurjak et al. (1994)[92]	RI ≤ 0.4	100	97.1	80	100	97.4

TVS, transvaginal ultrasonography.

overlap between vascular resistance in benign and malignant lesions. However, it is a fact that a difference in vascularity exists and blood vessels in malignant adnexal lesions show lower resistance to blood flow than in benign adnexal masses. Table 32.5 gives an overview of pulsed Doppler results in terms of resistance (RI) or pulsatility (PI) indices. We believe that the major problem with the observed overlap is due to variation of RI and PI results within the same tumor. It was suggested in several reports that such a variation exists in adnexal tumors[27–29,39,80,83] and it was further stressed that the operator's responsibility is highly significant in the detection and recording of an appropriate blood vessel resistance when no standardization in pulsed Doppler measurement is

Table 32.5 Various authors have tried to reach best accuracy by combining morphological, Doppler or biochemical parameters

Authors	Criteria for malignancy	Sensitivity	Specificity	PPV	NPV	Accuracy
Hata et al.[30]	RI < 0.72	92.6	52.8	59.5	90.5	69.8
	RI < 0.40	25.9	94.4	77.8	63.0	65.1
	TVS	85.2	69.4	67.6	86.2	
Kurjak and Predanic[88]	RI < 0.41	96.6	94.7	96.6	94.7	95.8
	TVS	48.3	98.1	93.3	77.9	80.7
	Color flow +	93.1	64.8	58.7	94.6	74.7
	Doppler score	89.7	98.1	96.3	96.4	95.2
	TVS + Doppler score	89.7	96.3	89.7	96.3	94
Weiner et al.[27]	PI ≤ 1.0	94.1	97.2	94.1	97.2	96.2
	TVS	94.1	69.4	59.3	96.2	77.4
Schneider et al.[33]	RI ≤ 0.8	93.8	56.4	46.8	95.7	67.3
	RI ≤ 0.5	56.3	89.7	69.2	83.3	80
	RI ≤ 0.4	37.5	97.4	85.7	79.2	80
	TVS					
	Subjective	87.5	84.6	63.6	94.3	85.5
	Scoring	87.5	74.4	58.3	93.6	78.2
Timor-Tritsch et al.[34]	RI < 0.46	93.8	98.7	93.8	98.7	97.9
	PI < 0.62	87.5	97.4	87.5	97.4	95.7
	TVS scoring	93.7	87.1	60	99	88.3
Bromley et al.[40]	RI < 0.8	91.7	52.4	52.4	91.7	75.8
	RI < 0.6	66.7	81	66.7	81	66.7
	TVS scoring	91.7	52.4	52.4	91.7	66.7
Brown et al.[38]	PI < 1.0	100	46	–	–	57
	PI < 0.8	100	75	–	–	80
	PI < 0.6	67	96	–	–	90
	RI < 0.5	83	83	–	–	83
	RI < 0.6	100	54	–	–	63
	RI < 0.4	50	96	–	–	87
Jain et al.[35]	RI < 0.4	70	82.5	50	91.7	80
	TVS	90	95	81.8	97.4	94
Alcazar et al.[58]	RI$_{lowest}$ < 0.45	100	–	11.4	–	–
	Central vessel location	90	–	11.4	–	–
Leeners et al.[64]	PI < 0.69	79.6	58.2	–	–	–
	RI < 0.45	66.7	68.7	–	–	–
	Sassone sono-morphological scale	85.2	67.1	–	–	–
Guerriero et al.[63]	B-mode and PI ≤ 1	88	87	59	97	–
	B-mode and RI ≤ 0.4	58	95	70	92	–
	CA125 ≥ 35 U/ml	82	64	32	94	–
	CA125 ≥ 65 U/ml	67	81	42	92	–
	B-mode and CA125 ≥ 35 U/ml	82	92	68	96	–
	B-mode and CA125 ≥ 65 ml/U	67	96	76	93	–
	CDE* and CA125 ≥ 35 U/ml	82	95	77	96	–
	CDE* and CA125 ≥ 65 U/ml	67	97	81	93	–

CDE*, color Doppler energy = power Doppler.

present. Therefore, a good basic knowledge of Doppler physics is mandatory as well as skillfulness with the Doppler instrumentation. Furthermore, potential pitfalls and artifacts must be known before anyone begins to apply this technique to patients.

Blood-flow velocities

Several authors documented the presence of abnormal flow spectra at the periphery of malignant tumors in terms of high blood-flow velocities, establishing the hypothesis that such signals result from arteriovenous anastomoses,[93,94] which was later confirmed by several groups.[95–99] It was suggested that a cutoff value of 40 cm/s could be used to distinguish blood-flow velocities in malignant versus benign tumors.[100] However, such high blood-flow velocities and cutoff values established for breast malignant tumors have not been found in adnexal tumors.[25,80] It is of value to stress that only one study[42] reported a significant difference between blood-flow velocities of benign and malignant lesions, stating the superiority of this measurement over the resistance index.

Tailor and co-workers[57] used blood-flow velocity indices in an ultrasound based test to discriminate between malignant and benign adnexal tumors. The accurate measurement of blood-flow velocity requires knowledge of the angle of insonation to the blood vessel. This potential limitation has prevented wider acceptance of velocity measurements in ovarian tumors. However, the reluctance to use velocity parameters for the assessment of ovarian blood flow might be unjustified. According to these authors, the degree of overlap between benign and malignant tumors for the velocity parameters was less than that for the impedance parameters. Therefore, when used in isolation, velocity parameters were more useful than the PI or RI for the diagnosis of malignancy. These authors suggest that the sonographer should search for the highest velocity rather than the lowest impedance. The best diagnostic accuracy under these circumstances will be achieved by the combination of velocity and impedance parameters. This approach would ensure that the ubiquitous low-velocity, low-impedance signals would not be falsely classified as those arising from malignant tissue.

Surgical stage of malignant tumors

Angiogenesis is a common phenomenon in malignant ovarian neoplasms, but the intensity of neovascularization may depend on individual tumor characteristics.[12] Therefore, an incremental decrease of the impedance indices in adnexal tumors may reflect the increase in angiogenic intensity as an indication of malignant potential.[13] Animal models and clinical research showed that angiogenesis could be detected by Doppler ultrasound even in a small volume of malignant tumor when the carcinoma is well confined within the ovarian capsule or exhibiting only low malignant potential.[14–17] Occasionally, the color Doppler ultrasound features may suggest malignancy in morphologically non-suspicious masses.[16] This stresses the importance of the integration of

clinical and laboratory information with color Doppler ultrasound findings. The newly developed power or energy modes of color Doppler imaging afford depiction of even smaller vessels but, paradoxically, small intraparenchymal arterioles in benign and normal tissues may show a low impedance and low velocity blood-flow pattern, causing false-positive results. Since blood-flow parameters are not only a result of the relationship of blood vessels and their wall structure, but also the increased permeability of the analyzed vascular network, stasis of blood flow and short shunts with low impedance can occur in different parts of the tumor.[20] Increased interstitial pressure and occurrence of necrosis are parameters which may elevate vascular impedance, and ultrasonographers performing Doppler analysis should be aware of these findings.

False-positive results

Until now, we have showed that although significant differences in vascular characteristics between benign and malignant adnexal lesions exist, an overlap in findings can also be expected. An adequate knowledge of ultrasound physics and vascular changes through the menstrual cycle, as well as acknowledging morphological characteristics of certain adnexal tumors, can reduce this overlap in results. Furthermore, the sonographer should be aware that an overlap is characteristic of any biologic system. However, even an experienced ultrasonographer using sensitive equipment will not escape the occasional misinterpretation of the ultrasound and Doppler information in equivocal cases. False results can also be caused by increased vascularity in some physiological conditions. An increased blood flow and significantly decreased impedance to blood flow distal to the point of sampling can be seen in preovulatory follicles (Plate 5) and the corpus luteum (Plate 9), suggesting that *vascular information derived from the premenopausal ovary must always be related to the phase of the cycle.*[101]

A ring of angiogenesis around the dominant follicle is most prominent at the moment of the presumed ovulation. The velocity of the perifollicular blood flow tends to increase, while the resistance to blood flow decreases.[101] With the rupture of the follicle and formation of the corpus luteum, angiogenesis continues and further dilatation of the stromal ovarian vessels occurs. The physiologic corpus luteum and its variants are frequent false-positive conditions in distinguishing ovarian malignancy, because of abundant and prominent blood flow (Plate 9). Luteal vascularity, described as 'a ring of fire', is probably a consequence of marked dilatation of stromal ovarian blood vessels or 'vascular luteal conversion'[102] due to increased local levels of E_2 prostaglandins which are known to be potent vasodilators.[103,104] Additional confusion to the accurate assessment of luteal blood flow is due to its appearance—a cystic structure with irregular walls of various types and intracystic echoes. Therefore, irregular cystic structure with echogenic fluid within the cavity, increased blood-flow velocity, and decreased resistance to blood flow may lead the sonographer to an incorrect interpretation (Plate 10).

Accordingly, physiological ovarian angiogenic activity should be excluded by carrying out the examination during the early proliferative phase of the menstrual cycle. However, this seems not to be completely true, because some corpus luteum activity, and consequently increased ovarian vascularity, can be observed in first 5 days of the menstrual cycle.[105] Therefore, the corpus luteum and its blood flow should be carefully avoided as a false-positive of ovarian malignancy.

Ovarian lesions are a cause of great concern because of the limited ability to distinguish accurately between benign and malignant neoplasms prior to surgery. This is particularly true for bizarre structures such as cystadenomas, hemorrhagic cysts, ovarian fibromas, dermoid cysts, and endometriomas.

Serous and mucinous cystadenomas are a common cause of false-positive results, due to suspicious ultrasonic appearance. They are usually presented as multilocular cysts with internal septa and papillary projections. The vascular location and type of angiogenesis are important parameters in reducing the overlap with malignant tumors. The peripheral and/or intraseptal location of the vessels and elevated vascular resistance indicate the benign nature of the lesion (Plate 6).

Ovarian fibroma is a benign solid ovarian tumor, which is commonly interpreted as ovarian malignancy because of its echogenic appearance. These well-delineated tumors demonstrate central and/or peripheral vascularization with moderate impedance to blood flow.

The remainder of benign adnexal lesions that may cause false-positive results are pelvic inflammatory disease (Plate 11) and endometriomas. In both these entities rich vascularity is usually triggered by inflammation.[106,107] The addition of color Doppler capabilities to transvaginal transducers enables detection of vascularity within endometriomas.[38] These echogenic cysts with a semi-solid content of a 'parenclymatous' texture, representing a 'chocolate' paste-like fluid, are supported by already existing vessels within the ovarian hilus, showing moderate vascular impedance (Plate 12). If present, inflammatory changes may show alterations in perfusion that are characterized by a marked reduction in blood-flow resistance. This finding may be wrongly interpreted as due to ovarian malignancy. In addition, hormonal imbalances in overweight patients can produce blood-flow patterns with a low resistance index.

Three-dimensional power Doppler ultrasound of adnexal lesions

Three-dimensional ultrasound is a new, emerging technology that provides additional information for the evaluation of ovarian tumors. Multiplanar and volume-rendering display methods, combined with the ability to rotate volume data into standard orientations, are essential components of the current and future success of three-dimensional ultrasound (Plate 13).[108] Recent developments of real-time three-dimensional ultrasound imaging will further advance clinical applications, particularly in the assessment of pelvic tumors. Introduction of the three-dimensional power Doppler systems may improve the information available on ovarian tumor vascularity and speed up the entire patient management process.[11,109,110]

Morphological analysis of the blood-vessel system represents another approach to tumor diagnosis which, so far, has not been evaluated extensively. There is a distinct subjective impression that the distribution and branching pattern of blood vessels that supply fast-growing tumors differ from those of the normal blood supply to normal organs. This means that the blood-vessel distribution seems to carry additional information which is missed in present diagnostic approaches. However, describing branching structures, such as the blood-vessel tree, is a mathematically complicated task that calls for the most recent mathematical apparatus.

The branching pattern is a result of some principle (mathematical law) that acts repeatedly upon the blood vessels so that they branch out in similar ways at different scale factors. The process is, presumably, similar to processes that govern branching in actual trees.

Our initial hypothesis is that the general view of the pattern of branching of blood vessels within 1 cm^3 generally resembles that of the branching in 50 cm^3 of the same tissue.[11] Structures that look alike at different magnifications are fractal[111–113] and are found in natural geometric forms (trees, bird's feathers, etc.) as well as in the maps of the (apparently chaotic) outcomes of processes that have nothing to do with geometry (e.g. animal populations). The growth of blood vessels is likely to have these properties. The main property of a fractal is its fractal dimension. We postulate that blood-vessel trees are an example of fractal[112,113] geometry. The normal blood-vessel trees (arteries and veins) form branched structures with ever-smaller branches and diameters. They provide blood supply to the whole body while taking up less than 6% of the available space. The basic underlying proposition of our hypothesis is that there is a change in fractal dimension when the branching is no longer regulated by normal processes, i.e. when the ordered growth is replaced by disordered growth.

Three-dimensional modelling on a large scale is a mathematically and technologically very demanding task. One important aspect of this approach is the interplay of results obtained by reconstruction of blood-vessel geometry using ultra-thin histological sections and the resolution of diagnostic imaging methods, particularly three-dimensional ultrasound imaging. While ultrasound resolution has greatly improved over the years, it is physically impossible to obtain resolutions of the order of 10 μm with any non-invasive form of ultrasonic imaging or Doppler. Three-dimensional reconstruction with ultrasound imaging and Doppler is now feasible and takes us a step nearer to this mathematical evaluation, but the resolution problems are similar in two- and three-dimensional studies.[114,115]

Three-dimensional display allows the physician to visualize many overlapping vessels easily and quickly, as well as to assess their relationship to other vessels or other surrounding tissues. It permits the ultrasonographer to view structures in three dimensions interactively, rather than having to assemble the sectional images in his or her mind. Interactive rotation of power Doppler rendered images provides improved visualization of the tumor vasculature. Malignant tumor vessels are usually randomly dispersed within the stroma and periphery, sometimes forming several tangles or coils around the surface (Plates 14 and 15).

The higher detection rate of small vessels after injection of contrast agents may facilitate application of the mathematical models assessing three-dimensional vascular chaos and fractals (Plate 16).[116]

The role of color Doppler sonography in the assessment of the architecture of tumor vascularity seems clinically pertinent, justifying expanded research into this topic. This opinion is based on the discovery and molecular characterization of a diverse family of regulators of angiogenesis, both stimulators and inhibitors.[117] In the case of solid tumors a shift in the balance of stimulators and inhibitors can trip the angiogenetic switch, allowing tumors to recruit new blood vessels from the surrounding host vasculature, which provides them with a survival advantage. This process appears to be necessary for tumors to grow beyond microscopic size. It is the ultimate goal of most researchers of tumor angiogenesis to find ways of turning off the angiogenetic switch, as a form of cancer treatment.

Boehm and colleagues[118] have shown that three different mouse tumors regressed after treatment with repeated cycles of endostatin, a newly discovered angiogenesis inhibitor. The tumors did not become drug resistant and, after a characteristic number of treatment cycles, became dormant. Such a treatment strategy could help circumvent many of the problems associated with current chemotherapeutic regimens, such as acquired drug resistance, attributable to tumor cell genetic instability, or intrinsic resistance, due to poor penetration of certain drugs into the tumor parenchyma.[119] The results of cyclic endostatin therapy strongly suggest that drugs targeting angiogenesis and the tumor vasculature will become a major new tool for effective treatment and possibly prevention of human cancer. As with any new treatment procedure, there are a number of important questions for the future. Indeed, a pure angiogenesis inhibitor would be expected to block new blood vessel growth, leaving quiescent blood vessels intact. Such an inhibitor should stop neovascularization in a tumor and effect a static dormant state. The tumor should neither grow nor regress but should continue to be fed by its established vessels, remaining in a metastable state of proliferation balanced by apoptosis.[120]

Conclusion

Color and pulsed Doppler sonography provide information about the vascularity of an adnexal mass, revealing insight into tumor histology and metabolism. Therefore, blood-flow data should be considered to indicate the angiogenic intensity of tumor, rather than malignancy itself. It seems clear that initial attempts to classify ovarian tumors solely on the basis of their impedance to blood flow have been too simplistic. This problem has been solved partly by introduction of other 'vascular parameters', such as blood-vessel arrangement and location, shape of the pulsed Doppler and appearance of an early diastolic notch, as well as by assessment of blood-flow velocities. However, the difference in flow parameters between benign and malignant lesions may not always be a sufficient basis an which to make a firm diagnostic decision. A common criticism of color Doppler is that the operator is never blind to the B-mode image: there is a tendency to search harder for low-impedance blood-flow patterns in lesions with a malignant appearance rather than in simple adnexal cysts. However, when applied by expert operators and in a disciplined fashion, it may add significantly to diagnostic information about an adnexal mass and its morphological appearance. If blood-flow data are treated as an insight into the tumor's pathology, they give reassurance for those masses with benign appearance, while providing confirmation of malignancy in adnexal masses with suspicious morphological features.

The application of three-dimensional power Doppler ultrasound raises many new questions about the regulation of tumor angiogenesis, density of tumor vessels, and differences between vessel architecture in benign and malignant growths. In the future, we may hope to use integrated software for calculating the total extent of the vascularity of a whole mass in the three-dimensional perspective. Contrast agents are another possibility for enhancing the three-dimensional power Doppler examination, by increasing the detection rate of small vessels. Future development of the three-dimensional power Doppler program should also include three-dimensional gray-scale information and simultaneous Doppler shift spectrum information.

References

1. Folkman, J. (1989). What is the evidence that tumors are angiogenesis dependent? *J. Natl Cancer Inst.*, **82**, 4–6.
2. Rak, J.W., St. Croix, D.B., and Kerbel, R.S. (1995). Consequences of angiogenesis for tumor progression, metastatis and cancer therapy. *Anti-Cancer Drugs*, **6**, 3–18.
3. Skobe, M., Rockwell, P., Vosseler, S., and Fusenig, N.E. (1997). Halting angiogenesis suppresses carcinoma cell invasion. *Nature Med.*, **3**, 1222–7.
4. Weidner, N. (1995). Intratumor microvessel density as a prognostic factor in cancer. *Am. J. Pathol.*, **147**, 9–15.
5. Liotta, L., Kleinerman, J., and Saidel, F. (1974). Quantitative relationships of intravascular tumor cells, tumor vessels, and pulmonary metastases following tumor implantation. *Cancer Res.*, **34**, 997–1004.
6. Hanahan, D. and Folkman, J. (1996). Parameters and emerging mechanisms of the angiogenic switch during tumorigenesis. *Cell*, **86**, 353–4.
7. Kurjak, A., Kupesic, S., Ilijas, M. *et al.* (1998). Preoperative diagnosis of primary Fallopian tube carcinoma. *Gynecol. Oncol.*, **68**, 29–34.
8. Kurjak, A., Jukic, S., Kupesic, S., and Babic, D. (1997). A combined Doppler and morphopathological study of ovarian tumors. *Europ. J. Obstet. Gynecol. Reprod. Biol.*, **71**, 147–50.
9. Emoto, M., Iwasaki, H., Mimura, K. *et al.* (1997). Differences in the angiogenesis of benign and malignant ovarian tumors, demonstrated by analyses of color Doppler ultrasound, immunohistochemistry, and microvessel density. *Cancer*, **80**, 899–907.
10. Suren, A., Osmers, R., and Kuhn, W. (1998). 3D Color Power Angio™ imaging: a new method to assess intracervical vascularization in benign and pathological conditions. *Ultrasound Obstet. Gynecol.*, **2**, 133–8.
11. Kurjak, A., Kupesic, S., Breyer, B. *et al.* (1998). The assessment of ovarian tumor angiogenesis: What does 3D power Doppler add? *J. Ultrasound Obstet. Gynecol.*, **12**, 136–46.
12. Bourne, T.H. (1994). Should clinical decisions be made about ovarian masses using transvaginal color Doppler? *Ultrasound Obstet Gynecol.*, **4**, 257–60.
13. Wu, C.C., Lee, C.N., Chen, T.M. *et al.* (1994). Incremental angiogenesis assessed by color Doppler ultrasound in the tumorigenesis of ovarian neoplasms. *Cancer*, **73**, 1251–6.

14. Ramos, I., Fernandez, L.A., Morse, S.S. *et al.* (1988). Detection of neovascular signal in a 3-day Walker 256 rat carcinosarcoma by CW Doppler ultrasound. *Ultrasound Med. Biol.*, **14**, 123–6.

15. Bourne, T.H., Campbell, S., Steers, C.V. *et al.* (1989). Transvaginal colour flow imaging: a possible new screening technique for ovarian cancer. *Br. Med. J.*, **299**, 1367–70.

16. Kurjak, A., Shalan, H., Matijevic, R. *et al.* (1993). Stage I ovarian cancer by transvaginal color Doppler sonography: a report of 18 cases. *Ultrasound Obstet. Gynecol.*, **3**, 195–8.

17. Fleischer, A.C., Cullinan, J.A., Peery, C.V., and Jones III, J.W. (1996). Early detection of ovarian carcinoma with transvaginal color Doppler ultrasound. *Am. J. Obstet. Gynecol.*, **174**, 101–6.

18. Barnhill, R.L., Fandrey, K., Levy, M.A. *et al.* (1992). Angiogenesis and tumor progression of melanoma: quantification of vascularity in melanocytic nevi and cutaneous malignant melanoma. *Lab. Invest.*, **67**, 57–62.

19. Srivastava, A., Laidler, P., Davies, R.P. *et al.* (1988). The prognostic significance of tumor vascularity in intermediate thickness (0.76–4.0mm thick) melanoma: a quantitative histologic study. *Am. J. Pathol.*, **133**, 419–23.

20. Blood, C.H. and Zetter, B.R. (1990). Tumor interactions with the vasculature: angiogenesis and tumor metastasis. *Biochim. Biophys. Acta*, **1032**, 89–118.

21. Kurjak, A., Zalud, I., Jurkovic, D. *et al.* (1989). Transvaginal color Doppler of the assessment of pelvic circulation. *Acta Obstet. Gynecol. Scand.*, **68**, 131–6.

22. Hata, T., Hata, K., Senoh, D. *et al.* (1989). Doppler ultrasound assessment of tumor vascularity in gynecologic disorders. *J. Ultrasound Med.*, **8**, 309–14.

23. Bourne, T., Campbell, S., Steer, C. *et al.* (1989). Transvaginal color flow imaging: a possible new screening technique for ovarian cancer. *Br. Med. J.*, **299**, 1367–70.

24. Campbell, S., Royston, P., and Bhan, V. (1990). Novel screening strategies for early ovarian cancer by transabdominal ultrasonography. *Br. J. Obstet. Gynaecol.*, **96**, 304–11.

25. Fleischer, A.C., Rodgers, W.H., Rao, B.J. *et al.* (1991). Assessment of ovarian tumor vascularity with transvaginal color Doppler sonography. *J. Ultrasound Med.*, **10**, 563–8.

26. Kurjak, A., Zalud, I. and Alfirevic, Z. (1991). Evaluation of adnexal masses with transvaginal color ultrasound. *J. Ultrasound Med.*, **10**, 295–7.

27. Weiner, Z., Thaler, I., Beck, D. *et al.* (1992). Differentiating malignant from benign ovarian tumors with transvaginal color flow imaging. *Obstet. Gynecol.*, **79**, 159–62.

28. Kawai, M., Kano, T., Kikkawa, F. *et al.* (1992). Transvaginal Doppler ultrasound with color flow imaging in the diagnosis of ovarian cancer. *Obstet. Gynecol.*, **79**, 163–7.

29. Tekay, A. and Jouppila, P. (1992). Validity of pulsatility and resistance indices inclassification of adnexal tumors with transvaginal color Doppler ultrasound. *Ultrasound Obstet. Gynecol.*, **2**, 338–44.

30. Hata, H., Hata, T., Manabe, A. *et al.* (1992). A critical evaluation of transvaginal Doppler studies, transvaginal sonography, magnetic resonance imaging, and CA 125 in detecting ovarian cancer. *Obstet. Gynecol.*, **80**, 922–6.

31. Kurjak, A., Schulman, H., Sosic, A. *et al.* (1992). Transvaginal ultrasound, color flow, and Doppler waveform of the postmenopausal adnexal mass. *Obstet. Gynecol.*, **80**, 917–21.

32. Hamper, U.M., Sheth, S., Abbas, F.M. *et al.* (1993). Transvaginal color Doppler sonography of adnexal masses: Differences in blood flow impedance in benign and malignant lesions. *Am. J. Rad.*, **160**, 1225–8.

33. Schneider, V.L., Schneider, A., Reed, K.L., and Hatch, K.D. (1993). Comparison of Doppler with two-dimensional sonography and CA 125 for prediction of malignancy of pelvic masses. *Obstet. Gynecol.*, **81**, 983–8.

34. Timor-Tritsch, I.E., Lerner, J.P., Monteagudo, A., and Santos, R. (1993). Transvaginal ultrasonographic characterization of masses by means of

color flow-directed Doppler measurements and a morphologic scoring system. *Am. J. Obstet. Gynecol.*, **168**, 909–13.

35. Jain, K.A. (1994). Prospective evaluation of adnexal masses with endovaginal gray-scale and dupler and color Doppler US: Correlation with pathologic findings. *Radiology*, **191**, 63–7.

36. Weiner, Z., Beck, D., and Brandes, J.M. (1994). Transvaginal sonography, color flow imaging, computed tomography scanning, and CA 125 as a routine follow-up examination in women with pelvic tumor: Detection of recurrent disease. *J. Ultrasound Med.*, **13**, 37–41.

37. Levine, D., Feldstein, V.A., Babcook, C.J., and Filly, R.A. (1994). Sonography of ovarian masses: Poor sensitivity of resistive index for identifying malignant lesions. *Am. J. Rad.*, **162**, 1355–9.

38. Brown, D.L., Frates, M.C., Laing, F.C. *et al.* (1994). Ovarian masses: Can benign and malignant lesions be differentiated with color and pulsed Doppler US? *Radiology*, **190**, 333–6.

39. Valentin, L., Sladkevicius, P., and Marsal, K. (1994). Limited contribution of Doppler velocimetry to the differential diagnosis of extrauterine pelvic tumors. *Obstet. Gynecol.*, **83**, 425–33.

40. Bromley, B., Goodman, H., and Benacerraf, B.R. (1994). Comparison between sonographic morphology and Doppler waveform for the diagnosis of ovarian malignancy. *Obstet. Gynecol.*, **83**, 434–7.

41. Carter, J., Saltzman, A., Hartenbach, E. *et al.* (1994). Flow characteristics in benign and malignant gynecologic tumors using transvaginal color flow Doppler. *Obstet. Gynecol.*, **83**, 125–30.

42. Prompeler, H.J., Sauerbrei, W.M., Latternann, U., and Pfleiderer, A. (1994). Quantitative flow measurements for classification of ovarian tumors by transvaginal color Doppler sonography in postmenopausal patients. *Ultrasound Obstet. Gynecol.*, **4**, 406–13.

43. Chou, C.Y., Chang, C.H., Yao, B.L., and Kuo, H.C. (1994). Color Doppler ultrasonography and serum CA 125 in the differentiation of benign and malignant ovarian tumors. *J. Clin. Ultrasound*, **22**, 491–6.

44. Wu, C.C., Lee, C.N., Chen, T.M. *et al.* (1994). Factors contributin to the accuracy in diagnosing ovarian malignancy by color Doppler ultrasound. *Obstet. Gynecol.*, **84**, 605–8.

45. Zaneta, G., Vergani, P., and Lissoni, A. (1994). Color Doppler ultrasound in the preoperative assessment of adnexal masses. *Acta Obstet. Gynecol. Scand.*, **73**, 637–41.

46. Salem, S., White, L.M., and Lai, J. (1994). Doppler sonography of adnexal masses: The predictive value of the Pulsatility index in benign and malignant disease. *Am. J. Rad.*, **163**, 1147–50.

47. Sengoku, K., Satoh, T., Saitoh, S. *et al.* (1994). Evaluation of transvaginal color Doppler sonography, transvaginal sonography and CA 125 for prediction of ovarian malignancy. *Int. J. Gynecol. Obstet.*, **46**, 39–43.

48. Savicki, E., Spiewankiewicz, B., Cendrowski, K., and Stelmachow, J. (1995). Transvaginal Doppler ultrasound with colour flow imaging in benign and malignant ovarian lesions. *Clin. Exp. Obstet. Gynecol.*, **22**, 137–42.

49. Franchi, M., Beretta, P., Ghezzi, F. *et al.* (1995). Diagnosis of pelvic masses with trasabdominal color Doppler, CA 125 and ultrasonography. *Acta Obstet. Gynecol. Scand.*, **75**, 734–9.

50. Maly, Z., Riss, P., and Deutinger, J. (1995). Localization of blood vessels and qualitative assessment of blood flow in ovarian tumors. *Obstet. Gynecol.*, **85**, 33–6.

51. Stein, S.M., Laifer-Narin, S., Johnson, M.B. *et al.* (1995). Differentiation of benign and malignant adnexal masses: Relative value of gray-scale, color Doppler, and spectral Doppler sonography. *Am. J. Rad.*, **164**, 381–6.

52. Carter, J.R., Lau, M., Fowler, J.M. *et al.* (1995). Blood flow characteristics of ovarian tumors: Implications for ovarian cancer screening. *Am. J. Obstet. Gynecol.*, **172**, 901–7.

53. Fleischer, A.C., Cullinan, J.A., Peery, C.V., and Jones III, H.W. (1996). Early detection of ovarian carcinoma with transvaginal color Doppler ultrasonography. *Am. J. Obstet. Gynecol.*, **174**, 101–6.

54. Buy, J.N., Ghossain, M.A., Hugol, D. *et al.* (1996). Characterization of adnexal masses: Combination of color Doppler and conventional sonography compared with spectral Doppler analysis alone and conventional sonography alone. *Am. J. Rad.*, **166**, 385–93.

55. Rehn, M., Lohmann, K., and Rempen, A. (1996). Transvaginal ultrasonography of pelvic masses: Evaluation of B-mode technique and Doppler ultrasonography. *Am. J. Obstet. Gynecol.*, **175**, 97–104.

56. Predanic, M., Vlahos, N., Pennisi, J. *et al.* (1996). Color and pulsed Doppler sonography, gray-scale imaging, and serum CA 125 in the assessment of adnexal disease. *Obstet. Gynecol.*, **88**, 283–8.

57. Tailor, A., Jurkovic, D., Bourne, T.H. *et al.* (1996). Comparison of intratumoral indices of blood flow velocity and impedance for the diagnosis of ovarian cancer. *Ultrasound Med. Biol.*, **22**(7), 837–43.

58. Alcazar, J.L., Ruiz-Perez, M.L., and Errasti, T. (1996). Transvaginal color Doppler sonography in adnexal masses: which parameter performs best? *Ultrasound Obstet. Gynecol.*, **8**, 114–19.

59. Wheeler, T.C. and Fleischer, A.C. (1997). Complex adnexal mass in pregnancy: predictive value of color Doppler sonography. *J. Ultrasound Med.*, **16**, 425–8.

60. Reles, A., Wein, U., and Licthenegger, W. (1997). Transvaginal color Doppler sonography and conventional sonography in the preoperative assessment of adnexal masses. *J. Clin. Ultrasound*, **25**, 217–25.

61. Valentin, L. (1997). Gray scale sonography, subjective evaluation of the color Doppler image and measurement of blood flow velocity for distinguishing benign and malignant tumors of suspected adnexal origin. *Europ. J. Obstet. Gynecol. Reproduct. Biol.*, **72**(1), 63–72.

62. Takac, I. (1998). Analysis of blood flow in adnexal tumors by using color Doppler imaging and pulsed spectral analysis. *Ultrasound Med. Biol.*, **24**(8), 1137–41.

63. Guerriero, S., Ajossa, S., Risalvato, A. *et al.* (1998). Diagnosis of adnexal malignancies by using color Doppler energy imaging as a secondary test in persistent masses. *Ultrasound Obstet. Gynecol.*, **11**, 277–82.

64. Leeners, B., Funk, A., Schild, R.L. *et al.* (1998). Preoperative determination of the structure of pelvic tumors with color coded Doppler ultrasound and conventional transvaginal ultrasound. *Zentralblatt für Gynakologie*, **120**(10), 503–10.

65. Angeid-Backman, E., Coleman, B.G., Arher, P.H. *et al.* (1998) Comparison of resistive index versus pulsatility index in assessing the benign etiology of adnexal masses. *Clin. Imaging*, **22**(4), 284–91.

66. Brown, D.L., Doubilet, P.M., Miller, F.H. *et al.* (1998). Benign and malignant ovarian masses: selection of the most discriminating gray-scale and Doppler sonographic features. *Radiology*, **208**(1), 103–10.

67. Buckshee, K., Temsu, I., Bhatla, N., and Deka, D. (1998). Pelvic examination, transvaginal ultrasound and transvaginal color Doppler sonography as predictors of ovarian cancer. *Int. J. Gynecol. Obstet.*, **61**, 51–7.

68. Alcazar, J.L., Errasti, T., Zornoza, A. *et al.* (1999). Transvaginal color Doppler ultrasonography and CA125 in suspicious adnexal masses. *Int. J. Gynecol. Obstet.*, **66**(3), 255–61.

69. Valentin, L. (1999). Pattern recognition of pelvic masses by gray-scale ultrasound imaging: the contributon of Doppler ultrasound. *Ultrasound Obstet. Gynecol.*, **14**, 338–47.

70. Kurjak, A. and Kupesic, S. (1996). Color Doppler imaging for the detection of ovarian malignancy is reliable. *Ultrasound Obstet. Gynecol.*, **7**, 379–83.

71. Kurjak, A. and Kupesic, S. (1995). Transvaginal color Doppler and pelvic tumor vascularity—lessons learned and future challenges. *Ultrasound Obstet. Gynecol.*, **6**, 145–59.

72. Folkman, J. (1985). Tumor angiogenesis. *Adv. Cancer Res.*, **48**, 2641–5.

73. Folkman, J. and Cotran, R.S. (1976). Relation of vascular proliferation to tumor growth. *Int. Rev. Exp. Pathol.*, **16**, 207–12.

74. Folkman, J. and Klaysburn, M. (1987). Angiogenic factors. *Science*, **235**, 442–7.

75. Jaffe, R. and Warsof, S.L. (1991). Transvaginal color Doppler imaging in the assessment of uteroplacental blood flow in the normal first-trimester pregnancy. *Am. J. Obstet. Gynecol.*, **164**, 781–5.

76. Bourne, T.H., Jurkovic, D., Waterstone, J. *et al.* (1991). Intrafollicular blood flow during human ovulation. *Ultrasound Obstet. Gynecol.*, **1**, 215–19.

77. Jain, R.K. (1987). Transport of molecules across tumor vasculature. *Cancer Metastasis Rev.*, **6**, 559–61.

78. Folkman, J., Watson, K., Ingber, D., and Hanahan, D. (1989). Induction of angiogenesis during the transition from hyperplasia to neoplasia. *Nature*, **339**, 58–61.

79. Schulman, H., Conway, C., Zalud, I. *et al.* (1994). Prevalence in a volunteer population of pelvic cancer detected with transvaginal ultrasound and color flow Doppler. *Ultrasound Obstet. Gynecol.*, **4**, 414–20.

80. Kurjak, A., Predanic, M., Kupesic-Urek, S., and Jukic, S. (1993). Transvaginal color and pulsed Doppler assessment of adnexal tumor vascularity. *Gynecol. Oncol.*, **50**, 3–9.

81. Hata, K., Hata, T., Manage, A., and Kitao, M. (1992). Ovarian tumors of low malignant potential: transvaginal Doppler ultrasound features. *Gynecol. Oncol.*, **45**, 259–64.

82. Meyerowitz, C.B., Fleischer, A.C., Pickens, D.R. *et al.* (1996). Quantification of tumor vascularity and flow with amplitude color Doppler sonography in an experimental model: Preliminary results. *J. Ultrasound Med.*, **15**, 827–33.

83. Fleischer, A.C., Rodgers, W.H., Kepple, D.M. *et al.* (1993). Color Doppler sonography of ovarian masses: a multiparameter analysis. *J. Ultrasound Med.*, **12**, 41–8.

84. Shubik, P. (1982). Vascularization of tumors: a review. *J Cancer Res. Clin. Oncol.*, **103**, 211–19.

85. Hata, T., Hata, K., Senoh, D. *et al.* (1989). Doppler ultrasound assessment of tumor vascularity in gynecologic disorders. *J. Ultrasound Med.*, **8**, 309–14.

86. Fleischer, A.C., Cullinan, J., Jones III, H.W. *et al.* (1995). Serial assessment of adnexal masses with transvaginal color Doppler sonography. *Ultrasound Med. Biol.*, **21**, 435–43.

87. Parsons, A.K. (1994). Ultrasound of the human corpus luteum. *Ultrasound Quart.*, **12**, 127–66.

88. Kurjak, A. and Predanic, M. (1992). New scoring system for prediction of ovarian malignancy based on transvaginal color Doppler sonography. *J. Ultrasound Med.*, **11**, 631–8.

89. Kurjak, A. and Zalud, I. (1990). Transvaginal color flow imaging and ovarian cancer [Letter]. *Br. J. Med.*, **300**, 330.

90. Kurjak, A., Jurkovic, D., Alfirevic, Z., and Zalud, I. (1990). Transvaginal color Doppler imaging. *J. Clin. Ultrasound*, **18**, 227–34.

91. Kurjak, A., Zalud, I., Alfirevic, Z., and Jurkovic, D. (1990). The assessment of abnormal pelvic blood flow by transvaginal color and pulsed Doppler imaging for hemodynamic assessment of reproductive tract umors. *Int. J. Gynecol. Obstet.*, **16**, 437–42.

92. Kurjak, A., Shalan, H., Kupesic, S. *et al.* (1994). An attempt to screen asymptomatic women for ovarian and endometrial cancer with transvaginal color and pulsed Doppler sonography. *J. Ultrasound Med.*, **13**, 295–301.

93. Wells, P.N.T., Halliwell, M., Skidmore, R. *et al.* (1977). Doppler studies of the breast. *Ultrasound Med. Biol.*, **15**, 231–5.

94. Burns, P.N., Halliwell, M., Webb, A.J., and Wells, P.N.T. (1982). Ultrasonics Doppler studies of the breast. *Ultrasound Med. Biol.*, 127–43.

95. Shimamoto, K., Sakuma, S., Ishigaki, T., and Makino, N. (1987). Intratumoral blood flow: evaluation with color Doppler echography. *Radiology*, **165**, 683–5.

96. Jellins, J., Kossoff, G., Boyd, J., and Reeve, T.S. (1983). The complementary role of Doppler to the B-mode examination of the breast. *J. Ultrasound Med.*, **10**, 29–35.

97. Maniasan, M. and Bamber, J.C.A. (1983). A preliminary assessment of an ultrasonic Doppler method for the study of blood flow in human breast cancer. *Ultrasound Med. Biol.*, **8**, 257–61.

98. Taylor, K.J.W. and Morse, S.S. (1988). Doppler detects vascularity of some malignant tumors. *Diagnostic Imaging*, **10**, 132–6.

99. Taylor, K.J.W., Ramos, I., Carter, D. *et al.* (1991). Correlation of Doppler US tumor signals with neovascular morphologic features. *Radiology*, **166**, 57–62.

100. Dock, W., Grabanwoger, F., Metz, V. *et al.* (1991). Tumor vascularization: assessment with duplex sonography. *Radiology*, **181**, 241–4.

101. Kurjak, A., Kupesic, S., Schulman, H., and Zalud, I. (1991). Transvaginal color flow Doppler in the assessment of ovarian and uterine blood flow in infertile women. *Fertil. Steril.*, **56**, 870–3.

102. Merce, L.T., Kupesic, S., and Kurjak, A. (1999). Color Doppler assessment of implantation and early placentation. *Prenatal Neonatal Med.*, **4**, 94–112.

103. Alila, H.W., Corradino, R.A., and Hansel, W. (1988). A comparison of the effects of cyclooxygenase prostanoids on progesterone production by small and large bovine luteal cells. *Prostaglandins*, **36**, 259–70.

104. Raud, J. (1990). Vasodilatation and inhibition of mediator release represent two distinct mechanisms of prostaglandin modulation of acute mast cell-dependent inflammation. *Br. J. Pharmacol.*, **99**, 449–54.

105. Sladkevicius, P., Valentin, L., and Marsal, K. (1994). Blood flow velocity in the uterine and ovarian arteries during menstruation. *Ultrasound Obstet. Gynecol.*, **4**, 421–7.

106. Kupesic, S., Kurjak, A., Pasalic, L., and Benic, S. (1995). Transvaginal color Doppler in the assessment of pelvic inflammatory disease. *J. Ultrasound Med. Biol.*, **6**, 733–8.

107. Kurjak, A. and Kupesic, S. (1994). Scoring system for prediction of ovarian endometriosis based on transvaginal color and pulsed Doppler sonography. *Fertil. Steril.*, **62**, 81–8.

108. Bonilla Musoles, F., Raga, F., and Osborne, N.G. (1995). Three-dimensional ultrasound evaluation of ovarian masses. *Gynecol. Oncol.*, **59**, 129–35.

109. Downey, B.D. and Fenster, A. (1995). Vascular imaging with a three dimensional power Doppler system. *Am. J. Rad.*, 665–8.

110. Chan, L., Lin, W.M., Verpairojki, B. *et al.* (1997). Evaluation of adnexal masses using three-dimensional ultrasonographic technology: preliminary report. *J. Ultrasound Med.*, **16**, 349–54.

111. Mandelbrot, B. (1977). *Fractals: form, chance and dimension.* W.H. Freeman and Co.

112. Breyer, B. and Kurjak, A. (1995). Tumor vascularization Doppler measurements and chaos: what to do? *Ultrasound Obstet. Gynecol.*, **5**, 209.

113. Schoenfeld, A., Levavi, H., Tepper, R. *et al.* (1994). Assessment of tumor induced angiogenesis by three dimensional display: confusing Doppler signals in ovarian cancer screening? *Ultrasound Obstet. Gynecol.*, **4**, 516–18.

114. Kurjak, A., Shalan, H., Kupesic, S. *et al.* (1993). Transvaginal color Doppler sonography in the assessment of pelvic tumor vascularity. *Ultrasound Obstet. Gynecol.*, **3**, 137–54.

115. Kurjak, A. and Kupesic, S. (2000). Three-dimensional static and power Doppler improves the diagnosis of ovarian lesions. *Gynecol. Oncol.*, in press.

116. Kupesic, S. and Kurjak, A. (2000). Contrast enhanced three-dimensional power Doppler sonography for the differentiation of adnexal lesions. *Obstet. Gynecol.*, **96**, 452–8.

117. Hanahan, D. and Folkman, J. (1996). Parameters and emerging mechanisms of the angiogenetic switch during tumorigenesis. *Cell*, **86**, 29–34.

118. Boehm, T., Folkman, J., Browder, T., and O'Reilly, M.S. (1997). Antiangiogenic therapy of experimental cancer does not induce acquired drug resistance. *Nature* (London), **390**, 404–7.

119. Kerbel, R.S. (1991). Inhibition of tumor angiogenesis as a strategy to circumvent acquired resistance to anticancer therapeutic agents. *Bioessays*, **13**, 31–6.

120. Holmgren, L., O'Reilly, M.S., and Folkman, J. (1995). Dormancy of micrometastases: balanced proliferation and apoptosis in the presence of angiogenesis suppression. *Nature Med.*, **1**, 149–53.

33. CT and MRI of ovarian cancer

S.A.A. Sohaib and R.H. Reznek

Introduction

Although computed tomography (CT) and magnetic resonance imaging (MRI) are not used routinely to stage the disease in patients presenting with ovarian cancer, they have an important role in the evaluation such patients. They may be used to help make the diagnosis at presentation, to assess the extent of disease, to define residual disease, to assess response to treatment, and to detect recurrent disease.

Computed tomography (CT)

The advantages of CT are that it is widely available and allows the whole abdomen and pelvis to be surveyed accurately and rapidly. It is relatively accurate in the detection of intra-abdominal spread of disease and it is familiar to clinicians and radiologists.

Recently spiral CT has been introduced into clinical practice. Unlike conventional CT, spiral CT allows continuous volumetric data acquisition within a single breath-hold. This potentially offers improved lesion detection, optimization of contrast media enhancement, multiplanar or three-dimensional image reformation.[1] However, the role of spiral CT in imaging of the female pelvis has yet to be fully evaluated.[2]

Technique

Patients undergoing CT scan for ovarian cancer are required to have a full bladder and are given about 600–800 ml of dilute oral contrast medium starting an hour before the scan. Prior to scanning a vaginal tampon is inserted and rectal contrast medium given. The oral and rectal contrast media are to allow differentiation of bowel loops from adnexal and soft-tissue structures and detection of tumour invasion of the bowel.[2] The vaginal tampon helps in delineating the position of the vaginal vault and uterine cervix. Routine administration of intravenous iodinated contrast medium is recommended in evaluation of these patients as it improves tumour delineation and characterization and increases the conspicuousness of peritoneal deposits.[3,4] Intravenous iodinated contrast medium is contraindicated in patients allergic to iodinated contrast medium, and has to be used with caution in patients with impaired renal function. The abdomen and pelvis should be scanned routinely using contiguous sections from the dome of the diaphragm to below the pubic symphysis.

Magnetic resonance imaging

Magnetic resonance imaging (MRI) is the newest of the cross-sectional imaging modalities. It is being used increasingly to image the pelvis, and has an established role in imaging cervical and endometrial cancer.[5,6] The multiplanar imaging capability and high contrast resolution of MRI offer potential technical advantages. The absence of ionizing radiation and iodinated contrast agent are of benefit in certain patients. MRI has no known adverse effect on the fetus, embryo, or reproductive potential of the ovaries. As with any new imaging modality, MR imaging techniques continue to change and improve, so its role continues to evolve. The main limitations of MRI are the lack of availability, long scanning times, perceived expense,[7,8] and the lack of familiarity to clinicians and radiologists.[5]

In ovarian cancer, MRI is proving useful in characterizing adnexal masses and may have a role in defining the extent of ovarian tumours or in the detection of recurrent disease.[9]

Technique

Patients undergoing MRI examination for ovarian neoplasm need to lie in the tunnel of the magnet and usually have a torso coil wrapped around their abdomen and pelvis. The complete examination takes between 30 and 60 min. The machine makes loud noises during the imaging sequences due to switching of the magnetic field gradients. Ear plugs or music are provided to the patients to compensate for this noise and an intercom in the tunnel allows communication between the patient and the MR technologist. Most patients tolerate the examination without any difficulty but some patients suffer from claustrophobia and are unable to complete the investigation. Some of these patients find oral sedation helpful to overcome their anxiety.[10] Patients with a pacemaker, neurostimulator, or cochlear implant are unable to undergo MRI scans, as the magnetic field will interfere with the operation of these devices. Other contraindications are metallic foreign body in the eye and paramagnetic aneurysm clips. Most patents with a hip prosthesis can undergo MRI, but there may be artefacts.

Pelvic MRI should be performed with a moderately full bladder, and an antiperistaltic agent to reduce bowel motility is also recommended (e.g. glucagon or Buscopan). Some workers recommend the use of a vaginal tampon as a useful anatomical marker, but others believe that the placement of a tampon within the vagina distorts the anatomy.[11] The MR images should be obtained in at least two orthogonal planes, axial and sagittal planes should be used routinely, and the coronal plane may prove useful in some situations, such as identifying the organ of origin in some adnexal masses.

Both T1- and T2-weighted sequences are required for lesion characterization. Scanning from the level of the renal hilum to the symphysis pubis on T1-weighted images is needed to evaluate the retroperitoneum for lymphadenopathy and/or hydronephrosis. T1-weighted images provide the necessary contrast between tumour and adjacent pelvic fat. Also, T1-weighted images are necessary to characterize haemorrhagic and fat-containing lesions. The T2-weighted images best display the uterine and ovarian zonal anatomy.[12] This sequence is needed to distinguish between a uterine or adnexal origin of pelvic masses. The T2-weighted images also provide superior tissue characterization compared to that of T1-weighted images. Intravenous gadolinium-enhanced T1-weighted sequence should be used routinely, as it significantly improves lesion characterization and the detection of peritoneal and omental metastases.[9,13–16] Fat suppression sequences should be performed because of their value in distinguishing blood from lipid-containing lesions and in identifying small, high-signal endometriomas in amongst the pelvic fat.[17,18] Some authors recommend contrast-medium-enhanced T1-weighted fat-saturation sequences through the entire abdomen for the evaluation of possible peritoneal metastases.[19]

Characterization of ovarian tumours

In patients presenting with a pelvic mass, cross-sectional imaging techniques have a valuable role in confirming the presence of a mass, determining the organ of origin, and can provide some information on the character of the lesion. Ultrasound, CT, or MRI may all be used in this way. Ultrasound is the preferred technique, since it is a widely available, and a lower cost technique, than CT or MRI. However, if ultrasound is equivocal, then CT or MRI may be performed.

CT

CT has a high sensitivity in the detection of ovarian tumours and is able to characterize the size and nature of a lesion.[4] Soft tissue, cystic components, fat, and calcification are all well shown. The CT density of serous fluid approaches that of water. Fluid with proteinaceous material, debris, or blood will result in a higher CT density, approaching that of soft tissue, but unlike soft tissue will not enhance following intravenous injection of contrast media. Other components of ovarian tumours, such as septa, cyst wall, and solid portions, are best seen on contrast-enhanced scans.[4] CT features of an ovarian cancer vary widely according to pathology.

MRI

MRI has been widely used in evaluating adnexal masses.[9,14,20] It is of particular value because of its ability to distinguish and accurately diagnose the vast majority of uterine leiomyomas (Fig. 33.1), ovarian dermoids (Fig. 33.2), endometriomas (Fig. 33.3), small simple follicular cysts and ovarian fibromas.[21,22] Several studies have shown superior characterization of adnexal masses in pregnant patients by MR imaging compared to ultrasound, which prevented surgery or permitted delay until after parturition.[23,24]

On MRI, the signal intensities of an individual tumour depend upon the presence, nature, and extent of solid and cystic components of the mass. Cystic components have high signal on T2-weighted images and are usually of low signal intensity on T1-weighted images (Fig. 33.4). However, the signal intensity of the cystic component of an ovarian neoplasm will vary with its protein content, presence of blood-related products and cellular debris. Such variations in signal intensity are commonly seen in mucinous tumours and haemorrhagic cystic lesions. Fat within a lesion is well demonstrated on MRI (Fig. 33.2) and is of high signal intensity on T1-weighted and T2-weighted sequences. On fat-suppressed sequences, such as frequency-selective fat saturation, or on STIR (short-tau inversion recovery) sequences fat is

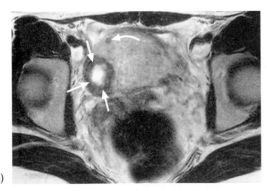
(a)

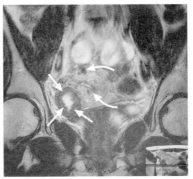
(b)

Fig. 33.1 A 34-year-old woman presenting with an adnexal mass. The (a) axial and (b) coronal T2-weighted scan shows that the adnexal mass (arrows) is arising from the uterine body. The mass has low signal around the periphery and central high signal, which would be in keeping with a degenerating fibroid. Other low-signal fibroids (curved arrow) can be seen within the in the myometrium.

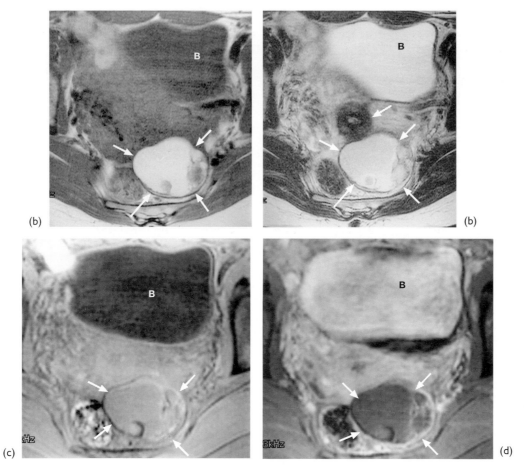

Fig. 33.2 Benign cystic teratoma in a 46-year-old woman. Axial (a) T1-weighted spin echo, (b) T2-weighted fast spin echo, (c) before and (d) after intravenous gadolinium enhanced fat-saturated spoiled gradient echo sequences show a mass (arrows) posterior to the cervix (small arrow). This is of high signal intensity on both the T1- and T2-weighted scans and shows loss of signal on the fat-saturated image. The signal intensity of the lesion follows that of intrapelvic and subcutaneous fat.

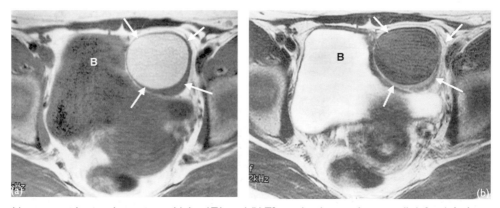

Fig. 33.3 A 48-year-old woman with an endometrioma. (a) Axial T1- and (b) T2-weighted scans show a well-defined thick-walled mass (arrow) lying anterior to the bladder (B). The central component of this is of high signal on T1- and of low signal on T2-weighted scans. These findings on this combination of sequences are typical of the appearance of the altered products of blood in an endometrioma.

of lower signal intensity. Calcification is not as well shown on MRI as on CT, but may appear as areas of low signal intensity on all sequences. As in CT, intravenous administration of contrast medium improves lesion characterization by increasing the con-spicuousness of vegetations, soft-tissue nodules (Fig. 33.5), fluid loculi, wall thickness, and presence of septae in complex adnexal masses (Fig. 33.6).[15,16,25–27] The signal intensity of the solid component varies, depending the composition of the material.

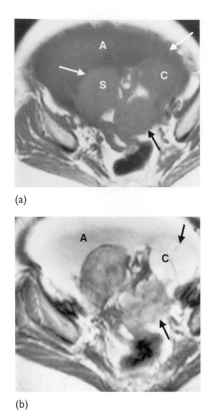

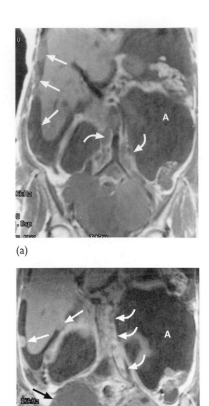

Fig. 33.4 A 50-year-old woman with an ovarian carcinoma. Axial
(a) T1-weighted spin echo and (b) T2-weighted fast spin echo scans
show a large, solid, cystic mass (arrow). There is ascites (A), seen as a
low signal on T1- and a high signal on the T2-weighted scans. The solid
components (S) are of low and intermediate signal intensity. The cystic
component (C) shows similar signal intensity as the ascitic fluid.

Fig. 33.6 A 49-year-old woman with advanced ovarian cancer.
(a) Before and (b) after intravenous gadolinium enhanced coronal
T1-weighted spin echo scans, showing a large mass arising out of the
pelvis. Ascites (A), peritoneal metastases (arrow) and lymph nodes
(curved arrow) can all be seen. The post-contrast-enhanced scan shows
the enhancing peritoneal nodules and that the pelvic mass has a solid
cystic nature.

Benign versus malignant

An important role of characterizing ovarian mass lesions is to distinguish between benign and malignant neoplasms. Both CT and MRI
have relied on morphological characteristics to distinguish benign
from malignant lesions. Findings suggestive of malignancy include
the detection of solid masses and partially solid/cystic masses, as well
as the presence of papillary projections into a cystic lesion and thick
septa (Figs 33.6, 33.7).[28] Secondary features of malignancy, such as
pelvic side-wall invasion, peritoneal, mesenteric, or omental involvement, and lymphadenopathy are readily detected indicators of
malignancy (Figs 33.6, 33.7, 33.8). Although suggestive of malignancy, the finding of pelvic ascites can also be seen in ovarian torsion, pelvic inflammatory disease, and benign ovarian fibroma, and
is therefore not specific.[2] Abdominal ascites alone, or the finding of
ascites anterior to the uterus, is highly suggestive of malignant
ascites.[2,4]

The accuracy of CT and MRI

The sensitivity of MRI in the detection of adnexal lesion is
87–100%, and that of CT 87–96%.[4,15,16,29–31] MRI and CT have an

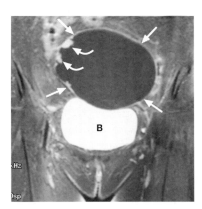

Fig. 33.5 A 30-year-old woman with a serious papillary tumour of low
malignant potential. The coronal fat-saturated spin echo T1-weighted
scan shows a large cystic mass (arrow) above the bladder (B). Some
enhancing nodules can be seen on the wall of this lesion (curved
arrows).

Fibrous tissue is of low signal on all sequences, and most neoplastic or inflammatory lesion are of intermediate to high signal
on the T2-weighted sequences.

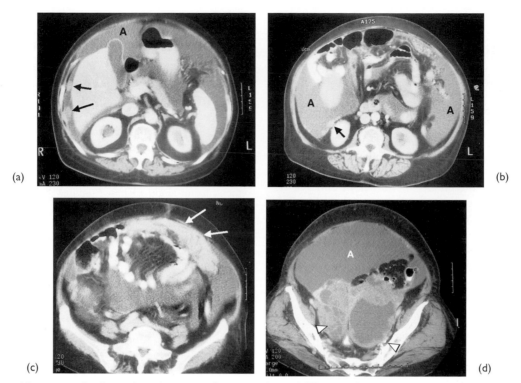

Fig. 33.7 A 79-year-old woman with advanced ovarian cancer. Contrast-enhanced CT scans of the abdomen and pelvis show ascites (A), peritoneal deposits (black arrows), and omental thickening (white arrows). A bilateral, large, solid, cystic mass (arrowheads) can be seen in the pelvis.

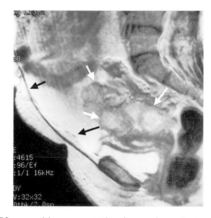

Fig. 33.8 A 50-year-old woman with advanced ovarian cancer. The sagittal T2-weighted fast-spin echo images show peritoneal deposits (black arrows) on the anterior abdominal wall against the high signal of ascitic fluid. Ovarian tumour mass (white arrows) is also well seen.

accuracy of 86–95%[2,15,32] and 66–94%,[4,33] respectively, in distinguishing a benign from a malignant lesion. The multiplanar imaging capability of MRI and the detailed depiction of uterine anatomy on the T2-weighted sequences allows uterine leiomyomas to be distinguished from other adnexal masses (Fig. 33.1).

MRI is the most sensitive imaging technique for imaging blood-related products. Characteristically an endometrioma shows a very high signal on T1- and a low signal on T2-weighted images (Fig. 33.3). Other signs on MRI of endometrioma are thick, low signal intensity wall, and adhesion to pelvic structures.[34] Consequently endometrioma can be diagnosed with high degree

of specificity on MRI.[34] However, some endometriomas may have a non-specific signal intensity and have to be distinguished from other cystic lesions, in particular haemorrhagic cyst lesions, simple cyst, corpus luteal cysts, and benign and malignant ovarian cystic neoplasms. The same morphological criteria as those used for non-haemorrhagic cystic lesions are used to distinguish benign from malignant haemorrhagic tumours.

CT and MRI characteristics of different ovarian tumours

Although definitive pathological characterization of the different ovarian neoplasms cannot be made with imaging, certain features may suggest a particular pathology

Epithelial tumours

Benign epithelial tumours, whether serous or mucinous cystadenomas, appear on CT and MRI as thin-walled cystic lesions without evidence of any soft-tissue components, irregular walls, or papillary projections.[2] Serous cystadenomas are most commonly uni- or bilocular; they may or may not show plaque-like calcification. Mucinous cystadenomas are typically multilocular.[35] Due to the serous nature of the fluid, CT density of the cyst content approaches that of water. Serous fluid on MRI is of high signal on T2-weighted and low signal on T1-weighted images. High-density fluid on CT without contrast enhancement, or high signal intensity fluid on T1- and T2-weighted images, indicates recent haemorrhage (especially in serous cystadenoma) or mucin (in mucinous cystadenoma). On MRI, characteristics specific for benign epithelial tumours, such as thin walls, minimal septation, and absence of papillary projections, are depicted with either T2-weighted images or, better still, with contrast-enhanced T1-weighted images.[4,15]

Cystadenocarcinomas are usually larger, more complex, multi-locular masses, which contain soft-tissue projections extending into the cystic spaces. Other epithelial neoplasms, such as endometrioid, clear cell cancers appear as complex solid–cystic lesions. Brenner tumours may appear as solid masses with or without calcification. On MRI their signal intensity pattern is similar to that of fibroma, thecoma, or uterine leiomyomas.

Tumours of low malignant potential are characterized by lack of invasive growth and have a more indolent course. They are most commonly of the serous or mucinous types. Morphologically, the features of these tumours are between those of benign tumours and their malignant counterparts (Fig. 33.5).

Germ cell tumours

Germ cell tumours include teratoma, dysgerminoma, endodermal sinus (yolk sac) tumours, embryonal tumours, and choriocarcinomas. Ovarian cystic teratomas may contain sebum, hair, epithelium, calcium, and other elements that give rise to their complex appearance. They have characteristic features on CT and MRI, such as a fat–fluid or hair–fluid level, often permitting definitive diagnosis on imaging. Fat is of low attenuation on CT and high signal on T1-weighted MR images. Fat on MRI is most effectively distinguished from high-signal blood-related products or proteinous material by frequency-selective presaturation, where loss of signal similar to that of abdominal fat is shown (Fig. 33.2).[17]

Dysgerminomas are solid masses, which may contain cystic areas representing haemorrhage or areas of necrosis.[36] A characteristic finding of dysgerminoma is fibrovascular septa within a solid mass, best seen on contrast-enhanced CT and MRI.[37]

Sex cord-stromal cell tumours

Sex cord-stromal cell tumours, such as granulosa cell tumours,[38] Sertoli–Leydig cell tumours, thecomas, and fibromas, have variable features on imaging and may therefore appear as small, solid masses on imaging or as large, multilocular cystic lesions similar to cyst adenocarcinomas.

Ovarian fibromas are well-circumscribed, solid tumours which demonstrate low signal intensity on both T1- and T2-weighted images. Fibromas show minimal enhancement.[39] The low signal intensity on T2-weighted images is also seen in leiomyoma. The multiplanar imaging on MRI allows one to differentiate an ovarian fibroma from a pedunculated leiomyoma or other tumour.[40,41]

Ovarian metastases

Metastases to the ovary may be solid, partially solid and cystic, or rarely as a multiloculated cystic lesion, on CT and MRI. They are usually bilateral, but on imaging alone they may be indistinguishable from primary ovarian tumours.[42] Kruckenberg tumours are

ovarian metastases with mucin-filled signet-ring cells. They are usually bilateral and solid and may have areas of haemorrhage and necrosis.

Staging

The role of cross-sectional imaging in pre-treatment evaluation of ovarian cancer is controversial. The most commonly used staging system for ovarian cancer is that of the International Federation of Gynaecology and Obstetrics (FIGO) (Table 33.1), which recommends a laparotomy for staging. Both CT and MRI have been shown to be less accurate than staging laparotomy. However, there are certain situations where preoperative abdominopelvic imaging with CT or MRI may be helpful.[33] These include: uncertain diagnosis; when the gynaecologist requires the overall assessment of the extent of disease; for guidance of percutaneous aspiration and biopsy or paracentesis; and to replace multiple other radiological techniques, such as barium studies and intravenous urography.

Table 33.1 FIGO staging

FIGO stage	TNM stage	Extent of disease
I	T1	Tumour limited to ovaries
Ia	T1a	Tumour limited to one ovary; capsule intact, no tumour on ovarian surface; no malignant cells in ascites or peritoneal washings
Ib	T1b	Tumour limited to both ovaries; capsule intact, no tumour on ovarian surface; no malignant cells in ascites or peritoneal washings
Ic	T1c	Tumour limited to one or both ovaries with any of the following: capsule ruptured, tumour on ovarian surface, malignant cells in ascites or peritoneal washings
II	T2	Tumour involves one or both ovaries with pelvic extension
IIa	T2a	Extension and/or implants on the uterus and/or tube(s); no malignant cells in ascites or peritoneal washings
IIb	T2b	Extension to other pelvic tissue; no malignant cells in ascites or peritoneal washings
IIc	T2c	Pelvic extension (IIa or IIb); malignant cells in ascites or peritoneal washings
III	T3 ± N1	Tumour limited to one or both ovaries with microscopically confirmed peritoneal metastasis outside the pelvis and/or regional lymph node metastasis
IIIa	T3a ± N1	Microscopic peritoneal metastasis beyond pelvis
IIIb	T3b ± N1	Macroscopic peritoneal metastasis beyond pelvis 2 cm or less in greatest dimension
IIIc	T3b ± N1	Peritoneal metastasis beyond pelvis more than 2 cm in greatest dimension and/or lymph node metastasis
IV	M1	Distant metastasis (excludes peritoneal metastasis)

Liver capsule metastasis is stage III/T3; liver parenchymal metastasis, stage IV/M1. Pleural effusion must have positive cytology for stage IV/M1.

The FIGO system of staging is based on the concept that ovarian cancer spreads first to sites within the pelvis and then to the peritoneal cavity, only metastasizing outside the peritoneal cavity in advanced disease. When interpreting CT or MRI, care should be taken to assess all the potential sites of metastatic disease, since small deposits of less than 1 cm can be overlooked easily, unless the areas of likely spread are scrutinized carefully.

Contiguous tumour spread from the ovary may occur along the Fallopian tube or involve the broad ligament and uterus directly. In more advanced disease direct tumour invasion of the rectum, sigmoid colon, bladder, and lateral pelvic wall is seen.

Transcoelomic spread occurs when the ovarian cancer breaks through the serosal epithelial surface of the ovary and tumour cells are shed into the peritoneal cavity. These cells may adhere to peritoneal surfaces, where aggregates of tumour cells grow into vascularized tumour deposits. The malignant cells, which are shed from the surface of the tumour, are carried around within the peritoneal fluid to the lymphatic vessels on the under surface of the diaphragm. Peritoneal metastases are therefore commonly seen in such sites as the under surface of the diaphragm, omentum, surfaces of the small and large bowel, surfaces of the liver, and pouch of Douglas. The right side of the diaphragm is affected more frequently than the left because peritoneal flow is impeded by the left phrenocolic ligament.[48,49]

Lymphatic-borne metastases result from direct invasion of ovarian lymphatics or by absorption into diaphragmatic lymphatic channels, as described above. The lymphatic drainage of the ovary is via lymphatic channels, which accompany the ovarian vessels along the anterior surface of the psoas muscles. On the right side, these lymphatic vessels fan out to drain into the pre-caval and lateral caval lymph nodes, which are situated between the right renal hilum and the aortic bifurcation. On the left, the lymphatic channels do not diverge from each other as extensively as on the right, and usually terminate in lymph nodes around the renal hilum. Accessory lymphatic channels extend laterally from the ovary, traversing the broad ligament to enter the upper external iliac lymph nodes. The regional lymph nodes for ovarian cancer are defined as follows: external iliac nodes, including hypogastric (obturator) nodes, lumbar (para-aortic) nodes and,

rarely, inguinal nodes. The frequency of lymph-node involvement increases with the stage of disease.[49a]

Haematogenous spread occurs late during the course of disease, and less than 1% of patients with epithelial cancers have parenchymal liver metastases at presentation.[50] However, the liver is a common site of haematogenous spread. Other sites of metastatic spread in the terminal stages include the lungs, pleura, kidney, and bone. Adrenal, bladder, and splenic deposits are also seen occasionally (Fig. 33.9).[48]

Although the majority of ovarian cancers spread according to the patterns described above, some tumours have a predilection for a particular route. For example, dysgerminomas spread to lymph nodes more frequently than epithelial tumours, but haematogenous spread is uncommon. However, the more aggressive endodermal sinus tumours, embryonal tumours, and choriocarcinomas metastasize predominantly by the haematogenous route.

CT staging

CT is the most frequently used imaging technique to define the extent of disease prior to treatment. As a method of staging, CT is useful in defining the extent of the primary, and for detecting tumour involvement of many intra-abdominal and pelvic structures, including small and large bowel, urinary tract, peritoneum and mesentery, liver, lymph nodes, ascites, and pseudomyxoma peritonei.

The detection of peritoneal tumour deposits is dependent on their size, location, and the presence of ascites.[3,29,51] On CT, peritoneal metastases may appear as rounded, plaque-like, stellate, or ill-defined masses (Fig. 33.7).[52] The soft-tissue nodules are seen along the peritoneum, or the whole of the peritoneal surface may be thickened. CT can identify psammomatous calcification in plaque-like peritoneal metastases from serous cyst adenocarcinoma, even if there is no associated soft-tissue component to the deposit.[53]

Peritoneal tumour deposits usually show contrast enhancement. In ovarian cancer, peritoneal infiltration is best seen in the right subphrenic space, the greater omentum, and pouch of Douglas.[3] The major limitation with CT in staging ovarian cancer is the inability to detect small (less than 1 cm) peritoneal deposits reliably, and the complete inability to identify microscopic lesions.

Intraperitoneal contrast media increases the detection of peritoneal tumour implants, and smaller tumour deposits of less than 5 mm in diameter can be identified, but the technique is seldom practical on a routine basis.[54] Compartmentalization of the peritoneal cavity may be apparent and it may also be possible to determine whether the lesion is intra- or extraperitoneal. This is useful for determining the utilization of intraperitoneal chemotherapy, which is sometimes used in patients with advanced intraperitoneal disease.

Omental tumour is seen as an increased soft-tissue density interspersed with fat within the omentum under the anterior abdominal wall, or as complete replacement of the omentum by a soft-tissue tumour mass (Fig. 33.7).

Small bowel wall thickening may be observed in advanced cases. This may cause intermittent chronic small bowel obstruction, with dilatation of small bowel loops intermingled with regions of stenosis.

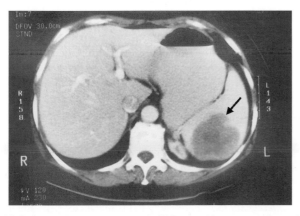

Fig. 33.9 Stage IV ovarian cancer in a 56-year-old woman with a splenic metastasis. The contrast-enhanced CT shows a large, poorly enhancing lesion (arrow) in the spleen.

Pelvic organ invasion by ovarian cancer may be difficult to diagnose accurately as the mass or masses may merely abut adjacent structures without infiltration. For example, uterine invasion is particularly difficult to diagnose because the parauterine fat plane may be lost without necessarily being due to invasion of the uterine serosa.[28] Indeed, in patients with large ovarian masses it may be difficult to identify the uterus, as it may be partially or completely surrounded by tumour. This is a common finding in postmenopausal women in whom the uterus is atrophied.

Spread to lymph nodes can be assessed with CT. Abnormal lymph nodes are diagnosed by size criteria only, and nodes larger than 1 cm in the retroperitoneum are considered pathological. It must be remembered that nodes that contain metastatic deposit but remain small will not be identified as abnormal on CT; conversely, nodes may be enlarged due to reactive hyperplasia rather than metastatic disease.

MRI in staging

There is only limited experience of the use of MRI in staging ovarian cancer, and therefore its role is not fully defined. MRI is able to define the extent of the primary tumour and spread into the uterus or adjacent organs such as the sigmoid colon, bladder, and rectum.[29]

Peritoneal deposits appear as thickening, nodularity, or focal masses involving peritoneal surfaces. These deposits are of intermediate to high signal intensity on T2-weighted sequences (Fig. 33.8). Peritoneal metastases may be better appreciated if oral contrast medium is used.[19,55] A negative contrast agent, such as supraparamagnetic iron oxide particles (e.g. Lumirem–Guerbet Ltd.) is preferable, since the bowel contents will then have a low signal intensity on T1-weighted images whereas enhancing tumour deposits have a high signal intensity.[19,27,55] Fat-suppression sequences may also increase the conspicuousness of enhancing peritoneal tumour deposits and omental disease by suppressing the signal from hyperintense fat in the abdomen and pelvis.[27]

Omental tumour involvement can be identified as an infiltrating mass lying beneath the abdominal wall, and finger-like projections of tumour may be seen spreading into the surrounding fat. Omental disease also shows enhancement following injection of intravenous contrast medium. Mesenteric masses replace normal high signal intensity mesenteric fat with low signal intensity tissue on T1-weighted sequences.

The MRI detection rate for pelvic and retroperitoneal lymph nodes is equal to that of CT.[56] As in CT, the only criterion of abnormality is enlargement. MRI signal characteristics cannot be used to distinguish between benign and malignant nodes; however, there have been early reports of the use of small iron oxide particles in distinguishing benign from malignant lymph nodes.[57] Malignant lymph nodes do not take up the iron oxide particle and therefore remain of high signal.

Accuracy of staging

Laparotomy allows both surgicopathological staging and tumour debulking. Surgical staging is the gold standard for assessing the extent of disease in patients presenting with ovarian cancer.[28,33,56a] However, as many as 30–40% of patients may be understaged at

initial laparotomy, due to inadequate exploration.[56] A frequent reason for understaging is that the preoperative diagnosis is that of a benign tumour, resulting in an inappropriate abdominal incision which precludes the detection of upper abdominal disease.[58,59] Compared to surgical staging, the staging accuracy of CT ranges from 70 to 90%.[60,61] However, CT may identify disease missed at surgery, important sites being tumour deposits posteriorly in the right lobe of the liver or in a subcapsular location, and involved enlarged retroperitoneal and retrocrural lymph nodes.[51,62]

MRI and CT appear to be of equal accuracy in staging abdominopelvic disease.[25] Peritoneal deposits greater than 1 cm in diameter can be identified with a similar sensitivity and specificity by both MRI and CT.[9,15] However, disease within the mesentery or implants on the wall of the small and large bowel are better detected by CT, and calcified deposits, which are highly conspicuous on CT, are very difficult to recognize on MRI. Evaluation of disease within the pelvis is better demonstrated with MRI, but within the abdomen both techniques understage peritoneal tumour implants.[25] The detection of enlarged retroperitoneal lymph nodes is probably equal with both CT and MRI.[56]

Tumour resectability

Aside from staging ovarian cancer, pretreatment evaluation with CT or MRI may be helpful either in identifying patients with non-resectable disease or those patients who cannot under go optimum cytoreduction. Criteria for non-resectable disease include tumour deposits larger than 2 cm in the porta hepatis, intersegmental fissure of the liver, diaphragm, lesser sac, or gastrosplenic ligament, presacral extraperitoneal disease, and lymph node enlargement at the level of the coeliac axis or above.[2,63,64] Both CT and MRI identify pathology in these sites extremely well and thus the accuracy of CT and MRI in predicting non-resectable disease is 93–96%.[32]

Assessment of residual disease, tumour response, and recurrence

CT or MRI are valuable for postoperative staging of patients with irresectable tumour or multiple sites of disease where optimum cytoreduction cannot be achieved. Furthermore, CT or MRI may be used in conjunction with clinical examination and serum marker measurements to identify tumour response to treatment, to detect disease progression, and to determine treatment end-

Table 33.2 Comparisons of CT and MRI for staging and re-staging ovarian cancer

	Accuracy (%)	Sensitivity (%)	Specificity (%)	References
CT	66–85	40–67	93–100	19,43–47
MRI	59–86	62–81	40–93	19,25,46

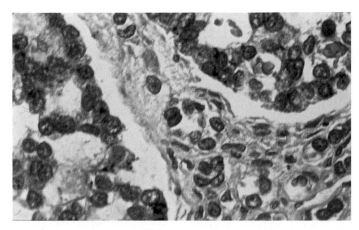

Plate 1 Immunohistochemistry for vascular endothelial growth factor (VEGF) in ovarian cancer.

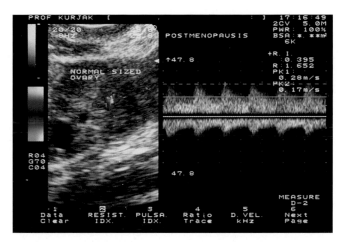

Plate 2 Abundant color flow within the central part of the ovary measuring 3 × 3 × 2 cm in a postmenopausal patient. Low resistance index value (RI = 0.40) indicated ovarian malignancy which was confirmed by histopathology.

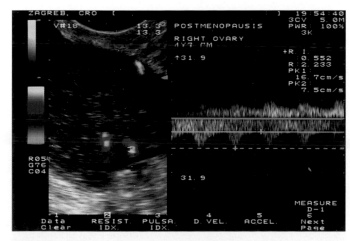

Plate 3 A slightly enlarged ovary (4 × 3 cm) detected in a postmenopausal patient. Blood-flow signals obtained from the peripheral vessels show moderate vascular resistance (RI = 0.55) typical of pre-existing vessels with a normal wall structure.

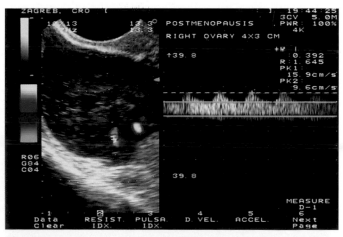

Plate 4 In the same patient as in Plate 3, the pulsed Doppler sonogram (right) displayed from the richly vascularized area only a few millimeters below the place of previous sampling demonstrates a low resistance index (RI = 0.39). Stage Ia ovarian carcinoma was confirmed by histopathology.

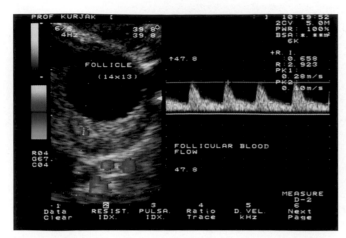

Plate 5 A transvaginal sonogram of the ovary containing a growing follicle. Color flow imaging facilitates the detection of a small vascular area surrounding the dominant follicle. The pulsed Doppler waveform analysis of the intraovarian blood flow shows a resistance index of 0.66.

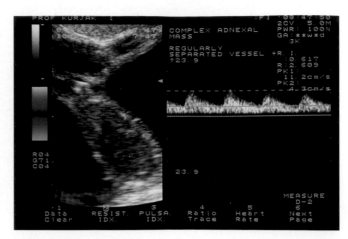

Plate 6 A transvaginal color Doppler scan of a multilocular ovarian tumor. Blood-flow signals obtained from a regularly separated septal vessel demonstrate moderate vascular resistance (RI = 0.62), typical for a benign lesion. Serous cystadenoma was proved by histopathology.

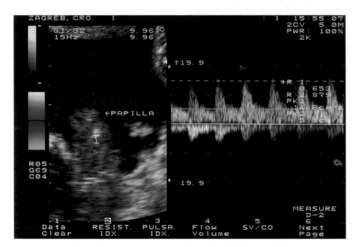

Plate 7 A complex adnexal tumor containing a papillary projection. Moderate- to high-resistance signals
(RI = 0.65) are depicted from the color-coded area at the base of the papilla. The benign nature of the lesion was confirmed by histopathology.

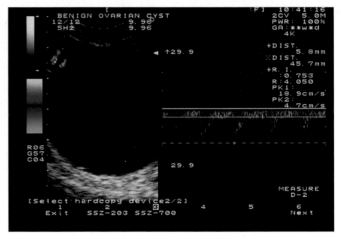

Plate 8 A transvaginal color Doppler scan of a solitary ovarian cyst. Color Doppler imaging demonstrates pericystic flow characterized by high vascular resistance (RI = 0.75).

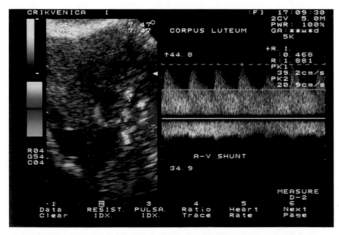

Plate 9 An increased blood flow velocity and decreased resistance index (RI = 0.47) represent typical signs of corpus luteum formation.

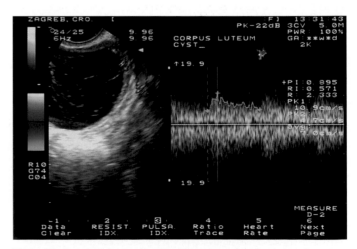

Plate 10 A transvaginal color Doppler sonogram of a corpus luteum cyst. Blood-flow signals obtained from the pericystic area demonstrate moderate vascular resistance (RI = 0.57), typical of a benign lesion.

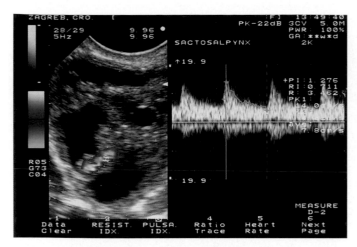

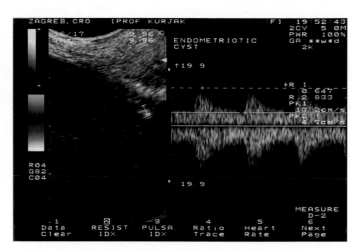

Plate 11 A complex adnexal mass containing thick septa in a patient with chronic pelvic inflammation. Pulsed Doppler waveform analysis demonstrates high resistance flow (RI = 0.71). Chronic salpingitis was proved by laparoscopy.

Plate 12 An ovarian endometrioma. Note the homogeneous high-level internal echoes and peripheral vascularization. Pulsed Doppler analysis shows moderate resistance flow (RI = 0.65) during the follicular phase of the menstrual cycle.

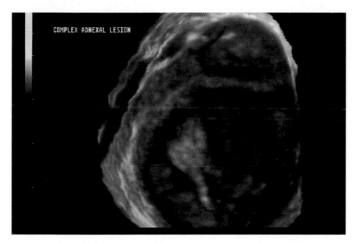

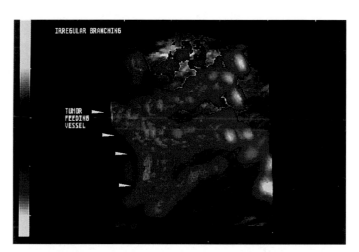

Plate 13 Three-dimensional view of the cystic-solid adnexal mass. Note the thick septa and papillary projection protruding into the tumoral cavity. Ovarian adenocarcinoma was confirmed by histopathology.

Plate 14 Chaotic vessel arrangement in a malignant ovarian neoplasm as seen by three-dimensional power Doppler ultrasound. Note irregular course and complicated branching of the tumoral vessels.

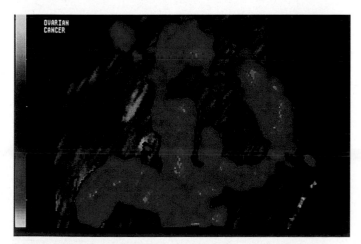

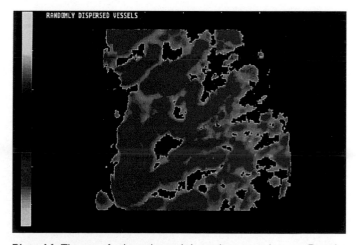

Plate 15 Three-dimensional power Doppler scan of an ovarian carcinoma. Malignant neovascularization arises from venous vessels that have a relatively poor tone. Focal areas of stenosis, blind-ending 'ponds', and shunting are clearly illustrated.

Plate 16 The use of echo-enhanced three-dimensional power Doppler imaging facilitates evaluation of tumoral perfusion. The use of contrasts enables high detection rate of tiny tumoral vessels, which may increase the sensitivity and specificity of the procedure.

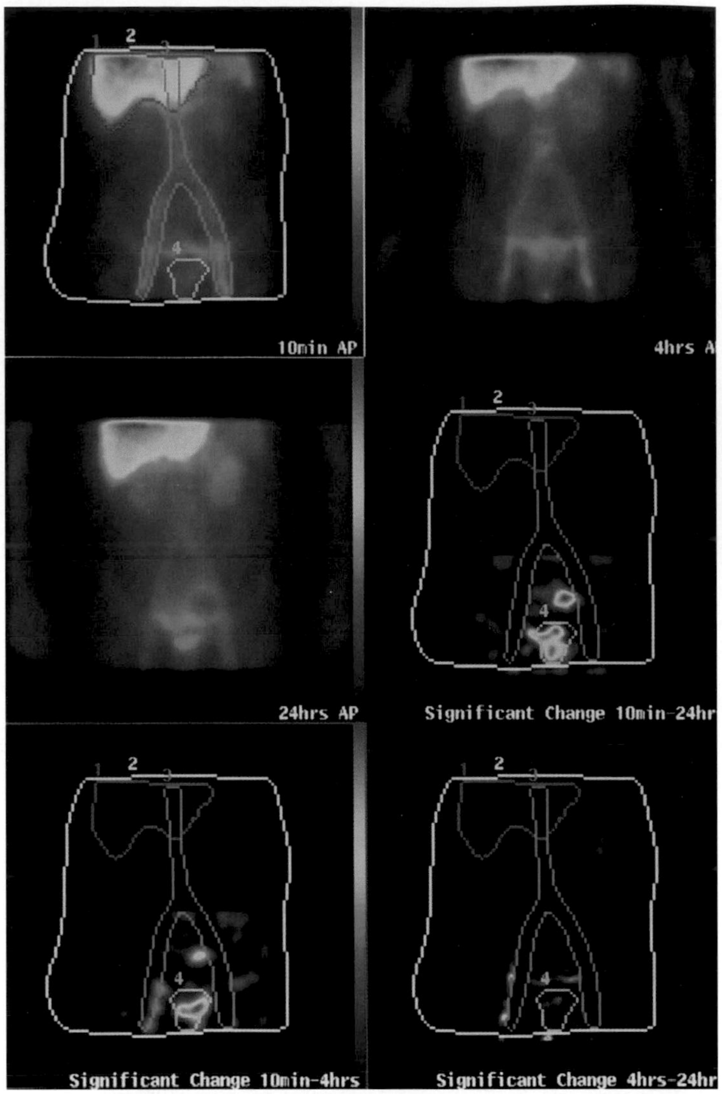

10min AP

4hrs A

24hrs AP

Significant Change 10min-24hr

Significant Change 10min-4hrs

Significant Change 4hrs-24hr

Plate 17 Radio-immunoscintigraphy of the pelvis with [^{99}Tc^m]SM3. Anterior images of the abdomen at 10 minutes, 4 hours, and 24 hours—top left, top right, and middle left. Change-detection images: centre right, comparison of the 10-minute image and the 24-hour image; bottom left, 10-minute and 4-hour images; and bottom right, 4- and 24-hour images. The colours now represent significance values: red, $P < 0.001$; orange, $P < 0.01$; green, $P < 0.05$. It can be seen on the 10-minute to 24-hour comparison and the 10-minute to 4-hour comparison, that there is significant uptake in the pelvis, indicating ovarian cancer. Conclusion: ovarian cancer.

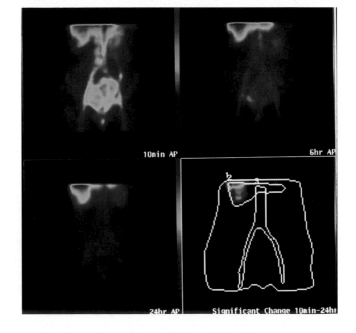

10min AP

6hr AP

24hr AP

Significant Change 10min-24hr

Plate 18 Radio-immunoscintigraphy of a pelvic mass with [^{99}Tc^m]SM3. Anterior abdominal views. Top left: 10-minute planar image shows irregular increased uptake in the pelvis. Top right: 6-hour planar image shows less uptake in the pelvis. Bottom left: 24-hour planar image shows no abnormal uptake in the pelvis. Change-detection analysis (bottom right): this compares the 10-minute and 24-hour planar images and presents the data as a probability map, where the P values are colour coded. No significant uptake is seen in the pelvis. Conclusion: there is no evidence of ovarian cancer. The mass was a tubovarian abscess, with high uptake on the early image due to its vascularity, fading with time as the blood level falls. There is no specific uptake of the antibody.

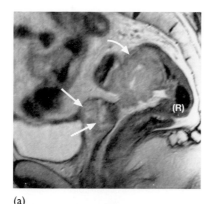

(a)

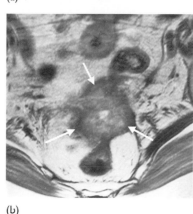

(b)

Fig. 33.10 Recurrent carcinoma of the ovary in a 73-year-old woman who had previously undergone total abdominal hysterectomy and bilateral salpingo-oophorectomy for ovarian carcinoma, presenting with a pelvic mass and rising CA125. (a) Sagittal and (b) axial and T2-weighted fast spin echo show a soft-tissue mass at the vaginal vault (arrow), which is distorting the parametrial tissues. The mass (curved arrow) extends posteriorly to involve the rectum (R).

point. The overall accuracy, sensitivity, and specificity of CT and MRI in re-staging ovarian cancer is shown in Table 33.2.

CT is frequently used to assess residual or recurrent disease. Sites of recurrence in addition to the peritoneal distribution of metastases include the vaginal vault and deep within the pelvis. Due to the transaxial plane of imaging on CT, tumour deposits in the region of the vaginal vault, in the cul-de-sac, and at the bladder base may be difficult to assess. These areas are better assessed with MR imaging in the sagittal plane (Fig. 33.10). Postoperative changes hamper the assessment of residual or recurrent disease. The generalized increased density within the mesentery and peritoneum may result from oedema, inflammation, fibrosis, and/or tumour infiltration. Also, unopacified bowel loops may be mistaken for tumour recurrence. The sensitivity for detecting recurrence is related to tumour size and improves for recurrent or residual disease larger than 2 cm.[13] Sites at which deposits are frequently overlooked include: the mesentery, omentum, peritoneum, anterior abdominal wall, distal ileum, sigmoid colon, mesocolon, infundibulopelvic ligament, and the surface of the liver.[28] As in the assessment of pretreated disease, the presence of ascites improves the detection of peritoneal disease and the use of oral bowel contrast medium and intravenous contrast medium facilitates tumour detection.[25,46]

The MRI findings in recurrent ovarian cancer are similar to those of CT; hence similar difficulties are encountered. Studies that have compared CT with MRI directly have shown that MR is similar to CT in the detection of recurrence.[25,46]

Summary

CT and MRI have a very limited role in the detection of ovarian pathology. Increasingly, the excellent tissue characterization of MRI has resulted in an increasing role in the evaluation of indeterminate masses detected clinically and on ultrasound. Although less accurate than a laparotomy in staging ovarian malignancy, both CT and MRI can be used to predict the feasibility of debulking or resection, and both will show disease in areas difficult to evaluate surgically. CT and MRI have broadly the same accuracy in detecting recurrence, assessing the extent of residual disease, and monitoring response to therapy. However, CT, because of its relatively wide availability and speed, is the investigation of choice in providing information in the clinical situation.

References

1. Heiken, J.P., Brink, J.A., and Vannier, M.W. (1993). Spiral (helical) CT. *Radiology*, **189** (3), 647–56.
2. Forstner, R., Hricak, H., and White, S. (1995). CT and MRI of ovarian cancer. [Review]. *Abdom. Imag.*, **20** (1), 2–8.
3. Buy, J.N., Moss, A.A., Ghossain, M.A. *et al.* (1988). Peritoneal implants from ovarian tumors: CT findings. *Radiology*, **169** (3), 691–4.
4. Buy, J.N., Ghossain, M.A., Sciot, C. *et al.* (1991). Epithelial tumors of the ovary: CT findings and correlation with US. *Radiology*, **178** (3), 811–18.
5. Bragg, D.G. and Hricak, H. (1993). Imaging in gynecologic malignancies. *Cancer*, **71** (Suppl. 4), 1648–51.
6. Hricak, H. (1997). Widespread use of MRI in gynecology: a myth or reality? *Abdom. Imag.*, **22** (6), 579–88.
7. Lessler, D.S., Sullivan, S.D., and Stergachis, A. (1994). Cost-effectiveness of unenhanced MR imaging vs contrast-enhanced CT of the abdomen or pelvis. *Am. J. Rad.*, **163** (1), 5–9.
8. Schwartz, L.B., Panageas, E., Lange, R. *et al.* (1994). Female pelvis: impact of MR imaging on treatment decisions and net cost analysis. *Radiology*, **192** (1), 55–60.
9. Outwater, E.K. and Dunton, C.J. (1995). Imaging of the ovary and adnexa: clinical issues and applications of MR imaging. *Radiology*, **194** (1), 1–18.
10. Murphy, K.J. and Brunberg, J.A. (1997). Adult claustrophobia, anxiety and sedation in MRI. *Magn. Reson. Imag.*, **15** (1), 51–4.
11. McCarthy, S. (1992). Magnetic resonance imaging of the normal female pelvis. *Radiol. Clin. North Am.*, **30** (4), 769–75.
12. Outwater, E.K. and Mitchell, D.G. (1996). Normal ovaries and functional cysts: MR appearance. *Radiology*, **198** (2), 397–402.
13. Forstner, R., Hricak, H., Powell, C.B. *et al.* (1995). Ovarian cancer recurrence: value of MR imaging. *Radiology*, **196** (3), 715–20.
14. Komatsu, T., Konishi, I., Mandai, M. *et al.* (1996). Adnexal masses: transvaginal US and gadolinium-enhanced MR imaging assessment of intratumoral structure. *Radiology*, **198** (1), 109–15.
15. Stevens, S.K., Hricak, H., and Stern, J.L. (1991). Ovarian lesions: detection and characterization with gadolinium-enhanced MR imaging at 1.5 T. *Radiology*, **181** (2), 481–8.
16. Thurnher, S., Hodler, J., Baer, S. *et al.* (1990). Gadolinium-DOTA enhanced MR imaging of adnexal tumors. *J. Comput. Assist. Tomogr.*, **14** (6), 939–49.

17. Stevens, S.K., Hricak, H., and Campos, Z. (1993). Teratomas versus cystic hemorrhagic adnexal lesions: differentiation with proton-selective fat-saturation MR imaging. *Radiology*, **186** (2), 481–8.

18. Sugimura, K., Okizuka, H., Imaoka, I. *et al.* (1993). Pelvic endometriosis: detection and diagnosis with chemical shift MR imaging. *Radiology*, **188** (2), 435–8.

19. Low, R.N., Carter, W.D., Saleh, F., and Sigeti, J.S. (1995). Ovarian cancer: comparison of findings with perfluorocarbon-enhanced MR imaging, In–111-CYT–103 immunoscintigraphy, and CT. *Radiology*, **195** (2), 391–400.

20. Yamashita, Y., Torashima, M., Hatanaka, Y. *et al.* (1995). Adnexal masses: accuracy of characterization with transvaginal US and precontrast and postcontrast MR imaging. *Radiology*, **194** (2), 557–65.

21. Outwater, E.K. and Kressel, H.Y. (1992). Evaluation of gynae-cologic malignancy by MRI. *Radiol. Clin. North Am.*, **30** (4), 797–806.

22. Weinreb, J.C., Barkoff, N.D., Megibow, A., and Demopoulos, R. (1990). The value of MR imaging in distinguishing leiomyomas from other solid pelvic masses when sonography is indeterminate. *Am. J. Rad.*, **154** (2), 295–9.

23. Kier, R., McCarthy, S.M., Scoutt, L.M. *et al.* (1990). Pelvic masses in pregnancy: MR imaging. *Radiology*, **176** (3), 709–13.

24. Weinreb, J.C., Brown, C.E., Lowe, T.W. *et al.* (1986). Pelvic masses in pregnant patients: MR and US imaging. *Radiology*, **159** (3), 717–24.

25. Forstner, R., Hricak, H., Occhipinti, K.A. *et al.* (1995). Ovarian cancer: staging with CT and MR imaging. *Radiology*, **197** (3), 619–26.

26. Ghossain, M.A., Buy, J.N., Ligneres, C. *et al.* (1991). Epithelial tumors of the ovary: comparison of MR and CT findings. *Radiology*, **181** (3), 863–70.

27. Low, R.N. and Sigeti, J.S. (1994). MR imaging of peritoneal disease. *Am. J. Rad.*, **163**, 1131–40.

28. Walsh, J.W. (1992). CT of gynaecologic neoplasm. *Radiol. Clin. North Am.*, **30** (4), 826–30.

29. Amendola, M.A., Walsh, J.W., Amendola, B.E. *et al.* (1981). Computed tomography in the evaluation of carcinoma of the ovary. *J. Comput. Assist. Tomogr.*, **5** (2), 179–86.

30. Andreotti, R.F., Zusmer, N.R., Sheldon, J.J., and Ames, M. (1988). Ultrasound and magnetic resonance imaging of pelvic masses. *Surg. Gynecol. Obstet.*, **166** (4), 327–32.

31. Sugiyama, T., Nishida, T., Komai, K. *et al.* (1996). Comparison of CA 125 assays with abdominopelvic computed tomography and transvaginal ultrasound in monitoring of ovarian cancer. *Int. J. Gynecol. Obstet.*, **54** (3), 251–6.

32. Semelka, R.C., Lawrence, P.H., Shoenut, J.P. *et al.* (1993). Primary ovarian cancer: prospective comparison of contrast-enhanced CT and pre-and postcontrast, fat-suppressed MR imaging, with histologic correlation. *J. Magn. Reson. Imaging*, **3** (1), 99–106.

33. Johnson, R.J. (1993). Radiology in the management of ovarian cancer. [Review]. *Clin. Radiol.*, **48** (2), 75–82.

34. Togashi, K., Nishimura, K., Kimura, I. *et al.* (1991). Endometrial cysts: diagnosis with MR imaging. *Radiology*, **180** (1), 73–8.

35. Mawhinney, R.R., Powell, M.C., Worthington, B.S., and Symonds, E.M. (1988). Magnetic resonance imaging of benign ovarian masses. *Br. J. Radiol.*, **61** (723), 179–86.

36. Tanaka, Y.O., Kurosaki, Y., Nishida, M. *et al.* (1994). Ovarian dys-germinoma: MR and CT appearance. *J. Comput. Assist. Tomogr.*, **18** (3), 443–8.

37. Kim, S.H. and Kang, S.B. (1995). Ovarian dysgerminoma: color Doppler ultrasonographic findings and comparison with CT and MR imaging findings. *J. Ultrasound Med.*, **14** (11), 843–8.

38. MacSweeney, J.E. and King, D.M. (1994). Computed tomography, diagnosis, staging and follow-up of pure granulosa cell tumour of the ovary. *Clin. Radiol.*, **49** (4), 241–5.

39. Schwartz, R.K., Levine, D., Hatabu, H., and Edelman, R.R. (1997). Ovarian fibroma: findings by contrast-enhanced MRI. *Abdom. Imag.*, **22** (5), 535–7.

40. Outwater, E.K., Siegelman, E.S., Talerman, A., and Dunton, C. (1997). Ovarian fibromas and cystadenofibromas: MRI features of the fibrous component. *J. Magn. Reson. Imaging*, **7** (3), 465–71.

41. Troiano, R.N., Lazzarini, K.M., Scoutt, L.M. *et al.* (1997). Fibroma and fibrothecoma of the ovary: MR imaging findings. *Radiology*, **204** (3), 795–8.

42. Megibow, A.J., Hulnick, D.H., Bosniak, M.A., and Balthazar, E.J. (1985). Ovarian metastases: computed tomographic appearances. *Radiology*, **156** (1), 161–4.

43. Goldhirsch, A., Triller, J.K., Greiner, R., Dreher, E., and Davis, B.W. (1983). Computed tomography prior to second-look operation in advanced ovarian cancer. *Obstet. Gynecol.*, **62** (5), 630–4.

44. Kahn, O., Cosgrove, D.O., Fried, A.M., and Savage, P.E. (1986). Ovarian carcinoma follow-up: US versus laparotomy. *Radiology*, **159** (7), 111–13.

45. Moskovic, E., Fernando, I., Blake, P., and Parsons, C. (1991). Lympho-graphy —current role in oncology. *Br. J. Radiol.*, **64** (761), 422–7.

46. Payer, L.M., Kainz, C., Kramer, J. *et al.* (1993). CT and MR accuracy in the detection of tumour recurrence in patients treated for ovarian cancer. *J. Comput. Assist. Tomogr.*, **17**, 626–32.

47. Silverman, P.M., Osborne, M., Dunnick, M.R., and Bandy, L.C. (1988). CT prior to second-look operation in ovarian cancer. *Am. J. Roentgenol.*, **150** (4), 829–32.

48. Neal, C.E. and Meis, L.C. (1994). Correlative imaging with monoclonal antibodies in colorectal, ovarian, and prostate cancer. [Review]. *Semin. Nucl. Med.*, **24** (4), 272–85.

49. Steege, J.F. (1994). Laparoscopic approach to the adnexal mass. *Clin. Obstet. Gynecol.*, **37** (2), 392–405.

49a. Musumeci, R., De Palo, G., Kenda, R. *et al.* (1980). Retroperitoneal metas-tases from ovarian carcinoma: reassessment of 365 patients studied with lymphography. *AJR*, **134**, 449–52.

50. Dauplat, J., Hacker, N.F., Nieberg, R.K. *et al.* (1987). Distant metastases in epithelial ovarian carcinoma. *Cancer*, **60** (7), 1561–6.

51. Johnson, R.J., Blackledge, G., Eddleston, B., and Crowther, D. (1983). Abdomino-pelvic computed tomography in the management of ovarian carcinoma. *Radiology*, **146** (2), 447–52.

52. Megibow, A.J., Bosniak, M.A., Ho, A.G. *et al.* (1988). Accuracy of CT in the detection of persistent or recurrent ovarian car-cinoma: correlation with second-look laparotomy. *Radiology*, **166**, 341–5.

53. Mitchell, D.G., Hill, M.C., Hill, S., and Zaloudek, C. (1986). Serous carci-noma of the ovary: CT identification of metastatic calcified implants. *Radiology*, **158** (3), 649–52.

54. Halvorsen, R.A., Panushka, C., Oakley, G. *et al.* (1991). Intraperitoneal contrast material improves the CT detection of peritoneal metastases. *Am. J. Rad.*, **157**, 37.

55. Payer, L.M., Stiglbauer, R., Kramer, J. *et al.* (1993). Superparamagnetic particles as oral contrast medium im MRI of patients with treated ovarian cancer—Comparison with plain MRI. *Br. J. Radiol.*, **66**, 415–19.

56. Dooms, G.C., Hricak, H., Crooks, L.E. *et al.* (1984). MRI of lymph nodes: comparison with CT. *Radiology*, **153**, 719.

56a. Young, R.C., Perez, C.A., Hoskins, W.J. *et al.* (ed.) (1993). *Cancer: principle and practice of oncology*, (4th edn). J.B. Lippincott, Philadelphia.

57. Harisinghani, M.G., Saini, S., Slater, G.J. *et al.* (1997). MR imaging of pelvic lymph nodes in primary pelvic carcinoma with ultrasmall super-paramagnetic iron oxide (Combidex): preliminary observations. *J. Magn. Reson. Imaging*, **7** (1), 161–3.

58. Ozols, R.F., Fisher, R.I., Anderson, T. *et al.* (1981). Peritoneoscopy in the management of ovarian cancer. *Am. J. Obstet. Gynecol.*, **140** (6), 611–19.

59. Piver, M.S., Barlow, J.J., and Lele, S.B. (1978). Incidence of subclinical metastasis in stage I and II ovarian carcinoma. *Obstet. Gynecol.*, **52** (1), 100–4.

60. Sanders, R.C., McNeil, B.J., Finberg, H.J. *et al.* (1983). A prospective study of computed tomography and ultrasound in the detection and staging of pelvic masses. *Radiology*, **146** (2), 439–42.

61. Shiels, R.A., Peel, K.R., MacDonald, H.N. *et al.* (1985). A prospective trial of CT in staging of ovarian malignancy. *Br. J. Obstet. Gynecol.*, **92**, 407–12.

62. Blaquiere, R.M. and Husband, J.E. (1983). Conventional radiology and computed tomography in ovarian cancer: discussion paper. *J. R. Soc. Med.*, **76** (7), 574–9.

63. Meyer, J.I., Kennedy, A.W., Friedman, R. *et al.* (1995). Ovarian carcinoma: value of CT in predicting success of debulking surgery. *Am. J. Rad.*, **165** (4), 875–8.

64. Nelson, B.E., Rosenfield, A.T., and Schwartz, P.E. (1993). Preoperative abdominopelvic computed tomographic prediction of optimal cytoreduction in epithelial ovarian carcinoma. *J. Clin. Oncol.*, **11** (1), 166–72.

34. Radionuclide imaging

Keith E. Britton, Faria Nasreen, Hikmat Jan, and Marie Granowska

Introduction

Radionuclide imaging is part of nuclear medicine, an independent medical monospecialty embracing all applications of unsealed radioactive materials in the diagnosis or treatment of patients and in medical research.

The basis of each nuclear medicine technique is the administration of a very small amount of a chemical agent which is labelled with a tiny amount of a radioactive isotope, a radionuclide. These radiopharmaceuticals are designed to demonstrate the system, tissue or organ for which they are chosen. This may be by using a selected function or by using a property of the tissue to characterize it.

After administration of the radiopharmaceutical, usually by intravenous injection into a vein in front of the elbow, the patient typically lies on the couch and the imaging system—a gamma camera which may have one, two, or three heads—is placed over the relevant part or parts of the body to obtain images of the distribution of the injected radiopharmaceutical at one or more time points. Images of the whole body, or images of sections through the body (single photon emission tomography; SPET), may be undertaken. For the latter, the gamma camera heads are rotated around the patient. The principal radionuclide for imaging is technetium–99m ($^{99}Tc^m$), which is produced from a generator in the department of nuclear medicine on a daily basis. Alternative radionuclides for imaging are indium–111 and iodine–123. The decay rate of the radionuclide is given as a time to half its activity—its half-life, which is 6 hours for $^{99}Tc^m$, 13 hours for ^{123}I, and 67 hours for ^{111}In. An alternative imaging modality is to use a positron emitter such as fluorine–18 (half-life 100 minutes) with a tomographic system called positron emission tomography (PET). This is available in only a few centres, but hybrid SPET/PET systems are becoming available which should increase the use of positron emitters such as $[^{18}F]$deoxyglucose, FDG.

Radionuclides for therapy are iodine–131 and yttrium–90, which are β-particle (electron) emitters with half-lives of 8 days and 2.5 days, respectively. Iodine–131 gives γ-rays as well as β-particles and therefore inpatient treatment in a special side ward with contained shower and toilet is required. Yttrium–90 is a pure β-particle emitter, and therefore in principle the treatment can be given as an outpatient.

Radiation is a natural phenomenon and nuclear medicine started as part of the peaceful use of atomic energy. The radiation that the patients receive from the diagnostic use of radionuclides is of the same order as that which occurs naturally during the course of a year for $^{99}Tc^m$ compounds (typical annual radiation level 2 mSv), for example a typical bone scan gives 4 mSv. Indium–111 compounds give higher absorbed doses (24 mSv). Iodine–123 gives a dose similar to $^{99}Tc^m$. The received doses are generally less than those of the equivalent X-ray techniques and are considered to be of negligible risk by the International Commission of Radiological Protection. Nuclear medicine therefore may be delivered safely to patients of all ages with appropriate adjustment of dose for children.

Cancer

The detection of ovarian cancer depends primarily on clinical history and examination, serum markers, abdominal and transvaginal ultrasound and Doppler, followed by surgery. The physical properties of the cancer, size, shape, echogenicity, position, flow, and effect on adjacent organs help in the radiological assessment as to whether the mass is benign or malignant. This physical approach is not inherently cancer specific. The nuclear medicine approach differs fundamentally in that it attempts to use the subtle differences between cancer cells and normal cells to identify cancer.[1] These differences relate primarily to the oncogenic difference between the cancer cell and the normal cell. This may be expressed as differences in cell function or metabolism, which are not specific, or in differences in expression of surface receptors or antigens, which are much more specific. These may be upregulated in cancer, and a cancer cell may have 5000–50 000 antigens on its surface, giving a considerable amplification factor, for example when binding a radiolabelled antibody. The strength of binding and the residence time of the bound agent can also be important, as well as the strength of the signal from the radionuclide. In principle, a radioactive pinhead is detectable if it contains sufficient activity. The trend in radionuclide imaging of cancer is showed in Table 34.1.

Of the agents listed in Table 34.1, the most relevant to the diagnosis and therapy of ovarian cancer are the radiolabelled mono-

Table 34.1 Tumour characterization in malignant disease

Non-specific: tumour and inflammation	More specific: mainly tumours	Class specific: several tumours	Type specific: few tumours
Gallium-67	Thallium-201	Anti-CEA	Anti-CD20 for lymphoma PR1A3 for colon cancer
Bone scan [^{18}F]DG	[^{99}Tc^m]tetrofosmin [^{99}Tc^m]MIBI [^{123}I]-, [^{111}In]-, [^{99}Tc^m]octreotide	[^{123}I]MIBG [^{123}I]VIP	Anti-melanoma SM3 for ovarian cancer

DG, deoxyglucose; MIBI, methoxyisobutyl isonitrile; CEA, carcino-embryonic antigen; MIBG, metaiodobenzylguanidine; VIP, vasoactive intestinal peptide; CD, a surface antigen on lymphocytes; PR1A3, an antibody against colonic epithelium; SM3, stripped mucin antibody for ovarian cancer.

clonal antibodies which are described in detail. The bone scan is generally used to determine the presence of bone metastases in advanced ovarian cancer when there is bone pain or discomfort. FDG with positron emission tomography is used in other cancers to determine lymph node involvement, but has a limited role in ovarian cancer. [^{99}Tc^m]MIBI is able to identify pelvic masses as due to tumour but is not more specific.[2] Occasionally ovarian tumours have neural crest or neuroendocrine elements histologically, but they usually lack chromatin granules and are [^{123}I]MIBG negative or lack somatostatin receptors and are [^{111}In]octreotide negative. Radio-immunoscintigraphy (RIS) is the use of a radiolabelled monoclonal antibody to detect and image a tissue or disease, in this case ovarian cancer. Radio-immunotherapy (RIT) is the use of a radionuclide-labelled monoclonal antibody for treatment. The main indications for RIS are shown in Table 34.2.

The antigen and the antibody

The ideal antigen should be cancer specific, expressed in high density, present on all species of cells of a particular cancer, whether differentiated or undifferentiated, at a site that is accessible to a circulating antibody or its fragments. It should be structurally stable and arranged so that an antigen–antibody combination can occur efficiently and persist on the cell unmetabolized to aid detection. The antigen should preferably not be released into the circulation or lymphatics, where it may complex antibody remote from the tumour. In such a case, the presence of the antigen does not mean the presence of a cancer cell. Totally cancer-specific antigens that are absent from the corresponding normal tissue or benign tumour still await identification, but the

Table 34.2 The management of ovarian cancer with radiolabelled monoclonal antibodies

1. Evaluation of ultrasound-screened pelvic lesions as malignant or not
2. Evaluation of raised serum markers
3. Evaluation of pelvic masses after therapy as containing viable tumour or not
4. Reduction of second-look surgery
5. Evaluation of chemotherapy

somatic mutation oncogene hypothesis of malignant change through the production of specific oncoproteins encourages the hope that such antigens will be identified. Meanwhile, a number of strategies are used to make use of tumour-associated antigens which are also present in normal tissues.

The increased expression of dedifferentiation antigens—carcino-embryonic antigen, human choriogonadotrophic antigen, and α-fetoprotein—in malignant tissue over normal was first used to develop antibodies that would bind to cancer tissue, but these antigens are also released into the lymphatics and the circulation. An alternative approach is to seek fixed cell surface component antigens of the cancer. One aspect of this is to use antigens present on the epithelial surface of the appropriate normal tissue at which site the antigen is not normally exposed to the circulation. The architectural disruption of the malignant process then exposes such antigens in higher density to the circulation. The human milk fat globule (HMFG) antigen, a 600 kDa glycoprotein found in the lining cells of the breast lactiferous duct epithelium[3] and in breast milk, is a typical example. It is also found in the epithelial lining of the ovarian follicle and in the crypts of the colon. Antibodies against this class of epithelial antigens, such as HMFG1 and HMFG2, have been used for RIS of ovarian, colorectal, and breast tumours.[4] The surface of the normal cell contains many glycoproteins which are highly glycosylated, whereas in the cancer cell there is a degree of deglycosylation.[5] This exposes more of the mucin core protein. SM3 was developed against the stripped mucin core protein epitope of five amino acids, as compared with HMFG1 which reacts with just three of these.[6] Whereas the malignant to benign ratio of uptake for an HMFG antibody is about 8 : 1, that for SM3 is about 17 : 1 and therefore enables it to be used for distinguishing malignant from benign tumours as well as detecting the tumour.[7] Other types of antigen and their related monoclonal antibodies are listed in Table 34.1.

The raising of monoclonal antibodies has progressed from the now conventional hybridoma technique, which gives whole monoclonal antibodies which can be further fragmented by enzyme digestion to F(ab')$_2$ and Fab' fragments, to the development of genetically engineered antibody-like molecules. There are chimeric molecules whereby the frame of the mouse antibody is replaced by the human equivalent and CDR (complementary determinant region) grafting (also called human reshaped antibodies), where all but the six CDR sequences reacting with the antigen are replaced by the human equivalent.[8] Such antibodies labelled with indium–111[9] or technetium–99m[10] have been used in patients with ovarian cancer. Some adjustment of the amino acids around each CDR may increase the affinity and residence time of the antibody bound to the antigen. Human antibodies may be produced either by culturing exposed peripheral blood lymphocytes which have been transformed by Epstein–Barr virus[11] or by the transference of human genes for heavy and light chains through transgenic mice. The creation of totally new antibodies by recombinant libraries of human genes for heavy and light chains, using the phage synthesis technique, avoids the need for immunization altogether.[12] These antibodies are part of the phage protein coat and the phages can be selected out using a high affinity column containing the chosen antigen. Phages with antibodies with high affinity for the antigen can then be removed from the column, grown up in bacteria and reselected with a similar affinity column containing only a few antigens. Only those phages containing the highest affinity antibodies are then selected. These are grown up again in bacteria and the antibody harvested from the bacterial media. These new antibodies are the designer molecules of the future.

Radiolabelling of antibodies was originally with ^{131}I or ^{123}I but is currently with ^{111}In and [99]Tc[m]. It was shown that the optimum time for imaging antibody uptake is between 6 and 24 hours[13] and therefore [99]Tc[m] with its 6-hour half-life is an entirely appropriate radiolabel, giving a high signal, a low radiation dose, and a γ-ray emission appropriate to the modern gamma camera. Antibodies are either radiolabelled through a linker, which may be chelate or a macrocycle for indium–111, or through a direct reduction technique, using an agent such as 2-mercaptoethanol,[14] or through a linker for [99]Tc[m]. (Table 34.4)

Imaging protocol and probability mapping

A modern single- or dual-head gamma camera may be used. It is set with a low energy parallel hole collimator and peaked with a 15% window around 140 keV for technetium–99m. The patient has the test explained to her and signed consent to the study is obtained. Patients with an allergy to foreign protein, such as a reaction to antityphoid inoculation, are excluded, as are patients with severe allergies. Skin testing is not appropriate as it sensitizes the patient. The patient receives an injection of 600 MBq [[99]Tc[m]]SM3 and is taken to the imaging couch. The patient lies supine, blood pressure and pulse may be checked. Marks are made with an indelible marker over the symphysis pubis and the two iliac crests, and tiny cobalt–57 markers are strapped over these sites. The patient is then imaged for a couple of minutes and a transparent film is placed over the persistence scope and the marks of the positioning markers are made on the transparent film to aid reposition of the patient for the later images. The formal images are then collected for 800 k counts of the anterior and posterior pelvis, anterior and posterior abdomen. Single photon emission tomography may also be performed. The images are repeated at 4–6 hours, and at 18–22 hours the next day. On each occasion, the cobalt markers are placed over the indelible ink marks and the patient repositioned as best as possible, so the marker image is superimposed on the previous transparent film, and then similar images are collected for the same counts. Repositioning the patient accurately is not only beneficial for the subsequent change detection analysis but also means that roughly the same amount of liver appears in each image and thus the relative counts in the pelvis on each image are somewhat similar, to aid visual comparison.[15]

The change detection analysis[16,17] consists of two main parts: the repositioning protocol and the image comparison. First, the marker images are analysed so that the maximum count of each marker is assigned to a particular pixel and each marker image undergoes a translation rotation programme so that the markers are superimposed. This may be done with a rigid transform or occasionally, if the patient has twisted, an elastic transform is required. The images are then translated and rotated in the same way as the marker images and thereby superimposed. A 5 × 5 square is set over each pixel and moved pixel by pixel over the 10 minute image, similarly over the 4–6 hour image, and similarly over the 18–22 hour image. The count data are compared and each pixel tested for significance of difference. Where there is a significant difference between one image and another, that significance is colour coded: $P < 0.001$ in red, $P < 0.01$ in orange, $P < 0.05$ in green, and $P > 0.05$ in blue. Since specific uptake of the antibody increases with time, there will be very little tumour uptake seen on the first image, more on the second image, and most on the third image, and thus the probability map shows the sites of cancer in red. Conversely, non-specific uptake, due to vascularity in a fibroid, tube-ovarian abscess, or endometriosis or vascular corpus luteum cyst, for example, will show best on the first image and will decrease with time as the blood level of the antibody falls. The probability map will show no significant positive difference between the early and late images, and thus benign causes of pelvic masses may be excluded. Since there is some excretion of the metabolic products of the labelled antibody through the kidneys and into the bladder, care must be taken in interpreting these sites, and the planar images help in this.

Patient studies

The ability of ultrasound to detect pelvic masses in well women, in women with a higher risk of ovarian cancer through having relatives with ovarian cancer, or just the interpretation of the nature of a pelvic mass, has been one of the problems that radioimmunoscintigraphy has addressed. There has been an improvement in the distinction between pelvic masses not due to malignancy and those that are malignant through the evolution from transabdominal ultrasound to transvaginal ultrasound and Doppler studies. Nevertheless, there is no inherent specificity in the ultrasound approach. For the reasons outlined above, using [[99]Tc[m]]SM3 imaging after the detection of a pelvic mass should aid the distinction between non-malignant change and ovarian cancer. If the early encouraging results are supported by further studies, then this approach should save a number of women having 'unnecessary' operations for benign pelvic changes, some

Table 34.3 Kinetic analysis with probability mapping in ovarian cancer: blind prospective evaluation of 100 sites in 21 patients before second-look operation

Map	Biopsy	Histology
	Tumour	No Tumour
Tumour	35	17
No tumour	9	39
	$\chi^2 = 25.8$	$P < 0.01$
Sensitivity 80%	Specificity 70%	Accuracy 74%
Correct diagnosis of		
patients with disease	17/17	Sensitivity 100%
patients without disease	3/4	Specificity 75%

of which are self-limiting, such as the vascular corpus luteum cyst.

For this distinction, it is essential to apply the probability mapping technique. This was first undertaken by Granowska *et al.*[16] using [^{123}I]HMFG2 in patients studied after chemotherapy, to determine whether or not second-look laparatomy would show disease. The results were reasonably successful (Table 34.3), with

100% sensitivity and 75% specificity, although the numbers were small. This work followed a series of evaluations of patients with ovarian cancer using radiolabelled antibodies from 1982 onwards.[4,15–21] Forty-six studies using [^{99}Tc^m]SM3 in 45 patients suspected of having ovarian cancer showed a sensitivity of 35/35 (100%) and a specificity of 8/11 (73%).[21] Updating the change-detection technique using [^{99}Tc^m]SM3 showed, in the first 13 patients, an accuracy of 85%; a further 80 patients' data confirm this. Other radiolabelled antibodies that are successful for imaging ovarian cancer include MOV–18,[22–24] 170 H2,[25] B72.3,[26] OV-TL3,[27,28] and OC–125.[29,30]

The effects of chemotherapy may be assessed by radio-immunoscintigraphy after completing the chemotherapy courses, and thereby avoiding a second-look laparatomy, although the latter has fallen into disfavour. During operation for potential recurrence, the use of the peroperative probe may be beneficial.[26,31]

Examples of the use of radio-immunoscintigraphy in ovarian cancer are shown in Figs 34.1 and 34.2 and of probability mapping in the differentiation of benign and malignant disease in Plates 17 and 18.

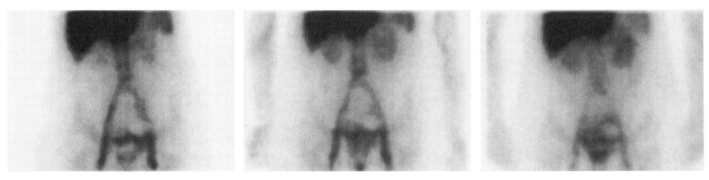

Fig. 34.1 Radio-immunoscintigraphy of ovarian cancer with [^{99}Tc^m]SM3. Images at 10 minutes, 4 hours, and 24 hours from left to right. Anterior views of the abdomen. At 10 minutes (left image): the liver, aorta, and iliac vessels are evident. There is a defect seen medial to the distal left iliac vessels. At 4 hours (central image): the kidneys are more evident and the defect remains. At 24 hours (right image): the defect is now surrounded by increased uptake. Conclusion: findings are typical of a malignant cystadenocarcinoma of the ovary.

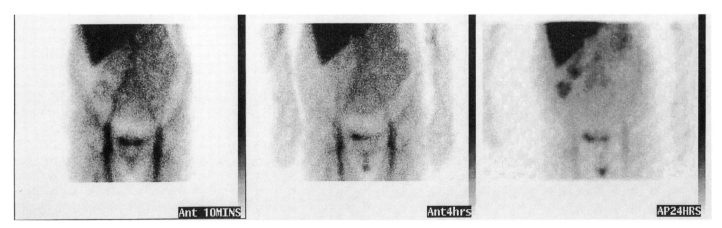

Fig. 34.2 Radio-immunoscintigraphy of the pelvis with [^{99}Tc^m]SM3. Images at 10 minutes, 4 hours, and 24 hours from top to bottom. Anterior images on the left. Posterior images on the right. Top left: some activity is seen in the anterior pelvis to the left side. Bottom left: this is clearly increased in intensity relative to the iliac vessels on the 24-hour image. The posterior views show renal and bladder activity but no definite abnormality. Conclusion: findings typical of an ovarian cancer.

Table 34.4 Ovarian cancer imaging with ^{99}Tc^m-labelled monoclonal antibodies

---

1. The ready availability, high count-rate signal, low absorbed radiation dose, and low cost of ^{99}Tc^m make it an excellent imaging agent

2. It is an ideal label for avid and effective monoclonal antibodies, such as HMFG1 and SM3, for ovarian cancer (sensitivity 100%)

3. Comparison of ^{111}In, ^{123}I, and ^{99}Tc^m as radiolabels for SM3 shows the superiority of ^{99}Tc^m

4. The ^{99}Tc^m radiolabel for radioimmunoscintigraphy allows the study to be completed within 24 hours of the request and thus the technique is applicable routinely in the general nuclear medicine department

---

References

1. Britton, K.E. (1997). Towards the goal of cancer specific imaging and therapy. *Nucl. Med. Commun.*, **18**, 992–1007.

2. Krolicki, L., Stelmachow, J., and Cwikla, J.B. (1998). Evaluation of Tc–99m MIBI uptake in patients with suspected ovarian cancer. *Eur. J. Nucl. Med.*, **25**, 1014.

3. Taylor-Papadimitrou, J., Peterson, J.A., Arkie, J. *et al.* (1981). Monoclonal antibodies to epithelium specific component of the human milk fat globule membrane, production and reaction with cells in culture. *Int. J. Cancer*, **28**, 17–21.

4. Epenetos, A.A., Britton, K.E. Mather, S.J. *et al.* (1982). Targeting of iodine–123 labelled tumour-associated monoclonal antibodies to ovarian, breast and gastrointestinal tumours. *Lancet*, **ii**, 999–1004.

5. Girling, A., Bartkora, J., Burchell, J. *et al.* (1989). A core protein epitope of polymorphic epithelial mucin detected by monoclonal antibody SM3 is selectively exposed in a range of primary carcinomas. *Int. J. Cancer*, **43**, 1072–6.

6. Burchell, S., J., Taylor-Papadimitrou, J., Boshell, M. *et al.* (1989). A short sequence, without the amino acid repeat of a cancer-associated mucin, contains immunodominant epitopes. *Int. J. Cancer*, **44**, 691–6.

7. Van Dam, P.A., Watson, J.V., Shepherd, J.H., and Lowe, D.G. (1990). Flow cytometric quantification of tumour-associated antigens in solid tumours. *Am. J. Obstet. Gynecol.*, **163**, 698–9.

8. Winter, G. and Milstein, C. (1991). Man made antibodies. *Nature*, **349**, 293–9.

9. Snook, D.E., Verheryen, M., Komas, C. *et al.* (1993). A preliminary comparison of a tumour associated reshaped human monoclonal antibody (Hu2 PLAP) with its murine equivalent (H 17E2). In *Monoclonal antibodies 2: applications in clinical oncology*, (ed. A.A. Epenetos), pp. 391–400. Chapman & Hall, London.

10. Granowska, M., Mather, S.J., and Britton, K.E. (1993). ^{99m}Technetium-labelled antibodies for radioimmunoscintigraphy. In *Monoclonal antibodies 2: applications in clinical oncology*, (ed. A.A. Epenetos), pp. 375–82. Chapman & Hall, London.

11. Hanna, M.G., Haspel, M.V., McCabe, R. *et al.* (1991). Development and application of human monoclonal antibodies. *Antibody Immunoconj. Radiopharm.*, **4**, 67–75.

12. Clackson, T., Hoogenboom, H.R., Griffiths, A.D., and Winter, G. (1991). Making antibody fragments using phage display libraries. *Nature*, **352**, 624–8.

13. Buraggi, G.L. Turrin, A., Cascinelli, N. *et al.* (1985). In *Immunoscintigraphy*, (ed. L. Donato and K.E. Britton), pp. 215–53. Gordon and Breach, London.

14. Mather, S.J. and Ellison, D. (1990). Reduction mediated Tc–99m labelling of monoclonal antibodies. *J. Nucl. Med.*, **31**, 692–7.

15. Granowska, M., Britton, K.E., and Shepherd, J. (1993). The detection of ovarian cancer using 123-I monoclonal antibody. *Radiobiol. Radiother. (Berlin)*, **25**, 153–60.

16. Granowska, M., Nimmon, C.C., Britton, K.E. *et al.* (1988). Kinetic analysis and probability mapping applied to the detection of ovarian cancer by radioimmunoscintigraphy. *J. Nucl. Med.*, **29**, 594–607.

17. Biassoni, L., Granowska, M., Carroll, M.J. *et al.* (1998). Tc–99m labelled SM3 in the pre-operative evaluation of axillary lymph nodes in primary breast cancer with change detection statistical processing as an aid to tumour detection. *Br. J. Cancer*, **77**, 131–8.

18. Granowska, M., Shepherd, J., Britton, K.E. *et al.* (1984). Ovarian cancer: diagnosis using I^{-123} monoclonal antibody in comparison with surgical findings. *Nucl. Med. Commun.*, **5**, 485–99.

19. Granowska, M., Mather, S.J., and Britton, K.E. (1991). Diagnostic evaluation of 111-In and Tc–99m radiolabelled monoclonal antibodies in ovarian and colorectal cancer: correlations with surgery. *Nucl. Med. Biol.*, **18**, 413–24.

20. Granowska, M. and Britton, K.E. (1991). Radioimmunoscintigraphy of ovarian cancer. *Dis. Mark.*, **9**, 191–5.

21. Granowska, M., Britton, K.E., Mather, S.J. *et al.* (1993). Radioimmunoscintigraphy with Technetium–99m-labelled monoclonal antibody, SM3, in gynaecological cancer. *Eur. J. Nucl. Med.*, **20**, 483–9.

22. Veggian, R., Fasolato, S., Menard, S. *et al.* (1989). Immunohistochemical reactivity of a monoclonal antibody prepared against human ovarian carcinoma on normal and pathological female genital tissues. *Tumori*, **75**, 510–13.

23. Crippa, F., Buraggi, G.L., Di Re, E. *et al.* (1991). Immunoscintigraphy of ovarian cancer with the MOVI8 monoclonal antibody. *Eur. J. Cancer*, **27**, 724–9.

24. Alexander, C., Villena-Heinsen, C.E., Trampert, K. *et al.* (1991). Radioimmunoscintigraphy of ovarian tumours with the MOV18 monoclonal antibody. *Eur. J. Cancer*, **27**, 724–9.

25. McEwan, A.J.B., MacLean, G.D., Hooper, H.R. *et al.* (1992). Mab 170H.82: an evaluation of a novel panadenocarcinoma monoclonal antibody labelled with Tc–99m and with In- lll. *Nucl. Med. Commun.*, **13**, 11–19.

26. Del-Vecchio, S., Camera, L., Petrillo, A. *et al.* (1991). Clinical studies with B72.3 in ovarian cancer and probe guided tumour localization. *Int. J. Rad. Appl. Instrum. B*, **18**, 85–7.

27. Massuger, L.F., Kenemans, P., Claessens, R.A. *et al.* (1990). Immunoscintigraphy of ovarian cancer with Indium-lll-labelled OV-TL 3 F(ab')^2 monoclonal antibody. *J. Nucl. Med.*, **31**, 1802–10.

28. Buist, M.R., Roos, J.C., Vermoken, J.B. *et al.* (1991). The diagnostic value of immunoscintigraphy using the monoclonal antibody OV-TL3 in patients with ovarian carcinoma. *Ned. Tijdschr. Geneeskd.*, **135**, 126–30.

29. Barzen, G., Mayr, A.C., Langer, M. *et al.* (1989). Radioimmunoscintigraphy of ovarian cancer with 131-Iodine labelled OC 125 antibody fragments. *Eur. J. Nucl. Med.*, **15**, 42–8.

30. Brokelmann, J., Bockisch, A., Vogel, J. *et al.* (1989). Immunoscintigraphy using CA125 antibodies in the management of ovarian cancer. *Arch. Gynecol. Obstet.*, **244**, 193–206.

31. Ind, T.E.J., Granowska, M., and Britton, K.E. (1994). Preoperative radioimmunodetection of ovarian carcinoma using a hand held gamma detection probe. *Br. J. Cancer*, **70**, 1263–6.

35. Telomerase in ovarian cancer: a possible diagnostic tool and therapeutic target?

G. Bea A. Wisman, Marco N. Helder, Steven de Jong, Elisabeth G.E. de Vries, and Ate G.J. van der Zee

Introduction

The enzyme telomerase is a ribonucleoprotein that synthesizes repetitive DNA sequences onto chromosomal ends (telomeres). Unique overexpression of telomerase in human cancers has raised great expectations with regard to possible diagnostic and therapeutic opportunities. In this chapter, the role of telomerase in immortalization of (pre)cancerous cells, current data on telomerase in ovarian tumours, and also the possible application of telomerase as a diagnostic tool and/or therapeutic target are discussed.

Immortalization model

Telomeres, present at the end of eukaryotic chromosomes, consist of highly conserved hexameric repeats, TTAGGG, with an average length of 10–15 kb in humans.[1,2] The physiological functions of telomeres are to provide chromosomes with stability and to protect them from recombination and end-degrading enzymes. Telomeres also play a role in solving the 'end replication problem'. In proliferating cells DNA polymerase produces new DNA from the 5′ end to the 3′ end during the replication of chromosomes. For the replication of the lagging strand the DNA polymerase uses short RNA fragments as starting points, thereby facilitating synthesis of DNA in this strand from the 5′ to the 3′ end. At the end of replication the RNA fragments are replaced by DNA, but at the 5′ end of the telomeres this fails, resulting in a loss of DNA (see ref. 3 for a review). This phenomenon is especially observed in somatic cells, where the telomeres shorten with every cell division.[4] It has been proposed that this telomere shortening acts as a mitotic clock. When at a certain point during proliferation a critical telomere length has been reached, upregulation of cell cycle proteins, such as p53 and pRb (retinoblastoma gene product) induces an irreversible growth-arrest, also called senescence or mortalization stage 1 (M1). However, some cells may overcome this M1 stage and will replicate further. Ability to pass this stage can be due to the absence of functional p53 and/or pRb, either by mutations or by increased breakdown.[5–8] In the absence of functional p53 and/or pRb, cells will continue to proliferate and, as a consequence, telomere shortening will continue. After approximately another 50 cell divisions the cell population enters a second mortalization (M2) phase, or 'crisis'. At this point most cells will die. However, some cells may overcome this 'crisis' and at this moment the enzyme telomerase may become activated, resulting in restoration of the length of chromosomal ends after every cell division. Therefore, the cell is now immortalized and has acquired an infinite life span.[3]

Telomerase

The enzyme telomerase is a ribonucleoprotein with an RNA template and protein components. Telomerase is able to synthesize repetitive sequences onto chromosomal ends. The integral RNA component of telomerase contains a short segment (11 nucleotides) functioning as a template for DNA synthesis.[9] The human telomerase RNA component (hTR) has been cloned by Feng *et al.*[10] Recently, protein components of human telomerase have also been identified, the telomerase-associated protein TP1,[11] and the catalytic subunit hTERT, initially called hTRT/hTCS1/hEST2.[12–14] Studies have shown that ectopic hTERT expression is sufficient to reconstitute enzymatic telomerase activity, to increase telomere length, and to extend cellular life span in cells already expressing the RNA component.[15–19] Thus, hTERT is presently considered to be the rate-limiting component in the formation of functional telomerase.

Besides the majority of malignant tumour cell lines and tumours, some normal cells, such as germ cells, lymphocytes, and basal layer cells of hair follicles, colonic crypts, and epidermis, exhibit telomerase activity.[20–25]

Assays for telomerase expression

Telomerase expression levels can be studied in several ways. Telomerase activity is nowadays determined using the telomeric repeat amplification protocol (TRAP).[26,27] This assay is based on primer elongation by telomerase and subsequent amplification of this product by polymerase chain reaction (PCR). The human RNA component, hTR, and the mRNAs of telomerase-associated protein and the catalytic subunit, TP1 and hTERT, can be detected by RNA blot analysis, reverse transcriptase PCR (RT-PCR),[10,12] or *in situ* hybridization.[28-30]

Assays for telomerase activity and (m)RNA levels (by RT-PCR) allow semi-quantitative determination of expression levels in homogenized samples, while *in situ* assays allow determination of expression of hTR and hTERT mRNA in individual cells. However, these *in situ* assays are difficult to quantitate. Recently, an *in situ* TRAP method has been developed by Ohyashiki *et al.*,[31] which visualizes telomerase activity in individual cells. The disadvantage of this method is that so far it can only be used in cell lines and cytological samples.

In conclusion, a variety of assays for telomerase expression are currently available. Which assay should be used in a diagnostic setting depends on the required application, and the nature (frozen, fresh, archival) and amount of clinical material available. The disadvantage of the TRAP and RT-PCR assays is that levels are determined in homogenized fresh or frozen material. For studying levels in single cells *in situ* hybridization in frozen or paraffin-embedded sections is required, but this assay is less sensitive in comparison to the TRAP and RT-PCR and more difficult to interpret. In the near future, with the development of antibodies against hTERT, immunohistochemistry may also be used to investigate the status of the catalytic subunit, hTERT, allowing determination of hTERT expression in individual cells. Current available data on diagnostic applications of telomeric level determination are discussed further below.

Telomerase in ovarian lesions

Table 35.1 summarizes studies on telomerase activity in ovarian specimens. In normal ovaries, no (or very weak) telomerase activity was detected, while between 80 and 100% of ovarian cancers were positive for telomerase activity. Although weakly expressed, 20–100% of benign ovarian cysts showed telomerase activity. However, two studies did not show any activity in a total of 13 benign tumours. Borderline tumours, also called tumours with low malignant potential, are interesting tumours to study as they can neither be characterized as benign nor as malignant tumours. Whereas telomerase activity in benign tumours is primarily weak, and activity in malignant carcinomas is high, for borderline tumours varying results have been reported. Some studies showed

60–100% of borderline tumours to be positive for telomerase activity, while others observed 17–20% positivity. However, the number of borderline specimens in the individual studies was rather small. In our own study, telomerase activity was detected in 6 of 13 borderline tumours. In general, the level of telomerase activity was low, with a level comparable to that of most ovarian cancers detected in only one tumour.

In malignant ovarian tumours there has been one study on hTR expression as determined by *in situ* hybridization. Six of the 34 (17%) cancers were positive for hTR.[41] Recently, Kyo *et al.* detected hTR and TP1 expression by RT-PCR in more than 80% of benign, borderline, and malignant tumours,[42] while hTERT was only detectable in the majority of ovarian cancers. Comparable results have been found in our own study (data not shown). It appears therefore, that hTERT is the rate-limiting determinant of telomerase activity in ovarian cancer, as has also been reported previously for other malignancies.

Determination of telomerase activity as diagnostic tool

Upregulation of telomerase activity in the majority of malignant ovarian tumours, versus no or weak telomerase activity in normal and benign tissue, presents detection of telomerase activity as a possible diagnostic tool. Several applications of telomerase activity determination can be envisaged:

Determination of telomerase activity in peritoneal fluids for preoperative diagnosis in patients with pelvic masses

In patients with pelvic masses, determination of telomerase activity by the TRAP assay in peritoneal fluids may be useful for preoperative diagnosis of malignancy. Three available studies on telomerase activity in peritoneal fluids show conflicting results (Table 35.2). One study reported a sensitivity of 88% for the TRAP assay and a sensitivity of 67% for cytology in ascites derived from patients with ovarian cancer, whereas another study showed a sensitivity of only 25% for the TRAP assay and 100% for cytology. However, the number of patients in this last study was small ($n = 8$) and no information on stage of the tumours was provided. Another group reported a 100% sensitivity for the TRAP assay. Ascites derived from patients with normal or benign ovaries were mostly negative for telomerase. Samples in this study that were positive in patients with no or benign disease contained

Table 35.1 Telomerase activity detected in frozen ovarian specimens

Normal	Benign	Borderline	Cancer	Reference
	3/3 (weak)	4/6 (75%) (weak)	18/21 (86%)	32
	5/24 (21%)	17/17 (100%)	20/20 (100%)	33
	2/10 (20%)	1/6 (17%) (weak)	23/25 (92%)	34
			14/16 (88%)	35
0/5		12/13 (92%)		36
1/12 (8%)	4/10 (40%)	1/5 (20%)	30/36 (83%)	37
0/3	0/4 (0%)	3/5 (60%)	33/41 (80%)	38
3/10 (30%)	6/15 (40%)		24/25 (96%)	39
	0/9 (0%)	6/13 (46%)	15/18 (83%)	40
Total				
4/25 (16%)	20/75 (27%)	32/52 (62%)	189/215 (88%)	

Table 35.2 Telomerase activity in peritoneal fluids

Normal	Cancer	Cytology	Reference
0/5	7/7 (100%)		43
2/43	37/42 (88%)	29/43 (67%)	44
0/4	2/8 (25%)	8/8 (100%)	36
Total			
2/52 (4%)	46/57 (81%)	37/51 (73%)	

inflammatory cells,[44] and it is known that these cells also may exhibit telomerase activity.[22,24]

In summary, it can be concluded that determination of telomerase activity by TRAP assay is applicable in peritoneal fluids and may be more sensitive than cytology for detection of malignant cells in primary disease. Whether other clinical applications (e.g. the TRAP assay for determination of residual disease after completion of chemotherapy) are useful in the clinic remains to be seen.

Determination of telomerase activity as a prognostic factor in gynaecological cancer

In other malignancies, e.g. leukaemias, breast cancer, and meningiomas, higher telomerase activity has been linked to a worse prognosis.[45–49] Presently available data do not suggest a role for telomerase activity, or the presence and/or upregulation of its components, as prognostic factors in ovarian cancer. However, the individual studies are, in fact, too small to properly evaluate a possible prognostic role, and therefore further, larger studies are needed for clarification of this issue.

Telomerase as therapeutic target

In initial reports[26,50] telomerase has frequently been described as an ideal cancer target, because telomerase activity is present at high levels in more than 85% of malignant tumours, while in contrast, benign tumours and normal tissues display no, or low, telomerase activities (see above). Due to the differences in telomerase activity in normal versus malignant cells, telomerase has been considered to be a highly specific molecular target, applicable for the treatment of a broad range of cancers. Inhibition of upregulated telomerase in tumour cells, resulting in further attrition of already short telomeres, might theoretically restore mortality to tumour cells that express this enzyme, leading to tumour cell death. However, recent findings have indicated that telomerase activity is also present at high levels in embryonic tissues and male germ cells,[20] and (albeit at much lower levels) in some self-renewing tissues with high regenerative potential (such as basal-layer cells of hair follicles, colonic crypts, epidermis, and endometrium). In addition, although somatic cells generally have much longer telomeres than most tumour cell populations,[51,52] it can be calculated that a relatively large number of cell divisions (>20 cell doublings) in most tumour cells is necessary for sufficient telomeric erosion to induce cell death.[53] Thus, tumour bulk may increase substantially before any growth inhibitory effects will become apparent. Moreover, tumours often contain relatively low percentages of proliferating cells, thus decreasing the effectiveness and increasing treatment duration time for anti-telomerase agents. Considering these problems with anti-telomerase therapies, it can be argued that premalignant and/or early malignant cells may be more suitable targets for these types of therapies. Such cells are near 'crisis' and thus have close to critically short telomere lengths and maximal chromosomal instability. Therefore, anti-telomerase treatment in these lesions may be more efficient, and should affect cells prone to immortalize or just

after immortalization with optimal efficiency. In advanced cancers, anti-telomerase treatment will probably be most effective following other forms of treatment, such as resection of tumour bulk, radiation therapy, and/or chemotherapy.

Various ways exist by which telomerase can be inhibited and/or telomeric attrition can be enhanced. In human carcinoma cell lines, downregulation of telomerase activity was found to be a general response to induction of differentiation by compounds such as retinoic acid derivatives, dimethyl sulphoxide, phorbol–12-myristate–13-acetate, and butyrates, implying (indirect) telomerase inhibition.[54–58] Some other ways of telomerase inhibition appear to be not very effective/specific yet. In particular, reverse transcriptase inhibitors. 3′-Azido–3′-deoxythymidine and dideoxyguanosine are the reverse transcriptase inhibitors most widely studied and have the greatest relative potency in telomerase inhibition *in vitro*.[59–64] However, no evidence of induction of senescence has been detected so far.[61–63]

Another way to inhibit telomerase activity is to follow an antisense strategy. The basic concept of the antisense strategy is straightforward: an antisense molecule recognizes complementary mRNA (or DNA) by sequence-specific base pairing, and hence prevents translation (or transcription), resulting in selective inhibition of protein synthesis. Interference with gene expression in cells at the molecular level may be accomplished in two ways. Either by *in situ* generation of mRNA from recombinant vectors, or by the exogenous introduction of synthetic antisense oligonucleotides.[65] In the case of hTR, antisense oligonucleotides directed against the active site of the telomerase template RNA may also inhibit telomerase functioning. hTR is, until now, the only component targeted by antisense technology. *In vitro* studies have shown that by transfecting antisense hTR-expressing vectors into telomerase-positive cells, telomerase activity can indeed be reduced markedly and telomeric attrition can be induced, ultimately resulting in cell death.[10,66] Nevertheless, it remains difficult to predict whether these gene transfer techniques may be applicable in anti-telomerase treatments protocols *in vivo*, as this type of therapy is unavoidably associated with all the pitfalls of gene therapy in general. In a more direct approach to telomerase inhibition, various (un)modified oligonucleotides targeted against the telomerase RNA template have been explored.[67–74] Antisense oligonucleotides containing a peptide-based backbone instead of a (deoxy)ribose backbone, the so-called peptide nucleic acids, are most effective when small (13-mer) oligonucleotides are used, whereas 'normal' diester and phosphorothioate oligonucleotides appear to require a longer length (16–20-mer) for maximal effect.

Instead of targeting the active site of the telomerase template RNA, one study described the use of a 19-mer antisense oligonucleotide complementary to the bases 76–94 of the hTR component. This oligonucleotide was linked to an RNase L-activating 2′,5′-tetraadenylate (2–5A) moiety, which directed the hTR RNA to RNase L-degradation. Treatment of glioma cell lines *in vitro* and subcutaneous xenografts *in vivo* resulted in an apoptosis-mediated 79% cell kill and 50% of initial tumour mass. Controls showed little or no cell death over this treatment period, which was far too short to induce relevant telomeric attrition.[74] Apparently, inhibition of telomerase activity in this model resulted in induction of apoptosis before critical telomere length was reached. In another study performed by Kondo *et al.*,[75] an anti-sense hTR-expressing vector was transfected in both cisplatin-sensitive and cisplatin-resistant glioblastoma cells, which respectively had no and high detectable telomerase activity. Interestingly, stable clones from cisplatin-resistant cells, having lost their telomerase activity, displayed increased susceptibility to cisplatin-induced apoptotic cell death. This suggests that telomerase inhibition might potentially represent a new way of chemosensitization for tumours resistant to anticancer drugs.[75] These studies imply that telomerase-targeted tumour cells could potentially be destroyed faster than expected by telomere attrition alone, and that treatment of some drug-resistant cancers may be improved by anti-telomerase therapy.

References

1. Morin, G.B. (1989). The human telomere terminal transferase enzyme is a ribonucleoprotein that synthesizes TTAGGG repeats. *Cell*, **59**, 521–9.
2. Moyzis, R.K., Buckingham, J.M., Cram, L.S. *et al.* (1988). A highly conserved repetitive DNA sequence, (TTAGGG)n, present at the telomeres of human chromosomes. *Proc. Natl Acad. Sci. USA*, **85**, 6622–6.
3. Rhyu, M.S. (1995). Telomeres, telomerase and immortality. *J. Natl Cancer Inst.*, **87**, 884–94.
4. Harley, C.B., Futcher, A.B., and Greider C.W. (1990). Telomeres shorten during ageing of human fibroblasts. *Nature*, **345**, 458–60.
5. Bond, J.A., Wyllie, F.S., and Wynford-Thomas, D. (1994). Escape from senescence in human diploid fibroblasts induced directly by mutant p53. *Oncogene*, **9**, 1885–9.
6. Shay, J.W., Pereira-Smith, O.M., and Wright, W.E. (1991). A role for both Rb and p53 in the regulation of cellular senescence. *Exp. Cell Res.*, **196**, 33–9.
7. Shay, J.W., Wright, W.E., and Werbin, H. (1991). Defining the molecular mechanisms of human cell immortalization. *Biochim. Biophys. Acta*, **1072**, 1–7.
8. Counter, C.M., Botelho, F.M., Wang, P. *et al.* (1994). Stabilization of short telomeres and telomerase activity accompany immortalization of Epstein–Barr virus transformed human B lymphocytes. *J. Virol.*, **68**, 3410–14.
9. Greider, C.W. and Blackburn, E.H. (1989). A telomeric sequence in the RNA of *Tetrahymena* telomerase required for telomere repeat synthesis. *Nature*, **337**, 331–7.
10. Feng, J., Funk, W.D., Wang, S.S. *et al.* (1995). The RNA component of human telomerase. *Science*, **269**, 1236–41.
11. Harrington, L., McPhail, T., Mar, V. *et al.* (1997). A mammalian telomerase-associated protein. *Science*, **275**, 973–6.
12. Nakamura, T.M., Morin, G.B., Chapman, K.B. *et al.* (1997). Telomerase catalytic subunit homologs from fission yeast and human. *Science*, **277**, 955–9.
13. Killian, A., Bowtell, D.D., Abud, H.E. *et al.* (1997). Isolation of a candidate human telomerase catalytic subunit gene, which reveals complex splicing patterns in different cell types. *Hum. Mol. Genet.*, **6**, 2011–19.
14. Meyerson, M., Counter, C.M., Eaton, E.N. *et al.* (1997). hEST2, the putative human telomerase catalytic subunit gene, is up regulated in tumor cells and during immortalization. *Cell*, **90**, 785–95.
15. Nakayama J., Tahara H., Tahara E. *et al.* (1998). Telomerase activation by hTRT in human normal fibroblasts and hepatocellular carcinomas. *Nature Genet.*, **18**, 65–8.
16. Beattie, T.L., Zhou, W., Robinson, M.O., and Harrington, L. (1998). Reconstitution of human telomerase activity *in vitro Curr. Biol.*, **8**, 177–80.
17. Weinrich, S.L., Pruzan, R., Ma, L. *et al.* (1998). Reconstitution of human telomerase with the template RNA component hTR and the catalytic protein subunit hTRT. *Nature Genet.*, **17**, 498–502.
18. Counter, C.M., Meyerson, M., Eaton, E.N. *et al.* (1998). Telomerase activity is restored in human cells by ectopic expression of hTERT (hEST2), the catalytic subunit of telomerase. *Oncogene*, **16**, 1217–22.
19. Bodnar, A.G., Ouellette, M., Frolkis, M. *et al.* (1998). Extension of life-span by introduction of telomerase into normal human cells. *Science*, **279**, 349–52.
20. Broccoli, D., Young, J.W., and De Lange, T. (1995). Telomerase activity in normal and malignant hematopoietic cells. *Proc. Natl Acad. Sci., USA*, **92**, 9082–6.
21. Counter, C.M., Gupta, J., Harley, C.B. *et al.* (1995). Telomerase activity in normal leukocytes and in hematologic malignancies. *Blood*, **85**, 2315–20.
22. Hiyama, K., Hirai, Y., Kyoizumi, S. *et al.* (1995). Activation of telomerase in human lymphocytes and hematopoietic progenitor cells. *J. Immunol.*, **155**, 3711–15.
23. Härle-Bachor, C. and Boukamp, P. (1996). Telomerase activity in the regenerative basal layer of the epidermis in human skin and in immortal and carcinoma-derived skin keratinocytes. *Proc. Natl Acad. Sci. USA*, **93**, 6476–81.
24. Wolthers, K.C., Wisman, G.B.A., Otto, S.A. *et al.* (1996). T cell telomere length in HIV–1 infection: no evidence for increased CD4+ T cell turnover. *Science*, **274**, 1543–7.
25. Yasumoto, S., Kunimura, C., Kikuchi, K. *et al.* (1996). Telomerase activity in normal human epithelial cells. *Oncogene*, **13**, 433–9.
26. Kim, N.W., Piatyszek, M.A., Prowse, K.R. *et al.* (1994). Specific association of human telomerase activity with immortal cells and cancer. *Science*, **266**, 2011–15.
27. Hiyama, K., Hiyama, E., Ishioka, S. *et al.* (1995). Telomerase activity in small-cell and non-small-cell lung cancers. *J. Natl Cancer Inst.*, **87**, 895–902.
28. Soder, A.I., Hoare, S.F., Muir, S. *et al.* (1997). Amplification, increased dosage and *in situ* expression of the telomerase RNA gene in human cancer. *Oncogene*, **14**, 1013–21.
29. Yashima, K., Litzky, L.A., Kaiser, L. *et al.* (1997). Telomerase expression in respiratory epithelium during the multistage pathogenesis of lung carcinomas. *Cancer Res.*, **57**, 2373–7.
30. Kolquist, K.A., Ellisen, L.W., Counter, C.M. *et al.* (1998). Expression of TERT in early premalignant lesions and a subset of cells in normal tissues. *Nature Genet.*, **19**, 182–6.
31. Ohyashiki, K., Ohyashiki, J.H., Nishimaki, J. *et al.* (1997). Cytological detection of telomerase activity using an *in situ* telomeric repeat amplification protocol assay. *Cancer Res.*, **57**, 2100–3.
32. Kyo, S., Kanaya, T., Ishikawa, H. *et al.* (1996). Telomerase activity in gynecological tumors. *Clin. Cancer Res.*, **2**, 2023–8.
33. Wan, M., Li, W.-Z., Duggan, B.D. *et al.* (1997). Telomerase activity in benign and malignant epithelial ovarian tumors. *J. Natl Cancer Inst.*, **89**, 437–41.
34. Murakami, J., Nagai, N., Ohama, K. *et al.* (1997). Telomerase activity in ovarian tumors. *Cancer*, **80**, 1085–92.
35. Zheng, P.S., Iwasaka, T., Yamasaki, F. *et al.* (1997). Telomerase activity in gynecologic tumors. *Gynecol. Oncol.*, **64**, 171–5.
36. Gorham, H., Yoshida, K., Sugino, T. *et al.* (1997). Telomerase activity in human gynaecological malignancies. *J. Clin. Pathol.*, **50**, 501–4
37. Kyo, S., Takakura, M., Tanaka, M. *et al.* (1998). Quantitative differences in telomerase activity among malignant, premalignant, and benign ovarian lesions. *Clin. Cancer Res.*, **4**, 399–405.
38. Oishi, T., Kigawa, J., Minagawa, Y. *et al.* (1998). Alteration of telomerase activity associated with development and extension of epithelial ovarian cancer. *Obstet. Gynecol.*, **91**, 568–71.
39. Yokoyama, Y., Takahashi, Y., Shinohara, A. *et al.* (1998). Telomerase activity in the female reproductive tract and neoplasms. *Gynecol. Oncol.*, **68**, 145–9.
40. Van de Meer, G.T., Wisman, G.B.A., De Vries, E.G.E. and Van der Zee, A.G.J. (1998). Telomerase activity (TA) in ovarian tumours. *Proc. Clin. Oncol. Soc. Aus.*, **25**, 88.

41. Soder, A.I., Going, J.J., Kaye, S.B., and Keith, W.N. (1998). Tumour specific regulation of telomerase RNA gene expression visualized by *in situ* hybridization. *Oncogene*, **16**, 979–83.

42. Kyo, S., Kanaya, T., Takakura, M. *et al.* (1999). Expression of human telomerase subunits in ovarian malignant, borderline and benign tumors. *Int. J. Cancer*, **80**, 804–9.

43. Counter, C.M., Hirte, H.W., Bacchetti, S., and Harley, C.B. (1994). Telomerase activity in human ovarian carcinoma. *Proc. Natl Acad. Sci. USA*, **91**, 2900–4.

44. Duggan, B.D., Wan, M., Yu, M.C. *et al.* (1998). Detection of ovarian cancer cells: comparison of a telomerase assay and cytologic examination. *J. Natl Cancer Inst.*, **90**, 238–42.

45. Norrback, K.F., Dahlenborg, K., Carlsson, R., and Roos, G. (1996). Telomerase activation in normal B lymphocytes and non-Hodgkin lymphomas. *Blood*, **88**, 222–9.

46. Zhang, W., Piatyszek, M.A., Kobayashi, T. *et al.* (1996). Telomerase activity in human acute myelogenous leukaemia: inhibition of telomerase activity by differentiation-inducing agents. *Clin. Cancer Res.*, **2**, 799–803.

47. Langford, L.A., Piatyszek, M.A., Xu, R. *et al.* (1997). Telomerase activity in ordinary meningiomas predicts poor outcome. *Hum. Pathol.*, **28**, 416–20.

48. Hoos, A., Hepp, H.H., Kaul, S. *et al.* (1998). Teloemrase activity correlates with tumor aggressiveness and reflects therapy effect in breast cancer. *Int. J. Cancer*, **79**, 8–12.

49. Clark, G.M., Osborne, C.K., Levitt, D. *et al.* (1996). Telomerase activity and survival of patients with node-positive breast cancer. *J. Natl Cancer Inst.*, **89**, 1874–81.

50. Morin, G.B. (1995). Is telomerase a universal cancer target? *J. Natl Cancer Inst.*, **87**, 859–61.

51. Shay, J.W., Werbin, H., and Wright, W.E. (1994). Telomere shortening may contribute to aging and cancer: A perspective. *Mol. Cell. Diff.*, **2**, 1–21.

52. Autexier C. and Greider C.W. (1996). Telomerase and cancer: revisiting the telomere hypothesis. *Trends Biochem. Sci.*, **21**, 387–91.

53. Kipling, D. (1995). Telomerase: immortality enzyme or oncogene? *Nature Genet.*, **9**, 104–6.

54. Reichman, T.W., Albanell, J., Wang, X. *et al.* (1997). Downregulation of telomerase activity in HL60 cells by differentiating agents is accompanied by increased expression of telomerase-associated protein. J. *Cell Biochem.*, **67**, 13–23.

55. Xu, D., Gruber, A., Peterson, C., and Pisa, P. (1996). Suppression of telomerase activity in HL60 cells after treatment with differentiating agents. *Leukemia*, **10**, 1354–7.

56. Albanell, J., Han, W., Mellado, B. *et al.* (1996). Telomerase activity is repressed during differentiation of maturation-sensitive but not resistant human tumor cell lines. *Cancer Res.*, **56**, 1503–8.

57. Miller, W.H. (1998). The emerging role of retinoids and retinoic acid metabolism blocking agents in the treatment of cancer. *Cancer*, **83**, 1471–82.

58. Bollag, W. (1994). Experimental basis of cancer combination chemotherapy with retinoids, cytokines, 1,25-dihydroxyvitamin D3, and analogs. *J. Cell Biochem.*, **56**, 427–35.

59. Melana, S.M., Holland, J.F., and Pogo, B.G. (1998). Inhibition of cell growth and telomerase activity of breast cancer cells *in vitro* by 3′-azido–3′-deoxythymidine. *Clin. Cancer Res.*, **4**, 693–6.

60. Pai, R.B., Pai, S.B., Kukhanova, M. *et al.* (1998). Telomerase from human leukemia cells: properties and its interaction with deoxynucleoside analogues. *Cancer Res.*, **58**, 1909–13.

61. Strahl, C. and Blackburn, E.H. (1996). Effects of reverse transcriptase inhibitors on telomere length and telomerase activity in two immortalized human cell lines. *Mol. Cell Biol.*, **16**, 53–65.

62. Gomez, D.E., Tejera, A.M., and Olivero, O.A. (1998). Irreversible telomere shortening by 3′-azido–2′,3′-dideoxythymidine (AZT) treatment. *Biochem. Biophys. Res. Commun.*, **246**, 107–10.

63. Yegorov, Y.E., Chernov, D.N., Akimov, S.S. *et al.* (1997). Blockade of telomerase function by nucleoside analogs. *Biochemistry Mosc.*, **62**, 1296–305.

64. Multani, A.S., Furlong, C., and Pathak, S. (1998). Reduction of telomeric signals in murine melanoma and human breast cancer cell lines treated with 3′-azido–2′–3′-dideoxythymidine. *Int. J. Oncol.*, **13**, 923–5.

65. Prins, J., De Vries, E.G.E., and Mulder, N.H. (1993). Antisense of oligonucleotides and the inhibition of oncogene expression. *Clin. Oncol.*, **5**, 245–52.

66. Kondo, S., Tanaka, Y., Kondo, Y. *et al.* (1998). Antisense telomerase treatment: induction of two distinct pathways, apoptosis and differentiation. *FASEB J.*, **12**, 801–11.

67. Pitts, A.E. and Corey, D.R. (1998). Inhibition of human telomerase by 2′-O-methyl-RNA. *Proc. Natl Acad. Sci. USA*, **95**, 11549–54.

68. Mata, J.E., Joshi, S.S., Palen, B. *et al.* (1997). A hexameric phosphorothioate oligonucleotide telomerase inhibitor arrests growth of Burkitt's lymphoma cells *in vitro* and *in vivo*. *Toxicol. Appl. Pharmacol.*, **144**, 189–97.

69. Norton, J.C., Piatyszek, M.A., Wright, W.E. *et al.* (1996). Inhibition of human telomerase activity by peptide nucleic acids. *Nature Biotechnol.*, **14**, 615–19.

70. Hamilton, S.E., Pitts, A.E., Katipally, R.R. *et al.* (1997). Identification of determinants for inhibitor binding within the RNA active site of human telomerase using PNA scanning. *Biochemistry*, **36**, 11873–80.

71. Glukhov, A.I., Zimnik, O.V., Gordeev, S.A., and Severin, S.E. (1998). Inhibition of telomerase activity of melanoma cells *in vitro* by antisense oligonucleotides. *Biochem. Biophys. Res. Comm.*, **248**, 368–71.

72. Kanazawa, Y., Ohkawa, K., Ueda, K. *et al.* (1996). Hammerhead ribozyme-mediated inhibition of telomerase activity in extracts of human hepatocellular carcinoma cells. *Biochem. Biophys. Res. Commun.*, **225**, 570–6.

73. Wan, M.S.K., Fell, P.L., and Akhtar S. (1998). Synthetic 2′-O-methyl-modified hammerhead ribozymes targeted to the RNA component of telomerase as sequence-specific inhibitors of telomerase activity. *Antisense Nucl. Acid Drug Dev.*, **8**, 309–17.

74. Kondo, S., Kondo, Y., Li, G. *et al.* (1998). Targeted therapy of human malignant glioma in a mouse model by 2–5A antisense directed against telomerase RNA. *Oncogene*, **16**, 3323–30.

75. Kondo, Y., Kondo, S., Tanaka, Y. *et al.* (1998). Inhibition of telomerase increases the susceptibility of human malignant glioblastoma cells to cisplatin-induced apoptosis. *Oncogene*, **16**, 2243–8.

36. Detection of circulating tumor cells in the peripheral blood and bone marrow of patients with ovarian cancer

Christian Marth, Hanne Høifødt, Lise Walberg, Janne Kærn, Ole Mathiesen, Marianne Andresen, Claes Tropé, and Øystein Fodstad

Introduction

Ovarian cancer has the highest lethality of all gynecological malignancies. The disease seems to be restricted for much of its course to the peritoneal cavity. The two most frequent sites for metastatic disease are pleural effusion and retroperitoneal lymph nodes, found in about 25% of the patients.[1,2] In contrast to this locoregional spread, hematogenous metastasis occurs to a minor extent. In view of this knowledge, local therapies such as intraperitoneal chemotherapy have been introduced. However, about 50% of the patients with a surgically documented complete intra-abdominal response later experience a recurrence. Moreover, 38% of the patients develop clinically manifest distant metastases, including bone metastases in a few cases (1.9%), during the course of their disease.[1] In this context, occult hematogenous micrometastasis, present at time of operation (a phenomenon common to most epithelial malignancies[3,4] but thus far ignored in ovarian cancer), might be one explanation for the progression of the disease.

In several clinical studies performed on samples from patients with different types of disease, the presence of tumor cells in bone marrow has been shown to be correlated to disease aggressiveness and also to be an independent prognostic parameter (see ref. 5 for a review). In most studies immunomorphological detection of tumor cells has been used, with antibodies recognizing cytokeratins or membrane-expressed tumor-associated antigens.[6,7] In other studies, reverse transcriptase polymerase chain reaction (RT-PCR) methods have been used for detecting mRNA of tissue-specific gene expression.[8] Although useful, these methods involve several methodological and interpretation problems.[9] Together with the fact that often very few (1–10) tumor cells are found in such examinations, the reliability of published data may vary. On the basis of this background, we wanted to apply a new immunomagnetic rosetting method[10,11] to blood and bone-marrow samples obtained from patients with ovarian cancer before initiation of chemotherapy, with the aim of determining the prevalence of the disseminated tumor cells.

Patients and methods

Patients

The study protocol was approved by the local ethics committee, and after receiving written, informed consent, patients with primary epithelial ovarian cancer were subjected to blood ($n = 85$) and bone-marrow aspiration ($n = 70$). The characteristics of the patients included in the study are shown in Table 36.1. Total abdominal hysterectomy, bilateral salpingo-oophorectomy, infracolic omentectomy, and pelvic plus para-aortic lymph-node dissection were performed when feasible. All metastatic lesions were confirmed by histology or cytology, reviewed at our Department of Pathology. Histological classification was based on criteria defined by the World Health Organisation.[12] Clear cell carcinomas were not graded.

Before initiation of adjuvant chemotherapy, 7–20 days after primary surgery, two bilateral bone-marrow samples were obtained from the patients under general anesthesia, through needle aspiration from the upper iliac crests. A volume of approximately 10 ml (ranging from 8.5 to 12 ml) per site was collected and mixed with a heparin-containing solution. Peripheral blood specimens (40 ml) were also obtained before initiation of anesthesia. Moreover, blood and marrow samples were obtained from healthy bone-marrow donors for specificity evaluation of our methods. The samples were brought immediately to the laboratory, stored on ice, and analyzed within 2 hours.

Monoclonal antibodies and immunobeads

MOC31 is an anti IgG1 class antibody that binds to an epithelial cluster 2 antigen in carcinoma cells[13,14] and was kindly donated by Dr L. de Leij, University of Groningen, The Netherlands. The antibody was conjugated directly to magnetic sheep—anti-mouse beads (SAM) IgG M450 Dynabeads, (Dynal, Oslo, Norway) as

Table 36.1 Patient characteristics

	Peripheral blood (n = 85)	Bone marrow (n = 70)
Age (years)		
median	59	59
range	32–82	32–82
FIGO stage		
I	16 (19%)	14 (20%)
II	6 (7%)	5 (7%)
III	45 (53%)	34 (49)
IV	18 (21%)	17 (24%)
Ascites		
yes	50 (59%)	39 (56%)
no	35 (41%)	31 (44%)
Pleural effusion		
yes	15 (18%)	13 (19%)
no	70 (82%)	57 (81%)
Histology		
serous	50 (59%)	40 (57%)
mucinous	3 (3%)	2 (3%)
endometrioid	5 (6%)	5 (7%)
clear-cell	11 (13%)	10 (14%)
not classified	10 (12%)	9 (13%)
mixed	2 (2%)	2 (3%)
borderline	4 (5%)	2 (3%)
Grade		
1	10 (12%)	8 (11%)
2	27 (32%)	21 (30%)
3	37 (43%)	31 (44%)
not graded	11 (13%)	10 (14%)
Karnofsky index		
100	44 (52%)	33 (47%)
90	16 (19%)	16 (23%)
80	12 (14%)	10 (14%)
<80	13 (15%)	11 (16%)
Operative treatment		
biopsy only	14 (16%)	13 (19%)
suboptimal procedure	15 (18%)	13 (19%)
optimal operation	56 (66%)	44 (62%)
Residual disease		
macroscopic negative	32 (38%)	27 (39%)
<2 cm	13 (15%)	9 (13%)
>2 cm	40 (47%)	34 (48%)
Chemotherapy		
none	14 (17%)	11 (16%)
carboplatin/paclitaxel	27 (32%)	20 (29%)
TEC	19 (22%)	17 (24%)
CAP	6 (7%)	6 (9%)
carboplatin	19 (22%)	16 (23%)

recommended by the manufacturer. SAM 450 Dynabeads were used unconjugated as a negative control.

Procedure for detection and separation of tumor cells

Briefly, the mononuclear cell fraction (MNC) was collected by standard density gradient centrifugation (Lymphoprep, Nycomed, Oslo, Norway), washed in phosphate-buffered saline (PBS), resuspended in PBS with 1% human serum albumin (HSA), and the number of cells counted by means of an electronic particle counter.

Magnetic immunobeads with or without conjugated antibody were added to the MNC at a ratio of 1 part beads to 2 parts MNC, and incubated with continuous rotation for 30 min at 4 °C. After incubation, cell suspensions were diluted with PBS + 1% HSA and put in a magnet holder for 1–2 min to separate bound ('rosetted') and unbound cells. The cells not bound to immunobeads were decanted. Rosettes were defined as at least five beads bound to a cell. Cells forming rosettes with immunobeads were counted under light microscopy by two independent observers.

Cell lines

The sensitivity of the immunobead method was evaluated by inclusion of various human ovarian carcinoma cell lines, namely SKOV6, SKOV8, HOC–7, and HTB77. The cells were maintained as monolayer cultures as previously described.[15] Following harvesting, increasing numbers of cells were mixed with blood and bone-marrow samples of healthy donors. These samples were then treated and examined similarly to samples from cancer patients.

Immunocytochemical staining

Cells detected by immunobead were confirmed to be epithelial by standard immunocytochemistry[9] in selected cases. On slides prepared as cytospins the indirect APAAP method with the anticytokeratin antibody AE1/AE3 was used, and the cells were counterstained with hematoxylin.

Statistics

Data were analyzed using the software package SPSS for Windows (SPSS Inc., Chicago, IL, USA) run on a personal computer. Differences between the groups were evaluated using by the χ^2 test for categorical data or the Wilcoxon U-test for nominal data. A P value of less than 0.05 was considered significant.

Results

The immunobead method, applying MOC31-coated beads or control beads (with SAM antibody only), was tested in peripheral blood and bone-marrow samples obtained from healthy donors. Rosettes were observed in none of the samples, although nonspecific binding of fewer than four beads to a few very small cells, apparently of lymphoid origin, was observed. These cells also bound the SAM control beads. No healthy donor was therefore classified as positive. This is in agreement with an earlier report demonstrating that antibody MOC31 does not bind to any cell type in the bone marrow.[16]

All the ovarian carcinoma cell lines tested expressed the antigen detected by the antibody MOC31, as demonstrated by flow cytometry. To test detection efficiency, 20 HTB77 cells were mixed with 2×10^6, 2×10^7, or 2×10^8 MNC, from which the immunobead method recovered 16 (80%), 14 (70%), and 12 (60%) ovarian cancer cells, respectively.

Table 36.2 Tumor cells in bone marrow and established prognostic factors

	Bone marrow		
	Negative	**Positive**	p^a
Number	56 (80%)	14 (20%)	
Peripheral blood			
negative	56 (92%)	5 (8%)	<0.0001
positive	0 (–)	9 (100%)	
FIGO stage			
I	13 (93%)	1 (7%)	
II	3 (60%)	2 (40%)	0.418
III	27 (79%)	7 (21%)	
IV	13 (76%)	4 (24%)	
Histology			
serous	33 (83%)	7 (17%)	
mucinous	2 (100%)	0 (–)	
endometrioid	4 (80%)	1 (20%)	
clear-cell	7 (70%)	3 (30%)	0.817
not classified	7 (78%)	2 (22%)	
mixed	1 (50%)	1 (50%)	
borderline	2 (100%)	0 (–)	
Grade			
1	8 (100%)	0 (–)	
2	19 (91%)	2 (9%)	0.037
3	22 (71%)	9 (29%)	
Pleural effusion			
yes	11 (85%)	2 (15%)	0.644
no	45 (79%)	12 (21%)	
Ascites			
yes	33 (85%)	6 (15%)	0.279
no	23 (74%)	8 (26%)	
Residual disease			
macroscopic negative	22 (82%)	5 (18%)	
<2 cm	6 (67%)	3 (33%)	0.561
>2 cm	28 (82%)	6 (18%)	
Age (years)			
median	58	65	0.297
quartile 1–quartile 3	51–71	52–74	
CA125 (U/ml)			
median	205	165	
quartile 1–quartile 3	37–640	27–692	0.364
n > 35 U/ml	46 (82%)	10 (73%)	
Hemoglobin (g/dl)			
median	12.6	12.6	0.562
quartile 1–quartile 3	12.0–13.4	11.2–13.4	
White cell count (10^9/l)			
median	6.95	7.55	0.467
quartile 1–quartile 3	5.68–8.18	5.95–8.85	
Platelet count (10^9/l)			
median	367	353	
quartile 1–quartile 3	263–454	257–450	0.977
n > 400	26 (47%)	6 (43%)	

[a] P-values were estimated by χ^2 test or by Wilcoxon U-test for categorical or nominal data respectively.

Bone-marrow samples from a total of 70 ovarian cancer patients were collected without any complications. In these, and in an additional 15 patients, peripheral blood samples were also drawn. We were able to detect tumor cells in 14/70 (20%) and 11/85 (13%) patients in bone marrow and peripheral blood, respectively (Table 36.2).

In 28 cases, immunocytochemical analyses on cytospins prepared from mononuclear cell fractions were also performed. The positivity of eight of these cases, as determined by the immunorosetting method, was in all cases confirmed, whereas the 20 remaining patients were negative by both methods. All patients with cancer cells in peripheral blood were also positive in the bone marrow. In five individuals, however, cancer cells were detected in the bone marrow alone.

When evaluating classical prognostic factors, only tumor grade correlated with the detection of tumor cells in bone marrow. It is necessary to mention that clear cell carcinoma, which are tumors with poor prognosis, were not graded but had a positivity rate similar to that of grade 3 tumors (30% and 29%, respectively). All other factors were not significantly associated with the presence of tumor cells in bone marrow or blood.

In three positive patients bone marrow was checked after three cycles of chemotherapy. These patients responded clinically with a reduction in residual disease as well as serologically with a decrease in CA125. Importantly, tumor cells disappeared from bone marrow and were no longer detectable using our method.

Conclusion and implications

In different types of cancer, studies on micrometastatic disease might help bring new insight into the metastatic process. Thus, the presence of hematogenous cancer cells has been reported in various solid tumor types, assessed either by immunocytochemistry or RT-PCR, commonly using cytokeratins as markers.[5,10] The detection rate of occult tumor cells in bone marrow in published studies varies between 8 and 49% in node-negative and 12 and 55% in node-positive breast cancer patients.[3,4,17,18]

Some antibodies used to detect minimal residual disease in breast cancers cross-react with normal hematopoietic cells,[19] and even with seemingly specific antibodies there is a risk of false-positive results.[9,10] Moreover, since in most patients only 1–10 tumor cells (per 2×10^6 normal bone-marrow cells) are detected by immunocytochemistry, more sensitive methods are warranted. Therefore, in order to improve the sensitivity, a larger number of bone marrow cells from each patient should be analyzed. However, standard immunocytochemistry methods are too time and resource demanding for analyzing larger numbers of cells.

One possibility is to use PCR, a technique that allows a target DNA sequence of interest to be amplified to millions of copies. This method has been applied most extensively to measure minimal residual disease in bone marrow and blood of the t(14;18)-carrying lymphomas and Philadelphia chromosome-positive chronic myelogenous leukemias. One major limitation of the PCR method is that most solid tumors of interest do not carry chromosomal translocations. Therefore, RT-PCR methods to detect the expression of tissue-specific and tumor-associated gene mRNA in bone marrow and blood have been developed. RT-PCR assays for cytokeratin 19 have been reported to be specific for detection of breast cancer cells in bone marrow.[8,20] However, some groups have experienced false-positive results when this method was used for tumor cell detection in bone marrow and peripheral blood. Thus, healthy volunteers may also express cytokeratins when sensitive PCR methods are used,[21] and there is also a risk of amplifying pseudogenes.[22] Therefore, as in the case of immunocytochemistry, RT-PCR assays may not have the specificity required for clinical use.

Based on previous experience with immunomagnetic bead cell separation techniques, a new immunomagnetic rosetting technique for the detection of micrometastatic cells has been developed.[6,10,11,23] We have adapted this technique to ovarian cancer and demonstrated in model experiments that using this method it was possible to detect 60–80% of tumor cells admixed to normal bone marrow cells. Although skeletal metastasis is extremely rare in ovarian cancer, micrometastatic cells were found in the bone marrow of 20% of the patients. It should be noted that this method has the advantage of increasing the sensitivity of tumor cell detection, since compared to immunocytochemistry a larger number of bone marrow cells ($\geq 2 \times 10^7$ MNCs) are screened. The monoclonal antibody applied on the immunobeads was MOC31, which binds well to ovarian carcinoma cell lines (data not shown), but not to cells derived from the normal bone marrow.[16] Our controls confirmed earlier findings with the immunobead method, indicating high sensitivity without reduced specificity.

In an immunocytochemical study Cain *et al.*[24] were unable to detect ovarian carcinoma cells at primary debulking using anti-cytokeratin antibodies. However, in follow-up at second- or third-look laparotomy, as well as in recurrent situations, these authors observed circulating tumor cells in up to 37% of patients. In contrast, our immunobead method permitted detection of tumor cells, even after primary surgery. There was good concordance between results in the peripheral blood and bone marrow. Thus, all patients with tumor cells in the peripheral blood were also bone-marrow positive, whereas in five individuals only the bone marrow was positive. This, however, indicates that only 60% of bone-marrow-positive patients are detected when using a blood sample. Therefore, peripheral blood should not be tested instead of bone marrow, although it would otherwise be preferable since collection is less invasive.

One very interesting finding of our study was the lack of a clear correlation between systemic disease and FIGO stage. Although more patients should be studied, it is surprising that tumors confined to the true pelvis seem to have access to peripheral circulation to the same extent as in more advanced stages. The follow-up period in our study was too short for evaluation of the prognostic value of circulating tumor cells. One could, however, expect that those stage I and II patients who seem to be biologically understaged represent poor survivors. This hypothesis is supported by findings for other solid tumors, where the presence of micrometastases in bone marrow at diagnosis was associated with an increased risk of systemic relapse.[3] In our study, patients with poorly differentiated tumors or clear cell carcinoma had the highest rate of bone-marrow involvement. It is possible that these tumor types are associated with poor prognosis because they are able to invade and enter the systemic circulation early. It is interesting that other prognostic factors, such as residual disease or tumor marker CA125 serum levels, were not correlated with circulating tumor cells.

In summary, with the sensitive immunomagnetic rosetting method, tumor cells were detected in peripheral blood, and to an even higher extent in bone-marrow samples, from ovarian cancer patients. The relationship between the presence of circulating tumor cells and tumor grade, as well as low tumor differentiation, seems to reflect biological factors involved in tumor spread. However, the lack of correlation with other clinically established parameters might indicate that the detection of micrometastatic cells can assist in prognostication. Indications were obtained that the method can be used as a surrogate marker for monitoring the effects of therapy. Together, the results exemplify the need for further exploration of the systemic spread of ovarian cancer.

References

1. Dauplat, J., Hacker, N.F., Nieberg, R.K. *et al.* (1987). Distant metastases in epithelial ovarian carcinoma. *Cancer*, **60**, 1561–6.
2. Burghardt, E., Girardi, F., Lahousen, M. *et al.* (1991). Patterns of pelvic and paraaortic lymph node involment in ovarian cancer. *Gynecol. Oncol.*, **40**, 103–6.
3. Funke, I. and Schraut, W. (1998). Meta-analyses of studies on bone marrow micrometastases: An independent prognostic impact remains to be substantiated. *J. Clin. Oncol.*, **16**, 557–66.
4. Kvalheim, G. (1996). Purging of autografts: Methods and clinical significance. *Ann. Med.*, **28**, 167–73.
5. Pantel, K., Cote, R.J., and Fodstad, Ø. (1999), Detection and clinical significance of micrometastatic disease. *J. Natl. Cancer Inst.*, **91**, 1113–24.
6. Fodstad, Ø., Høifødt, H.K., Rye, P.D. *et al.* (1996). New immunobead techniques for sensitive detection of malignant cells in blood and bone marrow. *Proc. Am. Assoc. Cancer Res.*, **37**, 214.
7. Fodstad, Ø., Trones, G.E., Forus, A. *et al.* (1997). Improved immunomagnetic method for detection and characterization of cancer cells in blood and bone marrow. *Proc. Am. Assoc. Cancer Res.*, **38**, 26.
8. Fields, K.K., Elfenbein, G.J., Trudeau, W.L. *et al.* (1996).Clinical significance of bone marrow metastases as detected using the polymerase chain reaction in patients with breast cancer undergoing high-dose chemotherapy and autologous bone marrow transplantation. *J. Clin. Oncol.*, **14**, 1868–76.
9. Borgen, E., Beiske, K.,Trachsel, S. *et al.* (1998). Immunocytochemical detection of isolated epithelial cells in bone marrow. Unspecific staining and contribution by plasma cells directly reactive to alkaline phosphatase. *J. Pathol.*, **185**, 427–34.
10. Pantel, K, Cote, R.J., Fodstad, Ø (1999). Detection and clinical importance of micrometastatic disease. *J. Natl. Cancer Inst*, **91**, 1113–24.
11. Forus, A., Høifødt, H.K. G.E.T. *et al.* (1999). Sensitive method for FISH characterisation of breast cancers in cells in bone marrow aspirates. *J. Clin. Pathol.: Molec. Pathol.*, **52**, 68–74.
12. Serov, S.F., Scully, R.E., and Sobin, L.H. (1973). *Histological typing of ovarian tumors*. International Histological Classification of Tumors No. 9. World Health Organisation, Geneva, pp. 17–18.
13. Beverley, P.C.L., Souhami, R.L., and Bobrow, L.G. (1988). Results of the central data analysis. Proceedings of the First International Workshop on Small Cell Lung Cancer, (ed. R.L. Souhami, P.C.L. Beverley, and L. Bobrow), Vol. 4, pp. 15–36. Elsevier Science Publishers, Amsterdam.
14. de Leij, Berendsen, H., Spakman, H. *et al.* (1988). Proceedings of the First International Workshop on Small-Cell Lung-Cancer Antigens. *Lung Cancer*, **4**, 1–114.
15. Marth, C., Zeimet, A.G., Widschwendter, M. *et al.* (1997). Paclitaxel- and docetaxel-dependent acitvation of CA125 expression in human ovarian carcinoma cells. *Cancer Res.*, **57**, 3818–22.
16. Myklebust, A.T., Beiske, K., Pharo, A. *et al.* (1991). Selection of anti-SCLC antibodies for diagnosis of bone marrow metastasis. *Br. J. Cancer*, **63**, 49–53.

17. Diel, I.J., Kaufmann, M., Costa, S.D. *et al.* (1996). Micrometastatic breast cancer cells in bone marrow at primary surgery: Prognostic value in comparison with nodal status. *J. Natl Cancer Inst.*, **88**, 1652–64.

18. Diel, I.J., Kaufmann, M., Solomayer, E.F. *et al.* (1997). Prognostische Bedeutung des Tumorzellnachweises im Knochenmark im Vergleich zum Nodalstatus beim primären Mammakarzinom. *Geburtsh u Frauenheilk*, **57**, 333–41.

19. Pantel, K., Schlimok, G., Angstwurm, M. *et al.* (1994). Methodological analysis of immunocytochemical screening for disseminated epithelial tumor cells in bone marrow. *J. Hematother.*, **3**, 165–9.

20. Datta, Y.H., Adams, P.T., Drobyski, W.R. *et al.* (1994). Sensitive detection of occult breast cancer by the reverse-transcriptase polymerase chain reaction. *J. Clin. Oncol.*, **12**, 475–82.

21. Krismann, M., Todt, B., Schröder, J. *et al.* (1995). Low specificity of cytokeratin 19 reverse transcriptase-polymerase chain reaction analyses for detection of hematogenous lung cancer dissemination. *J. Clin. Oncol.*, **13**, 2769–75.

22. Ruud, P., Fodstad, Ø., and Hovig, E. (1999). Identification of a novel cytokeratin 19 pseudogene that may interfere with reverse transcriptase-polymerase chain reaction assay used to detect micrometastic tumor cells. *Int. J. Cancer*, **80**, 119–25.

23. Rye, P.D., Høifødt, H.K., Øverli, G.E.T. *et al.* (1997). Immunobead filtration. A novel approach for the isolation and propagation of tumor cells. *Am. J. Pathol.*, **150**, 99–106.

24. Cain, J.M., Ellis, G.K. *et al.* (1990). Bone marrow involvement in epithelial ovarian cancer by immunocytochemical assessment. *Gynecol. Oncol.*, **38**, 442–5.

Part 6

Surgical treatment and organization of care

37. Overview of primary surgery for ovarian cancer

Thomas E.J. Ind and John H. Shepherd

Introduction

The history of primary surgery for ovarian cancer extends back to the late eighteenth century. In 1775, William Hunter recommended aspiration of ovarian cysts.[1] Ovarian excisions were performed by Johannes Theden and Samuel Hartman d'Escher, in 1771 and 1807 respectively.[1] The first published ovariotomy for ovarian cancer were reported by Ephraim McDowell in 1817.[2]

The modern approach to primary surgery was developed in the twentieth century. In the 1920s the cancer commission of the League of Nations initiated talks on classification which eventually led to the International Federation of Gynaecology and Obstetrics staging criteria.[1] The role of the omentum in tumour spread and the value of excision was first proposed by Pemberton in 1940[1] and in 1968, Christopher Hudson[3] described a technique of radical oophorectomy for removing malignant tumours fixed in the pelvis.

The function of primary surgery today involves diagnosis, staging, cytoreduction, and palliation (Table 37.1).

The role of primary surgery

Diagnosis

Providing tissue for a histological diagnosis is an important part of primary surgery for ovarian cancer. Numerous authors have reported the value of serological, radiological, and statistical tests for women with pelvic masses.[4-23] To date, none can predict ovarian carcinoma with 100% accuracy. A definitive diagnosis is rarely made prior to surgery and identification of histological type and differentiation may determine adjuvant therapy.

Table 37.1 The role of primary surgery for ovarian cancer

Diagnosis
Staging
Cytoreduction
Palliation

Staging

The International Federation of Obstetrics and Gynaecology stage (Table 37.2) influences survival.[24] Therefore, assessing the spread of malignancy is important for counselling patients of their prognosis. Furthermore, knowledge of the surgical stage is helpful when comparing treatments and assessing survival for audit.

The most important reason for determining the stage is in deciding the need for adjuvant treatment. The value of adjuvant therapy for advanced disease is well established.[25] However, none of the randomized controlled trials provide evidence that chemotherapy is of benefit for women with stage I tumours.[26-31] Therefore, accurate confirmation of stage I disease is essential if adjuvant therapy is to be omitted.

The staging laparotomy should be systematic, as often women with apparent 'early' ovarian cancer have tumour deposits outside the pelvis.[32-38] This was emphasized by Young et al.,[32] who 'upstaged' 28% of women with apparent stage I disease. In that study, histological grade was the most significant predictor of occult metastases.[32] The proportion of women with occult extrapelvic malignancy in apparent stage I disease is summarized in a meta-analysis by Berek.[38] The incidence of occult disease on the diaphragm was 7.3% (range 3.2–43.7%); para-aortic lymph node involvement occurred in 18.1% of cases (0–20.0%); pelvic lymph node involvement was present in 5.9% of cases (range 0–9.6%); occult omental involvement was present in 8.6% of cases (range 0–10.5%); and positive cytology existed in 26.4% of cases (range 10.0–36.0%).[38]

It is clear from the evidence above that a full staging laparotomy should include a thorough examination of the whole abdomen; biopsies of suspicious lesions; an omentectomy; and cytology of ascites or peritoneal washings. In the presence of obvious extraperitoneal disease, the presence of occult pelvic or para-aortic lymph node involvement would neither result in 'upstaging' nor influence the decision for subsequent adjuvant therapy. However, as there is clear evidence that some women have positive lymph nodes even when malignancy is apparently confined to the ovary, there is a potential role for lymphadenectomy in 'early' ovarian cancer. One retrospective study failed to demonstrate an improved outcome for pathological staging (including lymphadenectomy) for women with stage I and II

Table 37.2 International Federation of Obstetrics and Gynaecology stage classification for ovarian cancer

Stage I   Growth limited to the ovaries
  Stage Ia   Growth limited to one ovary
    No ascites containing malignant cells
    No tumour on the external surfaces
    Capsule intact
  Stage Ib   Growth limited to both ovaries
    No ascites containing malignant cells
    No tumour on the external surfaces
    Capsule intact
  Stage Ic   Tumour stage Ia or Ib but with tumour on the surface of one or both ovaries
    Or with the capsule(s) ruptured
    Or with ascites present containing malignant cells
    Or with positive peritoneal washings
Stage II   Growth limited to one or both ovaries with pelvic extension
  Stage IIa   Extension and/or metastases to the uterus and/or tubes
  Stage IIb   Extension to other pelvic tissues
  Stage IIc*   Tumour either stage IIa or IIb but with tumour on the surface of one or both ovaries
    Or with the capsule(s) ruptured
    Or with ascites present containing malignant cells
    Or with positive peritoneal washings
Stage III   Tumour involving one or both ovaries with peritoneal implants outside the pelvis and/or positive retroperitoneal or inguinal lymph nodes.
Superficial liver metastases equals stage III. Tumour is limited to the true pelvis but with histologically proven malignant extension to bowel or omentum
  Stage IIIa   Tumour grossly limited to the pelvis with negative nodes but with histologically confirmed microscopic seeding of abdominal peritoneal surfaces
  Stage IIIb   Tumour of one or both ovaries with histologically confirmed implants of abdominal peritoneal surfaces, none exceeding 2 cm in diameter. Nodes negative
  Stage IIIc   Abdominal implants > 2 cm in diameter and/or positive retroperitoneal or inguinal nodes
Stage IV   Growth involving one or both ovaries with distant metastases. If pleural effusion is present, there must be positive cytologic test results to allot a case to stage IV. Parenchymal liver metastases equals stage IV

* In order to evaluate the impact on prognosis of the different criteria for allotting cases to stage Ic or IIc, it would be of value to know if rupture of the capsule was (1) spontaneous or (2) caused by the surgeon, and if the source of malignant cells detected was (1) peritoneal washings or (2) ascites.

These criteria are based on findings at clinical examination and/or surgical exploration. The histological characteristics are to be considered in the staging, as are the results of cytological testing as far as effusions are concerned. It is desirable that a biopsy be performed on suspicious areas outside the pelvis.

disease.[39] However, no controlled trails have evaluated lymphadenectomy in early ovarian cancer.

Cytoreduction

The term 'cytoreduction' is often applied to surgery for ovarian cancer when the aim is to reduce the tumour bulk prior to adjuvant therapy. There are a number of theoretical advantages to cytoreduction. Skipper[40] proposed the *fractional cell kill hypothesis* that postulates that the proportion of tumour cells killed with each treatment is constant. Therefore, if the absolute number of cancer cells is lower at the initiation of chemotherapy, then the number of cycles required to eradicate the cancer would be less. Other scientific arguments also exist, based on tumour perfusion and immunological factors.[38]

A large number of studies have demonstrated the favourable prognostic effect of leaving minimal residual disease following primary surgery (Fig. 37.1). In a meta-analysis of 58 studies Hunter *et al.*[41] found the median increase in survival time to be 4.1% (95% Cl, 0.6–9.1). However, a statistically significant improvement in survival was demonstrated in two other meta-analyses.[42,43] No randomized studies exist comparing aggressive debulking with non-debulking of advanced disease. Therefore, some postulate that the apparent survival differences between

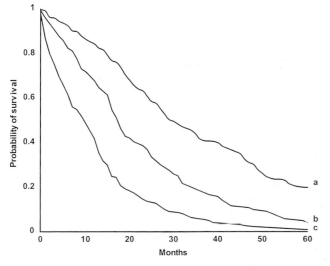

Fig. 37.1 Five-year survival in women with ovarian cancer and (a) less than 2 cm; (b) 2–5 cm; and (c) more than 5 cm residual disease following surgery. (Data from the North-East Thames Ovarian Cancer Series 1971–1981 by permission of Professor C. Hudson.)

optimally and suboptimally debulked disease is casual rather than causal, and related to the aggressive nature of disease when it cannot be surgically removed.

Venesmaa and Ylikorkala[44] reported that optimal cytological reduction, defined as leaving 2 cm or less of residual tumour, was achievable in 298 of 472 cases (63%). However, other authors define suboptimal debulking as resulting in less than 1.5 cm[45] and 0.5 cm[45] of residual disease. To achieve this, excision of bowel and other non-pelvic organs is sometimes required. In one series,[47] the small bowel was resected in 7.1%, the large bowel in 18.6%, and part of the urinary tract in 2.9% of cases. In that series, a stoma was formed in 8.6% of laparotomies.[47] Other series reported a rate of stoma formation as 0.5%[44] and 8.5%.[48]

It is the authors' opinion that the balance of evidence currently weighs in favour of cytoreductive surgery. Furthermore, 'aggressive' debulking is currently advocated by the United Kingdom National Health Service Executive.[25] However, further evidence is required from controlled studies, and the value must be assessed in context if new treatment protocols, such as interval debulking, find their way into clinical practice.

Palliation

Ovarian cancer is often asymptomatic at presentation. However, the bulk of tumour can cause bowel and urinary symptoms as well as pain. When significant ascites is present, a woman can also experience shortness of breath. Therefore, it is important to consider the possible palliative effects of primary surgery. Often ascites will disappear after removal of the primary tumour and omental cake. Furthermore, this may also alleviate nausea.[38] Removal of metastases in the bowel may relieve obstruction and improve bowel symptoms as well as improving the nutritional status of the patient.[38] There is little scientific evidence for the role of bowel surgery for palliation in primary therapy. However, in one series[49] bowel surgery led to palliation in 80% of woman with bowel obstruction from recurrent disease.

Primary laparotomy and cytoreduction for ovarian cancer

Preoperative assessment and preparation (Table 37.3)

The preoperative assessment should include a review of imaging, review of other investigations, and a multidisciplinary discussion (Fig. 37.2). This is essential to ensure that bowel and other tumours are considered as part of the differential diagnosis. Furthermore, investigations such as magnetic resonance imaging and computed tomography may assist in determining the spread of disease and therefore provide information necessary to obtain informed consent and for counselling. Specialist oncology nurses and specialist stoma nurses may also assist in preoperative counselling.

Informed consent is now considered an important part of any operation. Giving informed consent for primary surgery for ovarian cancer is complex as often the exact nature of the surgery depends on the operative findings. It is no longer acceptable for the most junior member of the medical team to ask a woman to sign a form with abbreviations such as 'TAH BSO'. Instead, a senior member of the team needs to explain all the possible surgical scenarios and give complication rates based on their own surgical practice. For cyto-reductive surgery it is unusual for this consent to take less than half an hour. Informed consent should include details of the suspected diagnosis; a description of the planned operation; an explanation of the intended goals of the operation; details of common side-effects that many women have postoperatively; important risks of the operation; alternative treatments possible; and a list of procedures that would be declined by the patient even if the surgeon thought them to be in the patients' best interest. 'Important risks' are those that may occur and would have permanent or severe implication for a woman's quality of life or that are common enough (more frequent than in 1 in 200 cases) to have a high likelihood of occurring. Consent should be signed and additional details should be clearly documented in the patient's notes.

A full history and examination should take place preoperatively and the stability of any chronic illnesses such as diabetes or hypertension assessed. Routine preoperative investigations should include a chest X-ray, an electrocardiogram, a full blood count, liver function tests, urea creatinine and electrolytes, and four units of packed red cells cross-matched. In addition, some surgeons prefer a limited intravenous urogram to assist location of the ureters.

Most surgeons use antibiotic prophylaxis prior to surgery. To advocate the use of prophylactic antibiotics in gynaecological surgery, seven criteria must exist.[50] The operation must carry a significant risk of postoperative site infection; the operation should cause significant bacterial contamination; the antibiotic used for prophylaxis should have laboratory evidence of effectiveness against some of the contaminating micro-organisms and demonstrate clinical effectiveness; the antibiotic should be present in the wound in effective concentration at the time of incision; a short-term low-toxicity regimen of antibiotics should be used; antibiotics needed to combat resistant infections should be reserved and not used for prophylaxis; the benefits of prophylactic antibiotics must outweigh the dangers of antibiotic use.[50]

The reported rate of pelvic infections following radical gynaecological oncology surgery varies from between 1.5% and 23.4%.[50] The wound infection rate ranges from 2.8% to 18.8%.[50]

Table 37.3 Preoperative preparation

Radiological review
Multidisciplinary discussion
Informed consent
Consultation with specialist nurse counsellor and specialist stoma nurse
Chest X-ray, ECG, LFTS, Us and Es, FBC
Cross-matching
Antibiotic prophylaxis
Thromboprophylaxis
Bowel preparation

ECG, electrocardiogram; LFTS, liver function tests; Us and Es, urea creatinine and electrolytes; FBC, full blood count.

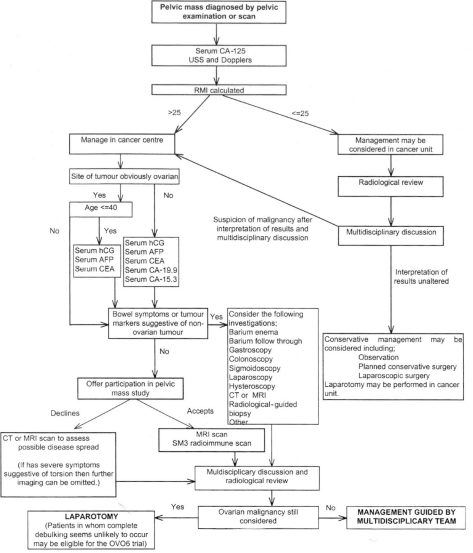

Fig. 37.2 An example of a preoperative diagnostic pathway used in a gynaecological cancer centre protocol.

For this reason, antibiotic prophylaxis must be considered for major gynaecological oncology cases. Data on the need for prophylactic antibiotics for primary cytoreductive surgery for ovarian cancer is controversial. In most prospective comparative studies the number of patients are small. However, when data from many prospective studies are combined, it appears that major postoperative infection is significantly reduced with prophylaxis.[51]

When compared with an antibiotic having a confined bacterial spectrum, a broad-spectrum antibiotic should provide enhanced protection, yet there is no strong evidence to support this in the literature. The timing of antibiotic prophylaxis is important. Classen *et al.*[51] reported that the most effective time to administer antibiotics was during the 2 hours before incision. Infection rates were significantly higher if antibiotics were administered more than 2 hours but less than 24 hours before surgery, and more than 3 hours but less than 24 hours after surgery.[52] The number of doses recommended is three, as there is evidence in the literature

that this is as effective as a longer course of prophylactic antibiotics.[53]

On the basis of the above evidence it is recommended that patients scheduled for major surgery should receive broad-spectrum antibiotic prophylaxis. They should receive their first dose on induction, to prevent the need for additional venepuncture, and should receive a total of three doses. As patients following radical gynaecological oncology surgery are rarely allowed to take oral preparations immediately postoperatively, the antibiotics should be administered intravenously. In the Gynaecological Cancer Centre at St. Bartholomew's Hospital, London we use cefuroxime (750 mg) and metronidazole (500 mg) on induction, and 6 and 12 hours postoperatively. In women with a type 1 sensitivity to penicillin, we substitute cefuroxime by vancomycin (1 mg).

The incidence of subclinical thromboembolic disease following major gynaecological oncology surgery is 22%.[54–57] However, the use of thromboprophylaxis agents, such as low molecular weight heparin, reduces this risk by 73%.[58] Therefore, the value of thromboprophylaxis outweighs the additional 3% risk of major haemorrhage it is associated with.[59] At present there are no adequate trials comparing pre-and postoperative initiation of low molecular weight heparin and dose scheduling.[58] Most North American studies gave the initial dose 12–24 hours postoperatively and on a twice-daily dose schedule. Most European studies gave the initial dose 12 hours preoperatively and on a once-daily dose schedule.[60] However, a meta-analysis concluded that preoperative initiation of heparin was significantly more effective and associated with less major bleeding when compared with postoperative initiation. As a result of this evidence, the protocol of the Gynaecological Cancer Centre at St. Bartholomew's Hospital advocates the usage of subcutaneous Clexane (40 mg) 12 hours preoperatively and daily until the woman is mobile. In addition, women receive throm-

boembolic disease stockings and utilize a calf compressor perioperatively.

Preoperative bowel preparation reduces the morbidity and mortality of bowel surgery.[62] Reduction in the incidence of wound infections and other septic complications have all been well documented.[63,64] Techniques for administrating bowel preparation vary and there is no evidence supporting one method. They tend to include the combination of a low residual diet, mechanical preparation and sometimes oral antibiotic prophylaxis. The complications of bowel preparation include electrolyte imbalance and overgrowth of antibiotic-resistant organisms. As a result, at the Gynaecological Cancer Centre at St. Bartholomew's Hospital, antibiotic preparation is not utilized and a gentle prophylaxis regime employed. This involves a 3-day low residual diet, two sachets of Picolax 24 hours prior to surgery, and a phosphate enema on the morning of surgery.

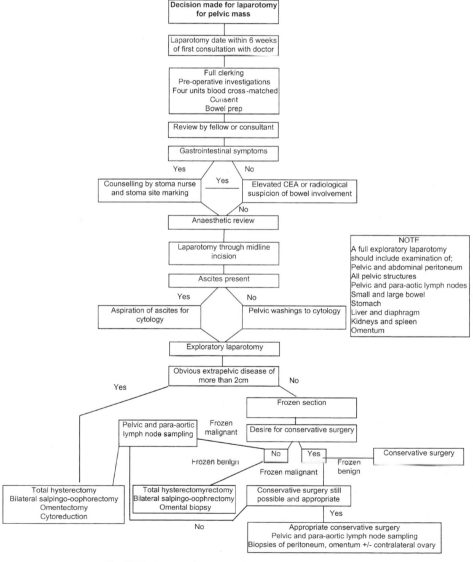

Fig. 37.3 A surgical pathway for women with pelvic masses.

Cytoreductive surgery

Cytoreductive surgery should be performed through a midline incision to allow proper examination of the upper abdominal organs in addition to the pelvis. Staging should include aspiration of free fluid or peritoneal washings, a systematic exploration of all intra-abdominal surfaces, biopsies of suspicious areas, an infra-colic omentectomy, and an exploration of the retroperitoneal spaces to evaluate pelvic and para-aortic lymph nodes. A pathway for primary surgery in a patient with suspected ovarian cancer is given in Fig. 37.3

Once the pelvis has been examined, the systematic exploration can be commenced by an examination of the small bowel and its mesentery, from the ileo-caecal junction to the ligament of Trietz. The omentum should also be inspected and eventually resected. The exploration should be continued by palpation in a clockwise manner from the caecum upwards along the right paracolic gutter and ascending colon to the right kidney. This should continue to the gall bladder, liver, and right hemidiaphragm. The exploration should proceed across the transverse colon to the left hemidiaphragm and along the descending colon and right paracolic gutter. The pelvic side wall should be entered and pelvic lymph nodes palpated. In addition, the surgeon should palpate for the presence of any obvious para-aortic lymph nodes.

It is important for the surgeon to bear in mind that the presence of any disease outside the ovary would result in a recommendation for adjuvant chemotherapy. In the presence of obvious extraovarian disease, a formal pelvic and para-aortic lymphadenectomy could not influence the decision for adjuvant chemotherapy. However, in the presence of an apparent stage I tumour a formal pelvic and para-aortic lymphadenectomy should be performed, in view of the evidence that 18% of women will have occult nodal disease.[38] To minimize the complications that might occur as a result of a lymphadenectomy, it may be necessary to request frozen sections during the procedure. This is as histologically confirmed disease which is extraovarian would result in a recommendation for chemotherapy, thus negating the need for a diagnosis of possible lymph node involvement. Furthermore, there is no therapeutic advantage in resecting non-bulky lymph nodes in women with high stage disease.[83]

The principles of cytoreductive surgery involve removable of both ovaries, the uterus and cervix, as well as excision of as much tumour as possible. Therefore, a bowel resection and subsequent stoma formation may be required. In most cases, the hysterectomy can be achieved in an extrafascial manner. However, if the tumour is fixed in the pelvis, the technique of a radical oophorectomy may be required.[3,65] This was described in 1968,[3] with the objective of increasing the operability of malignant tumours. It consists of a retroperitoneal mobilization of the pouch of Douglas as a 'false capsule' to a fixed tumour or one that has produced seedling deposits in the pouch. The uterus is then removed retrograde in continuity with the pelvic mass. The rectum must be mobilized from the hollow of the sacrum and the dissection is completed under direct vision and, if necessary, incising the rectum and attached viscera. The rectum is later allowed to fall back into the pelvis denuded of peritoneum.

Fertility-sparing surgery

The uterus and contralateral ovary can be left, thus preserving fertility in women with low-grade stage Ia disease, although it should be noted that recurrence rates are in the region of 5%.[66,67] Recurrence rates following conservative surgery for borderline ovarian cancer are also low[68–81] (Table 37.4), and a unilateral oophorectomy is all that is advocated in women with stage I disease in whom there is a desire to preserve fertility.[82] The presence of positive margins is a predictor of recurrence and should be considered carefully.[59]

As with low-stage epithelial tumours, the addition of a hysterectomy and contralateral oophorectomy does not not alter outcome in patients with stage Ia germ cell and stromal tumours.[84–88]

Postoperative care

The immediate postoperative care following cytoreductive surgery is best undertaken on a high-dependency surgical ward. Cardiovascular problems may arise due to depression in myocardial contractility, changes in the sympathetic tone induced by anaesthesia, and changes in intravascular volume from blood loss or third spacing. Pulmonary complications may arise due to pain, analgesic medication, and the supine position of nursing. This can result in a decrease in vital capacity, shallow rapid respiration with atelectasis, an alteration in ventilation/perfusion relationships with a decrease in arterial oxygen saturation, and a reduction in the clearance of pulmonary bacteria due to suppression of coughing from pain and impaired ciliary function. Therefore, great care should be taken to look for the early signs of cardiovascular and pulmonary complications in the immediate postoperative period. Cardiovascular changes may be monitored by carefully examining the pulse, blood pressure, and urinary output postoperatively, and central venous pressure measurements may assist in modifying the postoperative fluid regimen. A pulse oximeter should be used in the immediate postoperative period and regular examination of the patient's chest is advocated.

Table 37.4 Recurrence rates for stage I borderline tumours treated by cystectomy or unilateral oophorectomy (modified from NHS executive 2000[25])

Reference	n/N (%)
Tazelaar et al. (1985)[68]	3/20 (15.0)
Lim-Tan et al. (1988)[69]	4/33 (12.1)
Bell and Scully (1990)[70]	1/13 (7.7)
Rice et al. (1990)[71]	0/30 (0.0)
Sawada et al. (1991)[72]	1/5 (20.0)
Manchul et al. (1992)[73]	0/15 (0.0)
Casey et al. (1993)[74]	0/7 (0.0)
Trope et al. (1993)[75]	0/14 (0.0)
Chao et al. (1996)[76]	0/23 (0.0)
Chow et al. (1996)[77]	0/24 (0.0)
Darai et al. (1996)[78]	4/16 (0.0)
Kennedy and Hart (1996)[79]	2/18 (11.1)
Sykes et al. (1997)[80]	0/15 (0.0)
Chambers et al. (1998)[81]	2/10 (10.0)
Total	17/227 (7.5)

Other prophylactic measures to minimize complications post-operatively have already been discussed and involve efforts to minimize the risk of thromboembolic disease and the use of prophylactic antibiotics. Urinary catheters should be left *in situ* until a patient is mobile or, if the surgery has involved damage to the bladder, for at least a week. Furthermore, there is evidence that midnight removal of urinary catheters improves postoperative voiding, possibly due to a reduction in the sympathetic inhibition of the bladder produced by anxiety.[61] Care should be taken not to commence feeding too early and when bowel has been damaged or resected; a nasogastric tube should be used to aspirate gastric contents.

Complications of cytoreductive surgery

The operative mortality following cytoreductive surgery has been reported as being 1.1%,[44] 2.1%,[48] 2.9%,[47] and 4.0%[65] by four separate groups. Major complications include haemorrhage, cardiac failure, pneumonia, wound dehiscence, and thromboembolic disease.

Reports of the incidence of major haemorrhage vary from only 2.0%[48] in one series to 20.8%[44] in another. The need for a repeat laparotomy has been reported to be in the region of 1–2%.[48,47] In the series of Heintz *et al.*,[47] the incidences of postoperative cardiac failure and pneumonia were 7.1% and 11.4%, respectively. Wound dehiscence occurs in 3–4% of cases[47,48] and the incidence of pulmonary embolus has been reported as being 2.1%.[44]

For less serious complications, the incidence of urinary tract infection is in the region of 20%,[44] the risk of unexplained febrile morbidity ranges from 2 to 23%,[44,47,48] and prolonged ileus can occur in between 4 and 17% of cases.[47,48]

The role of minimal access surgery

The role of minimal access surgery in ovarian cancer is controversial. It is discussed in more detail in Chapter 40. However, the part that these techniques play in primary surgery should be discussed.

There is a theoretical advantage for employing endoscopic techniques, with magnification of visual fields and optimal light direction assisting the surgeon. Evidence from other conditions prove that operating times may be longer but recovery time shorter, with an overall reduction in minor complications. However, at present, with the absence of controlled studies and the concerns of tumour dissemination from the pneumoperitoneum, minimal access surgery for cytoreduction should be reserve for clinical studies.

There are some areas where minimal access techniques are beginning to find a place in primary surgery for ovarian cancer. When the risk of malignancy index[123] for ovarian cancer is low and the probability is that an ovarian cyst is benign, an endoscopic approach may be more suitable. A scenario where minimal access techniques can be employed in proven ovarian cancer is when an ovary or cyst has been removed in a young women and proven to be cancerous when previously thought benign. In this scenario an assumed diagnosis of stage Ia disease may exist but proper staging can be facilitated via the laparoscope. In such a situation an ovary may be removed and a contralateral ovary biopsied. In addition, omental and peritoneal biopsies should be performed along with pelvic washings and a pelvic and para-aortic lymphadenectomy. The procedure can be performed laparoscopically in an attempt to decide if 'up-staging' is required and adjuvant chemotherapy recommended.

There is a concern that laparoscopic surgery may promote tumour seeding and increase the risk of metastases. Numerous murine and porcine studies have hypothesized an adverse effect from trocars, eddy currents, and gas on the behaviour of tumour cells. However, there is little *in vivo* evidence to refute the hypothesis that port site recurrence is merely a different location for tumour growth rather than the presence of a tumour relapse itself. However, there is evidence to the contrary. A randomized controlled trial comparing open and closed procedures in colorectal cancer, where port site recurrence has been most reported, found no difference in the rate of relapse.[89]

The role of the gynaecological cancer centre

Surprisingly, there is still controversy as to whether primary surgery should be performed in a cancer centre or a local hospital. It is the author's opinion that the evidence weighs in favour of the former. The British National Health Service document *Improving outcomes in gynaecological cancers*[25] supports this opinion. The paper quotes unpublished data[90] from 1866 cases that demonstrate improved survival when surgery is performed by a trained gynaecological oncologist rather than a general gynaecologist. In that study there was a 25% reduction in the death rate when women with stage III disease were operated on by gynaecological oncologists.[90] Furthermore, differential use of chemotherapy only made a small impact on survival, suggesting that the main difference was due to the surgeon. In another study,[91] a survival benefit was demonstrated for stage I and II disease when surgery was performed by a subspecialist.

The reasons for poor outcomes when a general gynaecologist has been the primary carer are probably multiple. They may be related to understaging by general gynaecologists, an inability to obtain optimal cytoreduction, the absence of a multidisciplinary team, or the quality of histopathological analysis.

General gynaecologists, are more likely to understage ovarian cancer.[92] In one study, adequate staging for ovarian cancer was 97% for gynaecological oncologists, 52% for general gynaecologists, and 35% for general surgeons.[92] Understaging may result in the incorrect diagnosis of stage Ia disease, subsequent failure to administer adjuvant chemotherapy, and a consequential detrimental effect on survival.

Women in whom ovarian cancer has been optimally debulked live longer than those with residual disease (Fig. 37.1). Two studies have demonstrated that general surgeons were less likely to achieve complete debulking when compared to gynaecologists.[93,94] Furthermore, in these studies, survival was poorer for general surgeons.[93,94] It is possible that similar differences exist between general gynaecologists and gynaecological oncologists.

One benefit of management in a cancer centre is the presence of the multidisciplinary team. One study demonstrated that an independent prognostic factor for survival was follow-up at a multidisciplinary clinic.[95] Another study from Scotland demonstrated a poorer survival for patients treated in non-teaching hospitals compared to teaching hospitals.[96] In addition, cancer centres have expert histopathologists. Histopathological interpretation may influence treatment. In one study an expert review of slides found that an incorrect diagnosis was given in 10% of cases with a previous diagnosis of ovarian cancer.[97]

Conclusions

Cytoreduction remains the principal aim of primary surgery for ovarian cancer. This can be achieved in 70–90% of cases when surgery is performed by gynaecological oncologists.[46,47] There is a place for fertility-sparing surgery in young women with low-stage disease, yet this and other decisions concerning primary surgery are best made by a multidisciplinary team in a gynaecological cancer centre.

References

1. O'Dowd, M.J. and Philipp, E.E. (1994). Cancer of the ovary. In *The history of obstetrics and gynaecology*. Parthenon, Carnforth, UK.
2. McDowell, E. (1817). Three cases of extirpation of diseased ovarii. *Eclectic Repertory and Analytical Review*, 7, 242.
3. Hudson, C.N. (1968). A radical operation for fixed ovarian tumours. *J Obstet Gynaecol Brit Cwlth*, 75, 1155.
4. Maggina, G.T., Gadducci, A., D'Addario, V. *et al.* (1994). Prospective multicentre study on CA125 in postmenopausal pelvic masses. *Gynecol. Oncol.*, 54, 117.
5. Botta, G. and Zarcone, R. (1995). Transvaginal ultrasound examination of ovarian masses in premenopausal women. *Eur. J. Obstet. Gynecol.*, 62, 37.
6. Caruso, A., Caforio, L., Testa, A.C. *et al.* (1996). Transvaginal color Doppler ultrasonography in the presurgical characterization of adnexal masses. *Gynecol. Oncol.*, 63, 184.
7. Luxman, D., Bergman, A., Sagi, J. *et al.* (1991). The postmenopausal adnexal mass: correlation between ultrasonic and pathologic findings. *Obstet. Gynecol.*, 77, 726.
8. Finkler, N.J., Benacerraf, B., Lavin, P.T. *et al.* (1988). Comparison of serum CA125, clinical impression, and ultrasound in the preoperative evaluation of ovarian masses. *Obstet. Gynecol.*, 72, 659.
9. Franchi, M., Beretta, P., Ghezzi, F. *et al.* (1995). Diagnosis of pelvic masses with transabdominal color Doppler, CA125 and ultrasonography. *Acta Obstet. Gynecol. Scand.*, 74, 734.
10. Schutter, E.M.J., Kenemans, P., Sohn, C. *et al.* (1994). Diagnostic value of pelvic examination ultrasound, and serum CA125 in postmenopausal women with a pelvic mass. *Cancer*, 74, 1398.
11. Sengoku, K., Satoh, T., Saitoh, S. *et al.* (1994). Evaluation of transvaginal color Doppler sonography, transvaginal sonography and CA 125 for prediction of ovarian malignancy. *Int. J. Gynecol. Obstet.*, 46, 39.
12. Buy, J.-N., Ghossain, M.A., Hugol, D. *et al.* (1996). Characterization of adnexal masses: combination of color Doppler and conventional sonography compared with spectral Doppler analysis alone and conventional sonography alone. *Am. J. Rad.*, 166, 385.
13. Carter, J., Saltzmann, A., Hartenbach, E. *et al.* (1994). Flow characteristics in benign and malignant gynaecologic tumors using transvaginal color flow Doppler. *Obstet. Gynecol.*, 83, 125.
14. Leeners, B., Schild, R.L., Funk, A. *et al.* (1996). Colour Doppler sonography improves the preoperative diagnosis of ovarian tumors made using conventional transvaginal color Doppler. *Gynecol. Oncol.*, 61, 354.
15. Prömpeler, H.J., Madjar, H. and Sauerbrei, W. (1996). Classification of adnexal tumors by transvaginal color Doppler. *Gynecol. Oncol.*, 61, 354.
16. Rehn, M., Lohmann, K., and Rempen, A. (1996). Transvaginal ultrasonography of pelvic masses: evaluation of B-mode technique and Doppler ultrasound. *Am. J. Obstet. Gynecol.*, 175, 97.
17. Reles, A., Wein, U., and Lichtenegger, W. (1997). Transvaginal color Doppler sonography and convential sonography in the preoperative assessment of adnexal masses. *J. Clin. Ultrasound*, 25, 217.
18. Schneider, V.L., Schneider, A., Reed, K.L. *et al.* (1993). Comparison of doppler with two dimensional sonography and CA125 for prediction of malignancy of pelvic masses. *Obstet. Gynecol.*, 81, 983.
19. Stringini, F.A.L., Gadducci, A., Del Bravo, B. *et al.* (1996). Differential diagnosis of adnexal masses with transvaginal sonography, color flow imaging and serum CA125 assay in pre- and postmenopausal women. *Gynecol. Oncol.*, 61, 68.
20. Timor-Tritsch, I.E., Lerner, J.P., Monteagudon, A. *et al.* (1993). Transvagianl ultrasonographic characterisation of ovarian masses by means of color flow-directed Doppler measurements and a morphologic scoring system. *Am. J. Obstet. Gynecol.*, 168, 909.
21. Davies, A.P., Jacobs, I., Woolas, R. *et al.* (1993). The adnexal mass: benign or malignant? Evaluation of a risk of malignancy index. *Br. J. Obstet. Gynaecol.*, 100, 927.
22. Jacobs, I., Oram, D., Fairbanks, J. *et al.* (1990). A risk of malignancy index incorporating CA125, ultrasound and menopausal status for the accurate preoperative diagnosis of ovarian cancer. *Br. J. Obstet. Gynaecol.*, 97, 922.
23. Tingulstad, S., Hagen, B., Skeldestad, F.E. *et al.* (1996). Evaluation of a risk of malignancy index based on serum CA125, ultrasound findings and menopausal status in the pre-operative diagnosis of pelvic masses. *Br. J. Obstet. Gynaecol.*, 103, 826.
24. Ind, T.E.J., and Iles, R.K. (1998). Prognostic markers for epithelial ovarian cancer. *Cont. Rev. Obstet. Gynaecol.*, 3, 53.
25. NHS Executive (1999). *Guidance on commissioning cancer services. Improving outcomes in gynaecological cancers*. Department of Health. UK.
26. Bolis, G., Marsoni, S., and Chiari, N. (1995). Cooperative randomised clinical trial for stage I ovarian carcinoma. *Ann. Oncol.*, 6, 887.
27. Hreshchyshyn, M.M., Park, R.C., Blessiong, J.A. *et al.* (1980). The role of adjuvant therapy in stage I ovarian cancer. *Am. J. Obstet. Gynecol.*, 138, 139.
28. Sigurdsson, K., Johnsson, J.E., and Trope, C. (1982). Carcinoma of the Ovary, stages I and II. A prospective randomised study of the effects of postoperative chemotherapy and radiotherapy. *Ann. Chir. Gynecol.*, 71, 321.
29. Vergote, I.B., Vergote-De Vos, L.N., Abeler, V.M. *et al.* (1992). Randomized trial comparing cisplatin with radioactive phosphorus or whole-abdomen irradiation as adjuvant treatment of ovarian cancer. *Cancer*, 69, 741.
30. Trope, C., Kaem, J., Vergote, I. *et al.* (1997). Randomized trial on adjuvant carboplatin versus no treatment in stage I high risk ovarian cancer by Nordic Ovarian Cancer Group. *Proc. Ann. Meet. Ann. Soc. Clin. Oncol.*, 16, 1260 (abstract).
31. Young, R.C., Walton, L.A., Ellenberg, S.S. *et al.* (1990). Adjuvant therapy in stage I and stage II epithelial ovarian cancer. Results of two prospective randomised trials. *N. Engl. J. Med.*, 322, 1021.
32. Young, R.C., Decker, D.G., Wharton, J.G. *et al.* (1983). Staging laparotomy in early ovarian cancer. *J. Am. Med. Assoc.*, 250, 3072.

33. Buchsbaum, H.J., and Lifshitz, S. (1984). Staging and surgical evaluation of ovarian cancer. *Semin. Oncol.*, **11**, 227.

34. Yoshimuna, S., Scully, R.E., Bell, D.A., and Taft, P.D. (1984). Correlation of ascitic fluid cytology with histologic findings before and after treatment of ovarian cancer. *Am. J. Obstet. Gynecol.*, **148**, 716.

35. Piver, M.S., Barlow, J.J., and Lele, S.B. (1978). Incidence of subclinical metastasis in stage I and II ovarian carcinoma. *Obstet. Gynecol.*, **52**, 100.

36. Delgado, G., Chun, B., and Caglar, H. (1977). Para-aortic lymphadenectomy in gynaecologic malignancies confined to the pelvis. *Obstet. Gynecol.*, **50**, 415.

37. Guthrie, D., Davy, M.L.J., and Phillips, P.R. (1984). Study of 656 patients with 'early' ovarian cancer. *Gynecol. Oncol.*, **17**, 363.

38. Berek, J.S. (1994). Epithelial ovarian cancer. In *Practical gynecologic oncology*, (ed. J.S. and Berek N.F. Hacker). Williams & Wilkins, Baltimore, USA.

39. Hand, R., Fremgen, A., Chmiel, J.S. *et al.* (1993). Staging procedures, clinical management, and survival outcome for ovarian carcinoma. *JAMA*, **269**, 1119.

40. Skipper, H.E. (1978). Adjuvant chemotherapy. *Cancer*, **41**, 936.

41. Hunter, R.W., Alexander, N.D., and Soutter, W.P. (1992). Meta-analysis of surgery in advanced ovarian carcinoma: is maximum cytoreductive surgery an independent determinant of prognosis? *Am. J. Obstet. Gynecol.*, **166**, 504.

42. Marsoni, S., Torri, V., Valsecchi, M.G. *et al.* (1990). Prognostic factors in advanced epithelial ovarian cancer. *Br. J. Cancer*, **62**, 444.

43. Voest, E.E., Van Houwelingen, J.C., and Neijt, J.P. (1989). A meta-analysis of prognostic factors in advanced ovarian cancer with median survival and overall survival (measured with the log (relative risk)) as main objectives. *Eur. J. Cancer Clin. Care*, **25**, 711.

44. Venesmaa, P. and Ylikorkala, O. (1992). Morbidity and mortality associated with primary and repeat operations for ovarian cancer. *Obstet. Gynecol.*, **79**, 168.

45. Griffiths, C.T. (1975). Surgical resection of tumor bulk in the primary treatment of ovarian carcinoma. *Natl Cancer Inst. Monogr.*, **42**, 101.

46. Hacker, N.F. and Berek, J.S. (1986). Cytoreductive surgery in ovarian cancer. In *Ovarian cancer*, (ed. P.S. Albert and E.A. Surwit), pp. 53–67. Martinus Nijhoff, Boston.

47. Heintz, A.P.M., Hacker, N.F., Berek, J.S. *et al.* (1986). Cytoreductive surgery in ovarian carcinoma: Feasibility and morbidity. *Obstet. Gynecol.*, **67**, 783.

48. Hacker, N.F., Berek, J.S., Lagasse, L.D., Nieberg, R.K., and Elashoff, R.M. (1983). Primary cytoreductive surgery for epithelial ovarian cancer. *Obstet. Gynecol.*, **61**, 783.

49. Rubin, S.C., Hoskins, W.J., Benjamin, I. *et al.* (1989). Palliative surgery for intestinal obstruction in advanced ovarian cancer. *Gynecol. Oncol.* **34**, 16.

50. Hemsell, D.L., Bernstein, S.G., Bawdon, R.E. *et al.* (1989). Preventing major operative site infection after radical abdominal hysterectomy and pelvic lymphadenectomy. *Gynecol. Oncol.*, **35**, 55.

51. Classen, D.C., Evans, R.S., Pestotnik, S.L. *et al.* (1992). The timing of prophylactic administration of antibiotics and the risk of surgical-wound infection. *N. Engl. J. Med.*, **326**, 281.

52. Sevin, B.U., Ramos, R., Gerhardt, R.T., Guerra, L., Hilsenbeck, S., and Averette, H.E. (1991). Comparative efficacy of short-term versus long-term cefoxitin prophylaxis against postoperative infection after radical hysterectomy: a prospective study. *Obstet. Gynecol.*, **77**, 729.

53. Kingdom, J.C., Kitchener, H.C., and MacLean, A.B. (1990). Postoperative urinary tract infection in gynecology: implications for an antibiotic prophylaxis policy. *Obstet. Gynecol.*, **76**, 636.

54. Walsh, J.J., Bonnar, J., and Wright, F.W. (1974). A study of pulmonary embolism and deep leg vein thrombosis after major gynaecological surgery using labelled fibrinogen-phlebography and lung scanning. *J. Obstet. Gynaecol. Br. Commonw.*, **81**, 311.

55. Clarke-Pearson, D.L., Synan, I.S., Colemen, R.E., Hinshaw, W. and Creasman, W.T. (1984). The natural history of postoperative venous thromboemboli in gynecologic oncology: a prospective study of 382 patients. *Am. J. Obstet. Gynecol.*, **148**, 1051.

56. Clarke-Pearson, D.L., DeLong, E.R., Synan, I.S., and Creasman, W.T. (1984). Complications of low-dose heparin prophylaxis in gynecologic oncology surgery. *Obstet. Gynecol.*, **64**, 689.

57. Clarke-Pearson, D.L., DeLong, E.R., Synan, I.S., Coleman, R.E. and Creasman, W.T. (1987). Variables associated with postoperative deep venous thrombosis: a prospective study of 411 gynecology patients and creation of a prognostic model. *Obstet. Gynecol.*, **69**, 146.

58. Fifth ACCP Consensus Conference on Antithrombotic Therapy. (1998). *Chest*, **114**, (Suppl.), 531.

59. Kearon, C. and Hirsh, J. (1997). Management of anticoagulation before and after elective surgery. *N. Engl. J. Med.*, **336**, 1506.

60. Green, D., Hirsh, J., Heit, J., Prins, M., Davidson, B., and Lensing, A.W. (1994). Low molecular weight heparin: a critical analysis of clinical trials. *Pharmacol. Rev.*, **46**, 89.

61. Ind, T.E.J., Brown, R., Pyneandee, V.M., Swanne, M., and Taylor, J. (1993). What time of day is best for removal of urinary catheters. *Int. J. Urogynecol.*, **4**, 342.

62. Nichols, R.L., and Condon, R.E. (1971). Preoperative preparation of the colon. *Surg. Gynecol. Obstet.*, **132**, 323.

63. Coppa, G.F., Eng, K., Gouge, T.H., Ranson, J.H., and Localio, S.A. (1983). Parenteral and oral antibiotics in elective colon and rectal surgery. A prospective randomised trial. *Am. J. Surg.*, **145**, 62.

64. Condon, R.E. (1982). Bowel preparation for colorectal operations. *Arch. Surg.*, **117**, 265.

65. Hudson, C.N. and Chir, M. (1973). Surgical treatment of ovarian cancer. *Gynecol. Oncol.*, **1**, 370.

66. Zanetta, G., Chiari, S., Rota, S. *et al.* (1997). Conservative surgery for stage I ovarian carcinoma in women of childbearing age. *Br. J. Obstet. Gynaecol.*, **104**, 1030.

67. Marchetti, M., Padovan, P., Fracas, M. (1998). Malignant ovarian tumors: conservative surgery and quality of life in young patients. *Eur. J. Gynaecol. Oncol.*, **19**, 297.

68. Tazelaar, H.D., Bostwick, D.G., Ballon, S.C. *et al.* (1985). Conservative treatment of borderline ovarian tumors. *Obstet. Gynecol.*, **66**, 417.

69. Lim-Tan, S.K., Cajigas, H.E., and Scully, R.E. (1988). Ovarian cystectomy for serous borderline tumors: a follow-up study of 35 cases. *Obstet. Gynecol.*, **72**, 775.

70. Bell, D. and Scully, R. (1990). Ovarian serous borderline tumors with stromal microinvasion: a report of 21 cases. *Hum. Pathol.*, **21**, 397.

71. Rice, L., Berkowitz, R., Mark, S. *et al.* (1990). Epithelial ovarian tumors of borderline malignancy. *Gynecol. Oncol.*, **39**, 195.

72. Sawada, M., Yamasaki, M., Urabe, T. *et al.* (1991). Stage I epithelial ovarian tumors of low malignant potential. *Jpn J. Clin. Oncol.*, **21**, 30.

73. Manchul, L.A., Simm, J., Levin, W. *et al.* (1992). Borderline epithelial ovarian tumors: a review of 81 cases with an assessment of the impact of treatment. *Int. J. Radiat. Oncol. Biol. Phys.*, **22**, 867.

74. Cassey, A.C., Bell, D.A., Lage, J.M. *et al.* (1993). Epithelial ovarian tumors of borderline malignancy: long-term follow-up. *Gynecol. Oncol.*, **50**, 316.

75. Trope, C., Kaern, J., Vergote, B. *et al.* (1993). Are borderline tumors of the ovary overtreated both surgically and systemically? A review of four prospective randomised trials including 253 patients with borderline tumors. *Gynecol. Oncol.*, **51**, 236.

76. Chao, T., Yen, M., Chao, K. *et al.* (1996). Epithelial ovarian tumors of borderline malignancy. *Chung Hua I Hseub Tsa Chib*, **58**, 97.

77. Chow, S., Chen, C., Chen, Y. *et al.* (1996). Borderline malignant tumors of the ovary: a study of prognostic factors. *J. Formos. Med. Assoc.*, **95**, 851.

78. Darai, E., Teboul, J., Walker, F. *et al.* (1996). Epithelial ovarian carcinoma of low malignant potential. *Eur. J. Obstet. Gynecol. Reprod. Biol.*, **66**, 141.

79. Kennedy, A., and Hart, W. (1996). Ovarian papillary serous tumors of low malignant potential (serous borderline tumors). *Cancer*, **78**, 278.

80. Sykes, P., Quinn, M., and Rome, R. (1997). Ovarian tumors of low malignant potential: a retrospective study of 234 patients. *Int. J. Gynecol. Cancer*, **7**, 218.

81. Chambers, J.T., Merino, M.J., Kohorn, E.I. *et al.* (1998). Borderline ovarian tumors. *Am. J. Obstet. Gynecol.*, **159**, 1088.

82. Bostwick, D.G., Tazelaar, H.D., Ballon, S.C. *et al.* (1986). Ovarian epithelial tumors of borderline malignancy: a clinical and pathological study of 109 cases. *Cancer*, **58**, 2052.

83. Spirtos, N.M., Gross, G.M., Freddo, J.L., and Ballon, S.C. (1995). Cytoreductive surgery in advanced epithelial cancer of the ovary: the impact of aortic and pelvic lymphadenectomy. *Gynecol. Oncol.*, **56**, 345.

84. Norris, H.J., Zirken, H.J., and Benson, W.L. (1976). Immature (malignant) teratoma of the ovary: a clinical and pathologic study of 58 cases. *Cancer*, **37**, 2359.

85. Slayton, R.E. (1984). Management of germ cell and stromal tumors of the ovary. *Semin. Oncol.*, **11**, 229.

86. Thomas, G.M., Dembo, A.J., Hacker, N.F., and DePetrillo, A.D. (1987). Current therapy for dysgerminoma of the ovary. *Obstet. Gynecol.*, **70**, 268.

87. Bjorkholm, E., and Pettersson, F. (1983). Granulosa-cell and theca cell tumors: The clinical picture and long term outcome for the Radiumhemmet series. *Acta Obstet. Gynecol. Scand.*, **59**, 278.

88. Roth, L.M., Anderson, M.C., Govan, A.D. *et al.* (1981). Setoli-Leydig cell tumors: a clinicopathological study of 34 cases. *Cancer*, **48**, 187.

89. Lacy, A.M., Delgado, S., Garcia-Valdecasas, J.C. *et al.* (1998). Port site metastases and recurrence after laparoscopic colectomy. A randomised trial. *Surg. Endosc.*, **12**, 1039.

90. Junor, E.J. and Hole, D.J. (2000). Specialist gynaecologists and survival outcome in ovarian cancer: a Scottish National Study of 1866 patients. *Br. J. Obstet. Gynaecol.*, in press.

91. McGowan, L. (1993). Patterns of care in carcinoma of the ovary. *Cancer*, **71**, 628.

92. Mayer, A.R., Chambers, S.K., Graves, E. *et al.* (1992). Ovarian cancer staging: does it require a gynecologic oncologist? *Gynecol. Oncol.*, **47**, 223.

93. Kehoe, S., Powell, J., Wilson, S. *et al.* (1994). The influence of the operating surgeon's specialisation on patient survival in ovarian carcinoma. *Br. J. Cancer*, **70**, 1014.

94. Nguyen, H.N., Averette, H.E., Hoskins, W. *et al.* (1993). National Survey of ovarian carcinoma part V. *Cancer*, **72**, 3663.

95. Gillis, C.R., Hole, D.J., Still, R.M. *et al.* (1991). Medical audit, cancer registration, and survival in ovarian cancer. *Lancet*, **337**, 611.

96. Junor, E.J., Hole, D.J., Gillis, C.R. (1994). Management of ovarian cancer: referral to a multidisciplinary team matters. *Br. J. Cancer*, **70**, 363.

97. McGowan, L. and Norris, H.J. (1991). The mistaken diagnosis of carcinoma of the ovary. *Surg. Gynecol. Obstet.*, **173**, 211.

38. Interval debulking surgery significantly increases the survival and progression-free survival in advanced epithelial ovarian cancer patients: an EORTC Gynaecological Cancer Co-operative Group study

Maria E.L. van der Burg, Mat van Lent, Anna Kobierska, Maria Rosa Pittelli, Guiceppe Favalli, Angel J. Lacave, Mario Nardi, Guido Hoctin Boes, Ivana Teodorovic, and Sergio Pecorelli

Introduction

Cytoreductive surgery at primary laparotomy is well accepted as beneficial and considered as standard for patients with advanced epithelial ovarian cancer. Patients with an optimal tumour debulking (residual lesions smaller than 1 cm) have a significantly longer survival (almost two times the median survival) than patients with larger residual lesions.[1-5] This holds even for patients with FIGO stage IV tumours, regardless of the location of the extra-abdominal metatases.[6-9] Whether the improved survival is a result of the tumour reduction itself or whether it only reflects the biology of tumours with a good prognosis, which allow surgical cytoreduction, has never been investigated in a prospective randomized study. In a case-control study Eisenkop *et al.*[10] demonstrated that the excision of all tiny peritoneal lesions resulted in a significantly better survival compared to the survival of patients in whom these small lesions were left behind. This argues in favour of a positive effect of tumour reduction itself on survival. Hacker *et al.*,[11] Hoskins *et al.*,[12] and Vergote *et al.*,[13] on the contrary, reported that despite optimal tumour reduction the survival of patients with large preoperative intra-abdominal lesions had a significantly worse survival compared with patients with initial small tumours. These results indicate that, in addition to the residual tumour size, intrinsic biological tumour factors are of importance for survival.

The value of interval debulking surgery after induction chemotherapy is even more difficult to determine. Several studies indicated that optimal cytoreduction after induction chemotherapy significantly increased survival,[14-16] while others reported just the opposite.[2,17] All these studies of primary debulking surgery as well as intervention debulking surgery are hampered by the unavoidable, but serious, bias of comparing patients with different prognostic factors.

The question of whether cytoreduction has a significant effect on survival among patients with the same tumour size and the same prognostic factors can therefore only be answered in a prospective randomized study.

Rationale for cytoreduction

There is a sound rationale for cytoreductin surgery. Large tumours with areas having a relatively poor central blood supply and a low growth fraction, which are both rather insensitive to cytotoxic drugs,[18] are resected. In the better-perfused small residual lesions, the growth fraction is higher and the diffusion of cytotoxic drugs is increased, which both favour an increased cell kill by chemotherapy. In smaller tumour lesions, the probability of developing drug-resistant clones by spontaneous mutations is lower.[19] Smaller lesions require fewer chemotherapy cycles and therefore the chance of developing drug-induced resistance is lower. Moreover, a significant reduction in tumour volume improves the condition of the patient, resulting in a better performance status and better outcome.[2,20]

In 1987 the EORTC/GCCG activated the prospective randomized study of the value of cytoreductive surgery after induction chemotherapy in patients with residual lesions after primary debulking surgery. In 1995 we reported the first results.[21] After a follow-up of median 3.5 years, both the survival (median 26 months versus 20 months, $P = 0.012$) and progression-free survival (median 18 months versus 13 months, $P = 0.013$) were significantly lengthened in favour of the surgery group. We now report on the long-term results of interval cytoreduction in patients with suboptimal primary debulking surgery.[27,28]

Patient selection, study design, and evaluation methods

Patient selection

From March 1987 to May 1993, 425 patients were enrolled in the study. Eligible patients were those with epithelial ovarian carcinoma, FIGO stage IIb to IV, residual tumour lesions of more than 1 cm after primary cytoreductive surgery, a WHO performance status 0 to 2, an age of less than 75 years, and adequate bone-marrow and renal function.

The study design

After given informed consent, all eligible patients were registered centrally at the EORTC Data Centre before the start of chemotherapy. The chemotherapy had to start within 6 weeks after primary surgery. The chemotherapy consisted of cyclophosphamide/cisplatin (cyclophosphamide 750 mg/m^2, cisplatin 75 mg/m^2), once every 3 weeks. A clinical response evaluation was performed after the third cycle by means of gynaecological and general physical examination, CT scan and/or sonography, and serum CA125 measurement. Patients with progressive disease or a contraindication for surgery after the third cycle were removed from the study. All patients with stable disease or response were randomized between cytoreductive surgery and no surgery, after stratification for clinical response, performance status, and centre. Patients were stratified for centre to minimize any possible bias related to the extent of primary and intervention surgery between the institutes in this multicentre study. All randomized patients

were to receive a minimum of six cycles of cyclophosphamide/cisplatin unless clearly contraindicated. Continuation with chemotherapy after the sixth cycle was left to the policy of the individual institute.

At intervention debulking surgery, scheduled within 28 days after the third cycle, a maximal cytoreductive surgery and, if not performed previously, a bilateral salpingo-oophorectomy, hysterectomy, and infracolic omentectomy had to be performed if possible. The chemotherapy was to be resumed within 4 weeks from surgery. The endpoints of the study were overall survival and progression-free survival (Fig. 38.1).

Analyses

The endpoints of the study were overall survival and progression-free survival. Progression-free survival was calculated from the date of the outset of chemotherapy to the date of progression or death. Survival was calculated from the date of the outset of chemotherapy to the date of death, regardless of the cause of death. All randomized patients with some follow-up information were included in the analyses of progression-free survival and survival, which were performed strictly according to the intention to treat. Progression-free survival and survival curves were calculated for each treatment group using the Kaplan–Meier estimates[22] and compared using the logrank test.[23] Stratified analyses and Cox regression analyses were performed to adjust treatment comparisons for all known prognostic factors.[24]

Results

Recruitment and demographic characteristics of the patients

In the EORTC/GCCG study 425 patients have been registered. Seventy-five per cent of the patients have been randomized: 159 for interval debulking surgery and 160 for no surgery. Reasons for not randomizing 25% of the patients were: progression (10% of the patients), contraindication for surgery (6%), patient refusal (3%), early death (3%), lost to follow-up (1%), and ineligible (2%).

The age of the randomized patients ranged from 32 to 74 years, with an identical median of 59 years in both groups. In the randomized patients the percentage of the worst prognostic factors were: WHO grade 2, 17%; FIGO stage IV, 21%; tumour grade 3, 58%; tumour size greater than 2 cm, 91%; more than six tumour lesions, 64%; ascites, 77%; peritonitis, 80%; and ovaries still *in situ*, 30%. All prognostic characteristics of the randomized patients were well balanced between the two treatment groups. Furthermore, the number of patients responding to the three cycles of cyclophosphamide–cisplatin before randomization was identical: complete response, 17% each; partial response, 55% and 57%; and stable disease, 28% and 26%—for the surgery and no surgery group, respectively.

Treatment

The number of patients who received six cycles of cyclophosphamide and cisplatin was similar in both groups. Dose reduction

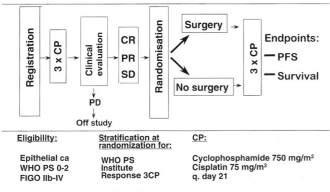

Fig. 38.1 Study design.

and postponement of chemotherapy cycles were comparable in both arms. In addition, the treatment duration from cycle 4 to cycle 6 was comparable. The interval cytoreductive surgery, therefore, did not interfere with adequate administration of the postoperative chemotherapy. The interval cytoreductive surgery increased the overall treatment duration, with a median of 4 weeks. The only difference in chemotherapy between the two treatment groups was the percentage of patients who received maintenance therapy after the sixth cycle. The percentage of patients who continued therapy was slightly higher in the no-surgery arm (56%) compared with the surgery arm (41%). If the maintenance therapy had any positive influence on survival, this would have been in favour of the no-surgery arm.

Surgical complications were minimal, neither death nor severe morbidity was associated with intervention debulking surgery. The morbidity and complications were comparable in kind and severity with those observed at primary surgery and reported in the literature.[25,26]

Cytoreduction at interval surgery

One hundred and forty-two patients had interval debulking surgery. In 28% of the patients the tumour was already reduced to less than 1 cm by the induction chemotherapy. In 47% of the 102 patients with lesions of more than 1 cm at laparotomy, the tumour was reduced to lesions of less than 1 cm by cytoreductive surgery. It should be stressed that in the patients with lesions of less than 1 cm prior to cytoreduction as well as in patients with residual lesions after cytoreduction, tumour lesions were totally or partially resected. After surgery, only 25% of the patients had lesions of more than 2 cm, despite tumour resection.

Benefit of cytoreductive surgery

A direct effect of cytoreductive surgery was observed in the final response rate. The clinical complete response rate in the surgery group was 62%, compared to 34% in the no-surgery group.[27,28] The survival ($P = 0.003$) and the progression-free survival ($P = 0.005$) were significantly increased in favour of the patients assigned to intervention cytoreductive surgery. After a median follow-up period of 6.3 years (maximum 9.4 years) the 5-year survival rate is 24% in the surgery group and 13% in the no-surgery group, the 5-year progression-free survival is 14% and 44%, respectively (Fig. 38.2).

There was significantly better survival among patients with minimal residual disease of less than 1 cm prior to (2-year survival, 77%) and after (2-year survival, 62%) cytoreductive surgery compared to the patients with residual lesions of more than 1 cm after cytoreduction (2-year survival, 41%; $P \leq 0.001$). The same held true for the progression-free survival. The 2-year progression-free survival was 38% and 41%, respectively, for patients with minimal residual disease prior to cytoreduction and after cytoreduction, compared to 16% for patients with residual lesions of more than 1 cm after cytoreduction ($P \leq 0.001$). More striking is the identical survival (2-year survival, 41%) and progression-free survival (2-year survival, 19%) of the whole no-surgery group with the worst prognostic group of patients (those with residual lesion > 1 cm) after interval cytoreductive surgery (Fig. 38.3).

Reduction of the risk of death

In the multivariate analyses with all prognostic factors, interval cytoreductive surgery was an independent factor for survival ($P = 0.0062$) and progression-free survival ($P = 0.0035$). The reduction of the risk of death unadjusted for prognostic factors was 44% ($P = 0.003$). Also, after adjustment for the different prognostic factors, the risk of death reduction varied from 38% for tumour size to 51% for response to induction chemotherapy ($P = 0.001$). When all prognostic factors were taken into account simultaneously in a Cox regression model, the reduction in the risk of deaths due to surgery was 49% ($P = 0.004$). Even when patients were subdivided into high-risk and low-risk groups, based on either individual prognostic factors or multivariate risk, there was no difference in the relative survival benefit between the two groups. Therefore it was not possible to identify a special subgroup of patients who did not benefit from intervention debulking surgery.

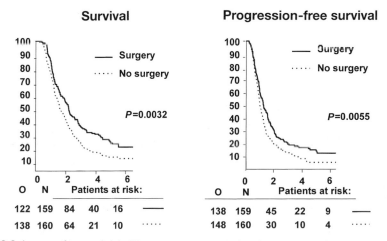

Fig. 38.2 Impact of interval debulking surgery on survival and progression-free survival.

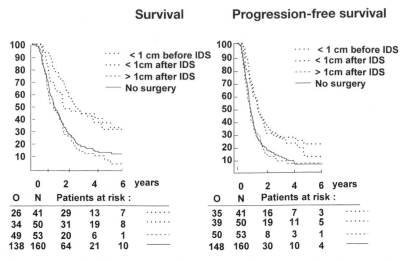

Fig. 38.3 Effect of interval debuling surgery and residual tumour volume on survival and progression-free survival.

Discussion

This is the first prospective randomized study to identify intervention debulking surgery as an independent prognostic factor for progression-free and overall survival.

Even after adjustment for all prognostic factors, the reduction of the risk of death was 49% ($P = 0.004$). The majority of studies in the literature compared the survival of patients with optimal cytoreductive surgery with that of patients with suboptimal tumor reduction.[1,15,16,20] All these studies are hampered by the unavoidable and serious bias inherent in the comparison of patients with different prognostic factors.

In the present study the progression-free and overall survival was significantly longer ($P = 0.001$) for patients with residual lesions of less than 1 cm before or after cytoreduction at intervention surgery compared with those of patients with larger residual lesions. None the less, the progression-free and overall survival of patients with suboptimal intervention debulking surgery—the patients with the worst prognosis—was no different from the progression-free and overall survival of the whole no-surgery group.

No subset of patients could be identified that did not benefit from intervention surgery. Surgery was not associated with death or severe morbidity; moreover, it did not interfere with postoperative chemotherapy. We believe that the increase in median progression-free and overall survival outweighs the morbidity associated with surgery. Interval cytoreductive surgery, however, cannot replace primary debulking surgery, which remains the gold standard in the management of ovarian cancer. Further investigations into the value of neoadjuvant chemotherapy in patients with advanced ovarian cancer are warranted. In the EORTC/GCCG a randomized study with neoadjuvant chemotherapy followed by interval debulking surgery versus primary cytoreductive surgery has recently been activated.

References

1. Neijt, J.P., ten Bokkel Huinink, W.W., van der Burg, M.E.L. *et al.* (1991). Long-term survival in ovarian cancer; Mature data from the Netherlands Joint Study Group for Ovarian Cancer. *Eur. J. Cancer.*, **27**, 1367–72.
2. Omura, G.A., Bundy, B.N., Berek, J.S. *et al.* (1989). Randomized trial of cyclophosphamide plus cisplatin with or without doxorubicin in ovarian cancer: a Gynecologic Oncology Group Study. *J. Clin. Oncol.*, **7**, 457–65.
3. Weber, A.M. and Kennedy A.W. 1994. The role of bowel resection in the primary surgical debulking of carcinoma of the ovary. *J. Am. Coll. Surg.*, **179**(4), 465–70.
4. Le, T., Krepart, G.V., Lotocti, R.J. *et al.* (1998). Does debulking surgery improve survival in biologically aggressive ovarian cancer? *Gynecol. Oncol.*, **67**, 208–14.
5. Michel, G., De Laco, P., Castaigne, D. *et al.* (1997). Extensive cytoreductive surgery in advanced ovarian cancer. *Eur. J. Gynecol. Oncol.*, **18**, 9–15.
6. Bristow, R.E., Montz, F.J., Lagasse, L.D. *et al.* (1999). Survival impact of surgical cytoreduction in stage IV epithelial ovarian cancer. *Gynecol. Oncol.*, **72**(3), 278–87.
7. Liu, P.C., Benjamin, I., Morgan, M.A. *et al.* (1997). Effect of surgical debulking on survival in stage IV ovarian cancer. *Gynecol. Oncol.*, **64**, 4–8.
8. Curtins, J.P., Malik, R., Venkatraman, E.S. *et al.* (1997). Stage IV ovarian cancer: impact of surgical debulking. *Gynecol. Oncol.*, **64**, 9–12.
9. Munkarah, A.R., Hallum, A.V., Morris, M. *et al.* (1997). Prognostic significance of residual disease in patients with stage IV epithelial ovarian cancer. *Gynecol. Oncol.*, **64**, 13–17.
10. Eisenkop, S., Nalick, R., Wang, H.J. *et al.* (1992). Peritoneal implant excision or ablation during cytoreductive surgery: The impact on survival. Abstract, *Gynecol. Oncol.*, **51**, 224–9.
11. Hacker, N.F., Berek, J.S., Lagasse, L.D., Nieberg, R.K., and Elashoff, R.M. (1983). Primary cytoreductive surgery for epithelial ovarian cancer. *Obstet. Gynecol.*, **61**, 413–20.
12. Hoskins, W.J., Bundy, B.N., Thipgen, T. *et al.* (1992). The influence of cytoreductive surgery on recurrence-free interval and survival in small-volume stage III epithelial ovarian cancer: a Gynecologic Oncology Group Study. *Gynecol. Oncol.*, **47**, 159–66.
13. Vergote, I., De Wever, I.W., Tjalma, W. *et al.* (1998). Neoadjuvant chemotherapy or primary debulking surgery in advanced ovarian carci-

noma: a retrospective analysis of 285 patients. *Gynecol. Oncol.*, **71**(3), 413–16.

14. Neijt, J.P., ten Bokkel Huinink, W.W., van der Burg, M.E.L. *et al.* (1984). Randomized trial comparing combination chemotherapy regimens (HEXA-CAF vs CHAP5) in advanced ovarian carcinoma. *Lancet*, **2**, 594–600.

15. Wils, J., Blijham, A., Naus, A. *et al.* (1986). Primary or delayed debulking surgery and chemotherapy consisting of cisplatin, doxorubicin, and cyclophosphamide in stage III–IV epithelial ovarian carcinoma. *J. Clin. Oncol.*, **4**, 1068–73.

16. Jacob, J.H., Gershenson, D.M., Morris, M. *et al.* (1991). Neoadjuvant chemotherapy and interval debulking surgery for advanced epithelial ovarian cancer. *Gynecol. Oncol.*, **42**, 146–50.

17. Neijt, J.P., ten Bokkel Huininck, W.W., van der Burg, M.E.L. *et al.* (1987). Randomized trial comparing two combination chemotherapy regimens (CHAP5 vs CP) in advanced ovarian carcinoma. *J. Clin. Oncol.* **5**, 1157–68.

18. Lawton, F.G., Redman, C.W.E., Luesley, D.M. *et al.* (1989). Neoadjuvant (cytoreductive) chemotherapy combined with intervention debulking surgery in advanced unresected epithelial ovarian cancer. *Obstet. Gynecol.*, **73**, 61–5.

19. Skipper, H. (1974). Thoughts on cancer chemotherapy and combination modality therapy. *J. Am. Med. Assoc.*, **230**, 1033–5.

20. Goldie, J.H. and Coldman, A.J. (1979). A mathematical model for relating the drug sensivity of tumors to their spontaneous mutation rate. *Cancer Treat. Rep.*, **63**, 1727–34.

21. Van der Burg, M.E.L., Van Lent, M., Buyse, M. *et al.* (1995). The effect of debulking surgery after induction chemotherapy on the prognosis in advanced epithelial ovarian cancer. *New Engl. J. Med.*, **332**, 629–34.

22. Kaplan, E.L. and Meier, P. (1958). Nonparametric estimation from incomplete observations. *J. Am. Stat. Assoc.*, **53**, 457–81.

23. Peto, R., Pike, M.C., Armitage, P. *et al.* (1976). Design and analysis of randomized clinical trials requiring prolonged observation of each patient. *Br. J. Cancer*, **35**, 1–39.

24. Cox, D.R. (1972). Regression models and life-tables. *J. R. Stat. Soc.*, **34**, 187–220.

25. Venesmaa, P. and Ylikorkala, O. (1992). Morbidity and mortality associated with primary and repeat operations for ovarian cancer. *Obstet. Gynecol.*, **79**, 168–72.

26. Ng, L.W., Rubin, S.C., Hoskins, W.J. *et al.* (1990). Aggressive chemosurgical debulking in patients with advanced ovarian cancer. *Gynecol. Oncol.*, **38**, 358–63.

27. Van der Burg, M.E.L. (2001). Debulking surgery in advanced ovarian cancer: the European study: In: *Recent advances in obstetrics and gynaecology* (ed J. Bonnar). Churchill Livingstone. ISBN 0-443-06022 3.

28. Van der Burg, M.E.L. (2001). Advanced ovarian cancer current treatment options *Oncology*, **2**, 109–18.

39. The role of surgery in relapse and palliation of ovarian cancer

Sean Kehoe and Christopher Mann

Introduction

As the majority of patients with ovarian cancer will succumb to the disease within 5 years from diagnosis, the role of surgery in relapsed disease and indeed palliation is important, albeit an area that has received relatively limited attention. When contemplating surgery, it is imperative that the objectives of the intervention are clearly defined. Curing patients with relapsed ovarian cancer is not a realistic goal, and hence the aims of surgery may be considered in two ways, to prolong survival or alleviate symptoms. Rarely, surgery may be performed for diagnostic purposes. Although much information regarding these aims is available within the medical literature, certain constraints exist rendering the interpretation of conclusions difficult because of the lack of randomized series, and small heterogeneous populations within those published.

Relapsed disease and surgical intervention

Patient selection

In order to discuss the therapeutic options it becomes necessary to define 'relapsed/recurrent' disease. This definition is variable, though most concur with a disease-free interval of at least 6 months from completion of primary chemotherapy. Within this period, evidence of disease is generally categorized as persistent in nature, and such patients may be considered for novel therapeutic strategies. Outside this period, platinum-based therapy is mainly used, vindicated by the response rate achieved. There is also a correlation between platinum efficacy and the duration of the disease-free interval.[1] Interestingly, the duration of the disease-free interval would also seem to correlate with surgical intervention and successful tumour debulking. Inevitably, the issues regarding tumour debulking, response to chemotherapy, and inherent tumour biology arise, and indeed a multivariate analysis on 704 women with recurrent ovarian cancer, does indicate the strong relationship between tumour load (<5 cm) and response to cytotoxics.[2]

Several factors influence both the decision to operate and the choice of procedure undertaken in recurrent disease. The most obvious is the patient's general physical well-being and capacity to withstand a general anaesthetic and laparotomy. Other factors include the sites of disease relapse, particularly if these are outside the abdominopelvic cavity. In ovarian cancer, recurrent disease tends to develop within the abdominopelvic cavity, although other sites are recorded. Vaccarello *et al.* (1995),[3] reviewed 57 patients with relapsed disease, noting that four had liver and three lung metastases. Corn *et al.* (1994),[4] treated 33 patients with relapsed disease, and although all had abdominopelvic-directed surgery, four had lung and three brain metastases. It has been reported[5] that in at least 10% of patients, relapsed disease develops in distant sites, making the logic of targeting surgery to the abdominal disease questionable. Indeed, whether patients with such disseminated disease at relapse should be considered for surgery at all is debatable. However, in stage IV disease there are advocates for primary debulking surgery[6] and opponents of it.[7] Nevertheless, caution is required when extrapolating the results of management undertaken in primary disease to relapsed disease.

Surgery for relapsed disease

As with primary surgery in ovarian cancer, the literature contains reports investigating the role of 'debulking' surgery at relapse, the premise for this approach being to enhance survival. Without the advantage of prospective randomized studies these reports must be assessed with this in mind. Furthermore, many series include patients who, according to the above definition, would be judged as having persistent disease. This accepted, such reports have permitted the elucidation of patient characteristics where 'debulking' surgery may enhance survival prospects (Table 39.1). The largest of these reports was by Segna *et al.* (1996).[8] This retrospective analysis involved 100 patients, all of whom had undergone attempted debulking surgery for relapsed disease detected clinically or radiologically. Survival outcome was best with optimum debulking (defined as <2 cm maximum diameter) at a median of 27.1 months, and the success rate correlated with the disease-free interval. Secondary debulking surgery was more likely to be achieved if the patient had undergone optimum primary surgery.

Table 39.1 Survival after debulking surgery for relapsed disease

Ref.	Number	Survival overall	Optimum vs non-optimum median survival
Segna et al.[8]	100	–	29 vs 9 months (P < 0.05)
Vaccarello et al.[9]	38	19 months (mean)	41 vs 23 months (optimum < 0.5 cm)
Janicke et al.[10]	30	18 months (median)	29 vs 9 months (P < 0.05)
Morris et al.[11]	30		18 vs 13 months (NS)
Eisenkop et al.[12]	22	–	43 vs 5 months (P < 0.003)

NS, not significant.

This compares with a median survival of only 9 months in patients with residual disease greater than 2 cm. Univariate analysis revealed that the cohort of patients most likely to have the best outcome was those with optimum primary debulking, a disease free interval of 12 months, and an age of less than 55 years.

A further study by Janicke et al. (1992)[10] reviewed 30 patients who underwent radical second operations in a relapse setting. The median recurrence-free interval was 16 months. Aggressive surgery achieved complete macroscopic clearance in 47% and optimum resection (<2 cm) in 40% of patients, although 63% of patients did require bowel resection to achieve this. Those with complete resection had a median survival time of 29 months, compared with 9 months for those with greater than 2 cm residual disease, P = 0.004. Using multivariate analysis, independent prognosticators of survival included residual disease after second surgery, the recurrence-free interval (at 12 months or more), and postoperative therapy. FIGO stage, tumour grade, and patient age were not significant determinants. In contrast to these studies, Morris et al. (1989)[11] described the outcome of patients with relapsed disease and at least 6 months disease-free interval from primary therapy, all of whom underwent secondary surgery. Optimum resection (<2 cm) was achieved in nearly 60% of patients, and though the trend was for a longer survival pattern in these women (median survival 18 months for <2 cm, 13.3 months for >2 cm), this was not a statistically significant difference.

Kuhn et al. (1998)[13] described an interesting prospective study in which patients were allocated treatment at relapse of either surgery and/or second-line chemotherapy. A total of 139 patients were recruited. Early relapse patients (defined as less than 12 months recurrence-free interval) were exposed to chemotherapy. Patients with relapse later than this were referred for surgery and tumour debulking. In these late-relapsing patients, those who had both surgery and chemotherapy had a longer median survival (38 months; P < 0.0001) compared to patients given only chemotherapy (at 12 months). However, a selection process was present for those in the surgical arm as not all patients with a recurrence-free interval larger than 12 months actually underwent surgery. The authors proposed that with late relapse combination modalities (surgery/chemotherapy) should be offered.

It would seem that certain patients treated by surgery and adjuvant chemotherapy have enhanced survival. Since these patients have survived 12 months from their primary disease a self-selection process is obvious. The true impact of debulking surgery can therefore only be determined within appropriately constructed randomized studies. Presently a European study (EORTC) is examining the role of debulking along with further interval surgery, compared with chemotherapy, based on the results of interval surgery in primary disease management (Chapter 38).[14] The outcome of this study will hopefully advance our knowledge with respect to the role of debulking at disease relapse.

Second-look and 'debulking surgery'

Debulking surgery has also been undertaken in patients with persistent disease found at second-look laparotomy (SLL). The largest report on this is by Williams et al. (1997)[15] who investigated 153 patients undergoing SLL: 124 had macroscopic and 29 microscopic disease. Of the 69 patients with greater than 1 cm disease, 15 were cytoreduced to microscopic residuum, and a further 15 to less than 1 cm residuum. Of 55 patients with 1 cm disease or less, 21 were cytoreduced to microscopic disease. Patients with more than 1 cm disease had the poorest survival pattern, and in all categories there was a significant improvement in survival with debulking. As the authors state, the question as to the beneficial effect of debulking for disease at SLL can only be answered by a randomized study. The proposal by Williams et al. of such a study is not novel; Hoskins et al. (1989)[16] nearly a decade earlier had published a similar study.

Palliation of bowel obstruction in relapsed disease

It is estimated that bowel obstruction occurs as a terminal event in up to 25–50% of patients with ovarian cancer. This has ramifications for patient care, in particular the decision to employ chemotherapy or surgery, and the impact this choice may have on duration and quality of life. Judicious clinical decisions are required as to which is the optimum mode of therapy. As with many interventions, there are no specific randomized studies to define the best therapeutic modality, and insurmountable ethical difficulties conceivably prevent such studies. Some clinicians advocate surgery, others chemotherapy. There are advantages and disadvantages with both approaches. Arguably, surgery affords a more instant alleviation of symptoms.

In patients' with bowel obstruction the primary objective is the relief of symptoms. Consideration must be given to the consequences of any intervention. For example, the relief of an obstruction achieved at the cost of inpatient care until death may not be the patient's desire, and so could be deemed a failure of therapy. Defining success and failure in this area can be extraordinarily complicated, as success defined by the physician may differ from that defined by the patient. Castaldo et al. (1981),[17] proposed a minimum survival after surgery of 60 days should be the standard for successful bowel diversion, and this is frequently employed in

Table 39.2 Median survival after surgery for bowel obstruction in ovarian cancer

Ref.	Number	Median survival (months)	Laparotomy only (%)
Jong et al.[19]	53	3.0	
Rubin et al.[20]	52	5.8	26.9
Redman et al.[21]	26	2.7	
Lund et al.[22]	26	2.3	26.9
Clarke-Pearson et al.[23]	49	5.7	
Mann et al.[24]	16	5.5	18.7
Larson et al.[25]	19	3.4	
Piver[26]	60	2.5	18.3
Krebs and Goplerud[27]	98*	3.1	12.0
Sun et al.[28]	23	3.2	26.0
Tunca et al.[29]	90	7.0	
Fernandes et al.[30]	34	35% at 12 months	
Gadducci et al.[31]	22	2.1	5
Total	567	3.85 (average)	19.1 (average)

118 procedures in 98 patients.

the literature. Other authors use discharge from hospital as a measure of successful outcome.

For some patients the most important information is the survival prospect and the failure rate of the proposed intervention. The median survival following surgery for bowel obstruction ranges from less than 3 to over 8 months, and from series involving over 500 procedures the average survival was reported as being 4 months (Table 39.2). Not unexpectedly the perioperative mortality (defined up to 30 days after surgery) is high, at 17%,[18] and equally important is the 'failed' procedure rate, of around 15–20%. Therefore approximately 66% of patients will have successful surgery as defined by resolution of bowel symptoms and survival over 60 days. Of course, this means that surgery in some cases could actually shorten the period of survival, and the need to identify those patients in whom surgery carries a reasonable chance of benefit is of paramount importance.

Developing prognostic factors for successful surgery in bowel obstruction

As previously alluded to, it is important to understand the restrictions of available studies. In particular, some studies involve patients with prior abdominal radiotherapy, which can increase the complication rates of surgery. As radiotherapy can result in bowel obstruction, it is important to confirm that the obstruction is secondary to recurrent disease. This problem relating to radiotherapy-induced bowel obstruction is less relevant in present practice.

Krebs and Goplerud (1983)[27] reported on 98 patients treated for bowel obstruction in ovarian cancer. Unsuccessful outcome was defined as death within 8 weeks of corrective surgery. The patient population was heterogeneous in nature, although most had exposure to either chemotherapy or radiotherapy. Analysis revealed that the patient's age (>65 years), poor nutritional status, tumour spread, and previous chemotherapy or radiotherapy were associated with a poorer outcome. Nutritional status was based on the recommendation of Dudrick et al. (1980),[32] involving a model which included body weight, serum albumin concentrations, and

Table 39.3 Scoring system for patients with bowel obstruction[27]

	Score 0	Score 1	Score 2
Age (years)	<45	45–65	>65
Nutritional deprivation	None	Moderate	Severe
Tumour status	Non-palpable	Abdominal	Liver/distant metastases
Ascites	None/mild	Moderate	Severe
Previous chemotherapy	None/inadequate	Failed (single)	Failed (combination)
Previous radiotherapy	None	To pelvis	To whole abdomen

Score of 6 or more indicates unlikely 'success' (i.e. survival <60 days) with surgery.

lymphocyte count. However, Krebs and Goplerud's series did not include logistic regression analysis for confounding variables, and importantly some patients underwent second bowel operations. Nevertheless, using the simple scoring system suggested by the group (Table 39.3) it is possible to predict 80% of patients who would survive more than 8 weeks after surgery.

More concise, statistically reliable indicators have been examined. A smaller prospective series by Fernandes et al. (1988)[30] investigated 62 patients with bowel obstruction, using 20 variables to define a prognostic model. Of these women, 45% received medical therapy and 58% surgical therapy for their obstruction. Univariate analysis revealed no survival difference whether medically or surgically managed, although inevitably there are certain inherent biases in the choice of treatment. Poorer-survival patterns were associated with patients older than 60 years, the presence of ascites, low serum albumin, elevated urea and alkaline phosphatase, lack of previous radiotherapy, advanced tumour stage, absence of obstruction on radiography, and a shorter diagnosis (primary) – obstruction interval. The 'absence' of definite obstruction on radiography, as a bad prognosis, was related to the fact that patients had widespread seedling disease at surgery. During the same period, Clarke-Pearson et al. (1988)[23] assessed variables in relation to surgical intervention for bowel obstruction which included those used by Krebs and Goplerud (1983),[27] along with other parameters. The aim was to define selective criteria that could predict survival for larger than 60 days. A total of 49 patients formed the study group and, in the model employed by these authors, the only independent significant prognosticators were preoperative serum albumin level and tumour status as determined clinically.

Zoetmulder et al. (1994)[33] reviewed 58 patients treated for bowel obstruction at their unit. In their review eight patients presented with bowel obstruction as the primary presentation of ovarian cancer. Using Cox regression analyses, both the interval from last treatment and the presence of ascites were variables associated with survival. However, 28 patients did not have surgery and all were treated conservatively prior to the selection of those for laparotomy. CA125 level did not prove to have a prognostic value in this series, and the criteria in making the decision for surgery were not defined. However, those who underwent surgery had a better overall outcome, as patients in poor physical condition were presumably not selected for operation. It is worth noting that one consistent prognostic variable seems to be nutritional status/albumin level, suggesting the potential benefits of pre-operative therapy. Although the most accurate methods on which to base clinical decisions preoperatively (for surgery or not) are still awaited, the proposals as shown in Table 39.3 give some guidance to the physician. Indeed, Larson et al. (1989)[25] applied this and concurred as to the practical value of such a scheme for clinical decision analysis.

Similarly, this approach was used by Gadduci et al. (1997),[31] whereby multivariate analysis revealed the Krebs and Goplerud score as an independent prognostic variable when applied to patients with bowel obstruction.

Alternatives to laparotomy

Some investigators have reported on the value of gastrotomies as an alternative treatment for terminal bowel obstruction. Cunningham et al. (1995)[34] used percutaneous gastrotomy for decompression purposes in 20 patients, 10 of whom had obstruction secondary to relapsed ovarian cancer. The patient population was selected on the basis that definitive surgical intervention was deemed inappropriate. The advantage of this approach is that general anaesthesia is avoided. Tube insertion was successful in all patients at first attempt, although 35% required tube replacement. From 20 patients 12 returned home for terminal care, and 18 patients had significant relief of symptoms. However, although surgery was considered not optional in these patients, two developed complete duodenal obstruction and underwent laparotomy. Campagnutta et al. (1996),[35] reported on 34 (29 ovarian cancer) patients using percutaneous endoscopic gastrostomy (PEG). Patients underwent endoscopy with mild sedation for tube placement. In two cases (5.4%) placement was unsuccessful, and in four cases transcutaneous placement of the catheter was undertaken. Symptomatic relief was achieved in 27 (84.4%) of cases and all patients were discharged from the hospital. Both these studies indicate the potential of alternative approaches to relief of symptoms in bowel obstruction without resort to laparotomy.

Quality of life

As in many cases, surgery in a relapse setting is primarily palliative, and thus the patient's quality of life should not be forgotten. The disease process and quality of life are intrinsically related, though quality of life is often ignored. Quality of life is often misunderstood or confused with side-effects of therapy. Although the sequelae of therapy impact on an individual's quality of life, it should always be borne in mind that there are many other factors that formulate quality of life. Without information on quality of life, it is only possible to evaluate morbidity and utilize this to facilitate decisions. An attempt at this was undertaken by Eisenkop et al. (1995).[12] In a cohort of 36 patients, all of whom had a 6-month interval from completion of chemotherapy, complete surgical excision of disease was achieved in 30 (83%) of patients. Surgical morbidity was 30% and mortality 2.8%. Of 27 women who had symptomatic relapsed disease, these symptoms were alleviated in 26 cases (96.2%). For those who survived for at least 6 months after surgery, an improvement in GOG (Gynecologic Oncology Group) scores (relating to mobility/ability to self-care) was detected. Further research is obviously warranted, although Eisenkop's study does suggest the potential quality of life benefits derived from surgical intervention for relapsed disease.

Conclusions

Many unanswered questions still remain when deciding on the clinical management of women with relapsed ovarian cancer. The clarification of the role of debulking in recurrent ovarian cancer should be forthcoming upon completion of relevant prospective trials. Until then the choice remains between surgery, chemotherapy or, indeed, non-intervention. Presently, it is only possible to select patients on an individual nature. There are exceptions to this, such as granulosa cell or borderline tumours, where second surgery is recommended at suspected relapse.

Regarding bowel obstruction, arguably, surgery affords the most rapid symptomatic relief and a reasonable outcome for a proportion of patients, although chemotherapy can be equally effective. Using clinical determinants, of known predictive variables, facilitates clinical decision making regarding the choice of patients for laparotomy. Other, less invasive methods are also available, such as gastrotomy tubes, which at least give an alternative to laparotomy. However, as in all aspects of interventions, patient choice is paramount, and possibly even more so when the survival time is limited.

References

1. Blackledge, G., Lawton, F., Redman, C., and Kelly, K. (1989). Response of patients in phase II studies of chemotherapy in ovarian cancer: implications for patient treatment and the design of phase II trials. *Br. J. Cancer*, 59, 650–3.
2. Eisenhauer, E.A., Vermorken, J.B., and van Glabbeke, M. (1997). Predictors of response to subsequent chemotherapy in platinum pretreated ovarian cancer: a multivariate analysis of 704 patients. *Ann. Oncol.*, 8, 963–8.

3. Vaccarello, L., Rubin, S.C., Vlamis, V. *et. al.* (1995). Cytoreductive surgery in ovarian carcinoma patients with a documented previously complete surgical response. *Gynecol Oncol.*, 57, 61–5.

4. Corn, B.W., Lanciano, R.M., Boente, M. *et al.* (1994). Recurrent ovarian cancer. Effective radiotherapeutic failure after chemotherapy failure. *Cancer*, 74, 2979–83.

5. Rose, P.G., Piver, M.S., Tsukada, Y., and Lau, T. (1989). Metastatic patterns in histologic variants of ovarian cancer. An autopsy study. *Cancer*, 64, 1508–13.

6. Liu, P.C., Benjamin, I., Morgan, M.A. *et al.* (1997). Effect of surgical debulking on survival in stage IV ovarian cancer. *Gynecol. Oncol.*, 64, 4–8.

7. Goodman, H.M., Harlow, B.L., Sheets, E.E. *et al.* (1992). The role of cytoreductive surgery in the management of stage IV epithelial ovarian cancer. *Gynecol. Oncol.*, 46, 367–71.

8. Segna, R.A., Dottino, P.R., Mandeli, J.P. (1993). Secondary cytoreduction for ovarian cancer following cisplatin therapy. *J. Clin Oncol.*, 11, 434–9.

9. Vaccarello, L., Rubin, S.C., Vlamis, V. *et al.* (1995). Cytoreductive surgery in ovarian carcinoma patients with a documented previously complete surgical response. *Gynecol. Oncol.*, 57, 61–5.

10. Janicke, F., Holscher, M., Kuhn, W. *et al.* (1992). Radical surgical procedure improves survival time on patients with recurrent ovarian cancer. *Cancer*, 70, 2129–36.

11. Morris, M., Gershenson, D.M., Wharton, J.T. *et al.* (1989). Secondary cytoreductive surgery for recurrent epithelial ovarian cancer. *Gynecol. Oncol.*, 34, 344–8.

12. Eisenkop, S.M., Friedman, R.L., and Wang, H.J. (1995). Secondary cytoreductive surgery for recurrent ovarian cancer. A prospective study. *Cancer*, 76, 1606–14.

13. Kuhn, W., Schmalfeldt, B., Pache, L. *et al.* (1998). Disease-adapted relapse therapy for ovarian cancer: results of a prospective study. *Int. J. Cancer*, 13, 57–63.

14. Van der Burg, M.E.L., van Lent, M., Buyse, M. *et al.* (1995). The effect of debulking surgery after induction chemotherapy on the prognosis in advanced epithelial ovarian cancer. *N. Engl. J. Med.*, 332, 629–34.

15. Williams, L., Brunetto, V.L., Yordan, E. *et al.* (1997). Secondary cytoreductive surgery at second-look laparotomy in advanced ovarian cancer. A gynecologic Oncology Group Study. *Gynecol. Oncol.*, 66, 171–8.

16. Hoskins, W.J., Rubin, S.C., Dulaney, E. *et al.* (1989). Influence of secondary cytoreductive surgery at the time of second-look laparotomy on the survival of patients with epithelial ovarian cancer. *Gynecol. Oncol.*, 34, 365–71.

17. Castaldo, T.W., Petrilli, E.S., Ballon, S.C., and Lagasse, L.D. (1981). Intestinal operations in patients with ovarian cancer. *Am. J. Obstet. Gynecol.*, 139, 80–4.

18. Hogan, W.M. and Boente, M.P. (1993). The role of surgery in the management of recurrent gynecologic cancer. *Semin. Oncol.*, 20, 462–72.

19. Jong, P., Sturgeon, J., and Jamieson, C.G. (1995). Benefit of palliative surgery for bowel obstruction in advanced ovarian cancer. *Can. J. Surg.*, 38, 454–7.

20. Rubin, S.C., Hoskins, W.J., Benjamin, I. *et al.* (1989). Palliative surgery for intestinal obstruction in advanced ovarian cancer. *Gynecol. Oncol.*, 34, 16–19.

21. Redman, C.W.E., Shafi, M.I., Ambrose, S. *et al.* (1988). Survival following intestinal obstruction in ovarian cancer. *Europ. J. Surg. Oncol.*, 14, 383–6.

22. Lund, B., Hansen, M., Lundvall, F. *et al.* (1989). Intestinal obstruction in patients with advanced carcinoma of the ovaries treated with combination chemotherapy. *Surg. Gynaecol. Obstet.*, 169, 213–18.

23. Clarke-Pearson, D.L., Delong, E.R., Chin, N. *et al.* (1988). Intestinal obstruction in patients with ovarian cancer. Variables associated with surgical complications and survival. *Arch. Surg.*, 123, 42–5.

24. Mann, C.H., Kehoe, S., Luesley, D.M. (1997). An audit of second-operations in relapsed ovarian cancer patients. *Br. J. Obstet. Gynaecol.*, 105, 963.

25. Larson, J.E., Podczaski, E.S., Manetta, A. *et al.* (1989). Bowel obstruction in patients with ovarian carcinoma: analysis of prognostic factors. *Gynecol. Oncol.*, 35, 61–5.

26. Piver, M.S., Barlow, J.J., Lele, S.B. *et. al.* (1982). Survival after ovarian cancer induced intestinal obstruction. *Gynecol Oncol.*, 13, 44–9.

27. Krebs, H.B. and Goplerud, D.R. (1983). Surgical management of bowel obstruction in advanced ovarian cancer. *Obstet. Gynecol.*, 61, 327–30.

28. Sun, X., Li, X., and Li, H. (1995). Management of intestinal obstruction in advanced ovarian cancer: an analysis of 57 cases. *Chinese J. Oncol.*, 17, 39–42.

29. Tunca, J.C., Buchler, D.A., and Mack, E.A. (1982). The management of ovarian cancer caused bowel obstruction. *Gynecol. Oncol.*, 12, 186–92.

30. Fernandes, J.R., Seymour, R.J., and Suissa, S. (1988). Bowel obstruction in patients with ovarian cancer: A search for prognostic factors. *Am. J. Obstet. Gynaecol.*, 158, 244–9.

31. Gadducci, A., Iacconi, P., Fanucchi, A. *et al.* (1997). Survival after intestinal obstruction in patients with fatal ovarian cancer; analysis of prognostic variables. *Int. J. Gynaecol. Cancer*, 8, 177–82.

32. Dudrick, S.J., Jensen, J.G., and Rowlands, B.J. (1980). Nutritional support: Assessment and indications. In *Nutrition in clinical surgery*, (ed. M. Deitel), pp. 19–27. Williams and Wilkins, Balitimore.

33. Zoetmulder, F.A.N., Helmerhorst, J.M.T., Coevorden, F.V., *et al.* (1994). Management of bowel obstruction in patients with advanced ovarian cancer. *Europ. J. Cancer*, 30A, 1625–8.

34. Cunningham, M.J., Bromberg, C., Kredenster, D.C. *et al.* (1995). Percutaneous gastrostomy for decompression in patients with advanced gynaecological malignancies. *Gynecol. Oncol.*, 59, 273–6.

35. Campagnutta, E., Cannizzaro, R., Gallo, A. *et al.* (1996). Palliative treatment of upper intestinal obstruction by gynaecological malignancy: The usefulness of percutaneous endoscopic gastrostomy. *Gynecol. Oncol.*, 62, 103–5.

40. The role of minimal access surgery in ovarian cancer

Robin A.F. Crawford

This chapter will address the following points:

(1) the operative procedure for laparoscopy for ovarian masses;
(2) laparoscopy and ovarian masses;
(3) should laparoscopy be used for the management of adnexal masses?
(4) the use of laparoscopy to assess operability in advanced disease
(5) second-look laparoscopy
(6) the risks of the pneumoperitoneum and the laparoscopic techniques on the spread of ovarian cancer; and
(7) prophylactic oophorectomy for at-risk patients.

The operative procedure for laparoscopy

Operative laparoscopy has progressed dramatically in the past 10 years, with most operative procedures now having an endoscopic equivalent. Gynaecological cancer has attracted the attention of the skilled laparoscopist because the laparoscopic equivalent of open radical surgery could potentially be performed without the apparent morbidity. In using the laparoscopic approach, there is improved exposure in the true pelvis and significant magnification of the structures examined by telescope, allowing more accurate dissection. There is a reduced incidence of ileus due to less bowel handling and postoperative analgesia requirements are reduced. These, in turn, reduce hospital stay. In addition, the cosmetic appearance of the laparoscopic operation is better than that of laparotomy. The disadvantage of the laparoscopic approach to gynaecological oncology is that it is technically more difficult and the theatre time required is longer. Complications have been reported, and the relatively high incidence of these may be related to a lack of appropriate training and expertise, as well as the difficulties encountered in developing a new procedure.

There is no consensus about performing laparoscopy in patients with suspected ovarian cancer. An information sheet for patients undergoing laparoscopic removal of a suspicious ovarian mass should inform them that there is a risk of finding an ovarian cancer. It is preferable to have a definite pathological result before proceeding with further surgery, and patients should be warned that they might need to undergo the definitive procedure some days after the laparoscopy under a separate anaesthetic.

The method of initial port entry will depend on the operator. For patients with ascites and advanced disease an open approach would be preferred (as there is a significant risk of visceral perforation due to disease) using a 10 mm operating laparoscope to provide a clear view. The initial inspection allows documentation of the extent of disease. The use of local anaesthetic (0.25% bupivacaine) prior to any port site insertion reduces postoperative pain significantly. After the initial port, all ports are inserted under direct vision. When operating on a suspicious adnexal mass it is important to take a sample of peritoneal fluid for cytology, using an aspirator–irrigator through a 5 mm accessory port. If there is no free fluid, then irrigation with saline will provide a sample. This sample can be collected conveniently in a trap fitted to the aspirator outflow.

As in open surgery, the anatomical landmarks are defined and the procedure carried out appropriately. If the adnexal mass is mobile, the ureter is defined in its course before any surgery. If there is any doubt with a fixed ovarian mass, it is appropriate to define the ureter by opening the retroperitoneum via the pelvic sidewall and retracting the ureter from the medial leaf of the peritoneum. This also allows clear identification of the ovarian vessels, which can be divided using bipolar diathermy then scissors. Bipolar diathermy causes less risk of thermal damage than does monopolar diathermy. The majority of diathermy-related bowel injuries in advanced laparoscopy (67%) have been in conjunction with monopolar usage.[1] Other methods of haemostasis include vascular clips, ties, or ultrasound dissector. To remove the adnexal mass, the suspect ovary should be placed in a waterproof bag. The cyst can then be deflated in the bag prior to removal through the umbilical port. An omental biopsy can be taken using diathermy or clips. An infracolic omentectomy is feasible laparoscopically. The port site used for retrieval can be enlarged to facilitate removal. A colpotomy has been used by some surgeons to allow tissue retrieval. When using larger ports (7 mm or greater) the sheath should be closed. This is especially important in the lateral ports to avoid herniation. Several devices are available to assist with this closure.

Laparoscopic transperitoneal pelvic lymphadenectomy has become a standard operation in less than a decade since it was first described by Professor Querleu (1991).[2] Two monitors are placed just beyond the patient's feet, allowing a comfortable operating position for the two surgeons. The bladder is kept empty with a Foley catheter. For the primary portal a 10 mm 0° laparoscope is inserted through an umbilical incision. Three further ports are used for manipulation, dissection, haemostasis, and specimen retrieval. Two 5 mm ports are used in the iliac fossae and a 10–12 mm port is used in the midline suprapubic area. The 5 mm ports are placed laterally to allow a good angle for operating on the contralateral pelvic sidewall. The larger midline port allows for specimen retrieval and the use of a clip applicator or linear stapler/cutter. The use of a clear port with a flap valve allows easy tissue retrieval as the lymph nodes can be observed as they are withdrawn from the abdomen. As usual for operative laparoscopy, a thorough inspection of the abdomen is performed. A steep Trendelenburg position allows the small bowel to fall out of the pelvis. The round ligament is divided with diathermy. The peritoneum is then retracted medially allowing access to the pelvic sidewall. If the lymphadenectomy is diagnostic and the uterus is being left *in situ*, the round ligament can be left intact. Using scissors and dissectors, the external iliac vessels are visualized. The temptation is to begin the dissection too laterally which leads to damage of the genito-femoral nerve and the psoas muscle. The paravesical and pararectal spaces are developed as in the open procedure. One may strip the external iliac vessels first but some operators clear the obturator fossa early as bleeding will stain the tissues, reducing the clarity of the picture. The obturator fossa is easily entered by slipping medially over the external iliac vein. Alternatively, access to this area can be obtained by dissecting behind the external iliac vessels and retracting them medially. Attention is paid to preserving the obturator nerve by identifying it before any sharp dissection or diathermy is performed. To retrieve the nodal tissue, a laparoscopic 10 mm Babcock forceps may be utilized. Alternatively, the three-pronged Ceolio-extractor (Lépine, Lyon, France) can be used. Further techniques include withdrawing the nodes into a reducing sleeve inside the 10 mm port or placing the nodes in a vaginal tube. The contamination of the port site with malignant tissue is a potential problem of more significance with ovarian cancer than cervical carcinoma. The nodal tissue from the external iliac vessels, adjacent to the internal iliac vessels, in and around the obturator fossa is easily removed. Troublesome bleeding can occur if the interiliac nodes are removed without careful dissection. Retraction of the ureter medially and the peritoneum cranially exposes the common iliac region, allowing removal of the nodal tissue from the lateral margin.

Laparoscopic para-aortic lymphadenectomy, described in 1992 by Childers[3] and then in 1993 by Querleu,[4] has a role in gynaecological cancer. The value of performing lymphadenectomy will be discussed elsewhere in this book. In advanced-stage epithelial disease, lymphadenectomy may form part of debulking surgery. However, it would be unusual to perform this debulking surgery laparoscopically. In early stage epithelial cancer, lymphadenectomy may allow complete staging. Querleu and LeBlanc (1994)[5] reported that it was feasible to perform lymphadenectomies up to the level of the renal vessels as a part of a restaging procedure in nine women who had a diagnosis of early ovarian cancer. Other authors[6,7] have reported case series of patients referred with incomplete staging. These centres have significant laparoscopic

experience and show that the operation is feasible using a laparoscopic approach. In women who are node negative early disease (i.e. true stage I), there are reports of survival without chemotherapy in excess of 90%.[8] In presumed early stage germ cell tumours, Charvolin and Querleu (1999)[9] suggest that there may be a survival advantage in those who undergo a complete infrarenal lymphadenectomy. The authors report that this may be done as secondary surgery using laparoscopy.

For transperitoneal para-aortic node dissection, the monitors are placed adjacent to the head of the patient. It is convenient to have the surgeon operating between the legs of the patient and the camera operator standing to the left of the patient. Identification of the landmarks is important, and steep Trendelenberg aids with displacement of the small bowel into the upper abdomen. On occasion, a further port can be useful for a fan retractor. An incision is made at the level of the bifurcation of the aorta over the common iliac artery. This allows the development of the retroperitoneal space and, at the same time, using the peritoneum to keep the small bowel from obscuring the field. As in open lymphadenectomy, the nodal tissue is identified by finding the adventitia of the aorta with sharp dissection and diathermy. The fat pad containing the lymph nodes is then removed. "Liga" clips can be useful for the perforating vessels. The vascular anatomy relating to the inferior vena cava as seen from the laparoscopic approach in gynaecological oncology is elegantly described by Possover *et al.* (1998).[10] Bipolar diathermy is used in preference to monopolar diathermy as it is more precise. Care must be taken in identifying the inferior mesenteric pedicle and the ureters. The Harmonic scalpel (Ultracision–Ethicon Endosurgery; an ultrasound cutting coagulating device) may be useful in performing the lymphadenectomy as it will reduce the changing of instruments during the procedure.

Fowler *et al.* (1993)[11] compared the yield from laparoscopic and open lymphadenectomies. In this study, between 62% and 97% of the total lymph nodes were sampled laparoscopically. It was noted that there was a significant learning curve for the techniques required for laparoscopic lymphadenectomy. Interestingly, no patient with negative nodes at laparoscopy had positive pelvic nodes at laparotomy. Learning the procedure on the pig model may reduce the morbidity and improve the outcomes when applied to humans. Querleu *et al.* (1998)[12] demonstrated that, after operating on seven pigs, a resident was capable of performing a unilateral pelvic lymphadenectomy in less than 30 minutes, removing more than 95% of the nodal tissue and without significant complications. The same level of competence was achieved for para-aortic node dissection after 14 operations. The same group showed that it required 10 porcine operations to learn the retroperitoneal technique.[13] Lanvin *et al.* (1997)[14] compared transperitoneal laparoscopic and open approaches for a complete lymphadenectomy in pigs. There was no difference in lymph node count, although the laparoscopic procedure took twice as long as the open procedure. There was significantly less adhesion formation with the laparoscopic approach.[15]

It is well documented that restaging of early ovarian cancer will lead to an upstaging in over 30% of cases.[16] The result of this upstaging leads to chemotherapy for those upstaged and a more accurate prediction of survival for those who are true early stage.

The criticism of laparoscopy is that there is no tactile sense associated with the minimal access approach. Possover *et al.* (1995)[17] showed that in a series of 223 patients with advanced ovarian cancer, visualization of the metastases in the omentum, bowel, and mesentery was possible and not compromised by the views obtained by laparoscopy. They concluded that in early ovarian cancer it was not therefore necessary to check the bowel manually for spread.

In conclusion, the gynaecological oncologist who has acquired the necessary laparoscopic skills is able to perform all the techniques needed for ovarian cancer management, using either the conventional or laparoscopic approach. The surgical technique used will obviously depend on the patient's presenting condition, as the laparoscopic approach may be possible in the woman with large masses involving bowel only to a few expert gynaecological oncological laparoscopists.

Laparoscopy and ovarian mass

The traditional teaching for the management of an ovarian mass or adnexal mass was surgical removal, as there was no clear way of determining whether or not it was malignant. It became increasingly obvious that a more selective approach to this management was required. A small ovarian cyst in a premenopausal woman does not have the same malignant potential as a persistent large adnexal mass in the postmenopausal woman. Ultrasound and tumour marker estimation allowed some element of selection, with the 'risk of malignancy' index.[18] If the removal of a benign adnexal mass using laparoscopic techniques allows the safe management of a woman with a short hospital stay, minimal pain, good cosmesis, and an early return to full function, then the technique is considered an advance. If, on the other hand, the laparoscopic management is associated with inadequate staging, the piecemeal removal of a potentially curable early cancer, the dissemination of a tumour with a possible worse outcome, then laparoscopy has no role in the ovarian cancer therapy. The incidence of finding a malignant cyst at laparoscopy where preoperative investigations suggested that the mass was benign (i.e. false negatives) ranges from 0.04% to 3.7%.[19–24] Canis *et al.* (1994)[24] advocated that women with adnexal masses showing extraovarian spread or suspicious cysts over 8 cm should be treated by laparotomy.

As operative laparoscopy became more widely used, instances of patients with ovarian cancer who had been inappropriately managed using laparoscopy were reported. Maiman *et al.* (1991)[25] surveyed the Society of Gynecologic Oncologists concerning the 'laparoscopic management of ovarian neoplasms subsequently found to be malignant'. Forty-two per cent of SGO membership replied to a questionnaire and 42 cases of ovarian cancer were reviewed. Of the cases reported, 31% were thought to be benign (showing the following characteristics: less than 8 cm; unilateral; cystic; and unilocular). Only 17% of the cases had an immediate laparotomy following the laparoscopy. The mean interval to a subsequent laparotomy was 4.8 weeks, with 16 of the 30 cases having their laparotomy within 2 weeks. Management of ovarian cysts by general gynaecologists using laparoscopic means was the third

most common indication for operative laparoscopy during this time period,[19] and one would expect more cases of ovarian cancer to have been assessed laparoscopically. Maiman[25] remarked that the reason that there were only 42 cases recorded in his survey was the limited population that he surveyed (gynecologic oncologists). As there was no denominator in the Maiman study, it is not possible to determine how frequently ovarian cancer was managed laparoscopically. The SGO survey highlighted that there was no clear way of determining which adnexal mass was malignant preoperatively. Secondly, even using selection criteria for benign lesions, nearly one-third of the masses were malignant on histological analysis.

Crawford *et al.* (1995)[26] performed a similar survey, asking members of the British Gynaecological Cancer Society (a multidisciplinary group with a specific interest in gynaecological cancer) about the management of adnexal masses with laparoscopic surgery in 1994. The aim was to construct guidelines for the use of minimal access surgery for adnexal masses for British gynaecologists. Fifty-one gynaecologists replied, representing 64.5% of the BGCS membership. These gynaecologists felt that adnexal masses with solid elements (87%), diameter greater than 8 cm (71%), multilocular (69%) or bilateral (65%) cysts, or those with increased blood flow on Doppler scanning (68%) should be operated on using conventional techniques. The criticism of constructing guidelines in this way is that it is not evidence based. These proposed guidelines need to be reviewed. Although there had been an increase in the tertiary referrals of ovarian cancer involving laparoscopy to the Royal Marsden Hospital, which prompted the 1994 Crawford survey, only 29 cases of ovarian cancer associated with, or managed by laparoscopy, were reported from the UK survey, including 10 from the Royal Marsden. The presented case histories highlighted problems such as delay in appropriate staging, limited initial surgery, and port site implantation. The delay in appropriate staging was 6.5 weeks. This is similar to data from America. Wenzl *et al.* (1996)[27] surveyed Austrian practice. This study covered over 16 000 laparoscopic procedures for adnexal masses and included 108 ovarian cancers. Twenty patients were treated with laparoscopy alone. In 22 cases, laparoscopy was followed by immediate laparotomy. A delayed laparotomy (3–1415 days) was performed in 54 cases. Staging revealed FIGO classifications from stages Ia to IV. Laparoscopic surgery on ovarian malignancies was rare (0.65% of all endoscopic surgeries on adnexal masses) in the Austrian setting. This relatively low frequency may be due to less frequent use of laparoscopy in assessing the suspicious adnexal mass, as well as underreporting, especially if it is felt to be poor practice to use a laparoscopic approach to patients with ovarian cancer. Wenzl *et al.* (1996)[27] suggested that in cases of malignancy, a laparotomy has to be performed to ensure optimal staging and treatment. Their survey did not address this question directly and only reported that there were some cases of ovarian cancer that were managed in a suboptimal fashion. Further investigation of these Austrian cases[28] compared patients receiving their primary surgical treatment (by laparotomy) within 17 days ($n = 24$ patients) to a group whose first therapeutic surgery was delayed by more than 17 days ($n = 24$ patients). Twenty-two cases had their definitive surgery immediately following the diagnostic laparoscopy and were therefore used as controls. In patients with borderline tumours who underwent laparotomy more than 17 days after laparoscopy, the odds ratio (OR) for FIGO stage IIb–IV disease was 5.3 (95% confidence interval (CI) 0.40, infinity), compared with patients undergoing immediate laparotomy. Patients with invasive ovarian cancer who underwent laparotomy more than 17 days after laparoscopy had an OR of 9.2 (CI 0.92, 481) for stage IIb–IV disease, compared with patients undergoing immediate laparotomy. In patients with borderline tumours, multivariate analysis showed that the timing of laparotomy is an independent prognostic factor for the stage of disease. A delay between laparoscopy and laparotomy may affect adversely the distribution of disease stage, although not at significant levels in this study. Unfortunately, it is not possible to ascertain the cause of the delay in these patients.

Therefore, the problem associated with ovarian cancer and laparoscopic management is probably related to delay. On balance of evidence, it is felt that if the tumour is entirely and immediately removed, the puncture of a stage I ovarian cancer has no influence on the prognosis (no effect for intraoperative cyst rupture, refs 29–34; or a detrimental effect of cyst rupture, refs 35,36). In contrast, the inadequate surgical management of an undiagnosed ovarian cancer may worsen the prognosis. The diagnosis is the key step. To be able to treat immediately and completely an ovarian cancer when managing an ovarian tumour surgically is the ideal. In an era of increasing subspecialization, not all gynaecologists will perform the appropriate surgery for women with ovarian cancer, whether diagnosed at laparoscopy or laparotomy. Therefore, it would be sensible for a pathway to be defined for these patients, involving the local cancer centre team, allowing rapid access to the appropriate management.

Should laparoscopy be used for the management of adnexal masses?

It is obvious that operative laparoscopy has been an advance in the management of benign adnexal masses.[37] The procedure is associated with a short hospital stay (even day case), low usage of analgesia, a good cosmetic result, and rapid return to function for the woman. Can we detect which adnexal mass is benign prior to surgery? The chance of finding a malignant cyst at laparoscopic surgery where preoperative investigations suggest a benign lesion ranges from 0.04% to 3.7%[19–24,38] Practitioners who use operative laparoscopy for 'benign' masses must have an arrangement for immediate intervention by a gynaecological oncologist if the mass is obviously malignant (confirmed on frozen section) or recourse to early management in the unlikely event of the histology showing malignancy. As the pathology result is benign in excess of 96% of cases, it is likely that there will be delay before further management for those women with a malignant diagnosis unless this pathway has been determined beforehand.

If all women with adnexal pathology are operated on using a laparoscopic approach regardless of the ultrasound or tumour marker findings, the likelihood of a malignant diagnosis rises from less than 4% to about 13%.[39,40] Most practitioners have excluded patients who have either ascites, gross metastatic disease,

fixed pelvic mass, or a pelvic mass extending above the umbilicus from primary laparoscopic management. van Dam et al. (1997)[41] used laparoscopy in advanced disease to determine whether aggressive surgery is feasible at the primary setting or in the interval setting; this will be discussed later.

The malignant potential of small, simple ovarian cysts (less than 5 cm diameter) in the postmenopausal group is very small (0.7%).[42] Therefore, these cysts can be managed safely using laparoscopic techniques if intervention is required. Dottino et al. (1999)[40] report that it is feasible to offer laparoscopic surgery for adnexal masses regardless of age. In their study, 13% of the group undergoing laparoscopy had a malignant diagnosis. Access to frozen section pathology was available although the concordance with subsequent pathology was only 97%. Canis et al. (1997)[43,44] undertook a prospective study of laparoscopic management of ovarian masses that appeared suspicious on ultrasound. Patients with general contraindications to laparoscopy, obviously disseminated ovarian cancer, and technically impossible laparoscopic treatment were excluded from the study. By using a protocol that allowed evaluation of the ultrasonically suspicious adnexal mass by laparoscopy, more than 80% of 323 suspicious cases were dealt with entirely laparoscopically as the adnexal mass was indeed benign.

Laparoscopic diagnosis is safe and reliable when used cautiously. The surgical diagnosis may, and should probably, be performed by laparoscopy whatever the ultrasonographic appearance of the tumour. Masses diagnosed as suspicious at surgery should be treated by appropriate methods. Washings should be taken for cytology. Biopsies should be taken of suspicious areas distant from the ovary. The ovary/adnexal mass should be removed intact in a specimen-retrieval bag. If these procedures cannot be completed laparoscopically without compromise, then a laparotomy should be performed. In young patients, conservative surgery is the main advantage of laparoscopy, and should be achieved for most benign masses. Frozen section can be used when treating highly suspicious masses, allowing immediate staging and avoiding the disadvantages of a second surgical procedure. However, there are problems associated with frozen section analysis, especially in relation to borderline tumours, and it may be more appropriate to obtain rapid processing of a paraffin section. This not only allows better usage of the operating time but the patient is also aware of the procedure that she will undergo, i.e. she will not have to consent to the open-ended '? proceed' operation. The patient is warned ahead of the first surgery that it may be necessary to perform a second operation rapidly after the first if malignancy is detected. Whenever a malignant tumour has been missed at laparoscopy, restaging is required and should be considered to be an oncological emergency.

Use of laparoscopy to assess operability in advanced disease

van Dam et al. (1997)[41] reported a study using laparoscopy to assess operability in advanced ovarian cancer. Patients with suspected advanced ovarian cancer underwent an open laparoscopy to obtain a tissue diagnosis and to assess whether surgery was technically feasible. Laparoscopy was not possible in 4% of cases. Malignancy was confirmed in 81% (67/83) and 58 patients had an ovarian primary. Operability was correctly confirmed in 91% of cases with ovarian cancer and there were six port-site implantations. Of the 58 with advanced ovarian cancer, 48% (28) had primary surgery, with 25 patients having no residual macroscopic disease. Twenty-four patients had interval debulking procedures and 12% (six patients) had progressive disease despite primary and secondary chemotherapy. By using laparoscopy to assess patients with presumed advanced ovarian cancer, laparotomy was avoided in 31% (26/83) patients with minimum morbidity. The authors concluded that, in combination with studies addressing primary versus interval debulking, laparoscopy needs to be studied further.

Second-look laparoscopy compares with laparotomy but what is the overall value?

A second-look procedure can be performed by laparoscopy in women with ovarian cancer. Originally, a laparoscopic approach was not felt to be helpful because of the complications seen in women who have had extensive prior surgery and because of the false-negative rate due to adhesions. A multicentre Italian study showed that the relative risk for a poor outcome related to laparoscopic second-look as opposed to laparotomy was 1.83.[45] The technical expertise available may now allow safe operative laparoscopy in these patients, but the evidence to show that a second-look procedure leads to a better outcome, is not persuasive.

Risk of pneumoperitoneum: is the operation using laparoscopy detrimental for the patient's health compared with the open procedure?

Multiple case reports have been published relating to malignant implantation in port sites following laparoscopic management of abdominal malignancy. Unfortunately, while case reports highlight a concern, they cannot give an this prevalence of the problem reported because there is no denominator. There have been several papers relating to the incidence of this occurrence. Childers et al. (1994)[46] reviewed the work at Tucson relating to laparoscopic surgery and ovarian cancer. They found 1% of cases developed abdominal wall tumour implantation. Kruitwagen et al. (1996)[47] reported on a series of 419 patients with ovarian cancer presenting between 1979 and 1991. Women having a paracentesis prior to surgery developed a tumour nodule at the entry site in 10% of cases, compared to 16% of women undergoing a diagnostic laparoscopy prior to surgery. All the women developing these nodules (whether related to paracentesis or laparoscopy) had stage III or IV disease, moderately or poorly differentiated tumours and

ascites. Interestingly, in 4% of those women with abdominal-wall metastases they were not associated with a wound (either paracentesis or port site). Although patients with port-site metastases had a shorter survival time, the difference was not significant compared to women without abdominal wall implants using a Cox proportional hazards model. It cannot be concluded that the patients with the abdominal-wall implants had a shorter survival due to the paracentesis or laparoscopy, as all these women had advanced disease with ascites. It may be features of a more aggressive tumour with a relative immunological deficiency in the patient that allow the tumour nodule to grow in the port site. van Damm et al. (1999)[48] reported that laparoscopy could be used safely in advanced ovarian cancer without significant risk of port-site implantation if the port site was closed in several layers, and that the definitive treatment was started early (within 1 week). The definitive treatment was cytoreductive surgery with excision of the port site or chemotherapy.

In view of the port-site metastasis problem, researchers looked at models to see whether the laparoscopic approach was a cause of these metastases and therefore should be contraindicated in ovarian cancer management. Animal models have been used to determine whether aspects of the pneumoperitoneum are adverse. Koster et al. (1996)[49] used a mouse model to compare tumour spread between animals that had undergone a CO_2-pneumoperitoneum and the control group which had no pneumoperitoneum. The mice with a CO_2-pneumoperitoneum had a significantly greater number and increased size of intra-abdominal metastases. The technique in this paper may be slightly questionable as the duration of the procedure (90-minute pneumoperitoneum) for the mice was similar or greater in length to that of the procedure used in humans, and therefore not proportional to the model. Canis et al. (1998)[50,51] used a rat model to observe tumour growth of ovarian cancer cells at the time of laparoscopy or laparotomy. Instilling malignant cells at the time of laparoscopy or laparotomy was intended to mimic the rupture of a malignant cyst. The rats underwent either a laparotomy or laparoscopy at several different insufflation pressures. The mean dissemination score ($\pm$ SD) (a semiquantitative measure of tumour spread at the time of animal sacrifice 2 weeks after the instillation of tumour cells), was 83.4 $\pm$ 12 in the laparotomy group and 67.3 $\pm$ 16 and 71.9 $\pm$ 17 in the 4 and 10 mmHg CO_2-pneumoperitoneum groups, respectively ($P <$ 0.01). The incidence of wound metastasis was 96% in the laparotomy group and 55% and 54% in the 4 mmHg and 10 mmHg pneumoperitoneum groups, respectively. The authors concluded that tumour growth was greater after laparotomy than after laparoscopy, but peritoneal tumour dissemination was more severe after the higher-pressure CO_2-pneumoperitoneum. It is not clear how this experiment would translate to the human setting. A further animal experiment, comparing laparotomy to CO_2 laparoscopy and gasless laparoscopy,[52] showed that the gasless approach was associated with less tumour implanatation. In both experiments with solid tumour implants and cell suspensions, the CO_2 laparoscopy was associated with significantly more peritoneal tumour growth and port-site implantation compared with the gasless laparoscopy. Laparoscopy was associated with a significantly smaller amount of peritoneal disease than laparotomy. The port site used for tumour extraction was associated with more deposits than the other ports sites. Bouvy *et al.* (1996)[52] came to the following conclusions: that direct contact between solid tumour and the port site enhances local tumour growth, that laparoscopy is associated with less intraperitoneal tumour growth than laparotomy, and that insufflation of CO_2 promotes tumour growth at the peritoneum and is associated with more abdominal-wall metastases than gasless laparoscopy. However, their final conclusion, that CO_2 promotes tumour growth at the peritoneum, is not valid from the presented data and requires further investigation. An Australian study[53] presented similar data and showed that CO_2 insufflation during laparoscopy resulted in widespread tumour dissemination and implantation, when compared with laparotomy and gasless laparoscopy.

The importance of the pneumoperitoneum may be less important when one considers the effect of tumour manipulation during surgery.[54] The operation (either laparotomy or laparoscopy in the rat model) did not affect spread *per se* but it was more related to the tumour manipulation.

Animal models used to investigate the problem with port-site implantation have not given consistent answers to the underlying cause of port-site implantation.[55] Pretreatment of port sites with antiseptic or antibiotic may reduce the implantation rate by virtue of interfering with the viable cancer cells.[56] Childers *et al.* (1994)[46] suggested that port-site wounds should be irrigated in order to reduce the likelihood of port-site recurrence. A literature review up to September 1996[57] suggested that risk factors for port-site recurrence included presence of ascites in addition to the diagnosis of ovarian cancer (as opposed to other cancers). A review of the experimental evidence for tumour dissemination[58] suggested that the evidence to date is not sufficiently clear for a decision on the property laparoscopic management of ovarian masses and cancer. The papers reviewed have inadequately described the methodology for the cancer model used and the power calculation to ensure statistical differences, as well as the surgical procedure.

Prophylactic oophorectomy by laparoscopy

A laparoscopic approach to prophylactic oophorectomy is entirely suitable. The procedure is quick and requires little time in hospital or off work. The patient who is at significant risk for ovarian cancer, as determined in a cancer genetics clinic, is offered initial screening according to the UK CCCR family history screening protocol. If she requests oophorectomy or the screen becomes abnormal, surgery is considered. The risks associated with the procedure (risk of damage to other organs and structures; risk of proceeding to an open procedure; risk of port-site herniation) are discussed. Consideration is given to the potential finding, either at laparoscopy or on histopathology report, of ovarian cancer. A protocol for the management of this eventuality allows rapid and appropriate management using the multidisciplinary approach. It is not suitable to discuss this for the first time after the event has occurred. The aim should be to offer definitive surgery in the case of an ovarian cancer within 1 week of the laparoscopic approach.

The decision to perform bilateral salpingo-oophorectomy alone or to include hysterectomy depends on the woman's individual situation. If there is an indication to perform the hysterectomy, laparoscopically assisted vaginal hysterectomy and bilateral salpingo-oophorectomy might be feasible. The additional morbidity of hysterectomy is not justified without uterine pathology. In women with a family history, it is appropriate to remove the Fallopian tubes as well as the ovarian tissue, as there is a suggestion that genetic predisposition may affect the tubal epithelium as well as the ovarian tissue.[59] Interestingly, Meiser *et al.* (1999)[60] demonstrated that breast/ovarian cancer anxiety, rather than objective risk, is the major factor that determines women's attitudes to prophylactic oophorectomy.

In a personal series of 30 women who have had prophylactic bilateral sphingo-oophorectomy (BSO) for genetic reasons, using laparoscopic techniques, that have seen no cases of unexpected carcinoma. The average operating time for BSO is 59 minutes, with an overnight stay (less than 24 hours). There was one case of laparotomy needed to complete the procedure due to significant adhesions and one case of small bowel obstruction which settled spontaneously. These figures are similar to other published figures.[61]

In all patients undergoing laparoscopic prophylactic bilateral salpingo-oophorectomy, thorough inspection of the peritoneum should be undertaken. Washings should be sent for cytology. The ovaries and tubes should be removed in their entirety in a bag (i.e. not piecemeal through the port) and sampled extensively by the pathologist.

The benefit in terms of life years gained by prophylactic oophorectomy may be from 0.3 to 1.7 years[62] and therefore a conservative approach to surgical excision should be encouraged. The low risk of the laparoscopic surgery and the minimal effect on the patient makes laparoscopic surgery the method of choice for these prophylactic operations.

References

1. Chapron, C., Pierre, F., Harchaoui, Y. *et al.* (1999). Gastrointestinal injuries during gynaecological laparoscopy. *Hum. Reprod.*, **14**, 333–7.
2. Querleu, D., Leblanc, E., and Castelain, B. (1991). Laparoscopic pelvic lymphadenectomy in the staging of early carcinoma of the cervix. *Am. J. Obstet. Gynecol.*, **164**, 579–81.
3. Childers, J.M., Hatch, K.D., Tran, A.N., and Surwit, E.A. (1993). Laparoscopic para-aortic lymphadenectomy in gynecologic malignancies. *Obstet. Gynecol.*, **82**, 741–7.
4. Querleu, D. (1993). Laparoscopic paraaortic node sampling in gynecologic oncology: a preliminary experience. *Gynecol. Oncol.*, **49**, 24–9.
5. Querleu, D. and LeBlanc, E. (1994). Laparoscopic infrarenal paraaortic lymph node dissection for restaging of carcinoma of the ovary or fallopian tube. *Cancer*, **73**, 1467–71.
6. Pomel, C., Provencher, D., Dauplat, J. *et al.* (1995). Laparoscopic staging of early ovarian cancer. *Gynecol. Oncol.*, **58**, 301–6.
7. Amara, D.P., Nezhat, C., Teng, N.N. *et al.* (1996). Operative laparoscopy in the management of ovarian cancer. *Surg. Laparosc. Endosc.*, **6**, 38–45.
8. Venesmaa, P. (1994). Epithelial ovarian cancer: impact of surgery and chemotherapy on survival during 1977–1990. *Obstet. Gynecol.*, **84**, 8–11.
9. Charvolin, J.Y. and Querleu, D. Relevance of surgical lymph node staging for malignant ovarian germ cell tumors [in French]. *Contracept. Fertil. Sex.*, **27**, 51–5.

10. Possover, M., Plaul, K., Krause, N., and Schneider, A. (1998). Left-sided laparoscopic para-aortic lymphadenectomy: anatomy of the ventral tributaries of the infrarenal vena cava. *Am. J. Obstet. Gynecol.*, **179**,1295–7.

11. Fowler, J.M., Carter, J.R., Carlson, J.W. *et al.* (1993). Lymph node yield from laparoscopic lymphadenectomy in cervical cancer: a comparative study. *Gynecol. Oncol.*, **51**, 187–92.

12. Querleu, D., Lanvin, D., Elhage, A. *et al.* (1998). An objective experimental assessment of the learning curve for laparoscopic surgery: the example of pelvic and para-aortic lymph node dissection. *Eur. J. Obstet. Gynecol. Reprod. Biol.*, **81**, 55–8.

13. Ocelli, B., Narducci, F., Lanvin, D. *et al.* (2000). Learning curves for transperitoneal laparoscopic and extraperitoneal endoscopic paraaortic lymphadenectomy. *J. Am. Assoc. Gynecol. Laparosc.*, **7**, 51–3.

14. Lanvin, D., Elhage, A., Henry, B. *et al.* (1997). Accuracy and safety of laparoscopic lymphadenectomy: an experimental prospective randomized study. *Gynecol. Oncol.*, **67**, 83–7.

15. Fowler, J.M., Hartenbach, E.M., Reynolds, H.T. *et al.* (1994). Pelvic adhesion formation after pelvic lymphadenectomy: comparison between transperitoneal laparoscopy and extraperitoneal laparotomy in a porcine model. *Gynecol. Oncol.*, **55**, 25–8.

16. Young, R.C., Decker, D.G., Wharton, J.T. *et al.* (1983). Staging laparotomy in early ovarian cancer. *JAMA*, **250**, 3072–6.

17. Possover, M., Mader, M., Zielinski, J. *et al.* (1995). Is laparotomy for staging early ovarian cancer an absolute necessity? *J. Am. Assoc. Gynecol. Laparosc.*, **2**, 285–8.

18. Jacobs, I., Oram, D., Fairbanks, J. *et al.* (1990). A risk of malignancy index incorporating CA 125, ultrasound and menopausal status for the accurate preoperative diagnosis of ovarian cancer. *Br. J. Obstet. Gynaecol.*, **97**, 922–9.

19. Peterson, H., Hulka, J., and Phillips, J (1990). American Association of Gynecologic Laparoscopists 1988 membership survey on operative laparoscopy. *J. Reprod. Med.*, **35**, 587–9.

20. Dreßler, F. (1991). Zur endoskopischen Therapie von zystischen Ovarialtumouren and Paraovarialzysten. *Geburtsh u Frauenheilk*, **51**, 474–80.

21. Lehmann-Willenbrock, E., Mecke, H., and Semm, K. (1991). Pelviskopische Ovarialchirurgie – eine retrospektive Untersuchung von 1016 operierten Zysten. *Geburtsh u Frauenheilk*, **51**, 280–7.

22. Hulka, J.F., Parker, W.H., Surrey, M.W., and Phillips, J.M. (1992). Management of ovarian masses: AAGL 1990 survey. *J. Reprod. Med.*, **37**, 559–602.

23. Nezhat, L., Nezhat, C., Welander, C.E., and Benigno, B. (1992). Four ovarian cancers diagnosed during laparoscopic management of 1011 women with adnexal masses. *Am. J. Obstet. Gynecol.*, **167**, 790–6.

24. Canis, M., Mage, G., Pouly, J.L. *et al.* (1994). Laparoscopic diagnosis of adnexal cystic massess: a 12-year experience with long term follow-up. *Obstet. Gynecol.*, **83**, 707–12.

25. Maiman, M., Seltzer, V. and Boyce, J. (1991). Laparoscopic excision of ovarian neoplasms subsequently found to be malignant. *Obstet. Gynecol.*, **77**, 563–5.

26. Crawford, R.A.F., Gore, M.E., and Shepherd, J.H. (1995). Ovarian cancers related to minimal access surgery. *Br. J. Obstet. Gynaecol.*, **102**, 726–30.

27. Wenzl, R., Lehner, R., Husslein, P., and Sevelda, P. (1996). Laparoscopic surgery in cases of ovarian malignancies: an Austria-wide survey. *Gynecol. Oncol.*, **63**, 57–61.

28. Lehner, R., Wenzl, R., Heinzl, H. *et al.* (1998). Influence of delayed staging laparotomy after laparoscopic removal of ovarian masses later found malignant. *Obstet. Gynecol.*, **92**, 967–71.

29. Ahmed, F.Y., Wiltshaw, E., A'Hern, R.P. *et al.* (1996). Natural history of prognosis of untreated stage 1 epithelial carcinoma. *J. Clin. Oncol.*, **14**, 2968–75.

30. Dembo, A.J., Davy, M., Stenwig, A.E. *et al.* (1990). Prognostic factors in patients with stage 1 epithelial ovarian cancer. *Obstet. Gynecol.*, **75**, 263–73.

31. Finn, C.B., Luesley, D.M., Buxton, E.J. *et al.* (1992). Is stage 1 epithelial ovarian cancer overtreated both surgically and systemically? Results of a five year cancer registry review. *Br. J. Obstet. Gynaecol.*, **99**, 54–8.

32. Sevelda, P., Dittrich, C., and Salzer, H. (1989). Prognostic value of the rupture of the capsule in stage 1 epithelial ovarian carcinoma. *Gynecol. Oncol.*, **35**, 321–2.

33. Sjövall, K., Nilsson, B., and Einhorn, N. (1994). Different types of ruptue of of the tumour capsule and the impact on survival in early ovarian carcinoma. *Int. J. Gynecol. Cancer*, **4**, 333–6.

34. Vergote, I.B., Kærn, J., Abeler, V.M. *et al.* (1993). Analysis of prognostic factors in stage 1 epithelial ovarian carcinoma: importance of degree of differentiation and deoxyribonucleic acid ploidy in predicting relapse. *Am. J. Obstet. Gynecol.*, **169**, 40–52.

35. Sainz de la Cuesta, R., Goff, B.A., Fuller, A.F. *et al.* (1994). Prognostic importance of malignant ovarian epithelial neoplasms. *Obstet. Gynecol.*, **84**, 1–7.

36. Webb, M.J., Decker, D.G., Mussey, E., and Williams, T.J. (1973). Factors influencing survival in stage 1 ovarian cancer. *Am. J. Obstet. Gynecol.*, **116**, 222–8.

37. Yuen, P.M., Yu, K.M., Yip, S.K. *et al.* (1997). A randomized prospective study of laparoscopy and laparotomy in the management of benign ovarian masses. *Am. J. Obstet. Gynecol.*, **177**, 109–14.

38. Rasmussen, C., Englund, K., and Lindblom, B. (1999). Management of cystic ovarian masses by laparoscopic surgery: results of 275 cases. *Gynaecol. Endosc.*, **8**, 35–9.

39. Childers, J.M., Nasseri, A., and Surwit, E.A. (1996). Laparoscopic management of suspicious adnexal masses. *Am. J. Obstet. Gynecol.*, **175**, 1451–7.

40. Dottino, P.R., Levine, D.A., Ripley, D.L., and Cohen, C.J. (1999). Laparoscopic management of adnexal masses in premenopausal and postmenopausal women. *Obstet. Gynecol.*, **93**, 223–8.

41. van Dam, P., Decloedt, J., Tjalma, W., and Vergote, I. (1997). Is there a role for diagnostic laparoscopy to assess operability of advanced ovarian cancer? *Int. J. Gynecol. Cancer*, **7**, 28.

42. Roman, L.D. (1998). Small cystic pelvic masses in older women: is surgical removal necessary? *Gynecol. Oncol.*, **69**, 1–2.

43. Canis, M., Mage, G., Wattiez, A. *et al.* (1997). [Operative laparoscopy and the adnexal cystic mass: where to set the limit?] *J. Gynecol. Obstet. Biol. Reprod. (Paris)*, **26**, 293–303.

44. Canis, M., Pouly, J.L., Wattiez, A. *et al.* (1997). Laparoscopic management of adnexal masses suspicious at ultrasound. *Obstet. Gynecol.*, **89**, 679–83.

45. Gadducci, A., Sartori, E., Maggino, T. *et al.* (1998). Analysis of failures after negative second-look in patients with advanced ovarian cancer: an Italian multicenter study. *Gynecol. Oncol.*, **68**, 150–5.

46. Childers, J.M., Aqua, K.A., Surwit, E.A. *et al.* (1994). Abdominal wall tumor implantation after laparoscopy for malignant conditions. *Obstet. Gynecol.*, **84**, 765–9.

47. Kruitwagen, R.F.P.M., Swinkels, B.M., Keyser, K.G.G. *et al.* (1996). Incidence and effect on survival of abdominal wall metastases at trocar or puncture sites following laparoscopy or paracentesis in women with ovarian cancer. *Gynecol. Oncol.*, **60**, 233–7.

48. van Dam, P.A., DeCloedt, J., Tjalma, W.A. *et al.* (1999). Trocar implantation metastasis after laparoscopy in patients with advanced ovarian cancer: can the risk be reduced? *Am. J. Obstet. Gynecol.*, **181**, 536–41.

49. Koster, S., Melchert, F., and Volz, J. (1996). Effect of CO_2 pneumoperitoneum on intraperitoneal tumor growth in the animal model [in German]. *Geburtshilfe Frauenheilkd*, **56**, 458–61.

50. Canis, M., Botchorishvili, R., Kouyate, S. *et al.* (1998). Surgical management of adnexal tumors [in French]. *Ann. Chir.*, **52**, 234–48.

51. Canis, M., Botchorishvili, R., Wattiez, A. *et al.* (1998). Tumor growth and dissemination after laparotomy and CO_2 pneumoperitoneum: a rat ovarian cancer model. *Obstet. Gynecol.*, **92**, 104–8.

52. Bouvy, N.D., Marquet, R.L., Jeekel, H., and Bonjer, H.J. (1996). Impact of gas(less) laparoscopy and laparotomy on peritoneal tumor growth and abdominal wall metastases. *Ann. Surg.*, **224**, 694–700.

53. Mathew, G., Watson, D.I., Rofe, A.M. *et al.* (1997). Adverse impact of pneumoperitoneum on intraperitoneal implantation and growth of tumour cell suspension in an experimental model. *Aust. NZ J. Surg.*, **67**, 289–92.

54. Mutter, D., Hajri, A., Tassetti, V. *et al.* (1999). Increased tumor growth and spread after laparoscopy vs laparotomy. Influence of tumor manipulation in a rat model. *Surg. Endosc.*, **13**, 365–70.

55. Paik, P.S., Misawa, T., Chiang, M. *et al.* (1998). Abdominal incision tumor implantation following pneumoperitoneum laparoscopic procedure vs. standard open incision in a syngeneic rat model. *Dis. Colon Rectum*, **41**, 419–22.

56. Wu, J.S., Pfister, S.M., Ruiz, M.B. *et al.* (1998). Local treatment of abdominal wound reduces tumor implantation. *J. Surg. Oncol.*, **69**, 9–13.

57. Wang, P.-H., Yuan, C.-C., Lin, G. *et al.* (1999). Risk factors contributing to early occurrence of port site metastases of laparoscopic surgery for malignancy. *Gynecol. Oncol.*, **72**, 38–44.

58. Lecuru, F., Robin, F., and Taurelle, R. (1999). Experimental studies on the effect of pneumoperitoneum on tumour dissemination: clarification is required. Results of experimental trials should be further assessed. *Gynaecol. Endosc.*, **8**, 267–70.

59. Zweemer, R.P., van Diest, P.J., Verheijen, R.H. *et al.* (2000). Molecular evidence linking primary cancer of the fallopian tube to BRCA1 germline mutations. *Gynecol. Oncol.*, **76**, 45–50.

60. Meiser, B., Butow, P., Barratt, A. *et al.* (1999). Attitudes toward prophylactic oophorectomy and screening utilization in women at increased risk of developing hereditary breast/ovarian cancer. *Gynecol. Oncol.*, **75**, 122–9.

61. Eltabbakh, G.H., Piver, M.S., Hempling, R.E. *et al.* (1999). Laparoscopic management of women with a family history of ovarian cancer. *J. Surg. Oncol.*, **72**, 9–13.

62. Schrag, D., Kuntz, K.M., Garber, J.E., and Weeks, J. (1997). Decision analysis – effects of prophylactic mastectomy and oophorectomy on life expectancy among women with BRCA1 or BRCA2 mutations. *N. Engl. J. Med.*, **336**, 1465.

41. The organization of care

H.C. Kitchener

Ovarian cancer presents the gynaecological oncologist's greatest challenges because, in the majority of cases, women do not present until the disease has advanced to a stage when it becomes essentially incurable. Advances in perioperative care mean that aggressive debulking surgery is now safer, and progress has been made in chemotherapy, with higher response rates which have led to increases in mean survival times. What has become clear during the past 10–20 years is that the optimal management of ovarian cancer requires multidisciplinary care, so that outcomes are improved where women are managed by expert teams. This means that the organization of health care for ovarian cancer matters, and it is desirable to achieve a situation where as many women as possible can access expert multidisciplinary care delivered using protocols based on the best available evidence. This chapter will focus on the expert multidisciplinary team and how it needs to function in order to deliver the optimal outcomes.

The expert multidisciplinary team

In considering a typical pathway for a woman with ovarian cancer; it begins with an anxious, often unwell woman being referred with an abdominopelvic mass. The initial consultation will require an honest, realistic idea of what will happen. There will be imaging and then a laparotomy. The laparotomy will stage and hopefully result in debulking the disease. Then an accurate pathological assessment is required. Considerable effort is required to counsel the patient, to try to alleviate fear of the unknown, and to try to make her understand what will happen. She will usually require chemotherapy, which may or may not achieve a response of 12–24 months. There then need to be decisions about second-line chemotherapy, and often control of persistent abdominal symptoms. Expert palliative care is often necessary. Throughout this 'cancer journey' there needs to be communication with the patient and her family, between members of the team, and between the hospital and the family doctor. It therefore seems obvious that such a complex, demanding condition should be treated by a multidisciplinary team, who are experienced and expert, and who meet to discuss management.

The incidence of ovarian cancer is such that the average gynaecologist might see between five and 10 cases per year, depending on the setting. Furthermore, the average gynaecologist may not have the type of surgical expertise that is required to undertake an adequate laparotomy and attempt to debulk ovarian cancer tumours, which will often be very difficult to dissect free of small or large bowel and bladder. Surgery therefore needs to be concentrated in the hands of competent, experienced pelvic surgeons. In some cases, there is an advantage in working with colorectal surgeons when there may be uncertainty as to primary site of the tumour or when decisions require to be made regarding resection of small or large bowel.

Initial surgery

The evidence for aggressive primary surgery will be presented elsewhere, but optimal debulking is still considered to be standard management. This means that when a gynaecologist who is inexperienced in such surgery or a general surgeon is faced by a large, complex malignant pelvic mass, he or she will sometimes feel that the safest thing is simply to take a biopsy and close the patient's abdomen. This may result in inadequate staging and may mean that the patient will have to undergo a second laparotomy in order to achieve staging and tumour resection. Therefore the best approach is for women who are assessed as being at high risk of having ovarian cancer to be referred to a gynaecological oncologist, rather than have treatment initiated by a less-experienced practitioner. Primary surgery for ovarian cancer brings with it anaesthetic challenges and risk of postoperative morbidity, which both mean that women are best managed in units where there is an infrastructure that is capable of managing these problems. In a number of gynaecological units, nurses are not used to managing women who have undergone major surgical procedures and may not be sufficiently experienced in managing patients who have fluid balance problems immediately postoperatively.

Multidisciplinary tumour board

Following the initial operation, key decisions need to be made about further management. These will be governed by the stage of the tumour, the pathology of the tumour, and the existence of residual disease. These are best undertaken at Tumour Boards, which are attended by the team, in order that consideration of all aspects of the case and future management can be considered jointly. This process encourages accurate prospective data collection, which is key to measuring outcomes. It also encourages the consistent use of evidence-based protocols and allows the opportunity for decisions to be made for entry into relevant trials. Such a co-ordinated approach reduces the potential for disjointed care, where a patient is referred from one hospital to another, with inadequate amounts of information being communicated from and to the referring consultant, and where increasing treatment delay and anxiety may also result. The Tumour Board should meet each week, without undue delay in pathology reporting, in order that management can be discussed with the patient. Delaying leads to uncertainty and anxiety. It is also important that the family doctor is made aware of the management plans.

The clinical nurse specialist

The role of the clinical nurse specialist (CNS) was first exemplified in the management of breast cancer, and now clinical nurse specialists are becoming firmly established as key members of the gynaecological oncology team. The emphasis of the gynaecological CNS is to provide support and information to the woman at all stages of the disease, but particularly at the early stage. It is extremely important that patients and carers really understand about the disease and the treatment, in order to try to minimize uncertainty and psychological distress. Clinical nurse specialists have both knowledge and the time that is required. Patients will often require to have more than one explanation about their condition and may have particular fears (for example, about toxicity of chemotherapy) that can be assuaged by explanations by the clinical nurse specialist. The clinical nurse specialist can also play a vital role in assisting communication between the patient and medical staff, who are sometimes unaware of particular aspects of concern to patients. A hospital-based clinical nurse specialist can also act as a liaison between the hospital and community support services.

Chemotherapy

All patients deserve to receive optimal chemotherapy; that is, chemotherapy which will produce the best response rates with the lowest incidence of severe toxic effects. Such chemotherapy requires to be given under the supervision of an oncologist who is very knowledgeable and experienced in the use of chemotherapy, specifically in the treatment of ovarian cancer, and should be administered in a setting suitable for the purpose. It is important that chemotherapy side-effects are minimized and that complications are managed promptly and competently. Where the management of ovarian cancer is too generalized, there is a danger that a number of women will not receive optimal chemotherapy, or indeed no chemotherapy, due to inexperience in its use. There is also the likelihood that entry to trials will be reduced because trial participation requires the type of infrastructure that tends to be found in expert centres.

Another key area of chemotherapy in ovarian cancer is the management of recurrent disease and decisions around second-line chemotherapy. This may involve repeating conventional chemotherapy, or there may be consideration given to entry into phase I and II trials. Such decisions require to be made in consultation with the patient, and by the practitioner who managed the primary chemotherapy.

Palliative care

Because the long-term prognosis for most patients with ovarian disease is so poor, it is inevitable that a large number of women will run into terminal problems. These will often involve pain, nausea, vomiting, ascites, and bowel obstruction. It is vital for the quality of life of these women that such difficult problems are managed meticulously. Sometimes these problems are managed in the more acute stage in a hospital setting, but they can often be managed at home. Sometimes there is a need for women to be admitted to hospices when symptom control is difficult. The key to good palliative care is appreciation of attention to detail and communication between the different professionals involved, to ensure that the patient's needs can be met. When active treatment is no longer appropriate, it is extremely important that the patient does not feel abandoned and that her suffering does not go unrelieved.

Evidence-based structure of care

If the care of women with ovarian cancer is to be achieved properly, it seems obvious that it requires expert, committed teamwork. Evidence to support this can be found from a number of sources. A long-term cohort study from Scotland has indicated clearly that expert teams deliver longer survival times with a reduction in the relative risk of dying at any point in time.[1] This study also showed that those who live in areas with subspecialists have a better outcome than those in which there are no subspecialists. This is independent of deprivation score and probably reflects the overall benefit of accessing an optimal care package. Data from south-east England has indicated that in teaching hospitals the outcomes from ovarian cancer are better than in isolated units with no oncology expertise on site.[2] It is also clear from hospital audits that, women are frequently not properly staged and do not receive optimal chemotherapy.[3] The evidence available therefore points to failures of process and poorer outcomes in non-specialist settings.

Women suspected of having ovarian cancer should, ideally, be referred initially to a specialist gynaecological oncologist who functions as a member of a team. Of course, such teams should demonstrate that women are being managed by evidence-based protocol. They should enter patients into important clinical trials and are also required to generate accurate and comprehensive databases which ensure that outcomes can be audited. This type of approach has been recommended in recent guidance by the Department of Health in England, but has been criticized by a number of general gynaecologists, who argue that it will require women and their carers to spend a lot of time far from their homes and that similar packages of care could be delivered at more local hospitals. The experience of those in expert centres is that patients will travel for expert care, and that this cannot be guaranteed in the generalized setting. In countries such as the United Kingdom, where outcomes in ovarian cancer are not as good as they should be, concentration of care in expert centres appears to offer the best prospect for improvement.

References

1. Junor, E.J. and Hole, D.J. (2000). Specialist gynaecologists and survival outcome in ovarian cancer: a Scottish National Study of 1866 patients. *Br. J. Obstet. Gynaecol.* in press.

2. Wolfe, C.D., Tilling, K., and Raju, K.S. (1997). Management and survival of ovarian cancer patients in south east England. *Eur. J. Cancer*, 33, 1835–40.

3. Woodman, C., Baghdady, A., Collins, S. *et al.* (1997). What changes in the organisation of cancer services will improve the outcome for women with ovarian cancer? 104, 135–9.

42. Patterns of care in ovarian cancer

Edward L. Trimble

Introduction

As we define optimal care for women with ovarian cancer, we must then ask whether women are receiving such care. The spectrum of care is broad, including the management of women with inherited risk, screening of the general population, the surgical approach to adnexal masses, the treatment of ovarian cancer once diagnosed, therapy for recurrent disease, and supportive care.

Healthcare systems differ radically between different countries. In some countries, such as the United States, the healthcare system, including cancer care, is fragmented. Obtaining data on healthcare delivery can be difficult. Ideally, one would like to be able to ascertain demographic information on each woman diagnosed with ovarian cancer, where she was treated, what surgery and chemotherapy she underwent, the training of her physicians, her cancer outcome, her quality of life, how she was treated if her cancer recurred, and the details of supportive care.[1] Even in countries with unified health systems and population-based cancer registries, much of these data are not available. We must glean the extant data and attempt to define the patterns of care. None the less, certain patterns begin to emerge, suggesting specific ways in which we can improve the care of women with ovarian cancer.

Women with inherited risk

Up to 5–10% of women with epithelial ovarian cancer inherit a susceptibility to cancer. The recent identification of the *BRCA1* and *BRCA2* genes have helped elucidate the genetics of ovarian cancer. Guidelines for the management of women who carry mutations of *BRCA1* and *BRCA2* have been published.[2] We have little data, however, on the absolute number of women screened for these and other mutations. In addition, we have only a few reports, mostly from single institutions, on how these women have been managed. Pooling data from all families identified with genetic mutations that put a woman at increased risk for ovarian cancer will help us to establish the patterns of care that these women have received, as well as to identify environmental and reproductive factors that may modify their cancer risks. De Silva *et al.* have suggested that breast cancer screening programs for the general population can be used to help identify women with family histories of breast cancer.[3]

Screening

The 1994 NIH Consensus Statement on Ovarian Cancer recommended against screening women in the general population outwith clinical trials.[4] Large screening trials evaluating transvaginal ultrasound and serum CA125 as potential screens for ovarian cancer are under way in the United States and Europe. Both these tests are available routinely. We do not know the extent to which they are used to screen women for ovarian cancer outside of clinical trials. The manufacturers of the serum CA125 test (Centocor, Inc.) reported that 4 million tests were performed in 1993, up from 1 million in 1989.[5] As Westhoff has commented, 'only a small fraction of these tests would be needed for the indicated use of monitoring progression of ovarian cancer during treatment; most of these tests are likely being performed for screening'.

Management of adnexal masses

A number of studies have examined the various factors that might predict malignancy in adnexal masses. Jacobs *et al.* have suggested that an index combining menopausal status, ultrasonographic appearance, and serum CA125 can help to discriminate between the mass that is likely to be benign and that which is likely to be cancer.[6] Tingulstad *et al.* have reported on the use of such a risk-of-malignancy index with triage of patients in three Norwegian counties, with a total population of 62 400.[7] Over a 2-year period, 365 women were enrolled and assessed using this criterion. Women with high risk-of-malignancy indices were referred to a gynecologic oncology unit, while those with low indices underwent surgery at local hospitals. The sensitivity and specificity to malignancy were 71% and 92% (Fig. 42.1). Of 28 stage II–IV ovarian cancers, 27 were identified correctly. The adherence to the study was acceptable. Sixty-five of 77 women (84%) with high indices were referred to the gynecologic oncology unit. Based on these data, such triage seems promising.

The surgical approach to an adnexal mass can be via laparoscopy or laparotomy. When physicians have the expertise both in laparoscopic surgery and the surgical management of gynecologic malignancies, a laparoscopic approach appears acceptable.[8,9] We do not know the extent of laparoscopic surgery in the diagnosis and management of ovarian cancer.

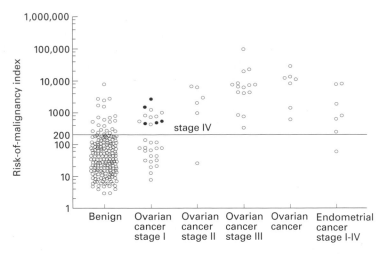

Fig. 42.1 Distribution of the risk-of-malignancy index in benign and malignant gynecologic pelvix masses. Closed circles = stage Ic ovarian cancer. (From Tingulstad *et al.* 1999.[7])

Guidelines for cancer management

Consensus statements on the management of ovarian cancer have been put forward in Europe and the United States.[4,10] Detailed guidelines for ovarian cancer management have been published in the United States by the National Comprehensive Cancer Network, a consortium of NCI-designated cancer centers, and the Society of Gynecologic Oncologists.[11,12] The Department of Health in the United Kingdom published a report on acceptable practices in ovarian cancer management in 1991.[13]

We have limited data as to how well these guidelines are followed. Grilli *et al.* evaluated the impact of guidelines for the management of ovarian cancer promulgated in Italy. First, in 1988, they surveyed physicians and found that only 44% were aware of the guidelines.[14] Next, they analyzed adherence to the guidelines among 100 consecutive newly diagnosed patients with epithelial ovarian cancer between 1986 and 1987. Information on residual tumor was available for only 45% of patients, and tumor grade for 30%. They found that stage I or II disease could only be confirmed after re-analysis in 1 of 4 cases. Only 34% of women with stage III–IV disease received multiagent chemotherapy.

Hogberg *et al.* analyzed the care given to 325 patients with epithelial ovarian cancer in the south-east Health Care Region of Sweden between 1984 and 1987.[15] Among these patients the 5-year survival was 49% for those who received recommended therapy versus 33% for those who did not receive such therapy. For women with stage III and IV ovarian cancer, the 5-year survival was 23% for those who received recommended therapy, and 11% for those who did not receive such therapy.

Junor *et al.* conducted a retrospective study of 479 patients with ovarian cancer diagnosed in Scotland in 1987.[16] In this study, the referral of a patient to a multidisciplinary clinic with expertise in the management of ovarian cancer was associated with increased survival. Similar data may be seen in the Norwegian experience between 1955 and 1994 (Fig. 42.2).[17] Patients referred to the Norwegian Radium Hospital had better survival than those treated in the community from 1969 to 1989. As gynecologic

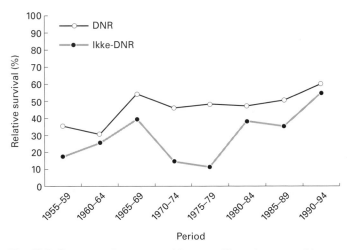

Fig. 42.2 Five-year relative survival for stage III ovarian cancer, Norway, 1955–94. DNR, women referred to the Norwegian Radium Hospital, Ikke-DNR, women not referred to the Norwegian Radium Hospital. (From Trope, personal communication.)

oncologists became available in regional hospitals, these survival differences resolved.

Wolfe *et al.* audited 118 cases of ovarian cancer diagnosed in 1991 in seven district health authorities in the United Kingdom.[18] Overall, 47 (43%) were managed appropriately. Appropriate management ranged from 66% in a teaching hospital, 45% in a non-teaching hospital with oncology support, and 28% in a non-teaching hospital without oncology support. In multivariate analysis, death was more likely among women who had been inappropriately managed.

Munoz *et al.* analyzed adherence to the staging and treatment recommendations made by the NIH Consensus Panel among 785 patients with ovarian cancer, diagnosed in 1991 and identified through the NCI's Surveillance, Epidemiology, and End Results (SEER) program.[19] They found that 10% of women with presumptive stage I and II disease, 71% of women with stage III disease, and 53% of women with stage IV disease received the recommended therapy. Treatment at a hospital with an approved residency program was associated with a greater likelihood that the patient would receive the recommended care. The presence of an approved residency program may be a proxy for the presence of a gynecologist or oncologist with expertise in ovarian cancer. Partridge *et al.* have reported on 5469 women with invasive ovarian cancer diagnosed in the United States in 1988 and another 7456 diagnosed in 1993. For these two periods, about three-quarters of patients were treated with surgery and chemotherapy. The type of chemotherapy was not disclosed.[20] Farrow *et al.*, who studied survival among 12 049 women with ovarian cancer diagnosed between 1983 and 1991 in the United States and included in the SEER registry, found no regional variation in survival between the SEER reporting sites.[21] This suggests that ovarian cancer may be treated similarly in the various geographic regions which comprise the SEER catchment areas.

Primary surgery

Staging

Women with ovarian cancer grossly confined to the pelvis often have microscopic disease in the upper abdomen or retro-peritoneum. For this reason, surgical staging should include assessment of both hemidiaphragms, all peritoneal surfaces, the large and small bowel, as well as the stomach, liver, gallbladder, and spleen. In addition, women with presumed early stage disease should undergo cytologic washings from either paracolic gutter, both hemidiaphragms, and the pelvis, as well as pelvic and para-aortic lymph node sampling. The ovarian lymphatics parallel the ovarian arteries and veins, which emerge from the central vasculature at the level of the renal arteries. Para-aortic lymph node sampling, therefore, should include resection of lymph nodes near the insertion of the ovarian vein into the vena cava on the right side and the renal vein on left side.

Several studies suggest that many women with presumed early stage ovarian cancer are not undergoing the recommended surgical staging. McGowan examined the adequacy of staging among 291 patients with epithelial ovarian cancer who underwent surgery in the Washington DC area between 1978 and 1981.[22] Overall, 54% had adequate surgical staging. The American College of Surgeons Commission on Cancer conducted a National Survey of Ovarian Cancer, focusing on 5156 women diagnosed in 1983 and 7160 patients in 1988.[23] Those women who underwent surgery by gynecologic oncologists had more biopsies performed than those whose surgery was performed by obstetrician-gynecologists and general gynecologists. In addition, gynecologic oncologists were more likely to use an upper and lower midline incision, while obstetrician-gynecologists and general surgeons favored a lower midline incision. Hand *et al.* performed a retrospective analysis of 2669 women diagnosed with ovarian cancer between 1983 and 1988 in the State of Illinois.[24] Of those with presumed stage I disease, only 30% had appropriate surgical and pathologic staging. In the Swedish study by Hogberg *et al.*, in which recommended staging did not include lymph node sampling, only 20%

of presumed stage I or II patients were considered adequately staged.[15] In the study by Munoz *et al.*, lymph node sampling was not performed in two-thirds of patients with presumed stage I and II disease.[19] Of note, tumor grade was also not assigned in 36% of women with stage I disease and 25% of women with stage II disease.

Debulking

Both retrospective and prospective studies suggest the impact of effective surgical debulking upon survival in women with stage III and IV ovarian cancer. Several retrospective population-based studies suggest that many women are not receiving a maximal effort at cytoreduction. In the American College of Surgeons Commission on Cancer study, optimal debulking rates were 40–45% among gynecologic oncologists and general gynecologists, compared to 25% among general surgeons.[23] Munoz *et al.* found that 90% of women with stage III disease did receive extensive surgery, compared to 64% of women with stage IV disease.[19] Older women and those with co-morbidities were less likely to receive extensive surgery.

Surgical specialty

Residency training in obstetrics and gynecology includes didactic teaching on ovarian cancer as well as exposure to the operative management of adnexal masses and ovarian cancer. Formal fellowship training in gynecologic oncology, as is now conducted in the United States, United Kingdom, and Australia, includes further didactics on ovarian cancer as well as training in the preoperative evaluation of women with suspected ovarian cancer, the operative management of women with ovarian cancer, the administration of chemotherapy for ovarian cancer, and supportive care. In a number of countries, gynecologists, gynecologic oncologists, and oncologists have established centers with expertise in the management of ovarian cancer.

In McGowan's study, the completeness of surgical staging was 97% for gynecologic oncologists, 52% for obstetrician-gynecologists, and 35% for general surgeons.[22] The American College of Surgeons National Cancer Commission on Cancer conducted a study of 5156 patients with ovarian cancer diagnosed in 1983 and reported to their National Survey of Ovarian Cancer.[23] Among these patients, obstetrician-gynecologists provided surgical care for 47%, gynecologic oncologists 17%, and general surgeons 24%. In their analysis, women with stages II, III, and IV ovarian cancer who underwent primary surgery conducted by a gynecologist or a gynecologic oncologist had significantly better survival than those whose surgery was conducted by a general surgeon (Fig. 42.3). There was no difference in survival for women with stage I disease. Overall, there was no difference in survival between women whose primary surgery was performed by an obstetrician-gynecologist and women whose surgery was performed by a gynecologic oncologist. The only exception was for women with stage IIb disease, among whom those whose surgery was performed by a gynecologic oncologist had better survival. As mentioned above, gynecologic oncologists were more likely to use an upper and lower midline incision and perform more biopsies that their

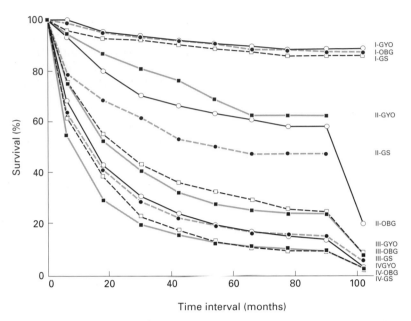

Fig. 42.3 Survival curves of 4260 women with ovarian cancer cared for by physicians of various specialities for different disease stages. I-GYO, patients with stage I cared for by a gynecologic oncologists. The same format is used for all abbreviations. I, stage I; II, stage II; III, stage III; IV, stage IV; GYO, gynecologic oncologist; OBG, obstetrician/gynecologist; GS, general surgeon. (From Nguyen *et al.* 1993.[23])

colleagues. The rate of optimal cytoreduction was 40–45% for both the gynecologic oncologist and the obstetrician-gynecologist, compared to 25% for the general surgeon. Data on adjuvant chemotherapy were not available in this study. Eisenkop *et al.* have reported a retrospective analysis of 263 patients with stage IIIc and IV epithelial ovarian cancer treated at 14 US hospitals between 1985 and 1988.[25] Optimal cytoreduction at the time of primary surgery and overall survival were both significantly associated with the specialty training of the operating surgeon (Fig. 42.4). In this study, surgeons were classified as gynecologic oncologists or other.

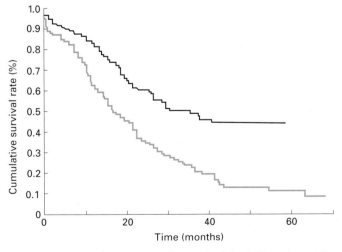

Fig. 42.4 Cumulative proportion of survival subdivided by subspecialty training of surgeons present. Solid line, gynecologic oncologist present. Dotted line, gynecologic oncologist absent. *P* < 0.0001. (From Eisenkop *et al.* 1992.[25])

In the UK, Kehoe *et al.* conducted a retrospective analysis of 1184 patients with ovarian cancer diagnosed between 1985 and 1987.[26] The median survival of patients under the care of a general surgeon was 9.87 months, compared to 29 months for those women under the care of a gynecologist. In multivariate analysis, the adverse prognostic factors included advanced-stage disease, increased age, bulky residual disease, and a general surgeon as the operator. In the Scottish study conducted by Junor *et al.*, gynecologists were significantly more likely to achieve optimal cytoreduction than general surgeons.[16] In addition, the 5-year survival rate for women whose initial surgery was performed by a gynecologist, after adjustment for age and stage, was 27%, compared to 19% for women whose initial surgery was performed by a general surgeon. Woodman *et al.* examined the influence of operator specialty among 691 women with ovarian cancer who underwent surgery in the North-west Region of the United Kingdom between 1991 and 1992.[27] In multivariate analysis, operation by a surgeon, rather than a gynecologist was found to have an adverse impact upon survival.

Age

The American College of Surgeons Commission on Cancer found that older patients were less likely to undergo major surgical procedures, to experience optimal cytoreduction, and to receive adjuvant chemotherapy, compared to younger patients.[28] Similar findings were reported by Ries, who analyzed treatment by age among 20 772 women with ovarian cancer diagnosed between 1973 and 1987.[29] Overall, younger women were more likely to receive surgery and multiagent chemotherapy than older women (Fig. 42.5). Over 40% of women older than age 85 years did not receive any treatment at all. In the subsequent SEER study conducted by Munoz *et al.*, younger women, who more commonly

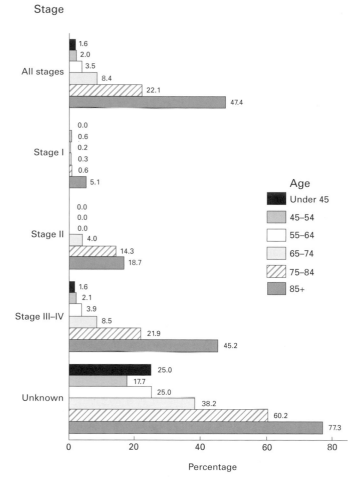

Fig. 42.5 Ovarian cancer: percentage untreated by age and stage, 1983–87. (From Ries 1993.[29])

had earlier stage disease, were less likely to receive appropriate staging.[19] Older women, particularly those with co-morbidity, were less likely to receive effective debulking surgery. In the Scottish study, older patients were less likely to see a gynecologist initially, to have surgery by a gynecologist, to undergo successful cytoreduction, to receive platinum-based chemotherapy, or to be referred to a multidisciplinary clinic.[16]

Adjuvant chemotherapy

Contemporary treatment recommendations for women with stage III and IV epithelial ovarian cancer include 6–8 courses of intravenous platinum–paclitaxel chemotherapy after primary surgery. The American College of Surgeons Commission on Cancer found that only 42% of women aged 80 years or older received chemotherapy, compared to 72% of those aged 60–79 years.[28] In the study by Munoz et al., which examined patterns of care before paclitaxel was available, 79% of women with stage III disease received surgery and platinum-based chemotherapy, compared to 61% of those with stage IV disease.[19] Women older than age 65 were less likely to get the combination of surgery and platinum-

based chemotherapy. Hand et al., in their study in Illinois, found that only three-quarters of patients with stage III disease received platinum-based chemotherapy after primary surgery.[24] In addition, older women with residual disease following primary surgery were significantly less likely to receive platinum-based chemotherapy than younger women. In the Scottish study, of women with stage III disease, 41% received platinum-based chemotherapy, 29% alkylating agents, and 30% no chemotherapy.[16] In the study by Woodman et al., women referred to an oncologist following primary surgery had significantly better survival than those who were not referred.[27] Data from Bristol-Myers Squibb suggest that over half of women with advanced ovarian cancer in the United States do receive paclitaxel as part of primary therapy.[30] In certain countries with national health programs, paclitaxel may not be routinely available.

Recurrence

Chemotherapy

A variety of drugs, with limited efficacy, are available to treat women with recurrent ovarian cancer. In the United States, for example, commercially available agents would include carboplatin, cisplatin, paclitaxel, taxotere, cyclophosphamide, ifosfamide, etoposide, 5-fluorouracil, tamoxifen, topotecan, hexamethylmelamine, gemcitabine, navelbine, and doxorubicin. Investigational approaches include intraperitoneal therapy, high-dose chemotherapy with hematologic support, and immunologic therapy. The Autologous Marrow Transplant Registry – North America recorded 390 women with ovarian cancer treated with high-dose chemotherapy between 1986 and 1989 in North America.[31] This registry is thought to capture data on half the transplants conducted in North America. We have limited, if any, data on patterns of care for recurrence otherwise.

Surgery

We do not know if debulking surgery at the time of recurrence will prolong survival. Surgery to relieve obstruction or improve quality of life appears reasonable. We have little or no data on the use of surgery in women with recurrent disease.

Supportive care

In the general cancer population, we know that pain management is often inadequate and that hospice services are underutilized.[32] Ovarian cancer patients commonly experience pain, fatigue, and psychological distress. This pain often interferes with activity, mood, enjoyment of life, sleep, and social relations.[33] We have limited, if any, data on control of pain among most ovarian cancer patients.[34]

In 1996, hospice services were provided to about half of all men and women dying of cancer.[35] Over 70% of dying cancer patients wanted to die at home, but only 20% were able to do so. It is likely that these patterns hold for ovarian cancer, although we have limited, if any, data specific to ovarian cancer.

Conclusions

Systems for collecting data on patterns of care clearly need improvement. Even in those countries with centralized healthcare and more effective data collection, we may need to conduct more intensive research on certain aspects of care for women with ovarian cancer. As mentioned above, we know little about the use of screening outside of research protocols, the use of laparoscopy in evaluating adnexal masses, intraoperative decision making, adjuvant chemotherapy, care for women with recurrent disease, and palliative care.

The existing patterns of care do point out some areas where we can make major improvements. Many women with advanced ovarian cancer do not have effective surgery initially. This may occur because effective surgery was not possible technically, or because the patient had too many co-morbidities, or because the properly trained surgeon was not present. None the less, the initiation of appropriate chemotherapy, followed by interval surgery, can improve the outlook for such patients. The data from the European Organization for Research on the Treatment of Cancer, Gynecologic Cancer Cooperative Group Suggests, that interval debulking enhances survival.[36] We must work to ensure that the appropriate chemotherapy is given and that the patient is followed by a multidisciplinary team with expertise in ovarian cancer. The window of time, while the patient is receiving this 'neoadjuvant chemotherapy' can be used to make the necessary arrangements. Once the woman with ovarian cancer has established a firm relationship with a such a team, then we have some assurances that she will receive appropriate cancer care for the rest of her life.

We need to focus physician and lay education on the importance of surgical staging. Through hospital tumor registries and tumor boards, we should be able to encourage physicians to increase the proportion of patients who have appropriate staging. With the development of laparoscopic techniques, this staging may be done as an outpatient or day-case procedure in most patients with presumed early stage disease. Widespread use of the risk-of-malignancy index for triage of women with adnexal masses would also facilitate both staging and cytoreduction.

How best to establish a comprehensive system of care for women with ovarian cancer will differ from region to region and from country to country. The characteristics of a model of excel-

Table 42.1 Characteristics of a model of excellence for cancer care (from Smith et al. 1999[37])

Co-ordinated care with one person in charge
Ease of access
Ready access to information, answers to questions, and psychosocial support
Multidisciplinary care with transparency for patients among the disciplines
Guidelines for patient management of all common problems
Full range of services from prevention to survivor follow-up and hospice care
Measurement of patient processes and outcomes to ensure good care
Accountability of healthcare providers to measured outcomes
Acceptable predetermined cost

lence have been described by Smith et al. (Table 42.1).[37] For women with ovarian cancer, the multidisciplinary care may well include gynecologists; gynecologic oncologists; medical, radiation, and nurse oncologists; psychologists; social workers; nutritionists; and physical therapists.

The patterns of care described above strongly suggest that an aggressive approach to multidisciplinary management can improve survival substantially for women with ovarian cancer. In addition, we need to focus efforts on collecting data more effectively, so that we can understand and improve patterns of care for women with ovarian cancer.

References

1. National Cancer Policy Board (1999). *Ensuring quality cancer care.* Institute of Medicine and Commission on Life Sciences, National Research Council. National Academy Press. Washington, DC.
2. Burke, W., Daly, M., Garber, J. *et al.* (1997). Recommendations for follow-up care of individuals with an inherited predisposition to cancer. BRCA1 and BRCA2. *J. Am. Med. Assoc.,* **277,** 997–1003.
3. de Silva, D., Gilbert, F., Needham, G. *et al.* (1995). Identification of women at high genetic risk of breast cancer through the National Health Service Breast Screening Program (NHSBSP). *J. Med. Genet.,* **32,** 862–6.
4. NIH Consensus Development Panel (1994). Ovarian cancer: screening, treatment, and follow-up. *Gynecol. Oncol.,* **55,** S4–S14.
5. Westhoff, C. (1994). Current status of screening for ovarian cancer. *Gynecol. Oncol.,* **55,** S34–S37.
6. Jacobs, I., Oram, D., Fairbanks, J. *et al.* (1990). A risk of malignancy index incorporating CA 125, ultrasound and menopausal status for the accurate pre-operative diagnosis of ovarian cancer. *Br. J. Obstet. Gynaecol.,* **97,** 922–9.
7. Tingulstad, S., Hagen, B., Skjeldestad, F.E. *et al.* (1999). The risk-of-malignancy index to evaluate potential ovarian cancers in local hospitals. *Obstet. Gynecol.,* **93,** 448–52.
8. Nezhat, F., Nezhat, C., Welander, C.E. *et al.* (1992). Four ovarian cancers diagnosed during laparoscopic management of 1011 women with adnexal masses. *Am. J. Obstet. Gynecol.,* **167,** 790–6.
9. Canis, M., Pouly, J.L., Wattiez, A. *et al.* (1997). Laparoscopic management of adnexal masses suspicious at ultrasound. *Obstet. Gynecol.,* **89,** 679–83.
10. Allen, D.G., Baak, J., Belpomme, D. *et al.* (1993). Advanced epithelial ovarian cancer: 1993 consensus statements. *Ann. Oncol.,* **4,** (suppl. 4), S83–S88.
11. Ozols, R.F. Update of the NCCN ovarian cancer practice guidelines. *Oncology – New York,* **11,** 95–106.
12. Society of Gynecologic Oncologists (1998). *Practice guidelines: ovarian cancer. Oncology – New York,* **12,** 129–33.
13. Report of a working group, Chairman, Professor J.S. Scott (1991). *Management of ovarian cancer. Current Clinical Practices.* Standing Subcommittee on Cancer of the Standing Medical Advisory Committee. Department of Health, United Kingdom.
14. Grilli, R., Alexanian, A., Apolone, G. *et al.* (1990). The impact of cancer treatment guidelines on actual practice in Italian general hospitals: the case of ovarian cancer. *Ann. Oncol.,* **1,** 112–18.
15. Hogberg, T., Carstensen, J. and Simonsen, E. (1993). Treatment results and prognostic factors in a population-based study of epithelial ovarian cancer. *Gynecol. Oncol.,* **48,** 38–49.
16. Junor, E.J., Hole, D.J., and Gillis, C.R. (1994). Management of ovarian cancer: referral to a multidisciplinary team matters. *Br. J. Cancer,* **70,** 363–70.
17. Trope, C., personal communication.

18. Wolfe, C.D.A., Tilling, Raju, K.S. (1997). Management and survival of ovarian cancer patients in South East England. *Eur. J. Cancer*, **33**, 1835–40.

19. Munoz, K.A., Harlan, L.C., and Trimble, E.L. (1997). Patterns of care for women with ovarian cancer in the United States. *J. Clin. Oncol.*, **15**, 3408–15.

20. Partridge, E.E., Phillips, J.L., and Menck, H.R. (1996). The National Cancer Data Base Report on Ovarian Cancer Treatment in United States Hospitals. *Cancer*, **78**, 2236–46.

21. Farrow, D.C., Samet, J.M. and Hunt, W.C. (1996). Regional variation in survival following the diagnosis of cancer. *J. Clin. Epidemiol.*, **49**, 843–7.

22. McGowan, L. (1993). Patterns of care in carcinoma of the ovary. *Cancer*, **71**, 628–33.

23. Nguyen, H.N., Averette, H.E., Hoskins, W. *et al.* (1993). National Survey of Ovarian Carcinoma Part V. The impact of physician's specialty upon patients' surrvival. *Cancer*, **72**, 3663–70.

24. Hand, R., Fremgen, A., Chmiel, J.S. *et al.* (1993). Staging procedures, clinical management, and survival outcome for ovarian carcinoma. *J. Am. Med. Assoc.*, **269**, 1119–22.

25. Eisenkop, S.M., Spirtos, N.M., Montag, T.W. *et al.* (1992). The impact of subspecialty training on the management of advanced ovarian cancer. *Gynecol. Oncol.*, **47**, 203–9.

26. Kehoe, S., Powell, J., Wilson, S. *et al.* (1994). The influence of the operating surgeons's specialisation on patient survival in ovarian carcinoma. *Br. J. Cancer*, **70**, 1014–17.

27. Woodman, C., Baghdady, A., Collins, S. *et al.* (1997). What changes in the organisation of cancer services will improve the outcome for women with ovarian cancer. *Br. J. Obstet. Gynaecol.*, **104**, 135–9.

28. Hightower, R.D., Nguyen, H.N., Averette, H.E. *et al.* (1994). National Survey of Ovarian Carcinoma IV: Pattersn of care and related survival for older patients. *Cancer*, **73**, 377–83.

29. Ries, L.A.G. (1993) Ovarian cancer. Survival and treatment differences by age. *Cancer*, **71**, 524–9.

30. Canetta, R., personal communication.

31. Horowitz, M.M., Stiff, P.J., Veum-Stone, J. *et al.* (1997). Outcome of autotransplants for advanced ovarian cancer. *Proc. Am. Soc. Clin. Oncol.*, **16**, 353a (abstract 1262).

32. Jacox, A., Carr, D.B., Payne, R. *et al.* (1994). *Management of cancer pain.* Clinical Practice Guideline Number 9. Agency for Health Care Policy and Research Publication No. 94–0592. Public Health Service. US Department of Health and Human Services.

33. Portnoy, R.K., Kornblith, A.B., Wong, G. *et al.* (1994). Pain in ovarian cancer patients; prevalence, characteristics, and associated symptoms. *Cancer*, **74**, 907–15.

34. Montazeri, A., McEwen, J., and Gillis, C.R. (1996). Quality of life in patients with ovarian cancer; current state of research. *Supportive Care in Cancer*, **4**, 169–79.

35. American Society of Clinical Oncology (1998). Cancer care during the last phase of life. *J. Clin. Oncol.*, **16**, 1986–96.

36. Van der Burg, M.E., van Lent, M., Buyse, M. *et al.* (1995). The effect of debulking surgery after induction chemotherapy on the prognosis in advanced epithelial ovarian cancer. Gynecological Cancer Cooperative Group of the European Organization for Research on the Treatment of Cancer. *N. Engl. J. Med.*, **332**, 629–34.

37. Smith, T.J., Desch, C.E. and Hillner, B.E. (1999). *The quality of cancer care: models of excellence.* National Cancer Policy Board.

Part 7

Adjuvant and palliative therapy for ovarian cancer

43. Current chemotherapy options in ovarian cancer

Martin Gore, Francisco Sapunar, and David Gibbs

Introduction

The incidence of ovarian cancer is similar in the United States and European Union, with 25 000 cases a year being reported.[1,2] The majority of patients present with advanced disease, and although response rates to chemotherapy are high, many patients eventually develop drug-resistant tumours and the 5-year mortality from ovarian cancer remains at 60–70%. In recent years, many new active agents have been developed and this has considerably widened the possibilities for treatment. The treatment options depend on whether a patient is being treated at first line or at relapse, with standard therapy or as part of an experimental protocol.

First-line therapy

Platinum drugs are the most active agents in untreated ovarian cancer and form the mainstay of any regimen for this disease (Table 43.1). The survival benefit for platinum therapy is particularly impressive in population-based studies although, interestingly, the effect of platinum on overall survival in individual randomized trials is not large.[2–5] This is almost certainly a function of the frequency of crossover in these randomized studies and the efficacy of platinum compounds in second-line therapy. This results in a degree of 'rescue' of patients who are randomized to the non-platinum-containing arms of these studies.

Table 43.1 Single-agent activity in previously untreated patients

	Number of studies	Number of patients	Response rate
Cisplatin	9+	686	58%
Paclitaxel	3[a]	269	46%
Anthracycline	3[b]	43	42%
Alkylating agents	10+	999	29%

+, Randomized data.

[a] 1/3 studies randomized.

[b] 2/3 studies randomized.

In the 1980s the main controversy was whether or not platinum should be given as a single agent, in combination with cyclophosphamide, or as part of a three-drug regimen with cyclophosphamide and Adriamycin (CAP). There were strong arguments for using single-agent platinum when carboplatin was developed because of its superior toxicity profile. However, there were benefits in terms of response rates to combination platinum-based therapy, but it was not until a meta-analysis by the Advanced Ovarian Cancer Trialists Group (AOCTG) in 1991 that a small but statistically significant survival benefit was demonstrated for combining other drugs with platinum ($P = 0.03$).[5] In practice, this meant a choice between cisplatin-cyclophosphamide or CAP. There was some evidence from two meta-analyses that the addition of Adriamycin was associated with a survival advantage, but recent data from a large randomized trial has failed to demonstrate any survival difference between single-agent carboplatin and CAP.[5–7]

Paclitaxel

In 1996, McGuire and colleagues from the Gynaecologic Oncology Group (GOG 111) described a significant survival benefit for cisplatin-paclitaxel over cisplatin-cyclophosphamide.[8] There were some criticisms of the data, in particular, the unusual finding that the increase in progression-free survival was not as great as the increase in overall survival. Some, including the present authors, argued that confirmatory data were required before the combination of a platinum compound and paclitaxel became standard therapy, because this result was counter-intuitive. These confirmatory data are now available, following presentation of the overall survival figures from a large multicentre collaborative trial in Europe, Scandinavia, and Canada (EORTC-GCCG, NOCOVA, NCIC-CTG and the Scottish Co-operative Group), this study is often referred to as the Intergroup trial.[9] There are differences between GOG 111 and the Intergroup studies in terms of patient eligibility (suboptimal disease only, as opposed to optimally and suboptimally debulked patients) and the schedule of paclitaxel; however, the striking feature of these two trials is the similarity of their results; median overall survival was increased from 24 months to 38 months in the GOG study and from 25 months to 35 months in the Intergroup trial. An analysis combining these two data sets demonstrates a survival advantage favouring cisplatin-paclitaxel, with a statistical significance rarely seen in cancer therapy trials ($P = 0.000001$).[10]

A third study from the GOG (132) randomized patients to single-agent cisplatin, single-agent paclitaxel, or a combination of the two. This study failed to show a survival advantage in favour of the combination, but the study has been widely criticised for the high percentage of patients who crossed over in the single-agent arms. In particular, almost half of the patients treated by single-agent cisplatin or paclitaxel received the other drug before progression was documented.[11] The results of GOG 132 allow speculation into the possibility of using sequential treatments as opposed to combination therapy.

Cisplatin-carboplatin equivalence

There are 12 randomized trials comparing cisplatin with carboplatin when administered either as single agents or in combination regimens. The results of these trials were part of the meta-analysis performed by the AOCTG which was recently updated.[12] The analysis included over 2000 patients and shows no difference in survival between patients treated with cisplatin or carboplatin. An important question is whether or not, in the context of paclitaxel, carboplatin can be substituted for cisplatin. The schedule used in GOG 111 is rather inconvenient, with paclitaxel being given over 24 hours. However, when paclitaxel was given over 3 hours in combination with cisplatin, as in the schedule reported by the Intergroup, there was a high incidence of serious neurotoxicity.[9] It has been argued that the results of the meta-analysis showing equivalence of cisplatin and carboplatin may not necessarily extend to platinum-paclitaxel combinations. Three randomized studies have now been performed which compare carboplatin-paclitaxel to cisplatin-paclitaxel. Early data from these trials have been presented and show a clear advantage for carboplatin—paclitaxel in terms of neurotoxicity, and from two of the trials there is a suggestion of equal efficacy, as assessed by response rates and progression-free survival.[13–15] However, mature data from these three studies are required before it is known whether overall survival is affected by substituting carboplatin for cisplatin in platinum-paclitaxel combinations (Table 43.2).

Platinum dose intensity

Dose intensity remains a subject for continuing debate. *In vitro* data suggest that increasing platinum concentrations in cultures of ovarian cancer cells increases cell kill,[16] but the majority of the 10 randomized trials that address this issue have been negative (reviewed in ref. 17). These trials increase the total dose or dose intensity of platinum by no more than a factor of 2. Only the two smallest trials showed benefit from the increase in dose intensity.[17,18] A large Scottish Co-operative Group trial initially reported a survival benefit when the dose of cisplatin was increased from 50 mg/m^2 to 100 mg/m^2 but on longer follow-up the advantage substantially reduced and, because of the increased toxicity of cisplatin at 100 mg/m^2, the authors recommended that cisplatin should be given at 75 mg/m^2.[19] The Danish Ovarian Cancer Co-operative group randomized patients to receive carboplatin at an AUC of 4 or 8 plus cyclophosphamide, and failed to demonstrate any survival benefit to doubling the dose of carboplatin.[20] A trial from the London Gynaecological Oncology Group showed a similar result when patients were randomized to receive single-agent carboplatin at an AUC of 6 for six cycles, compared to an AUC of 12 for four cycles.[21]

Conclusions

The overall conclusions from trials of first-line chemotherapy published in the 1990s are that carboplatin is considerably less oto-, neuro-, and nephrotoxic than cisplatin, and that in non-paclitaxel-containing regimens, it can be substituted safely for cisplatin. There is increasing evidence, although still not conclusive, that it can also be substituted safely for cisplatin within the context of paclitaxel-containing regimens. There appears to be no advantage to doubling the dose of platinum. In particular, cisplatin at a dose of 100 mg/m^2 every 21 days for six cycles, is associated with an unacceptably high rate of neurotoxicity and most trial groups now regard the standard dose of cisplatin to be 75 mg/m^2, every 21 days. The dose of carboplatin should always be determined by the AUC and doses within a range of AUC 5–8, every 21–28 days are standard. The method of calculating the dose in relation to renal function is not critical for standard therapy in patients who are of normal weight. Glomerular filtration can be calculated using the Cockcroft or Jelliffe formulae or measured directly by [^{51}Cr]EDTA clearance. The dose can then be estimated using the method described by Calvert and colleagues.[22–24]

Table 43.2 Randomized trials of carboplatin-paclitaxel versus cisplatin-paclitaxel

	AGO	GOG 158	Dutch/Danish
Cisplatin (mg/m^2)	75	75	75
Carboplatin (AUC)	6	7.5	5
Paclitaxel (mg/m^2, 3 h)	185	175	175
Patients			
Stage	IIB–IV	III	IIB–IV
Bulk	All	≤ I cm	All
n	798	792	190

Cycle 21 days.

Second-line therapy

Patients with relapsed ovarian cancer are incurable and one important option to consider is the one of best supportive care alone. In patients who receive chemotherapy, a balance needs to be struck between the oncological principle of avoiding unnecessary therapy in incurable (i.e. palliative) situations, and not delaying treatment for so long that the disease has progressed to an extent where response is unlikely. Patients need realistic information regarding the outcome of any intervention for relapsed disease.

Predictors of response

It has been known for some time that the interval between the end of first-line therapy and first relapse, or the treatment-free interval between subsequent relapses, is an important determining factor for response. Patients who relapse with treatment-free intervals of greater than 12 or 24 months have a good chance of responding to agents they have not previously received or a rechallenge with further platinum-based therapy.[25–27] An analysis by Eisenhauer and colleagues on 704 patients entered into 13 studies identified 11 predictive factors for response to second- and third-line treatment. A treatment-free interval of greater than 6 months was identified as one of the predictive factors, but it was not shown to be an independent predictor of response. A multivariate analysis showed that serous histology, number of disease sites, and tumour size, which was closely correlated with treatment-free interval, were the only independent predictors of response.[28]

Timing of treatment

The finding that the number of disease sites and the bulk of disease is an important predictor of response, when taken together with the fact that these patients are incurable, has important practical implications for standard practice, particularly in relation to the timing of treatment for relapsed disease.

A common problem is a rising CA125 with no clinical or CT evidence of disease in an asymptomatic patient. There is no justification for routinely treating such patients on the basis of a rising CA125 only, and an important MRC-EORTC trial has recently opened to accrual that sets out to answer this question of early versus delayed treatment. However, from Eisenhauer's multivariate analysis it appears that one can delay treatment too long, in that there is the potential for bulky, multisite disease to develop with time and hence reduce the patient's chance of response. Our relative lack of knowledge in this area makes the follow-up of patients difficult and the decision when to institute therapy for relapsed disease complex.

Active agents

A number of drugs are available to patients who relapse within 12 months of first-line therapy. Paclitaxel was the favoured treatment option at relapse, but is less so now that most patients receive this drug in the first line. There are, however, ongoing trials that examine different schedules of paclitaxel in the relapsed setting, in particular weekly administration.[29] Docetaxel has also been evaluated in the relapse setting and shown to have similar single-agent activity to paclitaxel, a 31% response rate in three trials involving 154 patients,[30–32] and it is now being evaluated as a first-line option in combination with carboplatin. Phase II studies of topotecan demonstrate response rates of 14–16%,[33,34] although, interestingly, when topotecan was compared to paclitaxel in a randomized trial, response rates were 20% and 13%, respectively.[35]

Table 43.3 Single-agent activity of new agents

	Number of studies	n	Response rate
Altretamine	7	308	21%
Gemcitabine	4	79	20%
Oxaliplatin	3	105	24%
Vinorelbine	2	59	30%

There has been renewed interest in the use of etoposide, particularly when given orally. The GOG has recently published a large phase II study of etoposide given at 50 mg/m^2/day for 21 days on a 28-day cycle, showing that in 41 patients with a treatment-free interval of 6 months the response rate was 27%, and in 41 patients with a treatment-free interval greater than 6 months the response rate was 34%.[36] Like etoposide, anthracyclines have been used for many years, and cumulative data from seven trials of doxorubicin involving 258 patients, and six trials of epirubicin involving 189 patients, show that response rates of 15% and 20%, respectively, are obtained.[37–48] Liposomal doxorubicin has been shown to result in a 26% response rate in patients previously being treated with platinum and paclitaxel.[49]

A number of new agents have become available in the past 5 years, including gemcitabine,[50–53] altretamine,[54–59] oxaliplatin,[31,60,61] and vinorelbine.[62,63] The data from these studies clearly show that these new agents have a similar activity to those drugs which have previously been shown to be active in relapsed ovarian cancer, namely paclitaxel, topotecan, anthracyclines, and etoposide (Table 43.3). As a result of these data, a large number of single-agent options have become available for the treatment of relapsed disease, and when deciding the most appropriate treatment for an individual patient consideration needs to be given to the toxicity, cost, and convenience of administration.

Combination regimens

There are data to suggest that higher response rates can be obtained in patients who relapse within 12 months of first-line chemotherapy if combination regimens are used. A combination of cisplatin, epirubicin, and infusional 5-fluorouracil (ECF) demonstrated a response rate of 38% in 37 patients,[64] weekly cisplatin combined with etoposide demonstrated a 67% response rate,[65] and, more recently, these latter authors reported very high response rate in relapsed patients treated with weekly cisplatin and paclitaxel.[66] A number of combinations involving drugs developed in the 1990s have been evaluated in relapsed patients, including cisplatin and irinotecan, which demonstrated a 40% response rate in 25 patients;[67] cisplatin plus oxaliplatin,[68] which demonstrated a response rate of 40% in 25 patients; and oxaliplatin plus paclitaxel, which demonstrated a 50% response rate in 23 patients.[69] In a randomized trial of paclitaxel versus paclitaxel plus epirubicin in patients relapsing within 6 months of first-line platinum-based chemotherapy, there was a doubling of the response rate from 17% to 34% with combination therapy, but this was not significant and there was no impact on overall survival.[70] A randomized study of CAP versus paclitaxel in patients relapsing after 12 months showed that there was a significantly higher complete remission rate and progression-free survival (PFS) with platinum-based re-challenge treatment than with single-agent paclitaxel (complete remission 32% versus 20%; median PFS 18.9% versus 7.3%). However, overall survival was not prolonged by the use of the combination, and it was more toxic.[71]

Conclusions

Guidelines regarding the institution of second- or third-line therapy should take known predictors of response into account. Patients with symptomatic disease who have a reasonable chance of responding to further chemotherapy based on these predictive factors should be offered further treatment. Patients with asymptomatic progressive disease defined by CA125 only should be carefully followed up, possibly with imaging investigations, and treatment instituted when there is other evidence of progression. However, this progression should not be so advanced as to compromise the patient's chances of a further response. Our practice is to perform CT scans on asymptomatic patients with rising serum CA125 levels and to institute treatment when there is measurable disease of about 2–3 cm. The preferred treatment option in patients who relapse should always be an offer to enter a clinical trial. Late-relapsing patients should be re-treated with platinum-based therapy, which can be a combination regimen if they are fit, and would include paclitaxel if this has not been used previously. The decision to advise a patient to stop having further lines of chemotherapy for their relapsed disease is difficult, as there are no trials that specifically address this issue. However, patients who are refractory to two lines of treatment or who relapse within 4 months of therapy on two occasions are unlikely to respond to further chemotherapy, and in our institution we would only rarely offer a third line of cytotoxic therapy to such a patient.

Research options

Patients with advanced ovarian cancer, whether they are being treated at presentation or for relapsed disease, should be offered entry into prospective studies. An important area of research is the targeting of patients for particular therapies, involving the examination of clinical factors, histopathological appearances and, perhaps more importantly, new molecular markers that can be used to predict response to a specific drug or combination of drugs. Therapeutic trials should aim to develop new regimens to either increase complete remission rate and/or consolidate them. There are four main strategies for developing new first-line therapies.

1. In the past, more cycles of standard therapy have been administered, but this has not been shown to benefit survival in previous studies involving platinum.[72–74] However, it remains an open question whether more cycles of platinum plus paclitaxel or some of the newer cytotoxics confer an advantage over the conventional six courses. It is important to generate such data because, increasingly, oncologists in some countries are treating patients with more than six courses of carboplatin-paclitaxel without randomized evidence that this is beneficial.

2. A second strategy is to increase the complete remission rate by increasing the dose of drugs given, either using high-dose chemotherapy with peripheral blood stem cell or bone-marrow rescue, or by utilizing the intraperitoneal route. Previously, we have reviewed the data on high-dose chemotherapy[17] and it is clear that initial therapy with multiple cycles of high-dose treatment, as described by Fennelly and colleagues,[75] is an important concept that should be evaluated. The use of intraperitoneal chemotherapy remains very controversial and a subject that induces great excitement in both exponents and detractors of this method of administration. It is clear that intraperitoneal therapy, either in the first-line or relapse setting, should only be considered for patients with disease of less than 1 cm diameter, and that great attention needs to be paid to the practicalities of the technique in terms of the placement of the catheters and their aftercare. There are two prospective randomized trials reporting these of intraperitoneal cisplatin as first-line therapy.[76,77] The results can best be summarized by stating that one shows a clear survival advantage to the use of intraperitoneal therapy, while the other shows a trend towards a survival advantage which just fails to reach statistical significance. There are no good randomized trials of intraperitoneal therapy given in the relapse setting. Our interpretation of the data is that intraperitoneal therapy is an important area for further investigation, but that this needs to be within the context of randomized trials and that intraperitoneal therapy should not be used routinely off-study.

3. Another method of increasing the remissions is to add more drugs to a basic platinum-paclitaxel combination. This can either be done by creating triple drug combinations, and such regimens are being developed with the addition of topotecan, gemcitabine, anthracyclines, or alkylating agents to platinum-paclitaxel. In addition, new two-drug combinations are being investigated, utilizing some of the cytotoxic agents that have been developed in the past 10 years; such combinations include cisplatin-topotecan, cisplatin-gemcitabine, and oxaliplatin-cyclophosphamide. These combinations could simply be compared to platinum-paclitaxel in randomized trials, but increasingly investigators are interested in using sequential therapies involving two-drug combinations. Such sequences might involve two platinum-containing regimens but with a change of non-platinum drug after 4–6 cycles, or initial platinum-paclitaxel therapy followed by a non-platinum-containing two-drug combination such as paclitaxel-anthracycline, topotecan-etoposide, etc.

4. Finally, future trials should attempt to consolidate the high remission rates that are seen with the new chemotherapy combinations by following six cycles of treatment with high-dose or intraperitoneal therapy. Alternatively, a 'maintenance' strategy can be adopted, using agents with non-cytotoxic mechanisms of action, such as immunotherapy, angiogenesis inhibitors, or metalloproteinase inhibitors. It is unclear how some of the entirely novel approaches to therapy, such as the correction of *p53* mutations using gene therapy techniques or genetically engineered viruses such as Onyx-015, will impact on patient management, but these are important areas of early investigation.

Conclusions

The chemotherapy options for patients with ovarian cancer have never been greater. There are now a large number of drugs and combinations that are clearly active both in the first-line and in the relapsed setting. Current data suggest that standard first-line therapy consists of a platinum compound in combination with paclitaxel, and increasingly it appears that it is safe to substitute carboplatin for cisplatin.

The treatment of relapsed disease is a complicated issue. Patients need to be involved closely in the decision of when to treat and which drug(s) to use, because therapy in this situation is palliative and therefore toxicity becomes a major concern. A fine balance needs to be struck between instituting treatment too early, when treatment may not be of benefit to the patient, or too late, when the chances of a response are reduced because of an increasing volume of disease and a deterioration in the patient's performance status. Gynaecological Oncology Units need to have a guideline to help them determine when it is appropriate to no longer offer patients chemotherapy because the disease is demonstrably chemoresistant.

The potential areas for clinical research are as numerous as the new agents that have appeared in the past 10 years. Investigators need to prioritize the available strategies, particularly in trials of first-line therapy. There are differences in philosophy between studies that use more drugs, or at higher doses or intensity, to existing regimens to increase the complete remission rate, and those that attempt to consolidate remissions by either high-dose chemotherapy/intraperitoneal therapy or agents with novel mechanisms of action suitable for maintaining remissions, such as angiogenesis inhibitors.

References

1. Cancer in the European Community (1992).
2. Landis, S.H., Murray, T., Bolden, S., and Wingo, P.A. (1998). *Cancer statistics, 1998*. *CA Cancer J. Clin.*, **48** (1), 6–29. [Published errata appear in *CA Cancer J. Clin.*, **48** (3), 192 and **48** (6), 329.]
3. Junor, E.J., Hole, D.J., and Gillis, C.R. (1994). Management of ovarian cancer: referral to a multidisciplinary team matters. *Br. J. Cancer*, **70**(2), 363–70.
4. Hunter, R.W., Alexander, N.D., and Soutter, W.P. (1992). Meta-analysis of surgery in advanced ovarian carcinoma: is maximum cytoreductive surgery an independent determinant of prognosis? [See comments.] *Am. J. Obstet. Gynecol.*, **166** (2), 504–11.
5. Advanced Ovarian Cancer Trialists Group (1991). Chemotherapy in advanced ovarian cancer: an overview of randomised clinical trials. Advanced Ovarian Cancer Trialists Group. [See comments.] *BMJ*, **303** (6807), 884 93.
6. A'Hern, R.P. and Gore, M.E. (1995). Impact of doxorubicin on survival in advanced ovarian cancer. *J. Clin. Oncol.*, **13**(3), 726–32.
7. The Icon Collaborators (1998). ICON2: randomised trial of single-agent carboplatin against three-drug combination of CAP (cyclophosphamide, doxorubicin, and cisplatin) in women with ovarian cancer. ICON Collaborators. International Collaborative Ovarian Neoplasm Study. [See comments.] *Lancet*, **352** (9140), 1571–6.
8. Piccart, M.J., K. Bertelsen, K. James, J. Cassidy *et al.*, (2000). Randomized intergroup trial of cisplatin-paclitaxel versus cisplatin-cyclophosphamide in women with advanced epithelial ovarian cancer: three-year results. *J. Natl. Cancer Inst.*, **92**(9), 699–708.
9. Stuart, G., Bertelsen, K., Mangioni, K. *et al.* (1998). Updated analsysis shows a highly significant improved overall survival (OS) for cisplatin-paclitaxel as first line treatment of advanced ovarian cancer. Mature results of the EORTC-GCCG, NOCOVA, NCIC CTG and Scottish Intergroup

trial. In *Thirty-Fourth Annual Meeting of the American Society of Clinical Oncology*, (ed. M.C. Perry). American Society of Clinical Oncology, Los Angeles, CA.
10. Adams, M., Calvert, A.H., Carmichael, J. *et al.* (1998). Chemotherapy for ovarian cancer-a consensus statement on standard practice [editorial]. [See comments.] *Br. J. Cancer*, **78**(11), 1404–6.
11. Muggia, F.M., P.S., Braly, M.F. Brady, G. Sutton *et al.* (2000). Phase III randomized study of cisplatin versus paclitaxel versus cisplatin and paclitaxel in patients with suboptimal stage III or IV ovarian cancer: a gynecologic oncology group study. *J. Clin. Oncol.*, **18**(1), 106–15.
12. Aabo, K., Adams, M., Adnitt, P. *et al.* (1998). Chemotherapy in advanced ovarian cancer: four systematic meta-analyses of individual patient data from 37 randomized trials. Advanced Ovarian Cancer Trialists' Group. *Br. J. Cancer*, **78**(11), 1479–87.
13. Neijt, J.P., Hansen, M., Hansen, S.W. *et al.* (1997). Randomized phase III study in previously untreated epithelial ovarian cancer FIGO stage IIB, IIC, III, IV, comparing paclitaxel-cisplatin and paclitaxel-carboplatin (Meeting abstract). In *Thirty-Third Annual Meeting of the American Society of Clinical Oncology*, (ed. M.C. Perry). American Society of Clinical Oncology, Denver, CO.
14. du Bois, A., Nitz, U., Schroder, W. *et al.* (1997). Cisplatin/paclitaxel versus carboplatin/paclitaxel as first-line chemotherapy in ovarian cancer: interim analysis of an AGO Study Group trial. [Meeting abstract] In *Thirty-Third Annual Meeting of the American Society of Clinical Oncology*, (ed. M.C. Perry). American Society of Clinical Oncology, Denver, CO.
15. Ozols, R.F., Bundy, B.N., Fowler, J. *et al.* (1999). Randomized phase III study of cisplatin (CIS)/paclitaxel (PAC) versus carboplatin (CARBO)/ PAC in optimal stage III epithelial ovarian cancer (OC): a Gynecologic Oncology Group Trial (GOG 158). In *Thirty-Fifth Annual Meeting of the American Society of Clinical Oncology*, (ed. M.C. Perry). p. 356a. American Society of Clinical Oncology, Atlanta, Georgia.
16. Alberts, D.S., Young, L., Mason, N., and Salmon, S.E. (1985). *In vitro*-evaluation of anticancer drugs against ovarian cancer at concentrations achievable by intraperitoneal administration. *Semin. Oncol.*, **12**(3 Suppl. 4), 38–42.
17. Gore, M.E. (1998). Overview—High-dose and intraperitoneal therapy. In *Ovarian Cancer 5*, (ed. F. Sharp, T. Blackett, J. Berek, and R. Blast), pp. 311–20. Isis Medical Media, Oxford.
18. Ngan, H.Y., Choo, Y.C., Cheung, M., *et al.* (1989). A randomized study of high-dose versus low-dose cis-platinum combined with cyclophosphamide in the treatment of advanced ovarian cancer. Hong Kong Ovarian Carcinoma Study Group. *Chemotherapy*, **35**(3), 221–7.
19. Kaye, S.B., Paul, J., Cassidy, J. *et al.* (1996). Mature results of a randomized trial of two doses of cisplatin for the treatment of ovarian cancer. Scottish Gynecology Cancer Trials Group. *J. Clin. Oncol.*, **14**(7), 2113–19.
20. Jakobsen, A., Bertelsen, K., Andersen, J.E. *et al.* (1997). Dose-effect study of carboplatin in ovarian cancer: a Danish Ovarian Cancer Group study. *J. Clin. Oncol.*, **15**(1), 193–8.
21. Gore, M., Mainwaring, P., A'Hern, R. *et al.* (1998). Randomized trial of dose-intensity with single-agent carboplatin in patients with epithelial ovarian cancer. London Gynaecological Oncology Group. *J. Clin. Oncol.*, **16**(7), 2426–34.
22. Calvert, A.H., Newell, D.R., Gumbrell, L.A. *et al.* (1989). Carboplatin dosage: prospective evaluation of a simple formula based on renal function. [See comments.] *J. Clin. Oncol.*, **7**(11), 1748–56.
23. Cockcroft, D.W. and Gault, M.H. (1976). Prediction of creatinine clearance from serum creatinine. *Nephron*, **16**(1), 31 41.
24. Jelliffe, R.W. (1973). Letter: Creatinine clearance: bedside estimate. *Ann. Intern. Med.*, **79**(4), 604–5.
25. Gore, M.E., Fryatt, I., Wiltshaw, E., and Dawson, T. (1990). Treatment of relapsed carcinoma of the ovary with cisplatin or carboplatin following initial treatment with these compounds. *Gynecol. Oncol.*, **36**(2), 207–11.
26. Markman, M., Reichman, B., Hakes, T. *et al.* (1991). Responses to second-line cisplatin-based intraperitoneal therapy in ovarian cancer: influence of a prior response to intravenous cisplatin. *J. Clin. Oncol.*, **9**(10), 1801–5.

27. Blackledge, G., Lawton, F., Redman, C., and Kelly, K. (1989). Response of patients in phase II studies of chemotherapy in ovarian cancer: implications for patient treatment and the design of phase II trials. *Br. J. Cancer*, **59**(4), 650–3.

28. Eisenhauer, E.A., Vermorken, J.B., and van Glabbeke, M. (1997). Predictors of response to subsequent chemotherapy in platinum pretreated ovarian cancer: a multivariate analysis of 704 patients. [See comments.] *Ann. Oncol.*, **8** (10), 963–8.

29. Fennelly, D., Aghajanian, C., Shapiro, F. *et al.* (1997). Phase I and pharmacologic study of paclitaxel administered weekly in patients with relapsed ovarian cancer. *J. Clin. Oncol.*, **15**(1), 187–92.

30. Francis, P., Schneider, J., Hann, L. *et al.* (1994). Phase II trial of docetaxel in patients with platinum-refractory advanced ovarian cancer. *J. Clin. Oncol.*, **12**(11), 2301–8.

31. Piccart-Gebhart, M., Green, A., Lacave, P. *et al.* (1998). A randomized phase II study of taxol or oxaliplatin in platinum-pretreated epithelial ovarian cancer (EOC) patients (Pts). In *Thirty-Fourth Annual Meeting of the American Society of Clinical Oncology*, (ed. M.C. Perry), p. 349a. American Society of Clinical Oncology; Los Angeles, CA.

32. Kavanagh, J.J., Kudelka, A.P., de Leon, C.G. *et al.* (1996). Phase II study of docetaxel in patients with epithelial ovarian carcinoma refractory to platinum. *Clin. Cancer Res.*, **2** (5), 837–42.

33. Creemers, G.J., Bolis, G., Gore, M. *et al.* (1996). Topotecan, an active drug in the second-line treatment of epithelial ovarian cancer: results of a large European phase II study. [See comments.] *J. Clin. Oncol.*, **14** (12), 3056–61.

34. Kudelka, A.P., Tresukosol, D., Edwards, C.L. *et al.* (1996). Phase II study of intravenous topotecan as a 5-day infusion for refractory epithelial ovarian carcinoma. *J. Clin. Oncol.*, **14**(5), 1552–7.

35. ten Bokkel Huinink, W., Gore, M., Carmichael, J. *et al.* (1997). Topotecan versus paclitaxel for the treatment of recurrent epithelial ovarian cancer. [See comments.] *J. Clin. Oncol.*, **15**(6), 2183–93.

36. Rose, P.G., Blessing, J.A., Mayer, A.R., and Homesley, H.D. (1998). Prolonged oral etoposide as second-line therapy for platinum-resistant and platinum-sensitive ovarian cancer: a Gynecologic Oncology Group study. *J. Clin. Oncol.*, **16**(2), 405–10.

37. De Palo, G.M., De Lena, M., and Bonadonna, G. (1977). Adriamycin versus adriamycin plus melphalan in advanced ovarian carcinoma. *Cancer Treat. Rep.*, **61**(3), 355–7.

38. Stanhope, C.R., Smith, J.P., and Rutledge, F. (1977). Second trial drugs in ovarian cancer. *Gynecol. Oncol.*, **5**(1), 52–8.

39. Barlow, J.J., Piver, M.S., Chuang, J.T. (1973). Adriamycin and bleomycin, alone and in combination, in gynecologic cancers. *Cancer*, **32**(4), 735–43.

40. Slavik, M. (1975). Adriamycin (NSC-123127) activity in genitourinary and gynecologic malignancies. *Cancer Chemother. Rep.*, **6**, 297–303.

41. Bolis, G., D'Incalci, M., Gramellini, F., and Mangioni, C. (1978). Adriamycin in ovarian cancer patients resistant to cyclophosphamide. *Eur. J. Cancer*, **14**(12), 1401–2.

42. Hubbard, S.M., Barkes, P., and Young, R.C. (1978). Adriamycin therapy for advanced ovarian carcinoma recurrent after chemotherapy. *Cancer Treat. Rep.*, **62**(9), 1375–7.

43. Trope, C., Christiansson, H., Johnsson, J.E. *et al.* (1982). A phase II study of 4'-epidoxorobucin in advanced ovarian carcinoma. In *Anthracyclines and cancer therapy*, pp. 216–21. Ronneby Brunn, Sweden.

44. Hurteloup, P., Cappelaere, P., Armand, J.P., and Mathe, G. Phase II clinical evaluation of 4'-epi-doxorubicin. *Cancer Treat. Rep.*, **67**(4), 337–41.

45. Simonsen, E., Bengtsson, C., Högberg, T. *et al.* (1987). A phase II study of the effect of 4' epi-doxorubicin, administered in high-dose 150 mg in 24 hours intravenous infusion in advanced ovarian carcinoma. In *ECCO*, p. 226.

46. Coleman, R., Towlson, K., Wiltshaw, E. *et al.* (1990). Epirubicin for pretreated advanced ovarian cancer [letter]. *Eur. J. Cancer*, **26**(7), 850–1.

47. Locatelli, M.C., D'Antona, A., Vinci, M. *et al.* (1990). Second-line chemotherapy with epirubicin (EDR) in ovarian carcinoma. (Meeting abstract.) *Ann. Oncol.*, **1**(15).

48. Vermorken, J.B., Kobierska, A., van der Burg, M.E. *et al.* (1995). High-dose epirubicin in platinum-pretreated patients with ovarian carcinoma: the EORTC-GCCG experience. *Eur. J. Gynaecol. Oncol.*, **16**(6), 433–8.

49. Muggia, F.M., Hainsworth, J.D., Jeffers, S. *et al.* (1997). Phase II study of liposomal doxorubicin in refractory ovarian cancer: antitumor activity and toxicity modification by liposomal encapsulation. *J. Clin. Oncol.*, **15** (3), 987–93.

50. Kaufmann, M., Bauknecht, T., Jonat, W. *et al.* (1995). Gemcitabine (Gem) in cisplatin-resistant ovarian cancer. In *Thirty-First Annual Meeting of the American Society of Clinical Oncology*, (ed. M.C. Perry), p. 272. American Society of Clinical Oncology, Los Angeles, CA.

51. Kudelka, A.P., Verschragen, C.F., Edwards, C.L. *et al.* (1998). A preliminary report of a phase 2 study of gemcitabine in women with platinum refractory Mullerian (ovarian, Fallopian tube and primary peritoneal) carcinoma. In *Thirty-Fourth Annual Meeting of the American Society of Clinical Oncology*, (ed. M.C. Perry), p. 367a. American Society of Clinical Oncology, Los Angeles, CA.

52. Lund, B., Hansen, O.P., Theilade, K. *et al.* (1994). Phase II study of gemcitabine (2', 2'-difluorodeoxycytidine) in previously treated ovarian cancer patients. *J. Natl Cancer Inst.*, **86**(20), 1530–3.

53. Millward, M.J., Rischin, D., Toner, G.C. *et al.* (1995). Activity of gemcitabine in ovarian cancer patients resistant to paclitaxel. In *Thirty-First Annual Meeting of the American Society of Clinical Oncology*, (ed. M.C. Perry), p. 277. American Society of Clinical Oncology, Los Angeles, CA.

54. Schink, J., Harris, J., Grosen, E. *et al.* Altretamine (Hexalen) an effective salvage chemotherapy after paclitaxel (Taxol) in women with recurrent platinum resistant ovarian cancer. In *Thirty-First Annual Meeting of the American Society of Clinical Oncology*, (ed. M.C. Perry). American Society of Clinical Oncology, Los Angeles, CA.

55. Manetta, A., MacNeill, C., Lyter, J.A. *et al.* (1990). Hexamethylmelamine as a single second-line agent in ovarian cancer. *Gynecol. Oncol.*, **36**(1), 93–6.

56. Fields, A., Schink, J., Miller, D. *et al.* (1991). Oral hexamethylmelamine: an effective salvage therapy for recurrent ovarian cancer. In *13th World Congress of Gynaecology and Obstetrics, Singapore*, p. 515.

57. Vergote, I., Himmelmann, A., Frankendal, B. *et al.* (1992). Hexamethylmelamine as second-line therapy in platin-resistant ovarian cancer. [See comments.] *Gynecol. Oncol.*, **47**(3), 282–6.

58. Moore, D.H., Valea, F., Crumpler, L.S., and Fowler, W.C., Jr. (1993). Hexamethylmelamine/altretamine as second-line therapy for epithelial ovarian carcinoma. *Gynecol. Oncol.*, **51**(1), 109–12.

59. Markman, M., Blessing, J.A., Moore, D. *et al.* (1998). Altretamine (hexamethylmelamine) in platinum-resistant and platinum-refractory ovarian cancer: a Gynecologic Oncology Group phase II trial. *Gynecol. Oncol.*, **69**(3), 226–9.

60. Chollet, P., Bensmaine, M.A., Brienza, S. *et al.* (1996). Single agent activity of oxaliplatin in heavily pretreated advanced epithelial ovarian cancer. *Ann. Oncol.*, **7**(10), 1065–70.

61. Dieras, V., Bougnoux, T., Petit, P. *et al.* (1998). Oxaliplatin (L-OHP) phase II study in platinum pretreated advanced ovarian cancer (AOC): preliminary results. In *Thirty-Fourth Annual Meeting of the American Society of Clinical Oncology*, (ed. M.C. Perry). American Society of Clinical Oncology, Los Angeles, CA.

62. Bajetta, E., Di Leo, A., Biganzoli, L. *et al.* (1996). Phase II study of vinorelbine in patients with pretreated advanced ovarian cancer: activity in platinum-resistant disease. *J. Clin. Oncol.*, **14**(9), 2546–51.

63. Burger, R.A., Burman, S., White, R. and DiSaia, P.J. (1996). Phase II trial of navelbine in advanced epithelial ovarian cancer. [Meeting abstract.] In *Thirty-Second Annual Meeting of the American Society of Clinical Oncology*, (ed. M.C. Perry). American Society of Clinical Oncology, Philadelphia, PA.

64. Ahmed, F.Y., King, D.M., Nicol, B. *et al.* (1995). Preliminary results of infusional chemotherapy (cisplatin, epirubicin and 5-fluorouracil) for refractory and relapsed epithelial ovarian cancer. In *Thirty-first Annual Meeting of the American Society of Clinical Oncology*, (ed. M.C. Perry), p. 281. American Society of Clinical Oncology.

65. van der Burg, M.E., Logmans, A., de Wit, R. *et al.* (1996). Six weeks of weekly high dose cisplatin (P) and daily oral vepesid (VP): a highly active regimen for ovarian cancer patients (pts) failing on or relapsing after conventional platinum containing combination chemotherapy. [Meeting abstract.] In *Thirty-Second Annual Meeting of the American Society of Clinical Oncology*, (ed. M.C. Perry). American Society of Clinical Oncology, Philadelphia, PA.

66. van der Burg, M.E.L., de Wit, R., Stoter, G., and Verweij, J. (1998). Phase I study of weekly cisplatin (P) and weekly or 4-weely taxol (T): a highly active regimen in advanced epithelial ovarian cancer. In *Thirty-Fourth Annual Meeting of the American Society of Clinical Oncology*, (ed. M.C. Perry), p. 355a. American Society of Clinical Oncology, Los Angeles, CA.

67. Sugiyama, T., Yakushiji, M., Nishida, T. *et al.* (1998). Irinotecan (CPT-11) combined with cisplatin in patients with refractory or recurrent ovarian cancer. *Cancer Lett.*, **128**(2), 211–18.

68. Soulie, P., Bensmaine, A., Garrino, C. *et al.* (1997). Oxaliplatin/cisplatin (L-OHP/CDDP) combination in heavily pretreated ovarian cancer. *Eur. J. Cancer*, **33**(9), 1400–6.

69. Kalla, S., Faivre, S., Bensmaine, M.A. *et al.* (1998). Paclitaxel (PXL)-oxaliplatin (L-OHP): a feasible active combination in heavily pretreated advanced ovarian carcinoma (ADOVCA) patients (PTS). In *Thirty-Fourth Annual Meeting of the American Society of Clinical Oncology*, (ed. M.C. Perry). American Society of Clinical Oncology; Los Angeles, CA.

70. Bolis, G., Scarfone, G., Villa, A. *et al.* (1996). A randomized study in recurrent ovarian cancer comparing the efficacy of single agent vs combination chemotherapy, according to time to relapse. [Meeting abstract.] In *Thirty-Second Annual Meeting of the American Society of Clinical Oncology*, (ed. M.C. Perry). American Society of Clinical Oncology, Philadelphia, PA.

71. Colombo, N., Marzola, M., Parma, G. *et al.* (1996). Paclitaxel vs CAP (cyclophosphamide, Adriamycin, cisplatin) in recurrent platinum sensitive ovarian cancer: a randomized phase II study. [Meeting abstract.] In *Thirty-Second Annual Meeting of the American Society of Clinical Oncology*, (ed. M.C. Perry). American Society of Clinical Oncology, Philadelphia, PA.

72. Bertelsen, K., Jakobsen, A., Stroyer, J. *et al.* (1993). A prospective randomized comparison of 6 and 12 cycles of cyclophosphamide, adriamycin, and cisplatin in advanced epithelial ovarian cancer: a Danish Ovarian Study Group trial (DACOVA). *Gynecol. Oncol.*, **49**(1), 30–6.

73. Hakes, T.B., Chalas, E., Hoskins, W.J. *et al.* (1992). Randomized prospective trial of 5 versus 10 cycles of cyclophosphamide, doxorubicin, and cisplatin in advanced ovarian carcinoma. *Gynecol. Oncol.*, **45**(3), 284–9.

74. Lambert, H.E., Rustin, G.J., Gregory, W.M., and Nelstrop, A.E. (1997). A randomized trial of five versus eight courses of cisplatin or carboplatin in advanced epithelial ovarian carcinoma. A North Thames Ovary Group Study. *Ann. Oncol.*, **8**(4), 327–33.

75. Fennelly, D., Vahdat, L., Schneider, J. *et al.* (1994). High-intensity chemotherapy with peripheral blood progenitor cell support. *Semin. Oncol.*, **21**(2 Suppl. 2): 21–5; quiz 26, 58.

76. Alberts, D.S., Liu, P.Y., Hannigan, E.V. *et al.* (1996). Intraperitoneal cisplatin plus intravenous cyclophosphamide versus intravenous cisplatin plus intravenous cyclophosphamide for stage III ovarian cancer. [See comments.] *N. Engl. J. Med.*, **335**(26), 1950–5.

77. Markman, M., Bundy, B., Benda, J. *et al.* (1998). Randomized phase 3 study of intravenous (IV) cisplatin (CIS)/paclitaxel (PAC) versus moderately high dose IV carboplatin (CARB) followed by IV PAC and intraperitoneal (IP) CIS in optimal residual disease ovarian cancer (OC): an Intergroup Trial (GOG, SWOG, ECOG). In *Thirty-Fourth Annual Meeting of the American Society of Clinical Oncology*, (ed. M.C. Perry), p. 361a. American Society of Clinical Oncology, Los Angeles, CA.

44. Chemotherapy for epithelial cancer of the ovary

Jonathan Shamash and Maurice Slevin

This chapter examines the role of chemotherapy in epithelial cancer of the ovary. Sex cord and germ cell tumours of the ovary are dealt with elsewhere.

Indications for chemotherapy

Early stage disease

Although the use of chemotherapy in the treatment of advanced epithelial carcinoma of the ovary is established (FIGO stages II–IV), the role of therapy in early stage disease remains uncertain. It would be helpful to be able to predict which patients with early stage disease are at the highest risk of relapse. It has become clear that the presence of peritoneal fluid with cancer cells (stage Ic) reduces survival.[1] However, the presence of a ruptured capsule (Ic), tumour involving both ovaries, a raised DNA S-phase fraction, and *p53* mutations in stage I disease have an uncertain predictive role. Information from the Gynaecologic Oncology Group (GOG)[2] suggests that stage I patients with well-differentiated tumours have 90% 5-year survival, while those with unfavourable features still have an 80% 5-year survival. In recent studies, the role of Ki67 and catenin have been investigated. Reduction of expression of α-catenin, which is required between E-cadherin (a *trans*-membrane protein required for cell adhesion) and the basement membrane, is associated with a poor prognosis and appears to be inversely related to Ki67 (a marker for cell proliferation).[3] In addition, decreased levels of the pro-apoptotic protein, Bax, have been associated with a poorer response and survival with paclitaxel-based therapy.[4]

Several adjuvant approaches have been suggested for this group of patients, although randomized trials have generally been inconclusive. Abdominopelvic radiotherapy intraperitoneal isotope therapy using ^{32}P (radioactive phosphorus), at the time of surgery—has been used. In a randomized trial comparing ^{32}P radiotherapy to melphalan, survival was similar.[1] Two studies comparing ^{32}P radiotherapy to cisplatin failed to show an advantage for either therapy.[2,5] Phosphorus–32 treatment appeared to be associated with an increased risk of abdominal pain and also chemical peritonitis.[6] Overall cytotoxic chemotherapy appears preferable because of lower toxicity than with ^{32}P or external-beam irradiation. Currently two trials comparing chemotherapy

to observation in stage I disease are ongoing, and the GOG 52 study (cisplatin/cyclophosphamide versus intraperitoneal ^{32}P) has been completed. Results from these trials are awaited.

Current evidence suggests that patients with well-differentiated tumours are candidates for observation, whereas those with poorly differentiated tumours with high Ki 67, low α-catenin, or low Bax, if they are fit and young, may wish to have adjuvant treatment, although proven evidence of benefit does not exist. The use of a regimen with efficacy in advanced disease would appear to be appropriate.

Advanced disease

Most patients with advanced disease will have undergone laparotomy, with an attempt at debulking surgery. Cytoreductive surgery appears important in achieving long-term survival, with the size of residual deposits having prognostic significance.[7] If chemotherapy is given, those with no macroscopic disease postoperatively have a progression-free survival of 42 months, versus 20 months for those with disease of 1 cm diameter or less.[8] These had an improved survival over those with disease greater than 1 cm in diameter. A majority of patients with stage III disease will still die from their disease, although combination chemotherapy has improved their survival, with 25–40% being alive at 5 years. Stage IV disease has a poor outcome, with a median survival of 12 months and only 5–10% alive at 5 years. In the absence of other life-threatening diseases making chemotherapy inappropriate, patients should be offered combination chemotherapy following their operation. Patients with stage IV disease are unlikely to be cured by current approaches, but significant palliation can be achieved and, if patients are fit enough, chemotherapy should be considered. Further surgery following initial chemotherapy can then be undertaken if there has been an adequate response to chemotherapy and interval debulking surgery has been shown to give a survival advantage.

Principles of chemotherapy: major drug classes and side-effects

Epithelial ovarian carcinoma has long been regarded as being a chemosensitive disease. Responses are seen to many drugs. Most cytotoxic drugs act by inducing damage at various points in the cell cycle; combining drugs with different activities may allow synergy and thus a greater anti-tumour effect, it may also increase toxicity to non-malignant tissues. Drugs act by either stopping cell division directly or, as is now being recognized particularly in resting (non-dividing) cells, by causing sufficient damage that the cells undergo apoptosis (programmed cell death, where the cells self-destruct). This may occur some time after chemotherapy has been given. Drugs are normally given on an intermittent basis to allow recovery of normal tissue. It is the inherent ability of normal tissue repair to exceed that of cancerous tissue that leads to reduction or elimination of tumours following chemotherapy.

Classes of drugs useful in ovarian cancer

Several classes of drugs are useful in the treatment of ovarian cancer. They include:

(1) the older alkylating drugs, many of which can be administered orally, e.g. melphalan, cyclophosphamide;
(2) the platinum co-ordination complexes, which also cause DNA damage, e.g. cisplatin, carboplatin, and oxaliplatin;
(3) the topoisomerase inhibitors, which are responsible for blocking the unwinding of DNA, e.g. etoposide, topotecan, irinotecan;
(4) the taxanes, which prevent microtubular disassembly, e.g. paclitaxel;
(5) gemcitabine—a new antimetabolite which is synergistic with platinum complexes; and
(6) vinorelbine—a vinca alkaloid which causes metaphase arrest.

The evolution of chemotherapy for ovarian cancer can be split into three phases: (1) use of non-platinum alkylating agents; (2) introduction of platinum complexes; and (3) platinum/taxane-based combination chemotherapy.

Following the observation that single agents such as melphalan were producing responses in 30–40% of patients (Table 44.1), combination treatments were developed. These often consisted of an alkylating drug with doxorubicin. Alternatively, fluorouracil and methotrexate were added (MMF).[9] The frequent finding was an increase in response rate without a major increase in survival. The introduction of the platinum complexes further boosted response rates and it was unclear how much non-platinum drugs were contributing. Complex, toxic regimes developed with high initial response rates.[10] A combination of cyclophosphamide, doxorubicin (Adriamycin), and cisplatin (CAP) became popular, and was eventually compared to single-agent carboplatin.[11] Carboplatin is renally excreted, and it is possible to derive equivalently myelosuppressive doses by calculating them based on renal function (area under curve dosing, AUC). The study showed that carboplatin dosed this way was equivalent to CAP and less toxic, with much less myelosuppression, nausea, vomiting, and alopecia.

The observation that a dose–response curve to platinum may exist encouraged many attempts to intensify carboplatin- and cisplatin-based therapies. One study compared standard-dose (AUC 6) to double-dose (AUC 12) carboplatin. In fact, dose intensity was only increased by a third because of delays in treatment due to thrombocytopenia.[12] No benefit from this intensification resulted. In another study, AUC 8 was compared to AUC 4,[13] this showed no benefit, even though AUC 4 is regarded by many as being suboptimal.

In cisplatin-treated patients, one large study[14] using cisplatin (100 mg/m^2) and cyclophosphamide (750 mg/m^2) every 3 weeks, versus 50 mg/m^2 cisplatin and same-dose cyclophosphamide showed initial benefit, with an increase in median survival (114 versus 69 weeks). However, over a 3–4-year period this benefit had disappeared. A study from Italy[15] showed that weekly cisplatin (50 mg/m^2), for nine courses given over 8 weeks, gave the same result as standard 3-weekly cisplatin (75 mg/m^2) and cyclophosphamide (750 mg/m^2). This meant that not only did the conventional treatment take longer to complete, but that the addition of cyclophosphamide did not appear necessary, as in both groups the total doses of cisplatin were the same and the toxicity was similar.

Controversy still surrounds the equivalence, or otherwise, of carboplatin and cisplatin. Prior to the introduction of paclitaxel, most studies suggested that in suboptimally debulked ovarian cancer they were equivalent, but that in optimally debulked cases there were suggestions that cisplatin might be superior.[16,17] Cisplatin is more readily combined with myelosuppressive drugs, although the combination with paclitaxel is more neurotoxic.[18]

The introduction of the combination paclitaxel and cisplatin has shown a survival advantage over conventional cisplatin and cyclophosphamide. This has now been demonstrated in two studies, with a median survival advantage of 14 and 10 months, respectively.[19,20] The increased, pathologically confirmed, complete remission supports this. In the first study, paclitaxel was given over 24 hours whereas, in the second, it was given over 3 hours, although the dose was higher in the latter (175 mg/m^2 versus 135 mg/m^2). There is some evidence that protracted infusions of paclitaxel may overcome resistance.[21]

Equivalence of carboplatin/paclitaxel has been confirmed in two studies, one using AUC 6,[22] and the other using AUC 7.5.[23]

Table 44.1 Single-agent activity in untreated ovarian cancer and treated ovarian cancer

	Untreated	Treated
Cisplatin	60–77%[15]	30–40% (if >6/12)[31]
Carboplatin	64%[12]	30–40% (if > 6/12)[31]
Oxaliplatin	–	29%[32]
Cyclophosphamide	22%[33]	–
Ifosfamide	–	10%[34]
Chlorambucil	20%[35]	–
Melphalan	34%[36]	
Etoposide	25% (IV)[37]	27% (oral)[38]
Topotecan/irinotecan	–	19%[39]
Paclitaxel	55%[40]	25%[41]
Docetaxel	–	35%[42]
Altretamine	42%[43]	15%[44]
Doxorubicin/epirubicin	33%[45]	20%[46]
Fluorouracil/folinic acid	–	19%[47]
Gemcitabine	–	19%[48]
Vinorelbine	–	21%[49]

Interestingly, paclitaxel appears to reduce thrombocytopenia due to carboplatin, and higher calculated doses (AUC 7.5) are required to produce the same degree of myelosuppression as AUC 5–6 when used as a single agent, suggesting a pharmacokinetic interaction between the two drugs.[24] One study, the results of which are at variance with the current enthusiasm for carboplatin/paclitaxel, is the recently reported ICON 3 study, comparing either single-agent carboplatin or CAP, to carboplatin (AUC 5) and paclitaxel. The preliminary results suggest no advantage in terms of progression-free or overall survival of the taxane arm,[25] but not enough events have occurred to come to any conclusions about this study. Other investigators are currently studying alternative combination regimens, e.g. paclitaxel and ifosfamide with or without cisplatin shows activity,[26,27] although with increased toxicity.

Combinations of cisplatin with other drugs with documented second-line activity, e.g. topotecan and etoposide, are being considered. The combination of cisplatin and topotecan has proved unexpectedly myelosuppressive.[28] Intensive therapies combining anthracyclines (epi- or doxorubicin) with a taxane and platinum are being considered in those with advanced disease,[29] as are those with carboplatin, gemcitabine, and paclitaxel.[30]

Other candidates for first-line therapy

Single-agent carboplatin (AUC 6) has the advantage of ease of administration, no alopecia, and mild myelosuppression. It is normally given every 3–4 weeks for six sessions. It is a reasonable choice in the elderly or those who are very frail. Many other regimens have been developed and a few are described in Table 44.2. Some appear to give response rates and overall survival that may appear superior to the current 'gold standard'; however, it must be remembered that these results are from single-centre phase II studies. Patient selection, the numbers of patients with residual disease, and the size of the study may vary considerably, making straight comparisons between such studies impossible.

Summary

Carboplatin and paclitaxel (AUC 5–7.5) remains the gold standard first-line therapy outside of a clinical trial. Combinations of carboplatin, altretamine, and etoposide, or carboplatin/gemcitabine/paclitaxel appear active and may even be superior. However, the current studies are small and these regimens should be confined to clinical trials.

Routes of administration: the role of intraperitoneal chemotherapy

As ovarian carcinoma spreads transcoelomically, intraperitoneal administration offers the possibility of much higher drug levels at the most likely site of metastatic disease, namely the peritoneum. This may be particularly helpful if residual disease is of small bulk. Many drugs seep into the circulation so the systemic side-effects may not be particularly reduced. One well-conducted randomized study using cisplatin and cyclophosphamide intravenously as control, with intraperitoneal cisplatin and intravenous cyclophosphamide in the same dosage schedule in the trial arm, showed a survival advantage, with a median survival of 49 months versus 41 in the standard intravenous versus therapy group.[50]

Neutropenia was more profound in the intravenous group, as was tinnitus and hearing loss, suggesting that systemic exposure to the cisplatin was less in the intraperitoneal group. Abdominal pain following administration of intraperitoneal cisplatin was worse. In this study, benefit extended to those whose residual disease consisted of masses greater than 0.5 cm in diameter.

Many intraperitoneal studies have been carried out using mitoxantrone,[51] etoposide,[52] and floxuridine.[53] In most of these cases there is no suggestion that relapse sites have changed, suggesting that the high dose delivered locally is still failing to prevent peritoneal relapse.

In one large, randomized study,[54] patients were randomized to receive cisplatin with or without intraperitoneal interferon. Unfortunately, no improvement in survival resulted; therefore, other than for one randomized study, the best combination of intraperitoneal therapy is difficult to determine.

In one study,[53] randomization between mitoxantrone and floxuridine in patients stratified for amount of residual disease showed that there was an advantage in terms of progression-free and overall reaction to floxuridine (69% versus 38% progression free at 1 year, and median survival 38 and 21 months, respectively). It is of interest that enlarged retroperitoneal nodes do not appear to be a contraindication to intraperitoneal chemotherapy.[55] Paclitaxel had been administered on a weekly schedule.[56] Peak levels of between 50 and 1273 mmol/l in this dose-escalating study were seen, compared with the 0.1 mmol/l required for cytotoxicity *in vitro*. At doses greater than 60 mg/m² levels were maintained for 4–7 days. Paclitaxel would appear to be a very suitable drug for intraperitoneal use as compared to other cytotoxic agents, as it has one of the lowest clearances from the peritoneal cavity.[56]

One further approach has been to try to reverse the multidrug-resistance phenotype, a common method of resistance.

Table 44.2 First-line therapy for ovarian cancer

Regimen	Patients	Objective response rate	Pathological CR
Cisplatin/paclitaxel[19]	184	73%	16%
Carboplatin[12]	110	64%	
Carboplatin/altretamine/etoposide[58]	29	92%	42%
Carboplatin/gemcitabine/paclitaxel[30]	24	100%	50%

Cyclosporin has been known to block the synthesis of the multidrug-resistant protein (MDR). Sufficient doses have been difficult to maintain *in vivo* because of toxicity; however, with intraperitoneal administration, a much higher level can be obtained. Thirty-four patients were treated with intraperitoneal cyclosporin and carboplatin. Five out of eight platinum-resistant patients responded symptomatically, but only 1/8 had an objective PR.[57]

Intraperitoneal chemotherapy has normally been administered on a single occasion, frequently in 2 litres of 0.9% NaCl, either via a Tenchkoff or port catheter.

Summary

Intraperitoneal chemotherapy offers a potential modest prolongation of survival in ovarian carcinoma at the cost of possible increased toxicity and practical difficulties in managing the peritoneal catheter. The optimal drugs schedule is unclear and the one randomized trial showing prolongation of life used as its control arm a regimen that would now be considered suboptimal (cyclophosphamide and cisplatin). Other than cisplatin, floxuridine and paclitaxel appear worthy of investigation, as does the attempt to reverse multidrug resistance in the peritoneum. Randomized studies using platinum and taxane combinations as the intravenous control are required, and further developments in drug preparations to enable them to persist longer in the peritoneal cavity may encourage the pursuit of this approach.

Chemotherapy for ovarian cancer on relapse

Many patients with stage III or IV ovarian cancer will relapse an average of 1–2 years following initial therapy. Most will never have responded completely to initial treatment. It has become the convention to consider relapse within 6 months of initial therapy as platinum resistant, as the response rate to further platinum on rechallenge is very low.[31] Beyond this period response rates are higher, and patients relapsing more than 1–2 years from initial therapy may have response rates to platinum-based treatment which are similar to those observed when initially treated.

Based on this, many recommend a platinum-based regimen on relapse after 6 months following platinum, whereas non-platinum-based chemotherapy may be recommended if relapse occurs within this period. However, to a certain extent the time to relapse represents the overall chemosensitivity of the tumour, and early relapses often respond poorly to all agents, with responses being short lived. In order to interpret clinical trials, it is important to know the initial response of the patients and how long it lasted. Second-line trials in which all patients relapse after more than 6 months from the end of primary therapy will have better results than those in which a proportion relapse sooner. It is clear that for some patients rapid relapse following front-line therapy can be retreated again with platinum-based treatment, confirming that the concept of platinum resistance is not absolute.[59]

For many patients, therapy is purely palliative, and in these cases it is reasonable to opt for a regimen that is of low toxicity

and convenient. Staging should include occasional ultrasound or CT, as an isolated metastasis may be seen, and in such cases laparotomy may be justified. Outside a clinical trial, single-agent platinum is a reasonable first choice if the relapse-free interval is longer than 6 months. There is a suggestion that following platinum, first-line cisplatin may be more effective than carboplatin[60] (34% response versus 9%), and only cisplatin produced responses in patients unresponsive to first-line treatment (3/12 months cisplatin, versus 0/11 carboplatin).

Additional drugs may improve the response rate, although combined treatment in this setting is more toxic. Carboplatin/paclitaxel has been used with a response rate of 90% (the median disease-free interval in this study was 10/12 months only, all were greater than 6 months); this demonstrates the responsiveness of a platinum-sensitive population on rechallenge.[61]

Oxaliplatin has been used on its own in a heavily pre-treated group of 34 patients. An objective response of 29% was seen. Three out of 11 patients who relapsed within 6 months responded to oxaliplatin.[32] The ease of administration of this drug and its low toxicity make it an ideal candidate to investigate in treatment of this tumour.

Both topotecan and irinotecan have activity in previously treated ovarian cancer. Topotecan has to be given over several days, which is inconvenient. Nausea, malaise, myelosuppression, and alopecia are common. In a large study it achieved an overall response rate of 14% (12% in platinum-resistant 19% in platinum-sensitive tumours).[39] The median time to progression was 18 weeks. In this study all patients had received first-line therapy with platinum and paclitaxel.

Irinotecan has been combined with cisplatin in the treatment of various tumours. Synergy with cisplatin occurs: cisplatin-induced damage to DNA requires topoisomerase–1 to help in its reversal, this is inhibited by irinotecan, leading to additional DNA damage. Twenty-five patients were treated with cisplatin 60 mg/m^2 on day 1 and with 60 mg/m^2 of irinotecan on days 8 and 15 of a 28-day cycle. All patients had received front-line platinum-based treatment. A response rate of 40% was seen (33% in platinum-resistant cases).[62] This appears to be a very active combination in this group of patients and warrants further investigation.

Despite disappointing results with intravenous etoposide, prolonged oral etoposide does appear to be active in ovarian cancer. In a study of 99 relapsing patients[38] (41 platinum resistant) an overall response rate of 34% was seen (27% in platinum-resistant cases), suggesting that there is no difference in sensitivity to etoposide between platinum-sensitive and platinum-resistant cases. The mean duration of response is 24–30 weeks. In view of its ease of administration, etoposide should certainly be considered as a first-line drug in platinum-resistant cases. Unfortunately, its bioavailability is variable, and it would not be suitable in the presence of subacute obstruction. Toxicity can be unpredictable. The initial suggested dose of 50 mg/m^2 for 21 days out of 28 is difficult to achieve, as the smallest capsule contains 50 mg. Alopecia is common.

Altretamine is enjoying a resurgence, since its main side-effects, nausea and vomiting, can be controlled with 5HT$_3$ antagonists. It is given for 14 days in a 28-day cycle. A response rate of 45% has been seen amongst platinum-sensitive patients.[63] Another report has shown that activity in those who have relapsed within 6 months of cisplatin treatment is substantial (24% response rate).[44] Neuropathy occurred in 36%, most often a mild sensory neuropathy. Toxicity appears to be slightly greater than with oral etoposide.

Response rates have been 15–30% for paclitaxel,[41] and 35% for docetaxel.[42] The tendency of docetaxel to cause fluid retention can be reduced by giving dexamethasone, 8 mg twice, starting 24 hours prior to and continuing for 3–5 days after administration of the taxane.

In platinum-sensitive patients the response rate to paclitaxel is 38%. Paclitaxel is well tolerated. The lack of evidence that it is superior to etoposide or altretamine, and its high cost, means that it is difficult to justify its use in the salvage setting as a single agent.

A dose–response curve for anthracyclines exists in ovarian cancer. High-dose epirubicin has significant activity. At doses of over 150 mg/m^2 every 21 days a response rate of 20% is seen.[46] An improvement in the toxicity profile has been seen by using liposomal doxorubicin.[64] In platinum-resistant disease, a response rate of 8% is seen. In platinum-sensitive disease, it was 19–45% (19% if 6–12 months platinum free; 45%, if more than 12 months platinum free).

Platinum-free combinations of paclitaxel and ifosfamide have been tried in relapsing ovarian cancer. These appear to be toxic and are unlikely to become established in this setting.[27]

Summary

In patients who are fit, who relapse after a non-taxane first-line treatment, carboplatin and paclitaxel would appear to be a suitable first choice. In those who had a platinum/taxane combination first, and a treatment-free interval of less than 6 months,

either single-agent etoposide or altretamine may be used. Beyond 6 months, single-agent cisplatin or carboplatin may be considered (Fig. 44.1). Alternatively, within a clinical trial, new combination therapy regimens could be used.

High-dose chemotherapy for ovarian cancer

The observation that ovarian cell lines show a dose response to cisplatin, and that high doses of chemotherapy may be possible if some form of bone-marrow rescue is used to prevent dose-limiting myelosuppression, has encouraged investigators to try such an approach in ovarian cancer. The doses of many alkylating drugs (e.g. melphalan, carboplatin, and thiotepa) may be escalated three- to fivefold if bone-marrow rescue is given before non-myeloablative toxicity supervenes. Rescue is in the form of either autologous stem cells or by autologous bone-marrow harvest. Following high-dose chemotherapy these cells are re-infused; blood counts recover after 10–20 days and a mortality of about 3–5% can be anticipated.

To try to appreciate the role of such a procedure, it is important to realize that many studies have different groups of patients—some with predominantly sensitive disease, some not,[65] and that comparisons are against historical controls, which tend to bias results.

High-dose chemotherapy in relapsing disease

These patients appear to be ideal candidates. They are incurable with standard therapy and yet, if they respond to further treatment, they may benefit from dose intensification. In one study,[66]

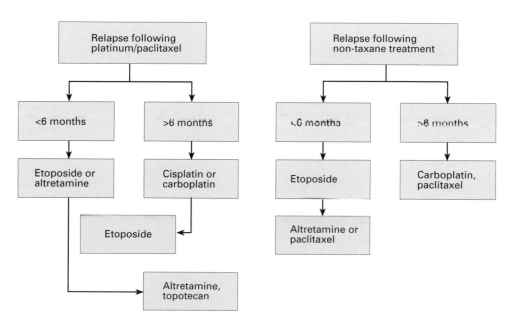

Fig. 44.1 Chemotherapy for ovarian cancer on relapse.

patients refractory to, or relapsing following, cisplatin-based treatment were treated with carboplatin (AUC 20–30) and mitoxantrone (75 mg/m^2) or melphalan (180 mg/m^2), mitoxantrone (75 mg/m^2), and paclitaxel (100 mg/m^2) over 48 hours.

Overall, 64% had a CR (radiological). There was 10% treatment-related death rate. The response rate was 88% (CR) in cisplatin-sensitive patients and 50% CR in cisplatin-refractory disease. However, remissions were short lived (5–7) months, although those with sensitive disease, with tumours or metastases less than 1.0 cm in diameter prior to high-dose chemotherapy, had a medium survival of 18 months.

High-dose chemotherapy in first remission

In a recent study,[67] 53 patients in first remission having had CAP pretreatment (19 of whom were in pathological CR) proceeded to high-dose melphalan (140 mg/m^2) or carboplatin (AUC 20–30) and cyclophosphamide (6.4 g/m^2).

The results showed 60% 5-year survival (24% progression-free at 5 years). This looked impressive, but the high number of patients in pathological CR shows the result for those with disease requiring debulking at second look, only 10% of whom were progression-free at 5 years. There was no suggestion that high-dose carboplatin was better than high-dose melphalan.

In another study,[68] patients with stage III or IV ovarian cancer had two cycles of intensive cisplatin induction chemotherapy, followed by a cycle of high-dose carboplatin-based treatment. Sixty per cent are alive at 5 years (51% progression-free). These results certainly appear better than expected; however, it can be seen that the median age was only 52 (28–55 years) and all had high performance status. In addition, most (80%) had residual tumour under 2 cm in diameter, making this a very select group of patients.

In a dose-intensity study,[69] with three repeated cycles of carboplatin (1 g/m^2) and cyclophosphamide (1.5 g/m^2) with stem cells, followed by single-agent paclitaxel, only 2 out of 14 patients responded with a pathological CR (14%). Again the median age was low.[45] The results do not support further development of this approach. Exact interpretation is difficult as some patients relapsed after a complete response. All were at least 6 months from primary therapy. Bone-marrow transplant registry data appear to back this finding, with the best results obtained in first CR (24 months median progression-free survival) versus only 9 months in second CR.[70]

Summary

High-dose chemotherapy, using either carboplatin or melphalan (or both), with autologous rescue is possible. It is difficult to show clear benefit due to patient selection. Overall benefit would appear to be greatest if performed during first remission, where residual disease is present, and the tumour is platinum sensitive. On relapse, disease-free survival is modest following high-dose chemotherapy. The variation in types of patients entering such studies makes its overall value difficult to ascertain. It should not be used outside a clinical trial at present.

Assessment of response

Assessment of response has previously been by second-look laparotomy, but this is no longer routine practice. Computed tomography (CT) scans are now the standard mode of assessment. Transvaginal ultrasound can be particularly useful in picking up isolated pelvic recurrences.

The use of CA125 (a glycoprotein produced by many ovarian carcinomas) has been gaining popularity as an alternative way to follow patients. It is easier, and indeed cheaper, than conventional scanning. In patients with elevated CA125 a 50% or 75% reduction can be shown to correlate with a PR on CT scanning. A 50% reduction can be defined as being a 50% reduction following two samples for CA125, this being confirmed by a fourth sample; and a 75% response can be defined as a serial reduction in CA125 levels of 75%, occurring over three samples. In both cases the final sample has to be taken at least 28 days after the previous one.[71]

In a subsequent study of oral altretamine, the use of these criteria correctly predicted the CT response, with a 40% objective response rate being seen as derived from CA125 values, and a 39% response rate when using CT criteria.[63]

The use of CA125 to monitor response, particularly following relapse, would appear to be justified, particularly if no further cytoreductive surgery is planned. At present the best predictor of a durable remission is a pathological complete remission confirmed at laparotomy. Approximately 50% of these are durable.

Hormonal therapy for ovarian cancer

The use of hormonal agents in cancer is attractive, in that side-effects are mild and they are outpatient treatments. Hormonal therapy is of established value in some cancers, e.g. prostate and breast. Even if a major response is not achieved, stabilization of disease is possible, often for much longer than can be achieved with cytotoxic drugs.

In ovarian cancer, anti-oestrogens (e.g. tamoxifen), gonadotropin analogues (e.g. leuprorelin, triptorelin or decaptyl), and progestogens (e.g. medroxyprogesterone acetate) have all been used. These agents have usually been used following the failure of platinum-based chemotherapy. One study[72] randomized patients receiving platinum-based chemotherapy to additional triptorelin or placebo. The choice was continued throughout treatment, with luteinizing hormone and follicle stimulating hormone levels being monitored centrally. Patients continued therapy in remission and during any subsequent therapy. No benefit was seen in terms of progression-free or overall survival. On subsequent analysis, benefit was seen if residual disease was less than 2 cm in diameter. In patients treated following exhaustion of chemotherapy options, response rates of approximately 10% were seen. Leuprorelin in 32 relapsed patients[73] gave a response rate of 13%, with a median survival of 12 months. In addition, 16% had stable disease with a median survival of 5 months. Those who progressed had a median survival of only 3 months. In one study of decaptyl,[74] 57% achieved disease stabilization after a maximum of 7 months' therapy. The median progression-free interval was only 3 months.

Summary

These agents have minimal activity, although occasional dramatic responses are seen.

Conclusion

The management of ovarian carcinoma remains dependent on the stage at diagnosis. Patients who have stage Ia and Ib disease are generally managed without chemotherapy, unless there are adverse prognostic features. Many patients with stage Ic disease are given chemotherapy, although the value of this has never been compared in a randomized trial to a no-treatment control arm.

For patients with advanced disease (stage II and beyond) standard practice is to undertake maximum debulking surgery and follow this by systemic chemotherapy. Optimal chemotherapy for fit patients consists of carboplatin and paclitaxel. Normally six cycles of chemotherapy are given, the outcome is monitored using the tumour marker, CA125, and CT and ultrasound as appropriate.

Several additional manoeuvres may be useful. These include intraperitoneal treatment with either cisplatin, fluorouracil, or paclitaxel; interval debulking, where patients are subjected to a further attempt to debulking surgery following the first few courses of chemotherapy; and, in the context of clinical trials, high-dose chemotherapy consolidation of patients in first remission. Patients who develop progressive disease are frequently incurable. Many approaches have been attempted, and the timing of relapse is significant. It has been the convention to consider patients relapsing within 6 months of platinum-based chemotherapy as platinum refractory, whereas those who relapse beyond this point are likely to be platinum sensitive. For the platinum-refractory group, etoposide and topotecan have modest activity, and patients who have not received a taxane initially can be considered for paclitaxel. Beyond 6 months, rechallenge with a platinum drug is advisable, this may be as a single agent or in combination. High-dose chemotherapy on relapse appears to have a little value, as remissions are frequently short lasting.

The role of new cytotoxic drugs continues to be evaluated, in particular gemcitabine appears to have promise, and alternative combination chemotherapy regimens continue to be developed. An attempt to improve on the current gold standard will inevitably require large randomized controlled trials, as currently only modest improvements with available cytotoxic drugs can be anticipated and no clear alternative to their use is forthcoming at present.

References

1. Young, R.C., Walton, L.A., Ellenberg, S.S. et al. (1990). Adjuvant therapy in stage I and stage II epithelial ovarian cancer. Results of two prospective randomized trials. [See comments.] N. Engl. J. Med., 322 (15), 1021–7.
2. Bolis, G., Colombo, N., Pecorelli, S. et al. (1995). Adjuvant treatment for early epithelial ovarian cancer: results of two randomised clinical trials comparing cisplatin to no further treatment or chromic phosphate (^{32}P). GICOG: Gruppo Interregionale Collaborativo in Ginecologia Oncologica. [See comments.] Ann. Oncol., 6 (9), 887–93.
3. Anttila, M., Kosma, V.M., Ji, H. et al. (1998). Clinical significance of alpha-catenin, collagen IV, and Ki–67 expression in epithelial ovarian cancer. J. Clin. Oncol., 16 (8), 2591–600.
4. Tai, Y.T., Lee, S., Niloff, E. et al. (1998). BAX protein expression and clinical outcome in epithelial ovarian cancer. [See comments]. J. Clin. Oncol., 16 (8), 2583–90.
5. Vergote, I.B., Vergote-De Vos, L.N., Abeler, V.M. et al. (1992). Randomized trial comparing cisplatin with radioactive phosphorus or whole-abdomen irradiation as adjuvant treatment of ovarian cancer. Cancer, 69 (3), 741–9.
6. Bakri, Y.N., Given, F.T. Jr, Peeples, W.J., and Frazier, A.B. (1985). Complications from intraperitoneal radioactive phosphorus in ovarian malignancies. Gynecol. Oncol., 21 (3), 294–9.
7. Hoskins, W.J., Bundy, B.N., Thigpen, J.T., Omura, G.A. (1992). The influence of cytoreductive surgery on recurrence-free interval and survival in small-volume stage III epithelial ovarian cancer: a Gynecologic Oncology Group study. Gynecol. Oncol., 47 (2), 159–66.
8. Omura, G.A., Bundy, B.N., Berek, J.S. (1989). Randomized trial of cyclophosphamide plus cisplatin with or without doxorubicin in ovarian carcinoma: a Gynecologic Oncology Group Study. J. Clin. Oncol., 7 (4), 457–65.
9. Miller, A.B., Klaassen, D.J., Boyes, D.A. et al. (1980). Combination v. sequential therapy with melphalan, 5-fluorouracil and methotrexate for advanced ovarian cancer. Can. Med. Assoc. J., 123 (5), 365–71.
10. Neijt, J.P., ten Bokkel Huinink, W.W., van der Burg, M.E. et al. (1984). Randomised trial comparing two combination chemotherapy regimens (Hexa-CAF vs CHAP–5) in advanced ovarian carcinoma. Lancet, 2 (8403), 594–600.
11. Anonymous (1998). ICON2: randomised trial of single-agent carboplatin against three-drug combination of CAP (cyclophosphamide, doxorubicin, and cisplatin) in women with ovarian cancer. ICON Collaborators. International Collaborative Ovarian Neoplasm Study. [See comments]. Lancet, 352 (9140), 1571–6.
12. Gore, M., Mainwaring, P., A'Hern, R. et al. (1998). Randomized trial of dose-intensity with single-agent carboplatin in patients with epithelial ovarian cancer. London Gynaecological Oncology Group. J. Clin. Oncol., 16 (7), 2426–34.
13. Jakobsen, A., Bertelsen, K., Andersen, J.E. et al. (1997). Dose–effect study of carboplatin in ovarian cancer: a Danish Ovarian Cancer Group study. J. Clin. Oncol., 15 (1), 193–8.
14. Kaye, S.B., Lewis, C.R., Paul, J. et al. (1992). Randomised study of two doses of cisplatin with cyclophosphamide in epithelial ovarian cancer. [See comments.] Lancet, 340 (8815), 329–33.
15. Bolis, G., Favalli, G., Danese, S. et al. (1997). Weekly cisplatin given for 2 months versus cisplatin plus cyclophosphamide given for 5 months after cytoreductive surgery for advanced ovarian cancer. J. Clin. Oncol., 15 (5), 1938–44.
16. Lokich, J. and Anderson, N. (1998). Carboplatin versus cisplatin in solid tumors: an analysis of the literature. Ann. Oncol., 9 (1),13–21. [Published erratum appears in Ann. Oncol., 9 (3), 341.]
17. Go, R. (1999). Review of the comparative pharmacology and clinical activity of cisplatin and carboplatin. J. Clin. Oncol., 17 (1), 409–22.

18. Guastalla, J.P., Pujade-Lauraine, E., Weber, B. *et al.* (1998). Efficacy and safety of the paclitaxel and carboplatin combination in patients with previously treated advanced ovarian carcinoma. A multicenter GINECO (Group d'Investigateurs Nationaux pour l'Etude des Cancers Ovariens) phase II study. *Ann. Oncol.*, **9** (1), 37–43.

19. McGuire, W.P., Hoskins, W.J., Brady, M.F. *et al.* (1996). Cyclophosphamide and cisplatin compared with paclitaxel and cisplatin in patients with stage III and stage IV ovarian cancer. [See comments.] *N. Engl. J. Med.*, **334** (1), 1–6.

20. (Not located). Scandanavian study.

21. Seidman, A.D., Hochhauser, D., Gollub, M. *et al.* (1996). Ninety-six-hour paclitaxel infusion after progression during short taxane exposure: a phase II pharmacokinetic and pharmacodynamic study in metastatic breast cancer. *J. Clin. Oncol.*, **14** (6), 1877–84.

22. Bois, A.D., Luek, H., Meier, W. *et al.* (1999). Cisplatin/paclitaxel versus carboplatin/paclitaxel in ovarian cancer: update of an Arbeitsgemeinschaft Gynaekologische Onkologie (AGO) Study group trial. *Proc. ASCO*, Abstract 1374 (1899).

23. Ozols, R., Bundy, B., Fowler, J. (1999). *et al.* Randomised phase III study cisplatin/paclitaxel versus carboplatin/paclitaxel in optimal stage III epithelial ovarian cancer. (GOG Philadelphia PA). *Proc. ASCO*, Abstract 1373 (18).

24. Huizing, M.T., van Warmerdam, L.J., Rosing, H. *et al.* (1997). Phase I and pharmacologic study of the combination paclitaxel and carboplatin as first-line chemotherapy in stage III and IV ovarian cancer. *J. Clin. Oncol.*, **15** (5), 1953–64.

25. Harper, P. (1999). A randomised comparison of paclitaxel and carboplatin versus a control arm of single agent carboplatin or CAP.2075 patients randomised to the 3rd International collaborative of ovarian neoplasm study (ICON3). *Proc. ASCO*, Abstract 1375 (18).

26. Bunnell, C.A., Thompson, L., Buswell, L. *et al.* (1998). A Phase I trial of ifosfamide and paclitaxel with granulocyte-colony stimulating factor in the treatment of patients with refractory solid tumors. *Cancer*, **82** (3), 561–6.

27. Veldhuis, G.J., Willemse, P.H., Beijnen, J.H. *et al.* (1997). Paclitaxel, ifosfamide and cisplatin with granulocyte colony-stimulating factor or recombinant human interleukin 3 and granulocyte colony-stimulating factor in ovarian cancer: a feasibility study. *Br. J. Cancer*, **75** (5), 703–9.

28. Raymond, E., Burris, H.A., Rowinsky, E.K. *et al.* (1997). Phase I study of daily times five topotecan and single injection of cisplatin in patients with previously untreated non-small-cell lung carcinoma. *Ann. Oncol.*, **8** (10), 1003–8.

29. Bois, A.D., Luck, H., Baukenecht, T. *et al.* (1999). First line chemotherapy with epirubicin, paclitaxel and carboplatin for advanced ovarian cancer: A phase I/II study of the Arbeitsgemeinschaft Gynakologische Onkologie Ovarian Cancer Study Group. *J. Clin. Oncol.*, **17** (1), 46–51.

30. Hansen, S., Anderson, H., Boman, K. *et al.* (1999). Germcitabine, carboplatin and paclitaxel (GCP) as first line treatment of ovarian cancer FIGO stages IIb—IV. *Proc. ASCO*, Abstract 1379 (18).

31. Markman, M. (1998). 'Recurrence within 6 months of platinum therapy': an adequate definition of 'platinum-refractory' ovarian cancer? [Editorial] *Gynecol. Oncol.*, **69** (2), 91–2.

32. Chollet, P., Bensmaine, M.A., Brienza, S. *et al.* (1996). Single agent activity of oxaliplatin in heavily pretreated advanced epithelial ovarian cancer. *Ann. Oncol.*, **7** (10), 1065–70.

33. Anonymous (1981). Medical Research Council study on chemotherapy in advanced ovarian cancer. Medical Research Council's Working Party on ovarian cancer. *Br. J. Obstet. Gynaecol.*, **88** (12), 1174–85.

34. Markman, M., Kennedy, A., Sutton, G. *et al.* (1998). Phase 2 trial of single agent ifosfamide/mesna in patients with platinum/paclitaxel refractory ovarian cancer who have not previously been treated with an alkylating agent. *Gynecol. Oncol.*, **70** (2), 272–4.

35. Bell, D.R., Woods, R.L., Levi, J.A. *et al.* (1982). Advanced ovarian cancer: a prospective randomised trial of chlorambucil versus combined cyclophosphamide and cis-diamminedichloroplatinum. *Aust. NZ J. Med.*, **12** (3), 245–9.

36. Young, R.C., Canellos, G.P., Chabner, B.A. *et al.* (1974). Chemotherapy of advanced ovarian carcinoma: a prospective randomized comparison of phenylalanine mustard and high dose cyclophosphamide. *Gynecol. Oncol.*, **2** (4), 489–97.

37. Maskens, A.P., Armand, J.P., Lacave, A.J. et al. (1981). Phase II clinical trial of VP–16–213 in ovarian cancer. *Cancer Treat. Rep.*, **65** (3–4), 329–30.

38. Rose, P.G., Blessing, J.A., Mayer, A.R., and Homesley, H.D. (1998). Prolonged oral etoposide as second-line therapy for platinum-resistant and platinum-sensitive ovarian carcinoma: a Gynecologic Oncology Group study. *J. Clin. Oncol.*, **16** (2), 405–10.

39. Bookman, M.A., Malmstrom, H., Bolis, G. *et al.* (1998). Topotecan for the treatment of advanced epithelial ovarian cancer: an open-label phase II study in patients treated after prior chemotherapy that contained cisplatin or carboplatin and paclitaxel. *J. Clin. Oncol.* **16** (10), 3345–52.

40. Trope, C., Kaern, J., Kristensen, G. *et al.* (1997). Paclitaxel in untreated FIGO stage III suboptimally resected ovarian cancer. *Ann. Oncol.*, **8** (8), 803–6.

41. Mayerhofer, K., Kucera, E., Zeisler, H. *et al.* (1997). Taxol as second-line treatment in patients with advanced ovarian cancer after platinum-based first-line chemotherapy. [See comments.] *Gynecol. Oncol.*, **64** (1), 109–13.

42. Francis, P., Schneider, J., Hann, L. *et al.* (1994). Phase II trial of docetaxel in patients with platinum-refractory advanced ovarian cancer. *J. Clin. Oncol.*, **12** (11), 2301 8.

43. Wharton, J.T., Rutledge, F., Smith, J.P. *et al.* (1979). Hexamethylmelamine: an evaluation of its role in the treatment of ovarian cancer. *Am. J. Obstet. Gynecol.*, **133** (7), 833–44.

44. Manetta, A., MacNeill, C., Lyter, J.A. *et al.* (1990). Hexamethylmelamine as a single second-line agent in ovarian cancer. *Gynecol. Oncol.*, **36** (1), 93–6.

45. De Palo, G.M., De Lena, M., and Bonadonna, G. Adriamycin versus adriamycin plus melphalan in advanced ovarian carcinoma. *Cancer Treat. Rep.*, **61** (3), 355–7.

46. Vermorken, J.B., Kobierska, A., van der Burg, M.E. *et al.* (1995). High-dose epirubicin in platinum-pretreated patients with ovarian carcinoma: the EORTC-GCCG experience. *Eur. J. Gynaecol. Oncol.*, **16** (6), 433–8.

47. Look, K.Y., Muss, H.B., Blessing, J.A., and Morris, M. (1995). A phase II trial of 5-fluorouracil and high-dose leucovorin in recurrent epithelial ovarian carcinoma. A Gynecologic Oncology Group Study. *Am. J. Clin. Oncol.*, **18** (1), 19–22.

48. Lund, B., Hansen, O.P., Neijt, J.P. *et al.* (1995). Phase II study of gemcitabine in previously platinum-treated ovarian cancer patients. *Anticancer Drugs*, **6** (Suppl. 6), 61–2.

49. Bajetta, E., Di Leo, A., Biganzoli, L. *et al.* (1996). Phase II study of vinorelbine in patients with pretreated advanced ovarian cancer: activity in platinum-resistant disease. *J. Clin. Oncol.*, **14** (9), 2546–51.

50. Alberts, D.S., Liu, P.Y., Hannigan, E.V. *et al.* (1996). Intraperitoneal cisplatin plus intravenous cyclophosphamide versus intravenous cisplatin plus intravenous cyclophosphamide for stage III ovarian cancer. [See comments.] *N. Engl. J. Med.*, **335** (26), 1950–5.

51. Le Donne, M., Messina, G., Buda, C. *et al.* (1997). Intraperitoneal chemotherapy with mitoxanthrone in ovarian cancer. *Tumori*, **83** (5), 837–40.

52. Barakat, R.R., Almadrones, L., Venkatraman, E.S. *et al.* (1998). A phase II trial of intraperitoneal cisplatin and etoposide as consolidation therapy in patients with Stage II–IV epithelial ovarian cancer following negative surgical assessment. *Gynecol. Oncol.*, **69** (1), 17–22.

53. Muggia, F.M., Liu, P.Y., Alberts, D.S. *et al.* Intraperitoneal mitoxantrone or floxuridine: effects on time-to-failure and survival in patients with minimal residual ovarian cancer after second-look laparotomy–a randomized phase II study by the Southwest Oncology Group. *Gynecol. Oncol.*, **61** (3), 395–402.

54. Bruzzone, M., Rubagotti, A., Gadducci, A. *et al.* (1997). Intraperitoneal carboplatin with or without interferon-alpha in advanced ovarian cancer patients with minimal residual disease at second look: a prospective randomized trial of 111 patients. G.O.N.O. Gruppo Oncologic Nord Ovest. *Gynecol. Oncol.*, **65** (3), 499–505.

55. Barakat, R.R., Fennelly, D., Pizzuto, F. (1997). Salvage intraperitoneal therapy of advanced epithelial ovarian cancer: impact of retroperitoneal nodal disease. *Eur. J. Gynaecol. Oncol.*, **18** (3), 161–3.

56. Markman, M., Brady, M.F., Spirtos, N.M. et al. (1998). Phase II trial of intraperitoneal paclitaxel in carcinoma of the ovary, tube, and peritoneum: a Gynecologic Oncology Group Study. *J. Clin. Oncol.*, **16** (8), 2620–4.

57. Chambers, S.K., Chambers, J.T., Davis, C.A. et al. (1997). Pharmacokinetic and phase I trial of intraperitoneal carboplatin and cyclosporine in refractory ovarian cancer patients. *J. Clin. Oncol.*, **15** (5), 1945–52.

58. Frasci, G., Comella, G., Comella, P. et al. (1995). Carboplatin (CBDCA)–hexamethylmelamine (HMM)–oral etoposide (VP–16) first-line treatment of ovarian cancer patients with bulky disease: a phase II study. *Gynecol. Oncol.*, **58** (1), 68–73.

59. Markman, M., Kennedy, A., Webster, K. et al. (1998). Evidence that a 'treatment-free interval of less than 6 months' does not equate with clinically defined platinum resistance in ovarian cancer or primary peritoneal carcinoma. *J. Cancer Res. Clin. Oncol.*, **124** (6), 326–8.

60. Gore, M.E., Fryatt, I., Wiltshaw, E., and Dawson, T. (1990). Treatment of relapsed carcinoma of the ovary with cisplatin or carboplatin following initial treatment with these compounds. *Gynecol. Oncol.*, **36** (2), 207–11.

61. Rose, P.G., Fusco, N., Fluellen, L., and Rodriguez, M. (1998). Second-line therapy with paclitaxel and carboplatin for recurrent disease following first-line therapy with paclitaxel and platinum in ovarian or peritoneal carcinoma. *J. Clin. Oncol.*, **16** (4), 1494–7.

62. Sugiyama, T., Yakushiji, M., Nishida, T. et al. (1998). Irinotecan (CPT–11) combined with cisplatin in patients with refractory or recurrent ovarian cancer. *Cancer Lett.*, **128** (2), 211–18.

63. Rustin, G.J., Nelstrop, A.E., Crawford, M. et al. (1997). Phase II trial of oral altretamine for relapsed ovarian carcinoma: evaluation of defining response by serum CA125. *J. Clin. Oncol.*, **15** (1), 172–6.

64. Rose, P., Gordon, A., Granai, C. et al. (1999). Interim analysis of a non comparative multicentre study of doxil/caelyx in the treatment of patients with refractory ovarian cancer. *Proc. ASCO*, Abstract 1392(18).

65. Thigpen, J.T. (1997). Dose-intensity in ovarian carcinoma: hold, enough? [Editorial comment.] *J. Clin. Oncol.*, **15** (4), 1291–3.

66. Stiff, P.J., Dahlberg, S., Forman, S.J. et al. (1998). Autologous bone marrow transplantation for patients with relapsed or refractory diffuse aggressive non-Hodgkin's lymphoma: value of augmented preparative regimens – a Southwest Oncology Group trial. *J. Clin. Oncol.*, **16** (1), 48–55.

67. Legros, M., Dauplat, J., Fleury, J. et al. (1997). High-dose chemotherapy with hematopoietic rescue in patients with stage III to IV ovarian cancer: long-term results. [See comments.] *J. Clin. Oncol.*, **15** (4), 1302–8.

68. Benedetti-Panici, P., Greggi, S., Scambia, G. et al. (1995). Very high-dose chemotherapy with autologous peripheral stem cell support in advanced ovarian cancer. *Eur. J. Cancer*, **31A** (12), 1987–92.

69. Morgan, M.A., Stadtmauer, E.A., Luger, S.M. et al. (1997). Cycles of dose-intensive chemotherapy with peripheral stem cell support in persistent or recurrent platinum-sensitive ovarian cancer. *Gynecol. Oncol.*, **67** (3), 272–6.

70. Ledermann, J., Herd, R., Maraninchi, D. et al. (1999). High dose chemotherapy in ovarian cancer—an analysis of the experience of the European Group for blood and marrow transplant over 7 years. *Proc ASCO*, Abstract 1391 (18).

71. Bridgewater, J.A., Nelstrop, A.E., Rustin, G.J. et al. (1999). Comparison of standard and CA125 response criteria in patients with epithelial ovarian cancer treated with platinum or paclitaxel. *J. Clin. Oncol.*, **17** (2), 501–8.

72. Emons, G., Ortmann, O., Teichert, H.M. et al. (1996). Luteinizing hormone-releasing hormone agonist triptorelin in combination with cytotoxic chemotherapy in patients with advanced ovarian carcinoma. A prospective double blind randomized trial. Decapeptyl Ovarian Cancer Study Group. *Cancer*, **78** (7), 1452–60.

73. Marinaccio, M., D'Addario, V., Serrati, A. et al. (1996). Leuprolide acetate as a salvage-therapy in relapsed epithelial ovarian cancer. *Eur. J. Gynaecol. Oncol.*, **17** (4), 286–8.

74. Ron, I.G., Wigler, N., Merimsky, O. et al. (1995). A phase II trial of D-Trp–6-LHRH (decapeptyl) in pretreated patients with advanced epithelial ovarian cancer. *Cancer Invest.*, **13** (3), 272–5.

45. Neoadjuvant chemotherapy in advanced ovarian carcinoma: present and future prospects

Ignace Vergote

Introduction

Virtually all studies of advanced ovarian carcinoma demonstrated that the size of residual tumour prior to the initiation of chemotherapy was an important determinant of prognosis (stages III and IV).[1–8] Present practice in such situations in many institutions is to optimally 'debulk' the tumour. Unfortunately, no prospective randomized controlled trials concerning the role of *primary* cytoreductive surgery in advanced ovarian carcinoma have been performed.

In reports from the seventies, and in some more recent multicentre trials on different chemotherapeutic regimens, the rates of optimal primary cytoreductive surgery were 20–30%.[2,6,9–12] Where centres have a particular interest and expertise in debulking surgery, optimal cytoreduction is possible in 60–90 % of the patients.[13–19]

In the past 20 years the definition of 'optimal debulking' has changed many times, going from a largest residual tumour mass of 2 cm to less than 0.5 cm. Originally, Griffiths and Fuller[2] proposed that for optimal debulking the residual tumour mass should be less than 1.5 cm. Later it was shown in many studies that patients without residual tumour had a better survival than patients with less than 0.5 cm as largest residual mass, and that the latter group had a better prognosis than patients with 0.5–1.5 cm residual tumour.[4,5,13,15,20–22] In a study by the present author the survival was only significantly improved in patients with less than 1 g of total residual tumour load.[23] Based on our results we suggested that 'optimal' cytoreductive surgery should be defined as no, or less than 1 g, of total residual tumour load.

The problem still fiercely under debate is whether the observed survival benefits for cytoreduced patients are a function of tumour biology or surgical skill. Indeed, patients with good prognostic variables may be easier to debulk than other patients with poor prognosis. Indirect evidence is available that inherent tumour biology relates to resectability. For example, Heintz *et al.*[21] observed that cytoreduction was easier to achieve in young patients who had low-grade tumours, small metastases, and no ascites. Burghardt *et al.*[24] showed that women in whom optimal debulking was impossible had a higher number of positive pelvic and para-aortic lymph-node metastases. In addition, Friedlander *et al.*[25] reported that the size of the largest residual tumour mass was not an independent prognostic factor when newer prognostic variables such as DNA ploidy were included in the multivariate analyses.

In an analysis of the UCLA data, Hacker *et al.*[20] first reported that patients with extensive metastatic disease (>10 cm in diameter) prior to cytoreduction, or with clinical ascites, had a poor prognosis even if the disease was cytoreduced to an optimal status. In a later study from the same centre, it was shown that the only factors influencing resectability to optimal status were metastatic disease larger than 5 cm and the presence of more than 1-litre ascites.[13] Also in a study from The Netherlands, Heintz *et al.*[21] observed that the diameter of the largest metastasis before cytoreduction, and the presence of ascites or peritoneal carcinomatosis, influenced prognosis. Potter *et al.*[15] analysed 302 patients with ovarian carcinoma and concluded that the role of bowel resection should be questioned when residual disease remained at the completion of the operative procedure. In a study of the Gynecologic Oncology Group on 349 patients with optimally resected (<1 cm) disease, the multivariate analyses revealed that older age, poor degree of differentiation, and the presence of 20 or more residual lesions were independent unfavourable prognostic variables.[22] In our study, patients with stage IV disease or more than 1000 g of total metastatic tumour load had a poor survival despite primary debulking surgery.[23] In addition, the presence of uncountable peritoneal metastases was the most frequent reason why cytoreduction to less than 1 g total residual mass could not be achieved (57/65 patients). This is in concordance with the observation of Webb,[26] who reported that the tumours that were most difficult to debulk were those spreading by massive confluent nodules and plaques (15% of the patients). Farias-Eisner *et al.*[27] found that the number of residual peritoneal metastases was the most important prognostic factor in patients with less than 0.5 cm residual tumour. Other studies suggest that the elimination of all peritoneal implants might improve survival.[28,29]

Recently, neoadjuvant chemotherapy has been proposed in patients with established bulky disease[23,30–36] (total number of patients treated with neoadjuvant chemotherapy, $n = 413$). These studies suggest that the same survival with a lower operative morbidity can be obtained with neoadjuvant chemotherapy compared with primary cytoreductive surgery.

Results with neoadjuvant chemotherapy

We compared[23] retrospectively 112 patients with stage III or IV ovarian carcinoma, treated between 1980 and 1988, who all underwent primary debulking surgery, with 173 patients treated between 1989 and 1997 who were evaluated first to receive neoadjuvant chemotherapy or primary debulking surgery, depending on different variables such as the total metastatic tumour load, stage of disease, the ability to perform optimal debulking surgery (i.e. debulking to no macroscopic residual tumour), and performance status (Table 45.1).

All consecutive patients with invasive epithelial ovarian carcinoma stage III or IV ($n = 285$) were included in the study. In all patients selected for primary surgery, every possible effort was made to debulk the patient to no residual tumour. The total amount of metastatic tumour load removed was weighed in all patients and expressed in grams. When the tumours were not removed the total metastatic tumour load was, whenever possible, estimated and expressed as logs of grams (<1 g, 1–10 g, 10–100 g, 100–1000 g, >1000 g). In the first time period (1980–88), 82% of the patients were aggressively debulked to less than 0.5 cm largest residual tumour mass. In the second time period (1989–97), 43% of the patients were treated with primary chemotherapy. The prognostic variables were similar for both time periods. The actuarial crude survival was higher in the second time period than in

the first period (3-year crude survival of 26 ± 4.3% and 42 ± 4.6% for the first and second time period, respectively; log-rank: $P = 0.0001$) (Fig. 45.1). However, this study was a retrospective study which makes comparison difficult (e.g. because of the use of different chemotherapeutic regimens).

Selection of patients: place of laparoscopy as a tool to select patients

Nelson *et al.* proposed computed tomographic criteria to predict operability in patients with suspect ovarian masses.[37] However, we believe that open laparoscopy is a better examination than computed tomography to confirm the diagnosis and to evaluate the operability. From 1993 on, the decision to give neoadjuvant chemotherapy or to perform primary debulking surgery in patients with obvious metastatic disease on radiological examination was made, in our institution, with the help of an open laparoscopy ($n = 77$).[23] Primary debulking surgery was performed in 28 (36%) of this subgroup of patients. Interval debulking surgery was performed after three courses of chemotherapy in 31 (63%) out of the 49 patients in whom it was decided to give neoadjuvant chemotherapy, based on the laparoscopy findings. Six patients developed a subcutaneous metastasis at the site of one of the trocars. In all patients the site of the trocar was excised and examined histologically. In only two of the six patients with a trocar metastasis, this was also suspected clinically. In the patients who received chemotherapy, these trocar metastases disappeared during chemotherapy. Four of the patients were alive with evidence of disease (not at the trocar site) and one died of disease without evidence of disease at the trocar site. One patient had no

Table 45.1 Factors influencing the decision to give neoadjuvant chemotherapy in advanced ovarian carcinoma during the second time period 1989–97 (see text); in all other patients every possible effort was made to cytoreduce the patient to no residual tumour

---

1. Absolute indications for neoadjuvant chemotherapy:
   (a) stage IV disease; or
   (b) metastases of more than 1 g, at sites that made cytoreductive surgery to no residual tumour impossible (e.g. growth in the porta hepatis, superior mesenteric artery)

2. Relative indications[a] for neoadjuvant chemotherapy in patients with an estimated total metastatic tumour load of >100 g:
   (a) uncountable (>100) peritoneal metastases;
   (b) estimated total metastatic tumour load (intra- and retroperitoneal) of > 1000 g;
   (c) presence of large (> 10 g) peritoneal metastatic plaques (e.g. on the diaphragm);
   (d) large-volume ascites (>5 itres);
   (e) WHO performance status 2 or 3

---

[a] In these patients (>100 g metastatic tumour load) the relative indications for neoadjuvant chemotherapy (instead of primary surgery) were evaluated in each patient separately. Usually at least two of the relative indications had to be present for choosing neoadjuvant chemotherapy.

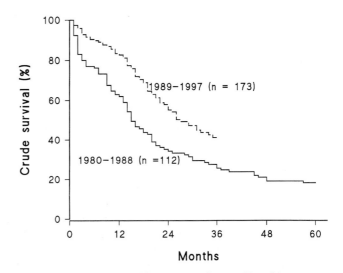

Fig. 45.1 Crude survival in 112 patients with stage III or IV ovarian carcinoma operated to less than 0.5 cm largest residual mass in 82% of the cases (period 1980–88), compared with 173 patients evaluated to receive neoadjuvant chemotherapy (43%) or primary debulking surgery (57%) (period 1989–97). The actuarial survival is better during the second time period (log-rank; $P = 0.0001$).

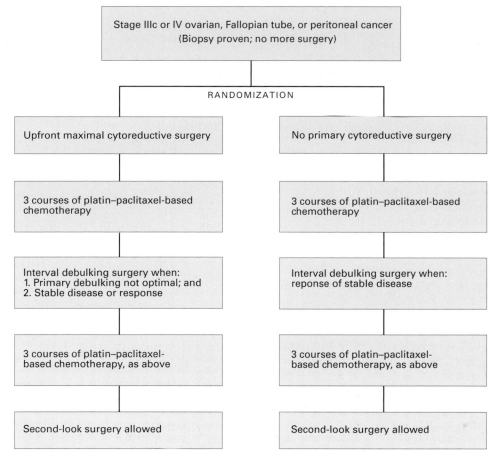

Fig. 45.2 EORTC 55971. Prospective randomized trial on neoadjuvant chemotherapy in advanced ovarian cancer.

evidence of disease. In another study we observed that the development of trocar-site metastases was associated with the presence of ascites, and that a careful closure of the peritoneum, rectus sheath, and skin decreased the number of trocar-site metastases.[38]

Randomized trials

Interval debulking surgery has been shown to increase progression-free and overall survival in a randomized trial performed by the European Organisation for Research and Treatment of Cancer–Gynaecological Cancer Co-operative Group (EORTC-GCCG).[39] The concept of neoadjuvant chemotherapy followed by interval debulking surgery clearly needs to be tested in a prospective randomized study. The EORTC–GCCG recently activated a prospective randomized trial, comparing the concept of neoadjuvant chemotherapy followed by interval debulking surgery with primary debulking surgery followed by chemotherapy and eventually interval debulking surgery (Fig. 45.2). The primary endpoint of this study is the overall survival. With an accrual time of 4 years and a minimum follow-up of 3 years, 704 patients are required in order to show equivalence with respect to survival between both arms.

Conclusion

Based on retrospective analyses, neoadjuvant chemotherapy seems to be a good alternative to primary debulking surgery in advanced ovarian cancer (especially in patients with a high total metastatic tumour load, e.g. >1000 g, stage IV disease, the presence of uncountable peritoneal metastases, or poor performance index). However, this concept needs to be tested in a prospective randomized study. The EORTC–GCCG has recently activated such a study.

References

1. Aure, J.C., Hoeg, K., and Kolstad, P. (1971). Clinical and histologic studies of ovarian carcinoma. Long-term follow-up of 990 cases. *Obstet. Gynecol.*, **37**, 1–8.
2. Griffiths, C.T. and Fuller, A.F. (1978). Intensive surgical and chemotherapeutic management of advanced ovarian cancer. *Surg. Clin. North. Am.*, **58**, 131–42.
3. Swenerton, K.D., Hislop, T.G., Spinelli, J. *et al.* (1985). Ovarian carcinoma: A multivariate analysis of prognostic factors. *Obstet. Gynecol.*, **65**, 264–70.
4. Redman, J.R., Petroni, G.R., Saigo, P.E. *et al.* (1986). Prognostic factors in advanced ovarian carcinoma. *J. Clin. Oncol.*, **4**, 515–23.

5. Neijt, J.P., ten Bokkel Huinink, W.W., van der Burg, M.E.L. *et al.* (1987). Randomized trial comparing two combination chemotherapy regimens (CHAP–5 v CP) in advanced ovarian carcinoma. *J. Clin. Oncol.*, **5**, 1157–68.

6. Gruppo Interegionale Cooperativo Oncologico Ginecologia (1987). Randomised comparison of cisplatin with cyclophosphamide/cisplatin and with cyclophosphamide/doxorubicin/cisplatin in advanced ovarian cancer. *Lancet*, **I**, 353–9.

7. Hogberg, T., Carstensen, J., and Simonsen, E. (1993). Treatment results and prognostic factors in a population-based study of epithelial ovarian cancer. *Gynecol. Oncol.*, **48**, 39–49.

8. Hoskins, W.J., McGuire, W.P., Brady, M.F. *et al.* (1994). The effect of diameter of largest residual disease on survival after primary cytoreductive surgery in patients with suboptimal residual epithelial ovarian carcinoma. *Am. J. Obstet. Gynecol.*, **170**, 974–80.

9. Smith, J.P. and Day, T.G. (1979). Review of ovarian cancer at the University of Texas Systems Cancer Center, M.D. Anderson Hospital and Tumor Institute. *Am. J. Obstet. Gynecol.*, **135**, 984–90.

10. Bertelsen, A., Jakobsen, A., Andersen, J.E. *et al.* (1987). A randomized study of cyclophosphamide ans cisplatinum with or without doxorubicin in advanced ovarian carcinoma. *Gynecol. Oncol.*, **28**, 161–9.

11. Voest, E.E., van Houwelingen, J.C., and Neijt, J.P. (1989). A meta-analysis of prognostic factors in advanced ovarian cancer with median survival and overall survival (measured with the log (relative risk)) as main objectives. *Eur. J. Cancer*, **25**, 711–20.

12. Hunter, R.W., Alexander, N.D., and Soutter, W.P. (1992). Meta-analysis of surgery in advanced ovarian carcinoma: is maximum cytoreductive surgery an independent determinant of prognosis? *Am. J. Obstet. Gynecol.*, **166**, 504–11.

13. Heintz, A.P.M., Hacker, N.F., Berek, J.S. *et al.* (1986). Cytoreductive surgery in ovarian carcinoma: Feasibility and morbidity. *Obstet. Gynecol.*, **67**, 783–8.

14. Piver, M.S., Lele, S.B., Marchetti, D.L. *et al.* (1988). The impact of aggressive debulking surgery and cisplatin-based chemotherapy on progression-free survival in stage III and IV ovarian carcinoma. *J. Clin. Oncol.*, **6**, 983–9.

15. Potter, M.E., Partridge, E.E., Hatch, K.D. *et al.* (1991). Primary surgical therapy of ovarian cancer: how much and when? *Gynecol. Oncol.*, **40**, 195–200.

16. Meerpohl, H.G., Sauerbrei, W., Schumacher, M., and Pfleiderer, A. (1991). Welche parameter beinflussen die Grosse des postoperativen Tumorrestes beim fortgeschrittenen Ovarialkarzinom. *Archives Gyn. Obstet.*, **250**, 174–5.

17. Tulusan, A.H., Neumann-Kleen, T., Adam, R. *et al.* (1991). Morbiditat der radikalen Krebschirurgie des Ovarial-Karzinoms. *Archives Gyn. Obstet.*, **250**, 171–2.

18. Rath, W., Meden, H., Brill, A., and Kuhn, W. (1991). Ergebnisse bei der operativen Primartherapie des Ovarialkarzinoms. *Archives Gyn. Obstet.*, **250**, 175–6.

19. Eisenkop, S.M., Spirtos, N.M., Montag, T.W. *et al.* (1992). The impact of subspeciality training on the management of advanced ovarian cancer. *Gynecol. Oncol.*, **47**, 203–9.

20. Hacker, N.F., Berek, J.S., Lagasse, L.D. *et al.* (1983). Primary cytoreductive surgery for epithelial ovarian cancer. *Obstet. Gynecol.*, **61**, 413–20.

21. Heintz, A.P.M., van Oosterom, A.T., Trimbos, J.B.M.C. *et al.* (1988). The treatment of advanced ovarian carcinoma (I): Clinical variables associated with prognosis. *Gynecol. Oncol.*, **30**, 347–58.

22. Hoskins, W.J., Bundy, B.N., Thigpen, J.T., and Omura, G.A. (1992). The influence of cytoreductive surgery on recurrence-free interval and survival in small-volume Stage III epithelial ovarian cancer: A Gynecologic Oncology Group Study. *Gynecol. Oncol.*, **47**, 159–66.

23. Vergote, I., de Wever, I., Tjalma, W. *et al.* (1998). Neo-adjuvant chemotherapy or primary debulking surgery in advanced ovarian carcinoma: A retrospective analysis of 285 patients. *Gynecol. Oncol.*, **71**, 431–6.

24. Burghardt, E., Girardi, F., Lahousen, M. *et al.* (1991). Patterns of pelvic and para-aortic lymph node involvement in ovarian cancer. *Gynecol. Oncol.*, **40**, 103–6.

25. Friedlander, M.L., Hedley, D.W., Swanson, C. *et al.* (1988). Prediction of long-term survival by flow cytometric analysis of cellular DNA content in patients with advanced ovarian cancer. *J. Clin. Oncol.*, **6**, 282–90.

26. Webb, M.J. (1989). Cytoreduction in ovarian cancer: achievability and results. *Ballière's Clin. Obstet. Gynecol.*, **3**, 83–94.

27. Farias-Eisner, R., Oliveira, M., Teng, F., and Berek, J. (1992). The influence of tumor distribution number and size after optimal primary cytoreductive surgery for epithelial ovarian cancer. *Gynecol. Oncol.*, **46**, 267.

28. Eisenkop, S.M., Nalick, R.H., Wang, H.J., and Teng, N.N.H. (1993). Peritoneal implant elimination during cytoreductive surgery for ovarian cancer: impact on survival. *Gynecol. Oncol.*, **51**, 224–9.

29. van Dam, P.A., Tjalma, W., Weyler, J. *et al.* (1996). Ultraradical debulking of epithelial ovarian cancer with the ultrasonic surgical aspirator: A prospective randomized study. *Am. J. Obstet. Gynecol.*, **174**, 943–50.

30. Lawton, F.G., Redman, C.W., Luesley, D.M. *et al.* (1989). Neoadjuvant (cytoreductive) chemotherapy combined with intervention debulking surgery in advanced, unresected epithelial ovarian cancer. *Obstet. Gynecol.*, **73**, 61–5.

31. Jacob, J.H., Gershenson, D.M., Morris, M. *et al.* (1991). Neoadjuvant chemotherapy and interval debulking surgery for advanced ovarian cancer. *Gynecol. Oncol.*, **42**, 146–50.

32. Lim, J.T. and Green, J.A. (1993). Neoadjuvant carboplatin and ifosfamide chemotherapy for inoperable FIGO stage III and IV ovarian carcinoma. *Clin. Oncol. Royal Coll. Radiol.*, **5**, 198–202.

33. Shimuzu, Y. and Hasumi, K. (1993). Treatment of stage III and IV ovarian cancer: Is neoadjuvant chemotherapy effective? *Nippon Sanka Fujinka Gakkai Zasshi*, **45**, 1007–14.

34. Onnis, A., Marchetti, M., Padovan, P., and Castellan, L. (1996). Neoadjuvant chemotherapy in advanced ovairan cancer. *Eur. J. Gynaecol. Oncol.*, **17**, 393–6.

35. Surwit, E., Childers, J., Atlas, M. *et al.* (1996). Neoadjuvant chemotherapy for advanced ovarian cancer. *International GCSI*, **6**, 356–61.

36. Schwartz, P.E., Rutherford, T., Chambers, J.T. *et al.* (1999). Neo-adjuvant chemotherapy for advanced ovarian cancer: long-term survival. *Gynecol. Oncol.*, **72**, 93–9.

37. Nelson, B.E., Rosenfeld, A.T., and Schwartz, P.E. (1993). Preoperative abdominopelvic computed tomographic prediction of optimal cytoreduction in epithelial ovarian carcinoma. *J. Clin. Oncol.*, **11**, 166–72.

38. Van Dam, P., Decloedt, J., Tjalma, W.A. *et al.* (1999). Trocar implantation metastasis after laparoscopy in patients with advanced ovarian cancer: can the risk be reduced? *Am. J. Obstet. Gynecol.*, **181**, 536–41.

39. Van der Burg, M.E.L., van Lent, M., Buyse, M. *et al.* (1995). The effect of debulking surgery after induction chemotherapy on the prognosis in advanced epithelial ovarian cancer. *N. Engl. J. Med.*, **332**, 629–34.

46. Randomized trials in epithelial ovarian cancer: the gynecologic oncology group studies

Jonathan S. Berek and Robert F. Ozols

Randomized clinical (phase III) trials performed by the Gynecologic Oncology Group have helped to define the optimal therapy for epithelial ovarian cancer. These studies have investigated the therapy for early stage disease, optimally resected advanced-stage disease, and suboptimally resected advanced-stage disease. Platinum-based combination therapy has emerged as the standard treatment for women with each of these categories. The inclusion of Taxol with platinum for advanced-stage malignancies has improved the survival of these patients. Future studies will evaluate the inclusion of new agents in the up-front treatment of ovarian cancer.

Introduction

The Gynecologic Oncology Group (GOG) has investigated the treatment of epithelial ovarian cancer in three separate series of prospective, randomized trials since 1983—those that evaluate the management of early stage ovarian cancer, those for optimally resected late stage, and those for suboptimally resected late-stage disease.

For early stage (stages I and II) epithelial cancers, there have been four randomized trials: protocols 7601, 7602, 95, and 157. For optimally resected stage III disease (for those patients whose maximum residual disease measures <1 cm), there have been five randomized trials: protocols 52, 104, 114, 158, and 172. For suboptimally resected patients, there have been six randomized trials since 1983: protocols 60, 97, 111, 132, 152, and 162 (Table 46.1).

Early stage epithelial ovarian cancer

For women with early stage disease after a comprehensive staging laparotomy, the principal question has been whether or not adjuvant therapy has an impact on the rate of relapse, as defined by disease progression-free survival, and an impact on overall survival.

The first two trials, protocols 7601 and 7602, were performed simultaneously on two separate groups of patients.[1–3] The first group (protocol 7601) included those who had low-risk disease, and the second protocol (protocol 7602) was for women whose disease was high-risk for relapse. Low-risk carcinomas were those

Table 46.1 Epithelial ovarian cancer, randomized GOG studies: early stage I–II disease

Protocol (ref.)	Randomization	Outcome	Conclusion
7601 (1)	Observation versus melphalan	Equal survival but drug-induced leukemia in melphalan-treated patients	Observation in low-risk patients has a better therapeutic index
7602 (1)	^{32}P versus melphalan	Equal survival but drug-induced leukemia in melphalan-treated patients	^{32}P in high-risk patients has a better therapeutic index
95 (3)	^{32}P versus cytoxan/cisplatin	31% reduction in risk of recurrence with cytoxan and cisplatin (P = 0.08)	Platinum-based therapy has some benefit
157	Carboplatin (AUC 6)/paclitaxel 3 versus 6 cycles	Too early	Too early

Table 46.2 Epithelial ovarian cancer randomized GOG studies: Optimal Stage III disease

Protocol (ref.)		Randomization	Outcome	Conclusion
52 (4)	Years accrual 1981–85	CP versus CAP	Equivalent end results with each treatment and both equitoxic	Doxorubicin in the dose and schedule used does not improve outcome
104 (6)	1988–92	i.v. Cytoxan and i.v. versus i.p. cisplatin	i.p. Cisplatin conferred 8 months survival advantage	i.p. Therapy seems to offer ? minimal improvement in outcome
114 (7)	1992–95	i.v. Cisplatin/paclitaxel versus moderate dose carboplatin × 2 then i.v. paclitaxel and i.p. cisplatin	i.p. Cisplatin conferred a 5 months improvement in DFI and survival	i.p. Therapy seems to offer ? minimal improvement in outcome
158 (8)	1995–98	i.v. Paclitaxel and cisplatin versus i.v. paclitaxel (day 1), i.p. cisplatin (day 2) and i.p. paclitaxel (day 8)	Carboplatin arm had 0.9 survival compared with standard arm	Carboplatin can supplant cisplatin in primary therapy
172	1998–	Taxol (135 mg/m^2) + cisplatin (75 mg/m^2) versus i.v. Taxol (135 mg/m^2, i.p. cisplatin (100 mg/m^2, i.p. Taxol	Too early	Too early

CP, Cisplatin/paclitaxel; CAP, cyclophosphamide/Adriamycin/platinum; DFI, disease-free interval.

that were either stage Ia or Ib, low tumor grade (grades 1 or 2) without evidence of capsular ingrowth, surface excrescence, or ascites. High-risk epithelial carcinomas are those of high-grade, stage Ic and II lesions, or those that have grown through the capsule of the ovary.

Protocol 7601 was a randomization of observation versus 12 cycles of single-agent oral alkylating therapy, i.e. melphalan. In this trial there was no difference between the disease progression-free survival and overall survival.[1] Therefore, in appropriately staged low-risk patients, no further adjuvant therapy with melphalan is warranted. While these trials did not use either a platinum compound or a taxane, the overall survival was about 94%, a result that is unlikely to improve regardless of the adjuvant therapy employed. Furthermore, there were two treatment-related deaths from leukemia.

In protocol 7602, the randomization was either to melphalan or the intraperitoneal administration of a single injection of radiocolloid with chromic phosphorus (^{32}P).[1] In this latter trial, there was also no difference in either disease progression-free survival or overall survival. Phosphorus-32 was the least toxic of the two treatments because of the melphalan-induced toxicity. However, this trial did not have an observation arm, so the impact on the natural history of the disease of either adjuvant therapy is uncertain.[2] The overall survival was about 80%, so there may be some potential for an improved survival if other adjuvant therapies were to be used.

To follow on these findings, patients with high-risk disease were randomized to either ^{32}P or three cycles of cisplatin (100 mg/m^2) plus cyclophosphamide (600 mg/m^2) (protocol 95). In this trial, the chemotherapy arm resulted in a 31% survival advantage compared with the ^{32}P.[3] Therefore, the use of platinum-based chemotherapy appeared to be superior adjuvant therapy in women with high-risk low-stage carcinomas.

In protocol 157, patients with high-risk early-stage disease are being treated with three cycles of carboplatin and paclitaxel and are then randomized to observation versus 26 weekly low-dose paclitaxel (40 mg/m^2) treatments. Carboplatin was substituted for cisplatin to reflect most common community practice, and paclitaxel replaced cyclophosphamide. The results of this trial are yet to be known as the protocol just completed accrual, and further follow-up will be necessary to determine the survival data.

Optimally resected stage III epithelial ovarian cancer

In optimally resected disease (Table 46.2), a randomization of cyclophosphamide/cisplatin with or without doxorubicin produced identical survivals in the two treatment groups.[4] Following this trial, the GOG attempted to conduct a study of whole abdominal radiation versus the three-drug combination; however, this

Table 46.3 Epithelial ovarian cancer randomized GOG studies: suboptimal disease stage III and stage IV

Protocol (ref.)		Randomization	Outcome	Conclusion
60 (10)	Years accrual 1982–86	Cytoxan/doxorubicin/ cisplatin ± BCG	No differnces in any outcome measures	BCG by scarification does not add to survival
97 (11)	1986–90	Cytoxan and cisplatin (500 mg/m²; 50 mg/m² × 8 versus cytoxan and cisplatin (1000 mg/m²; 100 mg/m² × 4	No differences in any outcome measures	Double dose intensity has no benefit
111 (12)	1990–92	Cytoxan and cisplatin versus paclitaxel and cisplatin	Paclitaxel/cisplatin adds 5 months to PFI and 14 months to median survival	Paclitaxel/cisplatin standard of care for suboptimal disease
132 (13)	1992–94	Cisplatin and paclitaxel or each single agent in higher dose	Paclitaxel inferior in response and PFI, cisplatin inferior in toxicity (neuro) but equal to combination in response and PFI; all equivalent in survival	Combination of taxane and platinum was better tolerated than sequential therapy
152	1994–99	i.v. Cisplatin and paclitaxel × 6 courses versus same × 3 courses, then interval debulking, then same × 3	Too early	Too early
162	1998–	Paclitaxel (135 mg/m²/24 h) and cisplatin (75 mg/m²) versus paclitaxel (140 mg/m²/96 h) and cisplatin (75 mg/m²)	Too early	Too early

PFI, Progression-free interval.

study was closed prematurely due to lack of sufficient accrual. Based on these findings and this circumstance, further studies of the Gynecologic Oncology Group, using doxorubicin in the front-line therapy for these patients, discontinued. Although there was a meta-analysis that suggested a slight survival advantage for the three-drug regimen over the two-drug regimen,[5] the GOG chose to pursue other avenues of investigation.

The next trial was a study of intravenous versus intraperitoneal chemotherapy (protocol 104), which was a study initiated by the Southwest Oncology Group. In this randomized trial, the ciplatin was given either intravenously or intraperitoneally, while the cyclophosphamide was administered intravenously in both arms.[6] Although there was a median survival advantage of 8 months (49 versus 41 months) in the group that received the intraperitoneal cisplatin, there were thought to be some statistical problems with the trial which suggested that the question remained open. The patients who were theoretically most likely to benefit from the intraperitoneal therapy were those women whose disease was less than 0.5 cm maximum diameter, but this group did not appear to have a survival advantage. Also, the apparent survival advantage

was less than that seen in suboptimally resected patients who had received paclitaxel instead of cyclophosphamide in their regimen.

Therefore, another trial of intraperitoneal therapy was conducted (protocol 114). In this study, intravenous cisplatin (100 mg/m²) plus paclitaxel (135 mg/m²) was randomly compared with two cycles of high-dose carboplatin (AUC = 9) followed by intravenous paclitaxel (175 mg/m²) and intraperitoneal cisplatin (100 mg/m²). In the intraperitoneal arm, 20% of the patients were not able to receive more than two cycles of carboplatin because of thrombocytopenia. However, there was a slight disease progression-free advantage observed in the group that received both the induction high-dose cyclophosphamide and the intraperitoneal cisplatin.[7] No advantage in overall survival was seen. It appears, therefore, that the more dose-intense regimen would not be the treatment of choice for these patients.

While the survival data for protocol 114 were still maturing, protocol 158 was initiated in order to compare the standard cisplatin/paclitaxel combination to the carboplatin/paclitaxel. In this trial, the survival of the two arms was nearly identical; the time to progression of patients receiving the carboplatin was 0.9 compared to those treated with cisplatin.[8] Also, the toxicity of the carboplatin/paclitaxel was in general lower and the regimen was better tolerated. Therefore, this trial, along with the data from the study in Germany, support the conclusion that carboplatin should supplant the use of cisplatin as the up-front therapy for these patients.[9]

Another trial of intraperitoneal versus intravenous therapy has been initiated (protocol 172). In this study, intraperitoneal paclitaxel and intraperitoneal cisplatin are being compared to both drugs administered intravenously. The intraperitoneal arm used intravenous paclitaxel (135 mg/m^2 over 24 hours) on day 1, intraperitoneal cisplatin (100 mg/m^2) on day 2, and intraperitoneal paclitaxel (60 mg/m^2) on day 8. This therapy is randomized to intravenous cisplatin (75 mg/m^2) and paclitaxel (175 mg/m^2) over 24 hours.

Suboptimally resected epithelial ovarian cancer

Protocol 60 studied the three-drug combination of cisplatin/cyclophosphamide/doxorubicin with or without BCG scarification (Table 46.3). There was no difference in survival between the two groups.[10]

Protocol 97 was a randomization of a lower dose of cisplatin/cyclophosphamide (50 mg/m^2; 500 mg/m^2) given for 8 cycles versus a higher dose (100 mg/m^2; 1000 mg/m^2) given for 4 cycles. There was no difference in survival.[11]

Protocol 111 was the first demonstration that paclitaxel and cisplatin was a superior combination to cyclophosphamide and cisplatin in those patients with epithelial ovarian cancer. There was a 39% overall survival advantage in the patients who received the paclitaxel arm.[12] As these data were confirmed in the EORTC trial, the combination of paclitaxel and platinum has become the standard treatment for advanced-stage epithelial ovarian cancer.

In protocol 132, suboptimally resected patients were randomized to one of three arms: cisplatin (100 mg/m^2), paclitaxel (175 mg/m^2), or the combination of the two drugs. The study permitted crossover to the other drug, so in essence, the study was a comparison between the combination of the two agents versus the sequential administration of the two drugs. The three survival curves were superimposable; however, the toxicity of the combination was somewhat lower and better tolerated.[13]

There is an ongoing trial that is seeking to confirm or refute the findings on the 'interval debulking' trial of the EORTC,[14] which was a positive trial in favor of the use of debulking surgery in these patients.[15] The randomization is between six cycles of cisplatin and paclitaxel versus three cycles, followed by an interval debulking, followed by three more cycles.

Another trial of prolonged infusion (96-hour) paclitaxel versus a 24-hour infusion is ongoing. This trial was initiated prior to the maturation of the results from protocol 158, so both regimens include cisplatin.

Future protocols

The Gynecologic Oncology Group phase II trials will focus on the incorporation of newer active chemotherapeutic agents into the front-line therapy of the disease. Non-cross-resistant agents that have been shown to be effective in phase I–II trials by the GOG will be incorporated into the frontline therapy, as either triplets or sequential doublets. Topotecan, doxil, etoposide, and gemcitabine have demonstrated sufficient activity to warrant inclusion in these trials.[16–20] The activity of these newer agents appears to be similar to those being used up-front, and the strategy will be to determine whether their addition to the standard therapy is any better than the paclitaxel and carboplatin combination standard therapy alone.

Triplet therapy may be more limited by toxicity, especially to the bone marrow. A more feasible strategy may be to use sequential combinations, e.g. alternating carboplatin/paclitaxel with topotecan/etoposide. Some doublets may have a better mechanistic rationale, i.e. the combination of platinum and gemcitabine to inhibit DNA repair, and topotecan plus etoposide plus doxil to upregulate topoisomerase levels followed by topoisomerase inhibition. In this manner, the non-cross-resistance of the combinations and their different mechanisms of interference with the cell cycle, as well as complementary toxicities, might augment the control of tumor growth.

References

1. Young, R.C., Walton, L.A., Ellenberg, S.S. et al. (1990). Adjuvant therapy in stage I and stage II epithelial ovarian cancer. Results of two prospective randomized trials. N. Engl. J. Med., **322**, 1021–7.
2. Berek, J.S. (1990). Adjuvant therapy for early-stage ovarian cancer. N. Engl. J. Med., **322**, 1076–8.
3. Young, R.C., Brady, M.F., Nieberg, R.M. (1999). Randomized clinical trial of adjuvant treatment of women with early (FIGO I–IIA high risk) ovarian cancer—GOG 95. Proc. Am. Soc. Clin. Oncol., Abstract 1376.
4. Omura, G.A., Bundy, B.N., Berek, J.S. et al. (1989). Randomized trial of cyclophosphamide plus cisplatin with or without doxorubicin in ovarian carcinoma: A Gynecologic Oncology Group study. J. Clin. Oncol., **7**(4), 457–65.
5. The Ovarian Cancer Meta-Analysis Project (1991). Cyclophosphamide plus cisplatin versus cyclophosphamide doxorubicin and cisplatin chemotherapy of ovarian carcinoma: a meta-analysis. J. Clin. Oncol., **9**(9), 1668–74.
6. Alberts, D.S., Lui, P.Y., Hannigan, E.V. et al. (1996). Intraperitoneal cisplatin plus intravenous cyclophosphamide versus intravenous cisplatin plus intravenous cyclophosphamide for state III ovarian cancer. N. Engl. J. Med., **335** (26), 1950–5.
7. Markman, M., Bundy, B., Benda, J. et al. (1998). Randomized phase 3 study of intravenous (IV) cisplatin (cis)/paclitaxel (PAC) versus moderately high dose IV carboplatin followed by IV PAC and intraperitoneal (IP) cis in optimal residual ovarian cancer: An Intergroup Trial (GOG, SWOG, ECOG). Proc. Am. Soc. Clin. Oncol., **17**, A, 1392.
8. Ozols, R.F., Bundy, B.N., Fowler, J. et al. (1999). Randomized phase III study of cisplatin/paclitaxel versus carboplatin/paclitaxel in optimal stage III epithelial ovarian cancer. A Gynecologic Oncology Group trial (GOG 158). Proc. Am. Soc. Clin. Oncol., Abstract 1373.
9. du Bois A., Lueck H.J., Meier W. et al. (1999). Cisplatin/paclitaxel versus carboplatin/paclitaxel in ovarian cancer: update of an Arbeitsgemeinschaft Gynaekologische Onkologie (AGO) Study Group trial. Proc. Am. Soc. Clin. Oncol., Abstract 1374.
10. Creasman, W.T., Omura, G.A., Brady, M.F. et al. (1990). A randomized trial of cyclophosphamide, doxorubicin, and cisplatin with or without bacillus Calmette–Guerin in patients with suboptimal stage III and IV ovarian cancer: A Gynecologic Oncology Group study. Gynecol. Oncol., **39**, 239–43.

11. McGuire, W.P., Hoskins, W.J., Brady, M.F. *et al.* (1995). Assessment of dose-intensive therapy in suboptimally debulked ovarian cancer: A Gynecologic Oncology Group study. *J. Clin. Oncol.*, **13**(7), 1589–99.

12. McGuire, W.P., Hoskins, W.J., Brady, M.F. *et al.* (1996). Cyclophosphamide and cisplatin compared with paclitaxel and cisplatin in patients with stage III and stage IV ovarian cancer. *N. Engl. J. Med.*, **334** (1), 1–6.

13. Muggia, F.M., Braly, P.S., Brady, M.F. *et al.* (2000). A Phase III randomized study of cisplatin versus paclitaxel in patients with suboptimal stage III or IV ovarian cancer: A Gynecologic Oncology group study. *J. Clin. Oncol.*, **18**, 106–15.

14. van der Burg, M.E.L., van Lent, M., Buyse, M. *et al.* (1995). The effect of debulking surgery after induction chemotherapy on the prognosis in advanced epithelial ovarian cancer. *N. Engl. J. Med.*, **332**, 629–34.

15. Berek, J.S. (1995). Interval debulking of ovarian cancer—an interim measure. *N. Engl. J. Med.*, **332**, 675–7.

16. Rose, P.G., Blessing, J.A., Mayer, A.R., and Homesley, H.D. (1998). Prolonged oral etoposide as second-line therapy for platinum-resistant ovarian carcinoma. A Gynecologic Oncology Group study. *J. Clin. Oncol.*, **16** (2), 405–10.

17. O'Reilly, S., Fleming, G.F., Baker, S.D. *et al.* (1997). Phase I trial and pharmacologic trial of sequences of paclitaxel and topotecan in previously treated ovarian epithelial malignancies: A Gynecologic Oncology Group study. *J. Clin. Oncol.*, **15** (1), 177–86.

18. Underhill, C., Parnis, F.X., Highley, M. *et al.* (1996). A phase II study of gemcitabine in previously untreated patients with advanced epithelial ovarian cancer. *Proc. Am. Soc. Clin. Oncol.*, **15**, A795.

19. Lund, B., Hansen, O.P., Neijt, J.P. *et al.* (1995). Phase II study of gemcitabine in previously platinum -treated ovarian cancer patients. *Anticancer Drugs*, **6** (Suppl. 6), 61–2.

20. Muggia, F.M., Hainsworth, J.D., Jeffers, S. *et al.* (1997). A phase II study of liposomal doxorubicin in refractory ovarian cancer: antitumor activity and toxicity modification by liposomal encapsulation. *J. Clin. Oncol.*, **15** (3), 987–93.

Part 8

Novel therapies: the future

47. Angiogenesis in epithelial ovarian cancer: an important biologic event and therapeutic target

Elise C. Kohn

What is angiogenesis?

Angiogenesis, or neovascularization, is the process of formation of new blood vessels.[1,2] This critical event can be both physiologic and pathologic, depending upon the time and context.[3,4] It occurs normally during embryogenesis and development, the ovulatory cycle, wound healing, and aging. Pathologic angiogenesis can occur also in wound healing, development, cardiovascular and peripheral vascular disease, and aging, and is found in a number of disease states, including immune disorders such as the collagen vasculitides and arthritides, diabetes, and neoplasias (both benign and malignant).[5-7]

The importance of angiogenesis in cancer and the invasive phenotype was described first and reduced to practice by Liotta[8,9] and Folkman[10] in the 1970s. They hypothesized that cancer progression was restricted by the requirement for angiogenesis for both nutritional needs and for tumor cell dissemination.[11] Nutritional diffusion was shown to be limited beyond a size of 0.125 mm^2. It has been demonstrated over the past several decades that hypoglycemia and hypoxia are two of the most potent stimuli for production of angiopromoting molecules.[12-14] This occurs within the local microenvironment, further underscoring the importance of angiogenesis as a micro-event. Liotta was the first to show that angiogenesis was critical in the metastatic, and now understood also to be invasive, phenotype.[8] Ovarian cancer is locally invasive and motile early, becoming locally and distantly metastatic later in its progression. Both components of ovarian cancer dissemination require neovascularization.

That new blood vessels develop from existing vascular trunks has long been known, but advances in the understanding of the molecular mechanisms of angiogenesis have led to new insights. Tumor neovascularization initiates from host vessels either as a sprout, as suggested by Folkman, or by branching, as described by Jain.[15-17] This initiation is in response to local elaboration of cytokines and growth factors produced by tumor and local stromal elements.[18-21] Basic fibroblast growth factor (bFGF) has been shown to be an autocrine growth factor for a number of tumor types but is also one of the most potent angiostimulatory factors.[22-24]

The process of vascular initiation requires endothelial cells at the site of new vessel sprouts to become activated. Under normal physiologic conditions, adult terminally differentiated endothelial cells are amongst the most quiescent cells in the body.[25] Upon receipt of an angiostimulatory message, endothelial cells turn on a proliferative and invasive phenotype. They become capable of new interactions with their underlying basement membrane, secrete proteolytic enzymes locally to degrade that scaffolding, and then migrate into the stroma in the process of new vessel germination. Proliferation is an associated and necessary event. Newly formed vascular buds, through the combination of local stromal remodeling and proliferation, form an extention that canalizes and anastamoses with opposing capillary structures to allow blood flow. This is demonstrated in the new model system in which a human skin graft is placed on a SCID or nude mouse.[26] Viability of the graft requires anastomosis of the human and mouse vessels. The final steps are the development and organization of a local basement membrane and recruitment of pericytes and smooth muscle cells for the larger vessels.[27] Pericytes are necessary for final maturation and are not seen on the vast majority of tumor-associated microvessels.[28] In tumor neovasculature, the basement membrane coating is not complete nor organized, and intraendothelial junctions are loose, both of which add to the leaky and tortuous vasculature seen in tumor vessels.[16]

Many have described the phenotype of neovessel formation as physiologic invasion. Indeed, the multiple steps outlined above involve most of the same cassette of proliferation and invasion genes used by invasive and metastatic tumor cells.[4] Additional angiogenesis-specific genes, most of which are quiescent in the mature endothelium, may be reactivated. Thus, neovascularization constitutes a unique set of molecular and biological events that can be targeted for diagnostic and therapeutic directions. A step-by-step protein or gene profile of the process of neovascular budding and vessel formation has not yet been done. We have initiated a project using microtechnology protein chips and gene arrays to analyze this process.

The recognition that the endothelium can be a dynamic organ has led to new investigations of the balance between the normal quiescence and the tumor-activated endothelia. Quiescent endothelium must first be awakened. If all of the required components are in place for the endothelium to activate angiogenesis, this process proceeds as described above. If critical parts are missing, the endothelial cell may recognize the message as one of cell death, stimulating apoptosis, as shown by the work of Holmgren and colleagues. They showed that maintenance of a balance between proliferation and apoptosis is a hallmark of 'quiescent' vasculature.[29] Where there is too much proliferative stimulation or too few apoptosis messages, there is angiogenesis. A shift in the balance by endogenous or exogenous molecules results in loss of vasculature and an off-switch for neovascularization. Under physiologic conditions, this balance is maintained. Many studies are focused upon identifying the critical components of this homeostasis for therapeutic targeting.

The role of angiogenesis in the ovary

Ovulation

The preovulatory follicle provides a unique physiologic example of rapid growth associated with neovascularization. Understanding this model may further our awareness of what happens in the development of ovarian cancer. The striking parallels between the angiogenic function during follicle development, ovulation, and involution of the corpora lutea may provide further support for a role of the surface and follicular cyst epithelium as a precursor for epithelial ovarian cancer. The preovulatory follicle is surrounded by a basement membrane, as is the ovarian parenchyma. Beginning immediately before ovulation and continuing through the development of the corpus luteum, there is a dramatic upregulation of proteins critical to angiogenesis and invasion. The preovulatory follicle has an increased density of vessels within the theca cell layers and the corpus luteum has a massive vascular component.[30,31] The behavior of the endothelial cells during the first third of the menstrual cycle is actively invasive and proliferative. Hypoxia has been shown to be the initial stimulation occurring during ovulation, inducing local vascular endothelial growth factor (VEGF) production through upregulation of hypoxia-inducing factor-1α.[12,13] Hypoglycemia is a secondary, though major, stimulus of angiogenesis. Confirming this, it has been shown that ovarian follicular cyst fluid is highly angiogenic[32] and that cultured endothelial cells respond by growth and migration to media conditioned by luteinized rat ovaries and from intact rabbit follicles.[33] In fact, Gospodarowicz and Thakral first suggested production of a local angiogenic stimulant during ovulation in 1978; this factor was later proven to be bFGF.[31,34] More recent data have indicated members of the angiopoietin family as well as VEGF and its receptors in the cyclic angiogenesis of corpus luteum development and luteolysis.[35] VEGF/VPF was initially identified by Dvorak and co-workers as a factor that stimulated the production of ascites in ovarian cancer xenografts.[36]

Later it was shown that VEGF plays an important role in these functions. VEGF expression is high within the thecal layer of healthy human follicles and in corpora lutea, but not in the atretic follicles or degenerating corpus luteum.[37] This selective regulation

of VEGF is also seen in the granulosa cells, where it has been proposed recently as a potential etiologic factor for ovarian hyperstimulation syndrome. VEGF transcription and translation was induced by human chorionic gonadotropin administration to women undergoing ovarian hyperstimulation for fertility.[38] Further support for a normal active regulation of angiogenesis in the ovary is given by the very recent demonstration of progesterone regulation of angiogenesis,[39] which shows that progesterone receptor activation is associated with slowing of aortic re-endothelialization in progesterone-receptor-competent mice but not in progesterone knockout mice. Progestins arrest endothelial cells in G_1, associated with altered expression of cyclins E and A and downregulation of retinoblastoma protein phosphorylation. VEGF is thus an important regulator of normal ovarian function. As will be discussed below, there is an important parallel between the normal physiology of angiogenesis in the ovary and angiogenesis activity occurring with ovarian cancer.

Evidence for angiogenesis in ovarian cancer

Several lines of evidence support the importance of angiogenesis in the process of ovarian cancer progression and suggest that it may be a critical factor in ovarian cancer development. This progress is based upon both *in vitro* and *in vivo* studies. The *in vitro* and xenograft studies have lagged behind our recognition of the importance of angiogenesis in clinical ovarian cancer. However, some seminal studies have been done. Neemann and colleagues hypothesized that there was a selective promoting event in the postmenopausal state[31,40] and demonstrated this to be regulation of VEGF, also known as vascular permeability factor (VPF).[36] They studied sham or ovariectomized mice implanted with ovarian cancer tumor spheroids. These spheroids require vascularization in order to form viable and proliferative tumors. The investigators showed that the take of the ovarian cancer spheroids in non-ovariectomized mice was diminished compared to the ovariectomized mice. They demonstrated that this was due to reduced VEGF production, with resultant blockade of neovascularization. They thus hypothesized that the postmenopausal state itself may be permissive for ovarian cancer by its associated release of the tight regulation of VEGF and other critical angiostimulatory cytokines, facilitating the progression of a transforming event. Together with the findings of progestin regulation of endothelial cell function described above, the dynamics of angiogenesis during normal ovarian cycling and the loss of physiologic regulation of angiogenesis occurring with menopause come together to show how neovascularization is a critical partner of the normal and malignant ovary. A misregulation of this partnership may be a simple first step in the promotion of ovarian cancer.

Several techniques have been developed to assess markers of vascularization in patient samples. Data provided are correlative and provide insight into the process but cannot be considered diagnostic nor definitive. While there are many such studies in the literature, none of these correlative biomarkers has been validated prospectively, nor have they been tested against an anti-angiogenic intervention for their predictive value. Technology and our understanding of the biology of neovascularization have both improved, providing newer techniques for these important correlative

Table 47.1 Autocrine and paracrine factors and their role in ovarian cancer

Cytokine	Physiologic role	Role in ovarian cancer	Ref.
Progesterone	Ovarian and endometrial cycle	Loss may release endothelial cells from cycle arrest	39
LH/FSH	Menstrual cycle; high in postmenopausal state	Induction of VEGF	40
bFGF	Produced by follicle development; involved in corpus luteum	Growth factor for ovarian cancer; proangiogenic factor	23, 31, 84–86
VEGF	Follicle development; Corpus luteum development	Promotes angiogenesis; may be a local autocrine growth factor	18, 31, 38, 40, 43, 44, 59
IFN	Immunoregulation; regulation of cytokine production	Regulation of angiogenic cytokines	45, 48, 87, 88

studies. Currently, several clinicolaboratory study approaches are used. Quantitation of high microvessel density and/or area within the tumor has been shown to correlate with poorer disease-free outcome in all cancers tested and with poor survival in some, including ovarian cancer.[2,6,7] Immunohistochemical staining of microvessels uses one of a number of antibodies that are relatively selective for neovessels or microvessels. This approach, first introduced by Weidner et al. in their seminal paper demonstrating a direct association between microvessel number and number of metastases in patients with advanced breast cancer,[41] is limited by the inability to stain all vessels, the nonspecificity of some antibodies, overlap with other antigens in selected tissues, and assumption that all stained segments are in some form a vessel. Most investigators use vascular hot spot tumor regions, containing the greatest number of detectable vessels, for their analysis, having found this to be the most reproducible and most reliable.

Many growth factors and cytokines have been identified that have growth stimulatory properties for ovarian cancer (Table 47.1).[31,42–45] Several, such as insulin-like growth factor-I, epidermal growth factor (EGF), and transforming growth factor-β (TGF-β) have been shown to form autocrine loops. Endothelial cells respond to many of the same growth stimulants as do the ovarian cancer cells, but in a paracrine fashion.[18,23,46–48] Amongst the most potent angiostimulatory agents are VEGF, acidic and basic FGFs, and then EGF and TGF-β. VEGF/VPF was initially identified by Dvorak and co-workers as a factor that stimulated the production of ascites in ovarian cancer xenografts.[36] Measurement of the elaboration or production of these proangiogenic growth factors has been done both qualitatively and quantitatively.[49–51] ELISA kits for bFGF and VEGF are available commercially and provide a reproducible format for assessments. Other markers of the invasive and angiogenic phenotype include matrix metalloproteinases, adhesion molecules, and newly described endogenous inhibitors, such as endostatin and angiostatin.[52,53] Antibodies and ELISA kits are available for many of these. Another approach for study of these proangiogenic cytokines and molecules is local assessment using immunohistochemical approaches or in situ hybridization. It has been shown using these latter techniques that the stroma plays an important role in the proangiogenic microenvironment in ovarian cancer and other cancers.

Hollingsworth and colleagues were the first to demonstrate a role for angiogenesis in ovarian cancer.[54] They assessed advanced microvessel area and number in advanced-stage epithelial ovarian cancer tissue samples from patients enrolled on two moderately platinum-dose-intense treatment regimens for which long-term follow-up was available. Immunohistochemical staining with anti-CD34, a pleiotrophic marker of stem cells including vascular cells,[55] antibody to Factor VIII and antibody to von Willebrand's factor was performed. The most reliable results were seen with anti-CD34, which stains immature vessels and some more mature small vessels. These investigators demonstrated a poorer outcome for those patients with high vascular density. Further, their data argued that patients with more vascular tumors are also more likely to have reduced overall survival. Schoell and colleagues addressed the predictive role of microvascular density with a different approach. They identified 14 patients with a greater than 5-year disease-free survival and matched them for histology, grade, age, extent of disease, and treatment with 14 patients with less than an 18-month survival.[56] Microvessel density was the unique phenotypic difference between the two groups within this tightly controlled but small cohort. Darai and co-workers studied microvessel density using anti-CD31, recognizing the intercellular adhesion marker PECAM-1, and measured soluble CD31 (sCD31) in the serum of patients.[57] They found a positive correlation between increasing CD31 expression and stage of disease, histologic subtype, degree of histologic differentiation, and survival of patients with invasive epithelial ovarian cancer, but not for those patients with low malignant potential disease. No correlation was found for sCD31. Similarly, Orre et al. found increased microvessel density in mucinous tumors using CD31 and CD34 expression.[58] Microvessel density was greater in mucinous tumors at all stages compared with serous tumors.

Other investigators have focused upon the elaboration of angiostimulatory cytokines in both early and late-stage ovarian cancer. Nguyen and colleagues measured bFGF in the urine of patients with varied cancers.[51] Ovarian cancer was a cancer with one of the highest concentrations of bFGF in the urine. While measurable in urine, bFGF has not been demonstrated to be either predictive of disease or outcome in ovarian cancer and other cancers. On the contrary, VEGF has been shown consistently in multiple tumors, including ovarian cancer, to be correlated with outcome. Paley and co-workers[59] assessed VEGF by *in situ* hybridization in a cohort of low malignant potential and stage I and II epithelial ovarian cancer patients. They found that VEGF expression was a statistically significant and independent predictor for shorter relapse-free survival and overall survival. Similar results were found in a small study by Hartenbach and colleagues, who found a median survival of 60 months for the advanced-stage serous histology ovarian cancer patients with low or negative VEGF, and a 28-month median survival for those patients who were positive for VEGF ($P = 0.058$).[60] More recently, investigators have measured circulating VEGF.[61] This has not of yet been demonstrated to provide useful clinical information in any solid tumor.

VEGF is reportedly selectively active on endothelial cells. However, *in situ* hybridization and immunohistochemical studies have identified epithelial ovarian cancer cells as capable of making and secreting VEGF to target local neovasculature.[44,59,62] This further supports the critical interactive role of angiogenesis in ovarian cancer progression. Interestingly, Boocock and colleagues reported the expression of flt and KDR, VEGF receptors, on the membrane of ovarian cancer cell lines. This suggests that VEGF may create an autocrine loop in ovarian cancer. Studies have not yet been reported that confirm this in patient samples.

A consistent message in these various studies is the potentially independent role of angiogenesis as a negative predictor for ovarian cancer patients with early and late-stage presentations. Further, they suggest that there is a critical local microenvironment program functioning in the normal ovary that is recapitulated or maintained during transformation and acquisition of the invasive phenotype of advanced epithelial ovarian cancer.

Angiogenesis as a novel therapeutic and diagnostic target

Considerable progress has been made in the treatment of epithelial ovarian cancer and improvement in survival has been seen in the past two decades. The improvement in survival cannot be attributed to early tumor detection or to an increase in early stage presentations, but appears to be due, in part, to optimal use of the platinum family members and the discovery of the activity of paclitaxel.[63–66] Improvement in overall survival has not been accompanied by an increase in the number of long-term survivors as yet. Thus, a critical objective in the field of ovarian cancer biology is identification of new targets that can be exploited for preventive, diagnostic, and therapeutic use. Angiogenesis is likely an early event in the progression of ovarian transformation and invasion, necessary for tumor nutrient delivery, and providing the conduits for dissemination to distant sites. Angiogenesis targets have been proposed logically in ovarian cancer treatment for several reasons, as described above: elaboration of and response to VEGF, production of invasion – and motility-associated cytokines, pronounced vascularity of the tumors, and the correlative relationships demonstrated between outcome and markers of invasion and angiogenesis. Current studies argue that it may be a potent prognostic factor for all stages of ovarian cancer, and its

dynamic biology suggests it a good target for therapeutic intervention.

Many putative anti-angiogenic agents are now under clinical investigation. Only two, taxanes and thalidomide, have received some form of approval by the US Food and Drug Administration. Paclitaxel, approved for and widely used in the initial treatment of ovarian cancer, has been shown to be angio-inhibitory by several investigators.[67,68] Taxotere has been reported in abstract form to facilitate inhibition of angiogenesis. Thalidomide, approved in the United States for use in leprosy, was shown to block corneal neovascularization in rabbits.[69] The bioactivity in leprosy or in cancer has not been definitively linked back to its ability to inhibit angiogenesis. However, its teratogenicity of blockade of bone growth and maturation may be due to loss or reduction of the very angiogenic region at the epiphyseal plate.[70] The remainder of the plethora of over 100 putative anti-angiogenic agents remain in clinical or preclinical testing.

Several common themes emerge when reviewing these agents. To date, most or many have demonstrated some activity in the inhibition of human xenograft cancer models or murine cancer models. Disease selectivity within the spectrum of cancers tested has not yet been a strong finding. This is logical, given that most, if not all, cancers require some component of angiogenesis, and for many at least one marker of angiogenic activity has been found to correlate with patient outcome. Only a handful of anti-angiogenic agents have been tested against ovarian cancer. BB-94 (Batimastat), a synthetic matrix metalloproteinase inhibitor, was shown by Davies and colleagues to decrease tumor burden and prolong survival in mice bearing ovarian cancer.[71,72] CAI (carboxyamido-triazole), an inhibitor of non-voltage calcium entry into cells, was shown to inhibit ascites formation, tumor burden, and to prolong survival in human ovarian cancer xenografts.[73,74] CAI is discussed in more detail below. While the family of anti-angiogenic agents has been shown to have marked activity *in vitro* and *in vivo* in xenografts or angiogenesis assays, rare complete responses have been demonstrated in the clinical trials. This may be due to activity against true neovessels, as are recruited during the short relative time course under which the animal models are run. Patient tumor vessels may be considerably older than the several weeks, at best, for the xenograft tumor vessels. The primary selection for anti-angiogenesis agent efficacy is xenografts, therefore selectivity against neovessels. It is unknown whether cancers have true neovessels with rapid turnover, or whether they have immature vessels that may be phenotypically similar to neovessels, given the methods of characterization that are in use. Many of the new anti-angiogenesis agents have been demonstrated in the laboratory to be cytostatic to endothelial cells, although some also have cytostatic activity against tumor cells. This might not be expected to yield a measurable disease reduction when given to patients, but might translate into disease stabilization, flattening of the tumor growth-rate curve, and improved progression-free and/or overall survival.

Many categories of anti-angiogenic agents have been proposed.[75,76] These usually focus upon those agents that are very selective to endothelial cells alone, and those that are anti-angiogenic within their framework as anti-invasive or anticancer agents. Alternatively, one can categorize agents according to mechanism

Table 47.2 Anti-angiogenic agents by functional category

Class/mechanism	Examples of agents	Phase
Matrix metalloproteinase inhibitors		
Hydroxamate	ex: BB-94/Marimastat	II/III
Non-hydroxamate	BAY 12–9566	I/III
Modified tetracyclines	Col 3, doxycycline	I/II
Integrin inhibition	$\alpha v\beta$ 3 peptide antagonists	I/II
	Antibody against $\alpha v\ \beta 3$ (LM609)	I/II
Ion-channel inhibition	Squalamine	I
	CAI	I/II/III
Growth-factor inhibition	Receptor kinase inhibitors ex: Su5416 (VEGFR)	I/II/III
	Anti-GF antibodies C225 anti-EGFR	I/II/III
Cytoskeleton inhibitors	Taxanes	I/II/III
Cell-cycle dysregulation	TNP-470 (putative mechanism)	I/II
Unknown/under study	Thalidomide	II/III
	2-methoxyestradiol	Preclinical

of action, as in Table 47.2. Many agents which are angio-inhibitory are anti-invasive agents. Some, such as the category of matrix metalloproteinases and CAI, were identified for their anti-invasive activity and later found to be anti-angiogenic.

CAI

We had posed the hypothesis that we could screen for anti-invasion agents using a simple tumor cell motility assay. This screen yielded CAI, carboxyamido-triazole, an agent inhibitory against human tumor cell lines and endothelial cell motility to several stimuli, including extracellular matrix and growth factors.[73,74,77–80] It was initially demonstrated to be cytostatic against multiple tumor cell types, including several ovarian cancer cell lines, and to have anticancer activity in nude mouse ovarian cancer xenografts. Oral administration of CAI abrogated distant metastatic dissemination in the OVCAR3 human ovarian cancer cell xenograft system. Further study showed it to be a broad anti-invasive agent, with inhibitory activity against adhesion, proteolysis, and migration, as well as against tumor and endothelial cell growth.[78,79,80,89] Studies showed that it reduced production, and thereby function, of matrix metalloproteinase-2 (gelatinase A), a key enzyme targeted in angiogenesis therapeutics. These observations were translated to the clinic in phase I and now phase II and III studies.[81–83] Oral administration of CAI results in plasma concentrations in the range targeted by the *in vitro* and *in vivo* laboratory studies. Daily oral treatment was found to cause disease stabilization ranging from 2 to greater than 15 months in patients with advanced cancers, and up to 15 months in women with advanced refractory ovarian cancer. In most patients, progression of disease occurred at existing sites of disease rather than at new metastatic sites.[81] CAI is generally well tolerated, with no hair loss, minimal gastrointestinal upset, and a less than 2% risk of reversible sensory peripheral neuropathy or cerebellar ataxia (grade 2). Prior neurotoxic chemotherapy administration does not seem to exacerbate the risk of peripheral neuropathy; however, we have not treated

women with active grade 2 or 3 neuropathy with CAI. The current phase II trial in women with ovarian cancer is open to accrual of women with minimal or measurable ovarian cancer who have had no more than three prior treatment regimens. Planned ancillary laboratory studies include measurements of microvessel counts in primary tumor samples and markers of angiogenesis, and measurement of a newly discovered CAI-associated gene, *CAIR-1*.[90] Other studies are under development by the Cancer Therapy Evaluation Program of the National Cancer Institute.

Evaluation of anti-angiogenesis therapy and when to use it

CAI is but one of an explosive number of new agents targeted against invasion and angiogenesis to reach clinical trial in the final decade of the twentieth century. Over 100 agents are under development, or at least in phase I clinical trial, at this writing. However, it is not yet clear how to use these agents optimally nor how to assess their benefit. Angiogenesis has been shown to be an early event in the development of malignancy (Fig. 47.1). Studies have shown it to precede invasion in carcinoma in situ of the breast, and to be evident in hyperplastic breast and prostate specimens prior to a detectable malignant change.[4] This would suggest that these agents, with the proper caveats for wound healing and pregnancy, may be useful prevention agents, as well as the therapeutic reasons for which they are currently under development. Critical questions remain:

1. When is the best time to use an anti-angiogenic agent?
2. How do we determine the balance between benefit and risk?
3. With what agents is this family of drugs best suited for combination therapy?
4. Are there cancers or patient subsets for whom these agents should be used as primary agents or in combination?

These questions require that the research physician has surrogate markers to identify which patient cohorts are more likely to benefit from this intervention, and as mechanisms to measure that benefit. As of now, no such markers have been validated.

Studies, such as those described above, have linked angiogenesis with outcome in many cancers, including ovarian cancer. These approaches are now being incorporated prospectively into clinical trials to validate their discrimination capacity. This conjecture would be supported if patients with high microvessel counts, high circulating VEGF, or high matrix metalloproteinase (MMP) serum concentrations were shown to respond to treatment with anti-invasive or anti-angiogenic agents with longer stabilization times or disease reduction. Angiogenesis is a microenvironmental event. It is likely that VEGF or MMPs may only be elevated in the local arena, and there may be intratumoral heterogeneity. Circulating cytokine or protease amounts may not correlate with the true activity of the agent or the cancer. New markers are needed that provide a mirror to the entire patient.

New clinical paradigms are being tested wherein anti-angiogenesis and anti-invasive agents are being used in the adjuvant mode. The

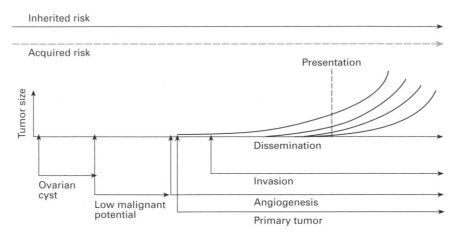

Fig. 47.1 Time course of gynecologic cancer progression. A hypothetical time course of ovarian cancer progression is shown. This paradigm shows where invasion and angiogenesis might fit in if there was a continuum of transformation and malignant progression. There is no molecular evidence at this time to confirm that this progression, from ovarian cysts to low malignant potential tumors, to invasive and disseminated epithelial ovarian cancer, occurs. Low malignant potential tumor is noninvasive to the ovarian stroma, but has some of the phenotypic changes of invasion in its ability to remove itself from the primary and adhere to other sites in the peritoneal cavity, to form disseminated nodules. The lack of stromal reaction does not negate the true metastatic nature of the implant, but does have a clinical impact on the less aggressive behavior that these tumors show. Angiogenesis has been demonstrated in a number of *in situ* cancers to occur locally in the stroma, while not yet invading the *in situ* carcinoma bed. It is shown, for that reason, as an early event, occurring at the transition between low malignant potential tumor and the primary invasive tumor. Acquired and inherited genetic events may be present at the earliest stages, or accumulate as the tumor grows and invades. The early introduction of angiogenesis and invasive potential in the process of epithelial ovarian cancer progression suggest that these events may be useful for the identification of tumor markers, treatment targets, and prognosticators.

prior conventional wisdom was that agents to be used in adjuvant treatment would only be active if the agent had produced clinical responses when used for active disease. This is not going to be the case for this new class of agents, as they do not cause marked disease reduction. The hypothesis underlying adjuvant testing is the capacity to maintain stabilization of disease and to reduce angiogenic and invasive potential. If cancer deposits can be maintained in the pre- or minimally vascularized and noninvasive state, patients may achieve a prolonged time to detectable relapse. Whether this translates into overall disease survival remains to be seen.

Conclusions

Angiogenesis is an ubiquitous process in cancer development and progression. It has been shown to be important in early and late-stage epithelial ovarian cancers and is a novel therapeutic target for ovarian cancer treatment. Understanding of the mechanisms underlying the physiologic invasion of angiogenesis and the genetic dysregulation that promotes angiogenesis has led to an explosion in the number of valid new targets. A striking number of new agents has reached the clinic and many have been targeted to ovarian cancer treatment cohorts. Current challenges include optimizing when and how to use these agents or combinations of anti-angiogenesis agents, and how to evaluate their benefit through the use of new or panels of surrogate markers. These agents, while not yet cytotoxic, have the capacity to stall or stop tumor cell invasion and growth by limiting vascular supply and access. A paradigm of chronicity of ovarian cancer may emerge with the well-timed use of this class of agents after initial debulking surgery and cytotoxic chemotherapy tumor reduction.

References

1. Fidler, I.J. (1998). Molecular determinants of angiogenesis in cancer metastasis. *Cancer J.*, **4**, S58–S66.
2. Folkman, J. (1997). Angiogenesis and angiogenesis inhibition: an overview. *Exs*, **79**, 1–8.
3. Brem, S.S., Jensen, H.M., and Gullino, P.M. (1978). Angiogenesis as a marker of preneoplastic lesions of the human breast. *Cancer*, **41**, 239–44.
4. Kohn, E.C. and Liotta, L.A. (1995). Molecular insights into cancer invasion: strategies for prevention and intervention. *Cancer Res.*, **55**, 1856–62.
5. Liotta, L.A. and Steeg, P.S. (1991). Cancer metastasis and angiogenesis: an imbalance of positive and negative regulation. *Cell*, **64**, 327.
6. Folkman, J. (1996). Clinical applications of research on angiogenesis. *N. Engl. J. Med.*, **333**, 1757–63.
7. Folkman, J. (1996). Fighting cancer by attacking its blood supply. *Sci. Am.*, 150–4.
8. Liotta, L.A., Kleinerman, J., and Saidel, G. (1974). Quantitative relationships of intravascular tumor cells: tumor vessels and pulmonary metastases following tumor implantation. *Cancer Res.*, **34**, 997–1003.
9. Liotta, L.A., Saidel, M.G., and Kleinerman, J. (1976). The significance of hematogenous tumor cell clumps in the metastatic process. *Cancer Res.*, **36**, 889–94.
10. Folkman, J. (1971). Tumor angiogenesis: Therapeutic implications. *N. Engl. J. Med.*, **285**, 1182–6.
11. Folkman, J., Hochberg, M., and Knighton, D. (1974). Self-regulation of growth in three dimensions: the role of surface area limitations. In *Control of proliferation in animal cells*, (ed. B. Clarkson and R. Bascrgn), pp. 833–42. Cold Spring Harbor, NJ.
12. Carmeliet, P., Dor, Y., Herbert, J.-M. *et al.* (1998). Role of HIF-alpha in hypoxia-mediated apoptosis, cell proliferation, and tumor angiogenesis. *Nature*, **394**, 485–90.
13. Shweiki, D., Neeman, M., Itin, A., and Keshet, E. (1995). Induction of vascular endothelial growth factor expression by hypoxia and by glucose deficiency in multicell spheroids: Implications for tumor angiogenesis. *Proc. Natl. Acad. Sci., USA*, **92**, 768–72.

14. Waleh, N.S., Brody, M.D., Knapp, M.A., *et al.* (1995). Mapping of the vascular endothelial growth factor-producing hypoxic cells in multicellular tumor spheroids using a hypoxia-specific marker. *Cancer Res.*, **55**, 6222–6.

15. Folkman, J., Karol, W., Ingber, D., and Hanahan, D. (1989). Induction of angiogenesis during the transition from hyperplasia to neoplasia. *Nature*, **339**, 58–61.

16. Jain, R.K. (1990). Vascular and interstitial barriers to delivery of therapeutic agents in tumors. *Cancer Met. Rev.*, **9**, 253–66.

17. Hanahan, D. and Folkman, J. (1996). Patterns and emerging mechanisms of the angiogenic switch during tumorigenesis. *Cell*, **86**, 353–64.

18. Neufeld, G., Cophen, T., Gengrinovitch, S., and Poltorak, Z. (1999). Vascular endothelial growth factor (VEGF) and its receptors. *FASEB J.*, **13**, 9–22.

19. Klein, S., Roghani, M., and Rifkin, D.B. (1997). Fibroblast growth factors as angiogenesis factors: new insights into their mechanism of action. *Exs*, **79**, 159–92.

20. Rosen, E.M. and Goldberg, I.D. (1995). Regulation of scatter factor (hepatocyte growth factor) production by tumor–stroma interaction. *Exs*, **74**, 17–31.

21. Pepper, M.S., Mandriota, S.J., Vassalli, J.D. *et al.* (1996). Angiogenesis-regulating cytokines: activities and interactions. *Curr. Top. Microbiol. Immunol.*, **213**, 31–67.

22. Burgess, W.H., and Maciag, T. (1989). The heparin-binding (fibroblast) growth factor family of proteins. *Annu. Rev. Biochem.*, **58**, 575–606.

23. Bikfalvi, A., Klein, S., Pintucci, G., and Rifkin, D.B. (1997). Biological roles of fibroblast growth factor-2. *Endocr. Rev.*, **18**, 26–45.

24. Furcht, L. (1986). Critical factors controlling angiogenesis: cell products, cell matrix, and growth factor. *Lab. Invest.*, **5**, 505–9.

25. Beck, L.J. and D'Amore, P.A. (1997). Vascular development: cellular and molecular regulation. *FASEB J.*, **11**, 365–73.

26. Brooks, P.C., Stromblad, S., Klemke, R. *et al.* (1995). Anti-integrin alpha v beta 3 blocks human breast cancer growth and angiogenesis in human skin. *J. Clin. Invest.*, **96**, 1815–22.

27. Benjamin, L., Golijanin, D., Itin, A. *et al.* (1999). Selective ablation of immature blood vessels in established human tumors follows vascular endothelial growth factor withdrawl. *J. Clin. Invest.*, **103**, 159–65.

28. Rosen, E.M., and Goldberg, I.D. (1997). Regulation of angiogenesis by scatter factor. *Exs*, **79**, 193–208.

29. Holmgren, L., O'Reilly, M.S., and Folkman, J. (1995). Dormancy of micrometastases: balanced proliferation and apoptosis in the presence of angiogenesis suppression. [See comments.] *Nature Med.*, **1**, 149–53.

30. Augustin, H.G., Braun, K., Telemenakis, I. *et al.* (1995). Ovarian angiogenesis: Phenotypic characterization of endothelial cells in a physiological model of blood vessel growth and regression. *Am. J. Pathol.*, **147**, 339–51.

31. Neeman, M., Abramovitch, R., Schiffenbauer, Y.S., and Tempel, C. (1997). Regulation of angiogenesis by hypoxic stress: from solid tumors to the ovarian follicle. *Int. J. Exp. Path.*, **78**, 57–70.

32. Rose, B.R. and Koos, R.D. (1988). The effect of human follicular fluid on endothelial cells: proliferation and DNA synthesis. *Biol. Reprod.*, **39**, 88–95.

33. Rone, J.D. and Goodman, A.L. (1990). Preliminary characterization of angiogenic activity in media conditioned by cells from luteinized rat ovaries. *Endocrinology*, **127**, 2821–8.

34. Gospodarowicz, D. and Thakral, K.K. (1978). Production of a corpus luteum angiogenic factor responsible for proliferation of capillaries and neovascularization of the corpus luteum. *Proc. Natl. Acad. Sci., USA*, **75**, 847–51.

35. Goede, V., Schmidt, T., Kimmina, S. *et al.* (1998). Analysis of blood vessel maturation processes during cyclic ovarian angiogenesis. *Lab. Invest.*, **78**, 1385–94.

36. Senger, D.R., Galli, S.J., Dvorak, A.M. *et al.* (1983). Tumor cells secrete a vascular permeability factor that promotes accumulation of ascites fluid. *Science*, **219**, 983–5.

37. Gordon, J.D., Mesiano, S., Zaloudek, C.J., and Jaffe, R.B. (1996). Vascular endothelial growth factor localization in human ovary and fallopian tubes: possible role in reproductive function and ovarian cyst formation. *J. Clin. Endocrinol. Metab.*, **81**, 353–9.

38. Neulen, J., Yan, Z., Raczek, S. *et al.* (1995). Human chorionic gonadotropin-dependent expression of vascular endothelial growth factor/vascular permeability factor in human granulosa cells: importance in ovarian hyperstimulation syndrome. *J. Clin. Endocrinol. Metab.*, **80**, 1967–71.

39. Vazquez, F., Rodriguez-Manzaneque, J.C., Lydon, J.P. *et al.* (1999). Progesterone regulates proliferation of endothelial cells. *J. Biol. Chem.*, **274**, 2185–92.

40. Schiffenbauer, Y.S., Abramovitch, R., Meir, G. *et al.* (1997). Loss of ovarian function promotes angiogenesis in human ovarian carcinoma. *Proc. Natl. Acad. Sci., USA*, **94**, 13203–8.

41. Weidner, N., Semple, J.P., Welch, W.R., and Folkman, J. (1991). Tumor angiogenesis and metastasis—correlation in invasive breast carcinoma. *N. Engl. J. Med.*, **324**, 1–8.

42. Aaronson, S.A. (1991). Growth factors and cancer. *Science*, **254**, 1146–53.

43. Abu-Jawdeh, G.M., Faix, J.D., Niloff, J. *et al.* (1996). Strong expression of vascular permeability factor (vascular endothelial growth factor) and its receptors in ovarian borderline and malignant neoplasms. *Lab. Invest.*, **74**, 1105–15.

44. Boocock, C.A., Charnock-Jones, S., Sharkey, A.M., *et al.* (1995). Expression of vascular endothelial growth factor and its receptors *flt* and KDR in ovarian carcinoma. *J. Natl Cancer Inst.*, **87**, 506–16.

45. Yoneda, J., Kuniyasu, H., Crispens, M.A. *et al.* (1998). Expression of angiogenesis-related genes and progression of human ovarian carcinomas in nude mice. *J. Natl Cancer Inst.* **90**, 447–54.

46. Ferrara, N., Houck, K., Jakeman, L., and Leung, D.W. (1992). Molecular and biological properties of the vascular endothelial growth factor family of proteins. *Endocr. Rev.*, **13**, 18–32.

47. Ferrara, N. (1995). The role of vascular endothelial growth factor in pathological angiogenesis. *Breast Cancer Res. Treat.*, **36**, 127–37.

48. Singh, R.K., Gutman, M., Bucana, C.D. *et al.* (1995). Interferons alpha and β down-regulate the expression of basic fibroblast growth factor in human carcinomas. *Proc. Natl. Acad. Sci., USA*, **92**, 4562–6.

49. Dirix, L.Y., Vermeulen, P.B., Pawinski, A. *et al.* (1997). Elevated levels of the angiogenic cytokines basic fibroblast growth factor and vascular endothelial growth factor in sera of cancer patients. *Br. J. Cancer*, **76**, 238–43.

50. Nguyen, M., Watanabe, H., Budson, A.E. *et al.* (1993). Elevated levels of the angiogenic peptide basic fibroblast growth factor in urine of bladder cancer patients. *J. Natl Cancer Inst.*, **85**, 241–2.

51. Nguyen, M., Watanabe, H., and Budson, A.E. (1994). Elevated levels of an angiogenic peptide, basic fibroblast growth factor, in the urine of patients with a wide spectrum of cancers. *J. Natl Cancer Inst.*, **86**, 356–.

52. O'Reilly, M.S., Boehm, T., Shing, Y. *et al.* (1997). Endostatin: an endogenous inhibitor of angiogenesis and tumor growth. *Cell*, **88**, 277–85.

53. O'Reilly, M.S., Holmgren, L., Chen, C., and Folkman, J. (1996). Angiostatin induces and sustains dormancy of human primary tumors in mice. *Nature Med.*, **2**, 689–92.

54. Hollingsworth, H.C., C. KE, Steinberg, S.M., Rothenberg, M.L., and Merino, M.J. (1995). Tumor angiogenesis in advanced stage ovarian carcinoma. *Am. J. Pathol.*, **147**, 9–19.

55. Asahara, T., Murohara, T., Sullivan, A., *et al.* (1997). Isolation of putative progenitor endothelial cells for angiogenesis. *Science*, **275**, 964–7.

56. Schoell, W.M., Pieber, D., Reich, O. *et al.* (1977). Tumor angiogenesis as a prognostic factor in ovarian carcinoma: quantification of endothelial immunoreactivity by image analysis. *Cancer*, **80**, 2257–62.

57. Darai, E., Bringuier, A.-F., Walker-Combrouze, F. *et al.* (1998). CD31 expression in benign, borderline, and malignant epithelial ovarian tumors: an immunohistochemical and serological analysis. *Gynecol. Oncol.*, **71**, 122–7.

58. Orre, M., Lofti-Miri, M., Mamers, P., and Rogers, P.A.W. (1998). Increased microvessel density inmucinous compared with malignant serous and benign tumors of the ovary. *Br. J. Cancer*, **77**, 2204–9.

59. Paley, P.J., Staskus, K.A., Gebhard, K. *et al.* (1997). Vascular endothelial growth factor expression in early stage ovarian carcinoma. *Cancer*, **80**, 98–106.

60. Hartenbach, E.M., Olson, T.A., Goswitz, J.J. *et al.* (1997). Vascular endothelial growth factor (VEGF) expression and survival in human epithelial ovarian carcinomas. *Cancer Lett.*, **121**, 169–75.

61. Kraft, A., Weindel, K., Ochs, A. *et al.* (1999). Vascular endothelial growth factor in the sera and effusions of patients with malignant and nonmalignant disease. *Cancer*, **85**, 178–87.

62. Olson, T.A., Mohanraj, D., Carson, L.F., and Ramakrishnan, S. (1994). Vascular permeability factor gene expression in normal and neoplastic human ovaries. *Cancer Res.*, **54**, 276–80.

63. Kohn, E.C., Sarosy, G.A., Davis, P.A. *et al.* (1996). Efficacy of addition of dose intense paclitaxel to cisplatin and cyclophosphamide for patients with newly diagnosed, advanced stage epithelial ovarian cancer. *Gynecol. Oncol.*, **62**, 181–91.

64. Reed, E., Sarosy, G., Kohn, E. *et al.* (1996). A Phase I study of paclitaxel and cyclophosphamide in recurrent adenocarcinoma of the ovary. *Gynecol. Oncol.*

65. Sarosy, G.A., Kohn, E.C., Stone, D.A. *et al.* (1992). Phase I study of taxol and granulocyte colony-stimulating factor in patients with refractory ovarian cancer. *J. Clin. Oncol.*, **10**, 1165–70.

66. McGuire, W.P., Hoskins, W.J., Brady, M.F. *et al.* (1996). Cyclophosphamide and cisplatin compared with paclitaxel and cisplatin in patients with stage III and stage IV ovarian cancer. *N. Engl. J. Med.*, **334**, 1–6.

67. Klauber, N., Parangi, S., Flynn, E. *et al.* (1997). Inhibition of angiogenesis and breast cancer in mice by the microtubule inhibitors 2-methoxyestradiol and taxol. *Cancer Res.*, **57**, 81–6.

68. Belotti, D., Vergani, V., Drudis, T. *et al.* (1996). The microtubule-affecting drug paclitaxel has antiangiogenic activity. *Clin. Cancer Res.*, **2**, 1843–9.

69. D'Amato, R., Loughnan, M., Flynn, E., and Folkman, J. (1994). Thalidomide is an inhibitor of angiogenesis. *Proc. Natl. Acad. Sci., USA*, **91**, 4082–5.

70. Vu, T.H., Shipley, J.M., Bergers, G. *et al.* (1998). MMP-9/gelatinase B is a key regulator of growth plate angiogenesis and apoptosis of hypertrophic chondrocytes. *Cell*, **93**, 411–22.

71. Davies, B., Brown, P.D., East, N. *et al.* (1993). A synthetic matrix metalloproteinase inhibitor decreases tumor burden and prolongs survival of mice bearing human ovarian carcinoma xenografts. *Cancer Res.*, **53**, 2087–91.

72. Taraboletti, G., Garofalo, A., Belotti, D. *et al.* (1995). Inhibition of angiogenesis and murine hemangioma growth by batimastat, a synthetic inhibitor of matrix metalloproteinases. *J. Natl Cancer Inst.*, **87**, 293–8.

73. Kohn, E.C. and Liotta, L.A. (1990). L651582, a novel antiproliferative and antimetastasis agent. *J. Natl Cancer Inst.*, **82**, 54–60.

74. Kohn, E.C., Sandeen, M.A. and Liotta, L.A. (1992). *In vivo* efficacy of a novel inhibitor of selected signal transduction pathways including calcium, arachidonate, and inositol phosphates. *Cancer Res.*, **52**, 3208–12.

75. Pluda, J.M. (1997). Tumor-associated angiogenesis: mechanisms, clinical implications, and therapeutic strategies. *Semin. Oncol.* **24**, 203–18.

76. Pluda, J.M. and Parkinson, D.R. (1996). Clinical implications of tumor-associated neovascularization and current antiangiogenic strategies for the treatment of malignancies of pancreas. *Cancer*, **78**, 680–7.

77. Kohn, E.C., Felder, C.C., Jacobs, W. *et al.* (1994). Stucture function analysis of signal and growth inhibition by carboxyamido-triazole, CAI. *Cancer Res.*, **54**, 935–42.

78. Kohn, E.C., Jacobs, W., Kim, Y.S. *et al.* (1994). Calcium influx modulates expression of matrix metalloproteinase-2 (72 kDa type IV collagenase, gelatinase A) expression. *J. Biol. Chem.*, **269**, 21505–11.

79. Kohn, E.C., Alessandro, R., Spoonster, J. *et al.* (1995). Angiogenesis: role of calcium-mediated signal transduction. *Proc. Natl. Acad. Sci., USA*, **92**, 1307–11.

80. Alessandro, R., Masiero, L., Liotta, L.A., and Kohn, E.C. (1996). The role of calcium in the regulation of invasion and angiogenesis. *In Vivo*, **10**, 153–60.

81. Kohn, E.C., Reed, E., Sarosy, G. *et al.* (1996). Clinical investigation of a cytostatic calcium influx inhibitor in patients with refractory cancers. *Cancer Res.*, **56**, 569–73.

82. Kohn, E.C., Figg, W.D., Sarosy, G.A. *et al.* (1997). Phase I trial of micronized formulation CAI in patients with refractory solid tumors: pharmacokinetics, clinical outcome and comparison of formulations. *J. Clin. Onc.*, **15**, 1985–93.

83. Berlin, J., Tutsch, K., Hutson, P. *et al.* (1997). Phase I clinical and pharmacokinetic study of oral carboxyamidotriazole, a signal transduction inhibitor. *J. Clin. Oncol.*, **15**, 781–9.

84. Mignatti, P., Tsuboi, R., Robbins, E., and Rivkin, D.B. (1989). *In vitro* angiogenesis on the human amniotic membrane: Requirement for basic fibroblast growth factor-induced proteinases. *J. Cell Biol.*, **108**, 671–82.

85. Sato, Y. and Rifkin, D.B. (1988). Autocrine activities of basic fibroblast growth factor: regulation of endothelial cell movement, plasminogen activator synthesis, and DNA synthesis. *J. Cell Biol.*, **107**, 1199–1205.

86. Westerlund, A., Hujanen, E., Puistola, U., and Turpeenniemi-Hujanen, T. (1997). Fibroblasts stimulate human ovarian cancer cell invasion and expression of a 72-kDa gelatinase A (MMP-2). *Gynecol. Oncol.*, **67**, 76–82.

87. Nastala, C.L., Edington, H.D., McKinney, T.G. *et al.* (1994). Recombinant IL-12 administration induces tumor regression in association with IFN-gamma production. *J. Immunol.*, **153**, 1697–706.

88. Fidler, I.J. and Hart, I.R. (1982). Biologic diversity in metastatic neoplasms–origins and implications. *Science*, **217**, 998–1001.

89. Masiero, L., Lapidos, K.A., Ambudkar, I., and Kohn, E.C. (1999). Regulation of the RhoA pathway in human endothelial cell spreading on type IV collagen: role of calcium influx. *Journal of Cell Science* **112**, 3205–13.

90. Price, J.T., Bonovich, M.T., and Kohn, E.C. (1997). The biochemistry of cancer dissemination. *Critical Reviews in Biochemistry and Molecular Biology.* **32**, 175–253.

48. Delivery of genes to ovarian cancer using targeted vectors based on self-assembling polymers

Kerry D. Fisher, Christopher M. Ward, Nigel Acheson, and Leonard W. Seymour

Existing treatments for ovarian cancer

Ovarian cancer results in the death of 4000 women annually in the UK, exceeding the figures of cancers of the cervix and endometrium combined. At first presentation more than two-thirds of these women have advanced disease. For these patients, despite the introduction of new chemotherapeutic agents, the poor 5-year survival of 10–20% has changed little over the past 30 years.[1] Attention is now beginning to focus on the rapid development of new techniques in molecular biology. Over the past few years this has led to the introduction of phase I clinical trials utilizing new approaches, and gene therapy strategies are emerging as among the most promising ways forward.[2–4]

Concept of gene therapy

In its purest form, somatic cell gene therapy involves correction or supplementation of cell phenotype by *in situ* expression of normal forms of genes that have become damaged and led to disease. A good example of this is in the treatment of cystic fibrosis, where researchers aim to deliver DNA encoding the cystic fibrosis transport regulator (CFTR) protein in order to restore normal ion transport.[5] Cancer is less amenable to such correction, since it is usually caused by cumulative dysfunction of several genes. However, there are suggestions that restoration of normal copies of genes for proteins such as the tumour suppressor p53 may, at least partially, inhibit tumour development.[6] At present, however, most forms of cancer gene therapy are based either on immunotherapy or suicide genes. In immunotherapy, cancer cells are engineered to become immunogenic, in the hope that the immune system will then mount a response, particularly a cytotoxic T-cell response, against the tumour.[7] So-called 'suicide genes' can encode agents such as the plant toxin, ricin, although more conventionally at present they encode enzymes capable of activating innocuous prodrugs *in situ* to potent chemotherapeutic agents. This approach is known as GDEPT (gene-directed enzyme–prodrug therapy).[8] Gene therapy is particularly attractive in this context since it combines great power (a result of the DNA–RNA–protein amplification, yielding many copies of the enzyme for every copy of DNA expressed in the tumour, and the activity of each enzyme molecule yielding many activated prodrugs) with great specificity (extracellular cell-selectivity, coupled with tissue-selective gene transcription, and the possibility that the agent produced will be selectively toxic to cancer cells). Hence, this approach marks, in principle, a major step forward in cancer treatment. In practice, results so far have been very disappointing, mainly because of poor efficiency of transgene expression within tumour cells.[9]

Vectors available for delivery of therapeutic genes to tumours

Viral vectors

Most approaches towards clinical application of gene therapy make use of viruses as the delivery vectors. Indeed, the greatest number of protocols evaluated clinically have employed retrovirus, closely followed by adenovirus. Experience has shown, however, that delivery of transgenes to tumours using these approaches is not adequate for therapeutic usefulness. There are many factors contributing to poor performance, but chiefly they include safety concerns (mainly for integrating viruses, but also in view of the possibility of generation of replication-competent forms following recombination with wild-type viruses), poor efficiency of infection (often caused by the presence of neutralizing antibodies in the serum of elderly patients), destruction of infected cells by the host immune system, and inappropriate tropisms.[10,11] Poor efficiency of transgene expression is an important factor contributing to the failure of any therapeutic gene transfer procedure to receive approval for licensing so far.

Non-viral vectors

Gene delivery vectors based on cationic lipids or simple self-assembling polyelectrolyte constructs are much safer and less immunogenic than viruses, and not subject to the complications of prior immunization.[12,13] However, they are usually significantly less efficient than viral vectors, at least *in vitro*, and rates of transfection of non-proliferating cells are particularly low. In addition, transfection using most simple non-viral vectors (such as poly(L-lysine)/DNA [pLL/DNA] or DOTAP/DNA) is significantly inhibited by the presence of serum proteins, probably as a result of neutralization of the positive charge that normally mediates non-specific association with the cell surface.[14,15] We have been developing means of counteracting both of these problems, described below.

Anatomical approaches to gene therapy for ovarian cancer

Ovarian carcinoma is a disease that normally remains mainly confined to the peritoneal compartment, with relatively rare metastasis to peripheral sites. Consequently, many treatment protocols have examined the usefulness of intraperitoneal administration of therapeutic agents, designed to increase the relative exposure of tumour cells to the agent while minimizing exposure of vulnerable normal cells. This approach is particularly valuable for delivery of agents to tumour cells within the ascites, and also for low molecular weight hydrophobic or amphipathic agents capable of diffusing into tumour masses. However, it is hard to conceive how such a delivery route could be valuable for a macromolecular system, such as a virus or polymer construct, where movement within tumour masses is likely to be governed by fluid convection rather than diffusion.[16–18] For gene therapy of established tumour masses, requiring penetration of the vector through several cell layers, delivery from the systemic circulation will be preferable, since the flow of interstitial fluid will enhance, rather than inhibit, penetration of the vector into the tumour. However, a major problem to realizing this concept is the absence of any delivery system capable of reaching the tumour following intravenous administration. One of our central aims is to develop a self-assembling polymeric delivery system capable of achieving tumour-selective gene delivery following intravenous administration.

Development of serum-stable vectors for targeted gene delivery

In order to overcome problems of protein binding and disruption of polyelectrolyte gene delivery vectors, we have developed a means to surface modify and crosslink preformed cationic polymer/DNA gene delivery vectors using hydrophilic polymers

such as poly-*N*-(2-hydroxypropyl)methacrylamide (HPMA).[19] The resulting polymer-coated complexes are stable to disruption by proteins and show low levels of non-specific interaction with cells and serum proteins. On the surface of the complexes, some of the reactive ester groups used to link the HPMA polymer to the polyelectrolyte complex are left unreacted, however, and these can be used for simple linkage of targeting agents on to the surface of the coated complexes. In this study we have evaluated the use of folic acid, basic fibroblast growth factor (bFGF), vascular endothelial growth factor (VEGF), transferrin, and various antibodies as targeting agents.

Evaluation of the folate receptor for targeted delivery of genes

Selective delivery of genes to ovarian cancer requires selection of cell surface markers that can be used as targets for gene delivery. There are several possible candidates; for example, the mucin CEA (carcino-embryonic antigen) is widely expressed on ovarian cancer cells. Its exploitation as a ligand for targeted delivery is compromised, however, as significant quantities of CEA are shed from the surface of tumours cells and can be detected in the serum. This will provide a sink for targeted vectors, decreasing the amount of material able to gain access to the target cells and inhibiting selectivity. Similar problems are anticipated with molecules such as CA–125 and CA 19–9.[20,21] However, one particularly promising ligand for gene delivery to ovarian cancer cells is the high-affinity receptor for folic acid.[22] This receptor is known to be significantly upregulated in malignant ovarian cancer cells, and

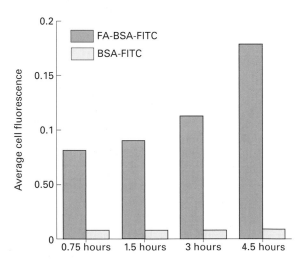

Fig. 48.1 FACS analysis of uptake of BSA-FITC and folic acid-BSA-FITC in HeLa cells. HeLa cells (50 000/well, 24-well plate) were grown overnight in folate-free Dulbecco's modified Eagle's medium supplemented with 10% fetal calf serum at 37°C/5% CO_2. Cells were washed with phosphate-buffered saline (PBS) and 1.0 ml fresh medium was added. Folic acid-BSA-FITC and BSA-FITC (both 10 μg/ml) were added to the cells and incubated for various lengths of time. Following incubation the medium was removed, trypsinized, and cell-associated fluorescence was determined using a Coulter EPICS XL flow cytometer using an argon laser set for excitation 488 nm, emission 520 nm.

undergoes internalization following ligand binding.[23,24] There are even suggestions that it delivers its ligand through to the cytoplasm of the cell, although the majority of the ligand seems to be restricted to vesicles in a perinuclear distribution.[25] We have shown that covalent linkage of folic acid to albumin–FITC results in perinuclear accumulation of the conjugate in HeLa cells after 12 h, suggesting this may be a useful means to deliver genes into tumour cells.

HeLa cells were grown in folate-free medium containing fetal calf serum (10%), seeded into 24-well plates, and incubated with either BSA–FITC or folate–BSA–FITC. Cells were acid-washed (to remove surface-bound materials) at various times and levels of uptake of FITC fluorescence was assessed by fluorescence-activated cell sorter (FACS). As shown in Fig. 48.1, conjugation of folic acid to the albumin–FITC promoted its uptake into cells, and the uptake mechanism shows no signs of saturation, even after 4 h. This enhanced uptake was mediated specifically by folic acid binding, since the interaction could displace [³H]folic acid from binding sites on the cell surface at 4 °C (data not shown). To determine whether folic-acid-mediated uptake could enhance the delivery of plasmids into cells, ³²P-labelled DNA was complexed with pLL, coated as described above, and retargeted with folate–albumin. Following incubation with HeLa cells, levels of DNA entering the cells were increased approximately fivefold

compared with controls (Fig. 48.2). This suggests that the folate receptor, despite its proposed caveolar internalization site, is capable of mediating uptake of DNA complexes. We are presently evaluating whether it distributes the DNA in a form and location suitable for transgene expression.

Angiogenesis and endothelium-associated markers

Access of gene vectors into solid tumours is likely to be restricted even when they are delivered from the bloodstream. Despite reports of enhanced vascular permeability in animal model tumours,[26–30] the size limitations reported in those model systems is approximately 100 nm.[32,33] Hence vectors larger than that size are likely to be excluded from animal model tumours. In addition, the permeability of the vasculature in human tumours is likely to be significantly less than in animal model systems.[34] Hence the practical feasibility of delivering gene vectors to tumour cells in human cancer remains to be established. There is a strong case to consider gene delivery to tumour-associated endothelial cells, partly because these cells are easily accessible from the bloodstream and partly because destruction of the vasculature is known to lead to an amplification of killing of the tumour parenchymal cells through anoxia.[35–37]

Tumour-associated endothelia express a range of molecules that may be useful for targeted gene delivery. In addition to expression of high levels of FGF receptors, VEGF receptors and Tie are thought to be upregulated in tumour endothelium.[38,39]

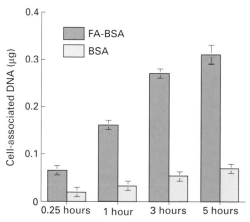

Fig. 48.2 Receptor-mediated uptake of DNA using folic acid-BSA as targeting ligand. Poly(L-lysine)/DNA (pLL/DNA) complexes were formed by adding pLL (34 kDa) to DNA (20 µg/ml calf thymus in water with a spike of 5 ng [³²P]DNA) at an N:P ratio of 2.0. The solution was mixed gently and left to stand for 1 h at room temperature. Folic acid-albumin (12.5 µg/ml) was added to 200 µg/ml reactive pHPMA copolymer in Hepes buffer (pH 7.5, 50 mM), mixed, and left to stand for 10 min. The folic acid-albumin-pHPMA solution was then added to the pLL/DNA complex solution (1:1, final DNA concentration of 10 µg/ml), mixed gently and left to stand overnight at room temperature. HeLa cells (50 000/well, 24-well plates) were grown overnight in folate-free Dulbecco's modified Eagle's medium supplemented with 10% fetal calf serum at 37°C/5% CO₂. Cells were washed with PBS and 900 µl fresh medium added. pLL/DNA complexes (100 µl) were added to the cells and incubated for various lengths of time. Following incubation the medium was removed, the cells washed in acid saline to remove any surface-bound pLL/DNA complexes, and dissolved in 1 M sodium hydroxide solution (30 min). Media and cell-associated radioactivity were measured in a Packard 1900TR liquid scintillation counter.

Targeting using transferrin, bFGF, and VEGF

pLL/DNA complexes were prepared by adding appropriate volumes of pLL solution (20 kDa, 2.5 mg/ml) to plasmid DNA (20 µg/ml) in water to achieve an N:P ratio of 2.0 (defined as the ratio of amino groups in the pLL to phosphate groups in the DNA). For coating with reactive polymer, the pLL/DNA complexes were allowed to stand for 1 h before addition of a polymer based on poly-N-(2-hydroxypropyl)methacrylamide (pHPMA) bearing 8.5 mol% reactive 4-nitrophenyl ester groups (200 µg/ml) in HEPES buffer (final concentration 50 mM, pH 7.5). Complexes were allowed to react for 1 h before addition of aminoethanol (1 µl/ml) to aminolyse any remaining paranitrophenyl ester groups. For linkage of targeting agents to the outside surface of coated complexes, the appropriate targeting ligand was added to complexes (final concentration 10–1000 µg/ml) 5 s following addition of pHPMA, and aminoethanol was added 1 h later, as above. No purification was necessary for binding experiments, although paranitrophenol was removed by dialysis (Tubulisers, cut-off 50 kDa, Spectrum Laboratories) for transfection studies. Recovery was checked in each case by trace labelling DNA with [³²P]dCTP.

For analysis of intracellular routing using fluorescence microscopy, ECV 304 cells were grown overnight on gelatin-pretreated cover slips at a density of 10 000 cells/cover slip. DNA complexes were prepared using Texas Red-labelled DNA and added to cells for 15 min pulse exposure (2.6 µg DNA/ml as a bubble on the cover slip). Cells were reincubated in full medium for 30 min or 3 h, washed in phosphate-buffered saline (PBS), fixed in paraformaldehyde (4%) in PBS, washed again, and mounted using Optimount containing DAPI (2 µg/ml). Cellular distribution of fluorescence was then determined by fluorescence microscopy, data captured using Improvision software and deconvoluted using OpenLab.

For analysis of transfection, cells were plated at 10 000 cells/well in 96-well plates and incubated overnight. DNA complexes were then added for 5 h at a final concentration of 2.6 µg DNA/ml. Cells were then washed, reincubated for a total of 48 h in the presence of antibiotics, and β-galactosidase gene expression was determined using Galactolight™ (Tropix, Cambridge, UK).

All targeting ligands (transferrin, bFGF, and VEGF) showed the ability to increase significantly the accumulation of targeted complexes within ECV 304 cells (Fig. 48.3). The uptake was shown to be receptor-mediated since it could be inhibited by the presence of excess competing ligand.[40] In addition, however, all targeted complexes were capable of achieving significantly increased levels of reporter gene expression (Fig. 48.4). This increased transfection was also mediated by specific receptor binding, since it was abolished if the ligands were simply added (not covalently linked) to the complexes. Importantly, the targeted transfection was completely resistant to disruption by serum proteins. In contrast, DOTAP and non-covalently assembled bFGF complexes showed greatly decreased transfection efficacy in the presence of serum, severely impairing their potential for application *in vivo*.

Analysis of intracellular DNA distribution using fluorescence microscopy showed elevated uptake for all targeting systems. However bFGF-targeted complexes showed a different pattern of distribution, demonstrating an unexpected nuclear accumulation of DNA (Fig. 48.5). The DNA appeared to become localized within a relatively small number of intranuclear sites, and their exact cellular significance remains to be established.

Implications and opportunities

There are several elegant strategies for tumour destruction following introduction of transgenes into tumour cells. These include gene-directed enzyme-prodrug therapy (GDEPT) and sophisticated immunological strategies, some of which could demonstrate powerful bystander killing of non-transfected tumour cells. However, in order to realize the potential of these approaches it is necessary to develop a means for successful expression of transgenes in a significant number of cells within the tumour, ideally cells of the tumour vasculature. The approach demonstrated in this study has several advantages over other vector systems for gene delivery. Significantly, it is not sensitive to disruption by the effects of serum, permitting its application *in vivo*. In addition to cell-selectivity that can be achieved by targeting specific receptors, the use of bFGF as targeting ligand promotes nuclear entry of DNA that should permit high levels of gene expression. The DNA is likely to be localized within stores previously reported for bFGF within the nucleus,[41] and future development of this approach will focus on gaining efficient transcription of the DNA following its entry into the nucleus of target cells.

Selective gene delivery to tumour-associated endothelium, coupled with gene activation regulated by specific tissue-associated

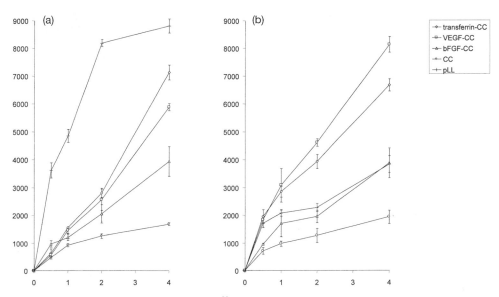

Fig. 48.3 Time-dependent association of complexes labelled with [³²P]DNA with ECV 304 cells (10 000 cells/, 96-well plates, incubated 24 h with 10% serum prior to experimentation) in the presence (a) and absence (b) of serum. The non-specific cell association of simple poly(L)lysine/DNA complexes (pLL) due to electrostatic interaction is decreased following addition of the hydrophilic coating polymer (CC). Restoration of cell association can be achieved by targeting the coated complexes using different ligands (transferrin, bFGF, and VEGF) in a manner that can be inhibited by the presence of excess unbound targeting ligand.

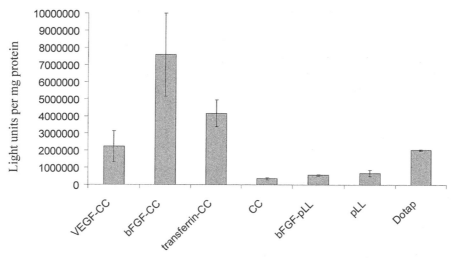

Fig. 48.4 Transfection of HUVE cells in the presence of serum. Proliferating HUVE cells well (10 000 cells/, 96-well plates, incubated 24 h with 10% serum prior to experimentation) were incubated in the presence of polymer-coated pLL/DNA complexes, surface modified with VEGF (VEGF-CC), bFGF (bFGF-CC), transferrin (transferrin-CC), non-targeted coated complexes (CC), simple pLL/DNA complexes (pLL), complexes formed using a self-assembling pLL-bFGF conjugate (bFGF-pLL) or DOTAP, in the presence of serum for 4 h. DNA final concentration was 2.8 μg/ml in each case. Cells were then washed, reincubated in fresh medium containing serum, and gene expression was evaluated 44 h later using a Galactolight™ kit and luminometry. Greatest levels of transfection were obtained using coated complexes retargeted with bFGF, and all materials that were not coated showed substantial inhibition due to the presence of serum (data not shown).

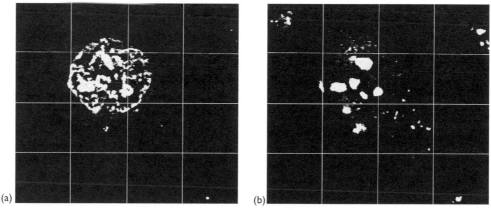

Fig. 48.5 ECV 304 cells were incubated with coated complexes containing Texas Red-DNA, surface modified with bFGF. Nuclei were visualized using DAPI (a). After 4 h incubation, deconvolution micrographs (63×) show nuclear deposition of Texas Red-labelled DNA (b). A more classical perinuclear distribution was seen with non-targeted complexes, or complexes targeted with VEGF or transferrin (data not shown). Delivery of DNA to the nucleus in this way resembles literature reports of bFGF deposition in endothelial cells.[41]

promoters, should lead to development of effective strategies for tumour ablation that could have significant therapeutic impact in the foreseeable future.

Acknowledgements

We are grateful to the Cancer Research Campaign, NHS Executive (West Midlands) Sheldon Fellowships Scheme, and the European Union for support.

References

1. Thomas, M. (1998). Cancer of the ovary: advances in chemotherapy. *Trends Urol. Gynaecol. Sex. Hlth*, **3**, 11–16.
2. Dorigo, O. and Berek, J.S. (1997). Gene therapy for ovarian cancer: Development of novel treatment strategies. *Int. J. Gynecol. Cancer*, **7**, 1–13.
3. Tait, D.L., Obermiller, P.S., Jensen, R.A., and Holt, J.T. (1998). Ovarian cancer gene therapy. *Hematol. Oncol. Clin. North Am.*, **12**, 539.
4. Tong, X.W., Kieback, D.G., Ramesh, R., and Freeman, S.M. (1999). Molecular aspects of ovarian cancer—Is gene therapy the solution? *Hematol. Oncol. Clin. North Am.*, **13**, 109.

5. Boucher, R.C. (1999). Status of gene therapy for cystic fibrosis lung disease. *J. Clin. Invest.*, **103**, 441–5.

6. Li, H.W., AlonsoVanegas, M., Colicos, M.A. *et al.* (1999). Intracerebral adenovirus-mediated p53 tumor suppressor gene therapy for experimental human glioma. *Clin. Cancer Res.*, **5**, 637–42.

7. Wollenberg, B., Kastenbauer, Mundl, H. *et al.* (1999). Gene therapy—Phase I trial for primary untreated head and neck squamous cell cancer (HNSCC) UICC stage II–IV with a single intratumoral injection of hIL–2 plasmids formulated in DOTMA/Chol. *Hum. Gene Ther.*, **10**, 141–7.

8. Hamstra, D.A. and Rehemtulla, A. (1999). Toward an enzyme/prodrug strategy for cancer gene therapy: Endogenous activation of carboxypeptidase A mutants by the PACE/furin family of propeptidases. *Hum. Gene Ther.*, **10**, 235–48.

9. Nevin, N.C. (1998). Experience of gene therapy in the United Kingdom. *Ann. NY Acad. Sci.*, **862**, 184–7.

10. Parasrampuria, D.A. (1998). Therapeutic delivery issues in gene therapy, part 1: Vectors. *Biopharm. Technol. Business Biopharmaceut.*, **11**, 38.

11. Putman, L. (1998). Debate grows on safety of gene-therapy vectors. *Lancet*, **351**, 808.

12. Li, S. and Huang, L. (1997). *In vivo* gene transfer via intravenous administration of cationic lipid–protamine–DNA (LPD) complexes. *Gene Ther.*, **4**, 891–900.

13. Remy, J.S., Abdallah, B., Zanta, M.A. *et al.* (1998). Gene transfer with lipospermines and polyethylenimines. *Adv. Drug Delivery Rev.*, **30**, 85–95.

14. Goula, D., Benoist, C., Mantero, S. *et al.* (1998). Polyethylenimine-based intravenous delivery of transgenes to mouse lung. *Gene Ther.*, **5**, 1291–5.

15. Li, S. and Huang, L. (1997). Protamine sulfate provides enhanced and reproducible intravenous gene transfer by cationic liposome/DNA complex. *J. Liposome Res.*, **7**, 207–19.

16. Boucher, Y., Brekken, C., Netti, P.A. *et al.* (1998). Intratumoral infusion of fluid: estimation of hydraulic conductivity and implications for the delivery of therapeutic agents. *Br. J. Cancer*, **78**, 1442–8.

17. Jain, R.K. (1996). 1995 Whitaker lecture: Delivery of molecules, particles, and cells to solid tumors. *Ann. Biomed. Engineer.*, **24**, 457–73.

18. Netti, P.A., Hamberg, L.M., Babich, J.W. *et al.* (1999). Enhancement of fluid filtration across tumor vessels: Implication for delivery of macromolecules. *Proc. Natl Acad. Sci., USA*, **96**, 3137–42.

19. Dash, P.R., Read, M.L., Fisher, K.D. *et al.* (2000). Decreased binding to proteins and cells of polymeric gene delivery vectors surface modified with a multivalent hydrophilic polymer and retargeting through attachment of transferrin. *J. Biol. Chem.*, **275**, 3793–802.

20. Keen, C.E., Szakacs, S., Okon, E. *et al.* (1999). CA125 and thyroglobulin staining in papillary carcinomas of thyroid and ovarian origin is not completely specific for site of origin [Full text delivery]. *Histopathology*, **34**, 113–17.

21. Kudoh, K., Kikuchi, Y., Kita, T. *et al.* (1999). Preoperative determination of several serum tumor markers in patients with primary epithelial ovarian carcinoma. *Gynecol. Obstet. Invest.*, **47**, 52–7.

22. Gabizon, A., Horowitz, A.T., Goren, D. *et al.* (1999). Targeting folate receptor with folate linked to extremities of poly(ethylene glycol)-grafted liposomes: *In vitro* studies. *Bioconjugate Chem.*, **10**, 289–98.

23. Reddy, J.A. and Low, P.S. (1998). Folate-mediated targeting of therapeutic and imaging agents to cancers. *Crit. Rev. Therap. Drug Carrier Syst.*, **15**, 587–627.

24. Wang, S. and Low, P.S. (1998). Folate-mediated targeting of antineoplastic drags, imaging agents, and nucleic acids to cancer cells. *J. Controlled Release*, **53**, 39–48.

25. Leamon, C.P. and Low, P.S. (1994). Selective targeting of malignant-cells with cytotoxin-folate conjugates. *J. Drug Target.*, **2**, 101–12.

26. Cabanes, A., EvenChen, S., Zimberoff, J. *et al.* (1999). Enhancement of antitumor activity of polyethylene glycol-coated liposomal doxorubicin with soluble and liposomal interleukin 2. *Clin. Cancer Res.*, **5**, 687–93.

27. Cabanes, A., Tzemach, D., Goren, D. *et al.* (1998). Comparative study of the antitumor activity of free doxorubicin and polyethylene glycol-coated liposomal doxorubicin in a mouse lymphoma model. *Clin. Cancer Res.*, **4**, 499–505.

28. Gabizon, A., Goren, D., Horowitz, A.T. *et al.* (1997). Long-circulating liposomes for drug delivery in cancer therapy: A review of biodistribution studies in tumor-bearing animals. *Adv. Drug Delivery Rev.*, **24**, 337–44.

29. Gabizon, A.A. (1995). Liposome circulation time and tumor targeting—implications for cancer-chemotherapy. *Adv. Drug Delivery Rev.*, **16**, 285–94.

30. Seymour, L.W., Ulbrich, K., Steyger, P.S. *et al.* (1994). Tumor tropism and anticancer efficacy of polymer-based doxorubicin prodrugs in the treatment of subcutaneous murine B16f10 melanoma. *Br. J. Cancer*, **70**, 636–41.

31. Dvorak, H.F., Nagy, J.A., Feng, D. *et al.* (1999). Vascular permeability factor vascular endothelial growth factor and the significance of microvascular hyperpermeability in angiogenesis. *Curr. Topic. Microbiol. Immunol.*, **237**, 97–132.

32. Seymour, L.W. (1992). Passive tumor targeting of soluble macromolecules and drug conjugates. *Crit. Rev. Therap. Drug Carrier Syst.*, **9**, 135–87.

33. Baban, D.F. and Seymour, L.W. (1998). Control of tumour vascular permeability. *Adv. Drug Delivery Rev.*, **34**, 109–19.

34. Amantea, M.A. and Gabizon, A. (1998). Pharmacokinetics (PKs) of Caelyx(R)/Doxil(R) (Stealth(R) liposomal doxorubicin) in patients with either breast or prostate cancer. *Ann. Oncol.*, **9**, 653.

35. Burrows, F.J. and Thorpe, P.E. (1994). Vascular targeting—a new approach to the therapy of solid tumors. *Pharmacol. Therapeut.*, **64**, 155–74.

36. Fan, T.P.D., Jaggar, R., and Bicknell, R. (1995). Controlling the vasculature—angiogenesis, anti-angiogenesis and vascular targeting of gene-therapy. *Trend. Pharmacol. Sci.*, **16**, 57–66.

37. Schnitzer, J.E. (1998). Vascular targeting as a strategy for cancer therapy. *N. Engl. J. Med.*, **339**, 472–4.

38. Brown, L.F., Harrist, T.J., Yeo, K.T. *et al.* (1995). Increased expression of vascular-permeability factor (vascular endothelial growth-factor) in bullous pemphigoid, dermatitis-herpetiformis, and erythema multiforme. *J. Invest. Dermatol.*, **104**, 744–9.

39. Hatva, E., Kaipainen, A., Mentula, P. *et al.* (1995). Expression of endothelial cell-specific receptor tyrosine kinases and growth-factors in human brain-tumors. *Am. J. Pathol.*, **146**, 368–78.

40. Fisher, D., Ulbrich, K., Subr, V. *et al.* (2000). A versatile system for receptor-mediated gene delivery permits increased entry of DNA into target cells, enhanced delivery to the nucleus and elevated rates of transgene expression. *Gene Ther.*, **7**, 1337–43.

41. Dellera, P., Presta, M., and Ragnotti, G. (1991). nuclear-localization of endogenous basic fibroblast growth-factor in cultured endothelial-cells. *Exp. Cell Res.*, **192**, 505–10.

49. Corporate drug discovery strategies

Mark P. Smith and
George R. P. Blackledge

Background

Companies exist primarily to provide a return on investment for their owners. Good companies will have other aims as well, but these will be secondary to their primary objective. All companies are different, but the most successful companies are effective because they focus on what they do well. In the case of a pharmaceutical company, it is critical that a successful company must discover, develop, and then sell a new drug to the highest levels of effectiveness. In order to do this, it is critical that the successful pharmaceutical company focuses on doable, profitable projects. The rest of this chapter reviews some of the issues.

Drug discovery

For a large pharmaceutical company there are a number of ways of identifying a potentially useful new chemical entity. The first is through the endeavours of in-house research, and the second is through identifying an interesting compound externally and licensing that compound from its owners. This second approach can enable close co-operation between the company and academic institutions or other external organizations. Collaborations recognize that no single institution has all the skills and knowledge that can lead to important discoveries, and that by working together there are greater opportunities for success.

There are a number of ways in which new agents are discovered as a result of in-house research. In general, companies will attempt to identify a target; for example, an enzyme that could be inhibited, a protein–protein interaction, or a higher-level, more complex target such as the proliferation of malignant cells. The techniques and approaches to the understanding of a target are common to all good scientific discovery, regardless of whether it is conducted within a pharmaceutical company or within an academic institution. Following as thorough an identification and understanding of the target as possible, companies will then put in place either a screening process to evaluate a large number of existing compounds against the target, or a programme of logical drug design using an understanding of the molecular structure or structures involved in the target, and altering the confirmation of potentially active molecules to obtain the maximum effect on the desired target. Increasingly, there is a move away from random screening of large numbers of compounds to a more structured strategy utilizing new technologies of genomics and proteomics, and evaluating these via effective bioformatics systems. In the area of cancer, there are still relatively crude screening processes in place, evaluating either cell lines or tumour xenografts. In an environment where an understanding of the biological mechanism of action of an agent is increasingly important, the law of diminishing returns now applies to these approaches.

Lead compounds may be identified from a number of sources. Compound libraries which exist within companies are the most common source for these, but, in the past, screening natural products has been a fertile source of cytotoxic agents, of which taxol, vincristine, and doxorubicin are all good examples.

Once a lead compound, or series of compounds, has been identified, it is likely that some chemistry effort will be employed to determine whether in an agreed set of tests, the therapeutic ratio for the agent can be improved. Finally, it is important that whatever compound is taken forward for further development is genuinely novel in origin, and that patent protection can be obtained, thus giving the company the ability to exploit their molecule fully.

Developing a molecule in the clinic

Three key factors need to be taken into consideration when a molecule is being evaluated and developed to become a useful drug. These are: time, risk, and cost. The three are completely interdependent. If the key objective of the development is to bring a drug to the market as quickly as possible, because of the competitive situation, then this is likely to cost more and have a higher risk. If the objective is to minimize the cost of development, then it is likely that it will take longer and will also be associated with higher risk, because fewer studies will be carried out, and this could limit the promotability of a new agent. Additional factors need to be considered; for example, when do the patent rights expire, will the treatment paradigms change during the development period, is the drug breaking new ground in terms of scientific, development, regulatory or marketing issues, and will the development and successful launch require such high levels of resource that other company opportunities will be at risk? It is, therefore, important that all aspects of a development programme are considered, and that a decision is made about which of the three factors—time, cost, and risk—needs to be optimized.

The standard development paradigms of sequential phase I, II, and III trials usually enable adequate evaluation of the drug's potential. It is not essential that this process is adhered to strictly, so long as the overall clinical trial programme satisfies regulatory authorities, who, in the main, reflect the clinical demands of the practising oncologist and his patient. The drug has, first and foremost, to be effective in the target population. In general, the toxicity profile has to be acceptable, although it may be different from other agents, providing that the overall benefit/risk profile is deemed to be appropriate to the patient. Other factors, such as convenience of schedule, route of administration, quality of life, health economics, and cost of treatment, have varying degrees of importance that depend upon personal preferences and healthcare systems that exist in different countries.

It is also important to be aware of the fact that there are many aspects of drug development beyond clinical trials. It is important that appropriate toxicology has been carried out, that the drug can be manufactured reproducibly, that its kinetics are understood, and that the data being produced will be satisfactory to regulatory authorities—a key prerequisite to marketing a new agent. For this reason, most pharmaceutical companies ensure that there is a cross-functional team with responsibility for the overall management of a drug development project.

For many anticancer agents, the potential for effective treatment goes beyond the initial development programme and approval, which may be in a second- or third-line advanced cancer population. Recent examples of limited approvals of potentially broad-spectrum anticancer agents include capecitabine, gemcitabine, irinotecan, oxaliplatin, raltitrexed, and topotecan. Factors that influence the choice of patient population for first approval include evidence of activity in preclinical and clinical models, ease of doing clinical trials, current standards of treatment, and opportunities to get accelerated approvals due to the high unmet medical need. Certain cancers have traditionally been more attractive than others because of the large patient numbers, e.g. colorectal, non-small cell lung cancer, and breast cancer, or because of the unmet medical need, e.g. refractory ovarian cancer or pancreatic cancer. It is important that the full potential of the new treatment is evaluated with a broad clinical trial programme that actively involves the collaboration of large numbers of clinicians, either as individuals or as collaborative groups, and the company. Trials will need to be conducted that examine the potential for combinations of agents and their effectiveness in new cancer populations. During this phase of development, the drug's future utility will be determined largely by local market needs, because of the variations in treatment patterns that exist from country to country and from clinic to clinic. Although the company's objectives will be to encourage widespread usage, it will also be desirable that new regulatory approvals are achieved in additional countries. These may be an extension of the first approval or genuine new indications. Often it is possible for the new indications to arise out of work and data generated from clinician-initiated trials.

The future

The above describes what may now be regarded as relatively conventional drug development. It is likely that there will be significant changes in the future. The first of these reflects a move away from conventional cytotoxics in the treatment of cancer to new mechanism-based therapies, which may require new diagnostics over and above a pathological diagnosis. The second is that as our understanding of different malignancies increases, then we are likely to be sub-setting current populations of patients on the basis of molecular diagnostics, and designing therapies which will be more specific to these. Both of these will produce new challenges for drug development processes. The use of surrogate endpoints for evidence of activity will become increasingly important, since new approaches that are thought to be cytostatic will be harder to evaluate in terms of clear objective responses. Other agents targeted at new mechanisms, such as epidermal growth factor (EGF) receptor antagonists such as ZD 1839 or anti-invasives such as matrix metalloproteinase inhibitors, may require new thinking as to the design of key clinical trials and dose-finding studies. Recruitment of patients to clinical trials may be more difficult unless closer relationships exist between the clinical centres and industry. Regulatory authorities may need to evaluate clinical data in new ways, although the ultimate judgement will, as always, be the overall clinical benefit to the patient.

Finally, there will be increasing cost pressures on all forms of healthcare, and it is therefore important that, in addition to demonstrating both the efficacy and safety of a new agent, the overall value in healthcare terms is also assessed. All of these factors will lead to new drug discovery and development strategies in the future, and it is likely that agents, or combinations of agents, very different from those that are utilized today will become more frequent over the next two decades.

50. DNA mismatch repair and drug resistance

Stephen B. Howell, Xinjian Lin, and Heung-Ki Kim

Introduction

The platinum-containing drugs cisplatin (DDP) and carboplatin (CBDCA) remain central to the primary chemotherapy of ovarian cancer. However, resistance to these agents emerges routinely and often quite rapidly during the treatment of ovarian cancer, and tumors that become nonresponsive to these drugs are frequently clinically resistant to a wide spectrum of other chemotherapeutic agents. This problem has been approached by trying to understand the mechanisms by which cells become resistant to DDP, but the biochemical changes that accompany resistance have been difficult to identify and clinically exploitable findings have been limited. Recently, we and others found that loss of DNA mismatch repair (MMR) directly produces resistance to DDP and CBDCA (reviewed in ref. 1). Among the multiple factors that can contribute to DDP resistance, this is the first for which the molecular mechanism has been identified. Information is rapidly accumulating to suggest that loss of MMR is a clinically important mechanism of resistance to DDP and CBDCA.

DNA mismatch repair

During the replication of DNA, misincorporation of a base or 'slippage' of DNA polymerase on the template can create a single base or short segment of mismatch. These types of errors are repaired by the MMR system. The products of at least five human genes participate in MMR, including hMSH2, hMSH3, hMSH6, hMLH1, and hPMS2. On the basis of genetic evidence, a sixth protein, hPMS1, is also believed to be important for MMR, although biochemical studies supporting its involvement in MMR are not yet available (reviewed in ref. 2). The first step involves the binding of a heterodimer of either hMSH2–hMSH6 or hMSH2–hMSH3 to the mismatched base. This is followed by binding of the hMLH1–hPMS2 heteroduplex, cutting of the daughter strand containing the mismatch, exonuclease-mediated removal of the segment between the nick and the mismatch, filling in the gap by DNA polymerase δ, and ligation that renders the strand whole again. The hMSH2–hMSH6 heteroduplex preferentially recognizes single-base mismatches, whereas the

hMSH2–hMSH3 heteroduplex has specificity for multibase mismatches and short loops.[3]

When MMR is lost, mismatches persist and become fixed as mutations at the next round of DNA synthesis. Loss of MMR results in the appearance of nucleotide additions or deletions, and transitions and transversions in both repetitive and nonrepetitive sequences scattered throughout the genome.[4,5] There is a marked increase in mutation rate, which reaches three orders of magnitude in some genes. Microsatellites are stretches of DNA in which the same sequence of two, three, or four bases is repeated many times. Microsatellite sequences are particularly prone to DNA polymerase slippage errors that create a mismatched base or short loop.[6] Variability in the length of such sequences is a hallmark of the loss of MMR,[7–9] and genes that contain microsatellites in their coding sequences are at particularly high risk of mutation. Increased mutation rates have been found in such important genes as *HPRT*,[4] *APC*,[10] type II *TGFβ* receptor,[11] and *BAX*.[12]

Subjects who carry a germline mutation that disables one of the genes having a product that plays an essential role in MMR are at increased risk for the development of cancer; this is the genetic basis for hereditary nonpolyposis colon cancer.[13] Most of these families have mutations in either *MSH2 or MLH1*.[14–16] While a single functional copy of one of these critical genes is sufficient to maintain normal MMR activity, loss of the second allele by somatic mutation commonly accompanies oncogenesis, and in such tumors MMR is completely lost.- However, loss of MMR function in at least some cells occurs frequently in many types of sporadic cancers, including endometrial, ovarian, pancreatic, and lung cancer.[17–19]

Loss of MMR causes resistance to DDP and CBDCA

In addition to recognizing mismatches, the MMR system recognizes the DNA adducts produced by a variety of chemotherapeutic agents, including the antimetabolite 6-thioguanine; the methylating agents procarbazine, temozolomide, and MNNG;[20–22] and the platinum-containing drugs DDP and CBDCA.[23,24] In each case, it appears that adduct recognition, and possibly processing, is accompanied by generation of a pro-apoptotic signal, since loss of MMR function results in less cell killing. The current paradigm is that the MMR system functions as a detector for these adducts. When MMR is disabled, the cell cannot detect the DNA damage and initiate apoptosis as readily, and thus the cell is phenotypically drug-resistant.

Loss of MMR results in 1.5- to fourfold resistance to DDP, irrespective of whether the disabling mutation is in *MLH1*, *MSH2*, or *PMS2*, suggesting that full assembly of the entire MMR complex is required for generation of a pro-apoptotic signal.[23,25] This phenomenon has been examined primarily in pairs of cells of the same genetic background that differ from each other in more ways than just the expression of a single MMR gene.[23,26] However, DDP resistance is also observed in cell pairs which differ only by the knockout of a single MMR gene.[25]

DDP treatment enriches for cells that have lost MMR

Even though loss of MMR produces relatively low-level resistance, one would predict that DDP treatment would gradually enrich for such cells when they are present as a minor component in a population of MMR-proficient cells. This has now been demonstrated directly using MMR-deficient cells genetically engineered to express green fluorescent protein (GFP).[27] As shown in Fig. 50.1, starting with a population containing 5% deficient cells, a single exposure to an IC_{50} concentration of DDP increased the MMR-deficient cells to 7.5% within 5 days, and an IC_{90} exposure enriched to 8.7%. Repeated cycles of exposure produced progressive enrichment for the MMR-deficient cells.

Enrichment has also been demonstrated *in vivo* using a xenograft model in which MMR-deficient Chinese hamster ovary

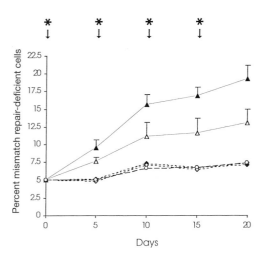

Fig. 50.1 Effect of loss of DNA mismatch repair on enrichment *in vitro* in a population containing 5% MMR-deficient GFP-expressing cells and 95% MMR-proficient HCT116+ch3 cells subjected to four cycles of a 1 h exposure (↓) to either cisplatin (△, 25 μM; ▲, 50 μM) or oxaliplatin (□, 25 μM; ◆, 50 μM). Each data point represents the mean of three experiments compared to the untreated control population (o). Bars = SD.

(CHO) clone B cells were engineered to express GFP.[28] Tumors were inoculated with a population of CHO cells containing a minority of MMR-deficient cells, and 48 hours later the mice were treated with a single LD_{10} dose of DDP. The tumors were harvested 14 days after inoculation, and the fraction of GFP-expressing MMR-deficient cells determined by flow cytometric analysis. Untreated tumors contained an average of 4.6 ± 2.3% (SD) MMR-deficient cells, whereas the DDP-treated tumors contained 6.8 ± 2.3% (SD) deficient cells ($P = 0.04$). Thus, a single exposure to DDP produced a 48% enrichment *in vivo*.

Loss of MMR causes hypersensitivity to the mutagenic effects of DDP

It has long been recognized that DDP is a mutagen in mammalian cells.[29–32] The most abundant lesions produced in DNA are guanine–guanine (65%) and adenine–guanine (25%) intrastrand adducts. While it appears difficult for most DNA polymerases to synthesize across the GG adduct when it is on the lagging strand, translesional bypass occurs to a significant extent on the leading strand during DNA replication. This results in the misincorporation of nucleotides opposite the intrastrand adduct.[33] Both the GG adduct itself and the lesion consisting of an adduct and a misincorporated base on the opposite strand are recognized, and possibly processed, by the MMR system.[34,35] Recently it was demonstrated that the probability of mutagenic bypass replication is increased in cells that have lost MMR,[26] suggesting that the recognition of the adduct by the MMR protein complex serves to protect against this form of genomic destabilization.

Consistent with this hypothesis, studies from this laboratory have documented that cells that have lost MMR are hypersensitive to the mutagenic effects of DDP (H.-K. Kim and S.B. Howell, unpublished). This was first demonstrated using clones of the human colon cancer cell line HCT116 that contains mutations in both alleles of *MLH1*. The HCT116+ch3 subline was rendered MMR-proficient by microcell transfer of chromosome 3 containing a wild-type copy of *MLH1*.[36] Chromosome 2 was transferred to other cells as a control, thus generating the HCT116+ch2 subline that remains MMR-deficient. These cells were exposed to increasing concentrations of DDP for 1 hour, and then allowed to grow in drug-free medium for 10 days, after which the number of putative HGPRT (hypoxanthine guanine phosphoribosyl transferase) mutants in the population was determined by culturing the cells in the presence of a high concentration of 6-thioguanine.

Figure 50.2 shows the number of 6-thioguanine-resistant colonies per 10^6 clonogenic cells as a function of DDP concentration for the two cell lines. In the absence of any DDP treatment, the spontaneous mutant frequency to 6-thioguanine resistance was 6.0 ± 7.0 (SD) per 10^6 clonogenic cells in the MMR-proficient cells and 14.9 ± 14.4 (SD) in the MMR-deficient cells. Increasing concentrations of DDP produced progressively higher mutant frequencies in both types of cells over the range tested (50 μM DDP killed approximately 99.9% of the HCT116+ch3 cells and 99% of the HCT116+ch2 cells). The slope of the linear regression curve for the MMR-deficient cells was 3.7 ± 1.3 (SD)-fold greater than

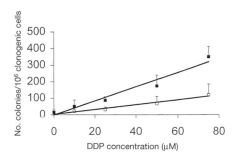

Fig. 50.2 Number of 6-thioguanine resistant colonies per 10^6 clonogenic cells as a function of DDP concentration for the MMR-proficient HCT116+ch3 (open squares) and MMR-deficient HCT116+ch2 cells (closed squares). Each data point is the mean (±SD) of four experiments for each concentration of cisplatin.

that for the MMR-proficient cells ($P < 0.05$, $n = 4$). Thus, for a given degree of exposure, DDP was more mutagenic to the MMR-deficient than the MMR-proficient cells for the HGPRT gene. It is noteworthy that higher mutant frequencies were observed at both low and high concentrations of DDP across the range of tumor cell kill that is anticipated for a clinically responsive tumor in patients.

There are several ways in which loss of MMR could augment the mutagenicity of DDP. First, loss of the ability of the cell to detect DDP adducts and trigger apoptosis may result in the survival of a cell with mutagenic lesions in its DNA that would have otherwise died. Secondly, the MMR system may repair a fraction of the mismatches that result from the misincorporation of an incorrect base opposite the adducted 1,2d(GpG) or 1,2d(ApG), thus preventing fixation of a mutation at the subsequent round of DNA synthesis. If the MMR system succeeds in correcting the mismatch despite persistence of the adduct, then the strand containing the mismatch will serve as a faithful template on the next round of DNA synthesis and the mutation will be avoided. A third possibility is that adduct recognition by the MMR proteins serves to prevent the mutagenic bypass replication in the first place. Recently Vaisman et al.[26] reported that loss of MMR is associated with an increased probability of bypass replication, suggesting that the MMR proteins, and specifically the hMSH2–hMSH6 heterodimer, play a role in signaling the polymerase to halt.

Loss of MMR increases the risk of development of cells resistant to other drugs following DDP exposure

Hypersensitivity to the mutagenic effect of clinically relevant exposures to DDP is of general concern because of the possibility that it will increase the risk of activation of oncogenes or inactivation of tumor or metastasis suppressor genes. Of more immediately concern, however, is the question of whether DDP can mutagenize tumor cells to drugs that are frequently used in combination with it in the treatment of ovarian cancer, and whether this propensity is augmented when MMR is lost.

Mutant frequency studies were carried out using the HCT116+ch3 and HCT116+ch2 cells as described above, but using etoposide (VP–16), topotecan (TPT), gemcitabine (GEM), or paclitaxel (TAX) as the selecting agent (X. Lin and S. B. Howell, unpublished observations). These drugs were chosen because of their frequent use in DDP-based combination therapy (VP–16 and TAX), or their promise as potentially useful DDP partners. The experiments measured the ability of DDP to generate cells in the population which were resistant to very high concentrations of the selecting drug that were sufficient to reduce clonogenic survival to 0.0002%. Even in the MMR-proficient cells, DDP exposure increased the number of cells in the population that were resistant to each of the four drugs tested in a DDP-concentration-dependent manner. As was the case for the generation of 6-thioguanine-resistant cells, the effect was apparent at even relatively modest DDP exposures. Table 50.1 shows that, for all four drugs, the slope of the number of resistant variants as a function of DDP concentration was statistically significantly higher for the MMR-deficient subline than for the MMR-proficient cells. The largest differential effect was observed for VP–16. Since TPT, GEM, and TAX are so often used concurrently with or sequentially following DDP, the ability of DDP to generate resistant clones has the potential of limiting the effectiveness of such combinations.

To determine whether the mutagenic hypersensitivity to DDP was limited to just the HCT116 system, or just the loss of MHL1 function, the experiments are being repeated using another pair of MMR-proficient and deficient cells. HEC59 cells have mutations in both alleles of *MSH2* that disable MMR, whereas the HEC59+ch2 cells, in which a wild-type copy of *MSH2* has been transferred on chromosome 2, are MMR-proficient.[37] Experiments have been completed with TPT, GEM, and TAX to date. Table 50.2 shows that the MMR-deficient subline was hypersensitive to this effect of DDP in the case of TPT and GEM, but not TAX. The magnitude of the effect for TPT and GEM was less than was observed in the HCT116 cell pair. Whether this reflects differences in residual MMR function due to mutations in hMSH2 versus hMLH1 awaits further analyses using true knockout cell pairs. It is possible that in hMLH1-deficient cells the MSH2–MSH6 heterodimer still recognizes and processes the DDP adduct in a manner that contributes to a mutagenic propensity that is even greater than that resulting from the simple failure to recognize the adduct that accompanies MSH2 loss.

Table 50.1 Ratio of the ability of DDP to generate resistant variants in MMR-deficient to MMR-proficient HCT116 cells

Drug	Slope ratio[a] (mean ± SD)	P value
6-Thioguanine	3.7 ± 1.3	<0.05
Etoposide	6.7 ± 0.8	<0.02
Topotecan	2.6 ± 0.3	<0.004
Gemcitabine	3.6 ± 0.9	<0.005
Paclitaxel	2.3 ± 0.1	<0.007

[a] Ratio of the slope of the number of resistant colonies per 10^6 clonogenic cells as a function of DDP concentration for the HCT116+ch2 cells to that for the HCT116+ch3 cells. N = 4 for all drugs.

Table 50.2 Ratio of the ability of DDP to generate resistant variants in MMR-deficient to MMR-proficient HEC59 cells

Drug	Slope ratio[a] (mean ± SD)	P value
Topotecan	1.4 ± 0.3	0.018
Gemcitabine	1.4 ± 0.4	0.037
Paclitaxel	1.1 ± 0.6	0.70

[a] Ratio of the slope of the number of resistant colonies per 10^6 clonogenic cells as a function of DDP concentration for the HEC59 cells to that for the HEC59 +ch2 cells. N = 6 for all drugs.

It is important to emphasize that these experiments did not establish that each of the surviving colonies was a true genetic mutant, nor that the putative mutant was phenotypically stable. However, from the point of view of the cancer chemotherapist, what is important is whether, at the time the second drug is injected, the population of tumor cells in the patient contains within it a larger number of cells capable of surviving exposure to the second drug. Such cells do not have to be true genetic mutants nor have a stable phenotype in order to contribute to the failure of treatment with these drugs.[38] No information is currently available on the kinetics of the appearance and possible subsequent disappearance of such resistant clones within the tumor, and it is conceivable that with enough time most of these revert to a more sensitive state. However, the current results suggest that, at least at 10 days after DDP exposure, such resistant variants are still present.

Anticipated effects of loss of MMR on the rate of development of resistance

The finding that DDP treatment enriches for MMR-deficient cells, and that such cells are hypersensitive to the ability of DDP to generate variants resistant to other drugs, is of substantial concern with respect to the development of clinical resistance. Although no information is available on how quickly enrichment occurs *in vivo*, or how many tumors contain biologically important numbers of MMR-deficient cells, these findings lead to several predictions that merit consideration.

One prediction is that, if MMR-deficient cells are present in the tumor, primary chemotherapy with either a DDP-based or CBDCA-based regimen will result in enrichment for MMR-deficient cells. The prediction extends to both drugs since loss of MMR results in equal degrees of enrichment in tissue culture experiments with both agents.[39] The prediction is supported by the observation that DDP enriches for MMR-deficient cells both *in vitro* and *in vivo* at relatively low levels of drug exposure.[27] The fact that primary chemotherapy for ovarian cancer consists of repeated cycles of drug exposure favors such enrichment because, under these circumstances, even small enrichment factors can have major consequences.[38] In the tissue culture experiments, an IC_{50} exposure resulted in enrichment by a factor of 1.4–1.5,[27,39] and a single LD_{10} dose in the xenograft model also increased the fraction of MMR-deficient cells in the tumor by a factor of 1.5.[28] If an enrichment factor of this magnitude occurs in patients with ovarian cancer, and it remains constant with each cycle of drug exposure, then six cycles of DDP or CBDCA-based chemotherapy would result in a tenfold enrichment for MMR-deficient cells. Two clinical studies suggest that such enrichment may in fact be common. Both studies examined the extent of MLH1 expression in ovarian cancers before and after therapy, as measured by immunohistochemical staining,[28,40] and both found that staining was significantly reduced following treatment with a platinum drug-containing regimen, consistent with reduction in MMR activity.

A second prediction that emerges from these findings is that clinical resistance should develop more rapidly in tumors that start out with a large fraction of MMR-deficient cells. At the present time there is no method available to quantify precisely the fraction of cells that are MMR-deficient. There is a very high probability that at least 15–20% of ovarian cancers contain a significant fraction of MMR-deficient cells, because microsatellite instability, a genetic hallmark of loss of MMR, is found in this percentage of tumors.[41,42] However, microsatellite instability is a fairly crude indicator of the presence of MMR-deficient cells. Since at diagnosis stage III/IV ovarian carcinomas often contain 10^{11}–10^{12} cells (approximately 100–1000 g), and mutation rates in tumors are frequently in excess of 10^{-6}, there is a high probability that a much larger fraction of such tumors contain at least some MMR-deficient cells prior to the start of treatment. Despite the limitations of microsatellite instability measurements, it may be possible to detect differences in survival in carefully crafted clinical trials.

A third prediction that emerges from these studies is that tumors that contain a large fraction of MMR-deficient cells will be at higher risk for the development of cross-resistance to VP–16, TPT, GEM, and TAX than those that contain few such cells, and that treatment with DDP will increase the risk of developing cross-resistance. This prediction is in general agreement with clinical observation that the greater the DDP resistance, as reflected by either lack of response to primary DDP or CBDCA chemotherapy or early relapse, the lower the probability of response to other types of chemotherapeutic agents. However, head-to-head comparisons of the response to any of these drugs following primary treatment with DDP or CBDCA versus a drug regimen that does not enrich for MMR-deficient cells are not available.

The final prediction is based on the observation that loss of MMR results in resistance to the topoisomerase II inhibitors doxorubicin (1.7-fold) and etoposide (2.0-fold) as well as to DDP and CBDCA.[39] Although currently less thoroughly documented, this would suggest that enrichment for genomically unstable MMR-deficient cells may accompany primary chemotherapy with regimens containing these drugs as well.

The observation that loss of MMR results in resistance to DDP has now been documented in many laboratories, using a variety of cell systems. The potential significance of loss of MMR for the development of drug resistance during chemotherapy is amplified by the observation that such MMR-deficient cells are hypersensitive to the ability of DDP to generate variants resistant to drugs often used in combination with DDP and CBDCA. Little information is currently available as to the actual clinical significance of this particular mechanism of resistance, and it would be premature to diverge from the use of DDP or CBDCA in the primary chemotherapy of ovarian cancer. However, the available observations do permit formulation of specific predictions, and some of these can be addressed with tools currently in hand. Clearly, a method for measuring MMR activity in individual cells obtained from patient tumor samples would greatly facilitate this effort.

Strategies for overcoming the development of clinical resistance due to loss of MMR

If loss of MMR is an important factor in the development of clinical resistance, is there any way to circumvent this process? One approach would be to use drugs that do not enrich for MMR-deficient cells. Interestingly, MMR-deficient cells are not resistant to oxaliplatin and other DDP analogs that contain carrier ligands other than just the ammine groups found in DDP.[23,26] For example, oxaliplatin does not enrich for MMR-deficient cells in tissue culture experiments.[27] Thus, one would predict that resistance to oxaliplatin would emerge more slowly than resistance to DDP. Oxaliplatin, as well as later generations of DDP analogs, may find utility in the primary chemotherapy of ovarian cancer for this reason, as well as for their ability to overcome other mechanisms of DDP resistance.

Another approach to circumventing the development of resistance due to enrichment for MMR-deficient cells would be to combine DDP or CBDCA with a drug that is more effective at killing MMR-deficient than proficient cells. Studies by Aquilina et al.[43] using human cells defective in hMLH1 function in tissue culture have suggested that MMR-deficient cells are two- to fivefold hypersensitive to the cytotoxic effects of lomustine (CCNU). Although this effect was observed only in cells with low O^6-methylguanine-DNA-methyltransferase activity, this observation provides a starting point in the search for agents that could offset the enriching effect of DDP and CBDCA.

Acknowledgements

This work was supported in part by grant CA78648 from the National Institutes of Health and a grant from Sanofi Research. It was conducted in part by the Clayton Foundation for Research, California Division. Drs Howell and Lin are Clayton Foundation Investigators.

References

1. Fink, D., Aebi, S., and Howell, S.B. (1998). The role of DNA mismatch repair in drug resistance. *Clin. Cancer Res.*, **4**, 1–5.
2. Kolodner, R. (1996). Biochemistry and genetics of eukaryotic mismatch repair. *Genes Develop.*, **10**, 1433–42.
3. Acharya, S., Wilson, T., Gradia, S. *et al.* (1996). hMSH2 forms specific misrepair-binding complexes with hMSH3 and hMSH6. *Proc. Natl Acad. Sci., USA*, **93**, 13629–34.
4. Bhattacharyya, N.P., Skandalis, A., Ganesh, A. *et al.* (1994). Mutator phenotypes in human colorectal carcinoma cell lines. *Proc. Natl. Acad. Sci., USA*, **91**, 6319–23.
5. Modrich, P. (1991). Mechanics and biological effects of mismatch repair. *Ann. Rev. Genet.*, **25**, 229–53.
6. Kunkel, T.A. (1993). Slippery DNA and diseases. *Nature*, **365**, 207–8.
7. Ionov, Y. (1993). Ubiquitous somatic mutations in simple repeated sequences reval a new mechanism for colonic carcinogenesis. *Nature*, **363**, 558–61.
8. Thibodeau, S.N., Bren, G., and Schaid, D. (1993). Microsatellite instability in cancer of proximal colon. *Science*, **260**, 816–18.
9. Strand, M., Prolla, T.A., Liskay, R.M. *et al.* (1993). Destabilization of tracts of simple repetitive DNA in yeast by mutations affecting DNA mismatch repair. *Nature*, **365**, 274–6.
10. Huang, J., Papadopoulos, N., McKinley, A.J. *et al.* (1996). *APC* mutations in colorectal tumors with mismatch repair deficiency. *Proc. Natl Acad. Sci., USA*, **93**, 9049–54.
11. Markowitz, S., Wang, J., Myeroff, L. *et al.* (1995). Inactivation of the type II TGF-β receptor in colon cancer cells with microsatillite instability. *Science*, **268**, 1336–8.
12. Rampino, N., Yamamoto, H., Inonv, Y. *et al.* (1997). Somatic frameshift mutations in the BAX gene in colon cancers of the microsatellite mutator phenotype. *Science*, **275**, 967–9.
13. Fishel, R. and Kolodner, R.D. (1995). Identification of mismatch repair genes and their role in the development of cancer. *Curr. Opin. Genet. Develop.*, **5**, 382–95.
14. Leach, F.S., Nicolaides, N.C., Papadopoulos, N. *et al.* (1993). Mutations of a mutS homolog in hereditary nonpolyposis colorectal cancer. *Cell*, **75**, 1215–25.
15. Papadopoulos, N., Nicolaides, N.C., Wei, Y.-F. *et al.* (1994). Mutation of a mutL homolog in hereditary colon cancer. *Science*, **263**, 1625 9.
16. Nicolaides, N.C., Papadopoulos, N., Liu, B. *et al.* (1994). Mutations of two *PMS* homologues in hereditary nonploypois colon cancer. *Nature*, **371**, 75–80.
17. Han, H.-J., Yanagisawa, A., Kato, Y. *et al.* (1993). Genetic instability in pancreatic cancer and poorly differentiated type of gastric cancer. *Cancer Res.*, **53**, 5087–9.
18. Risinger, J.I., Berchuck, A., Kohler, M.F. *et al.* (1993). Genetic instability of microsatellites in endometrial carcinoma. *Cancer Res.*, **53**, 5100–3.
19. Merlo, A., Mabry, M., Gabrielson, E. *et al.* (1994). Frequent microsatellite instability in primary small cell lung cancer. *Cancer Res.*, **54**, 2098–101.
20. Kat, A., Thilly, W.G., Fang, W.-H. *et al.* (1995). An alkylation-toleration, mutator human cell line is deficient in strand-specific mismatch repair. *Proc. Natl. Acad. Sci., USA*, **90**, 6424–8.
21. Griffin, S., Branch, P., Xu, Y.Z. *et al.* (1994). DNA mismatch binding and incision at modified guanine bases by extracts of mammalian cells: implications for tolerance to DNA methylation damage. *Biochemistry*, **33**, 4787–93.
22. Liu, L., Markowitz, S., and Gerson, S.L. (1996). Mismatch repair mutations override alkyltransferase in conferring resistance to temozolomide but not to 1,3-bis(2-chloroethyl)nitrosourea. *Cancer Res.*, **56**, 5375–9.
23. Fink, D., Nebel, S., Aebi, S. *et al.* (1996). The role of DNA mismatch repair in platinum drug resistance. *Cancer Res.*, **56**, 4881–6.
24. Friedman, H.S., Johnson, S.P., Dong, Q. *et al.* (1997). Methylator resistance mediated by mismatch repair deficiency in a glioblastoma multiforme xenograft. *Cancer Res.*, **57**, 2933–6.
25. Fink, D., Nebel, S., Aebi, S. *et al.* (1997). Loss of DNA mismatch repair due to knockout of MSH2 or PMS2 results in resistance to cisplatin and carboplatin. *Intl J. Oncol.*, **11**, 539–42.
26. Vaisman, A., Varchenko, M., Umar, A. *et al.* (1998). Defects in hMSH6, but not in hMSH3, correlate with increased resistance and enhanced replicative bypass of cisplatin, but not oxaliplatin, adducts. *Cancer Res.*, **39**, 159.
27. Fink, D., Zheng, H., Nebel, S. *et al.* (1997). *In vitro* and *in vivo* resistance to cisplatin in cells that have lost DNA mismatch repair. *Cancer Res.*, **57**, 1841–5.

28. Fink, D., Nebel, S., Norris, P.S. *et al.* (1998). Enrichment of DNA mismatch repair-deficient cells during treatment with cisplatin. *Intl J. Cancer*, **77**, 746.

29. Yarema, K.J., Lippard, S.J., and Essigmann, J.M. (1995). Mutagenic and genotoxic effects of DNA adducts formed by the anticancer drug cis-diamminedichloroplatinum(II). *Nucleic Acids Res.*, **23**, 4066–72.

30. Johnson, N.P., Hoeschele, J.D., Rahn, R.O. *et al.* (1980). Mutagenicity, cytotoxicity, and DNA binding of platinum (II)- chloroammines in Chinese hamster ovary cells. *Cancer Res.*, **40**, 1463–8.

31. Wiencke, J.K., Cervenka, J., and Paulus, H. (1979). Mutagenic activity of anticancer agent cis-dichlorodiammine platinum-II. *Mutat. Res.*, **68**, 69–77.

32. Turnbull, N.C., Popescu, J.A., DiPaolo, J.A. *et al.* (1979). *cis*-platinum (II) diamine dichloride causes mutation, transformation, and sister-chromatid exchanges in cultured mammalian cells. *Mutat. Res.*, **66**, 267–75.

33. Hoffmann, J.S., Pillaire, M.J., Lesca, C. *et al.* (1997). Fork-like DNA templates support bypass replication of lesions that block DNA synthesis on single-stranded templates. *Proc. Natl Acad. Sci., USA*, **93**, 13766–9.

34. Duckett, D.R., Drummond, J.T., Murchie, A.I.H. *et al.* (1996). Human mutSa recognizes damaged DNA base pairs containing O^6-methylguanine, O^4-methylthymine, or the cisplatin- d(GpG) adduct. *Proc. Natl Acad. Sci., USA*, **93**, 6443–7.

35. Yamada, M., O'Regan, E., Brown, R. *et al.* (1997). Selective recognition of a cisplatin-DNA adduct by human mismatch repair proteins. *Nucleic Acids Res.*, **25**, 491–5.

36. Koi, M., Umar, A., Chaudan, D.P. *et al.* (1994). Human chromosome 3 corrects mismatch repair deficiency and microsatellite instability and reduces N-methyl-N'-nitro-N-nitroguanidine tolerance in colon tumor cells with homozygous hMLH1 mutation. *Cancer Res.*, **54**, 4308–12.

37. Umar, A., Koi, M., Risinger, J.I. *et al.* (1997). Correction of hypermutability, N-methyl-N'-nitro-N-nitrosoguanidine-resistance and defective DNA mismatch repair by introducing chromosome 2 into human tumor cells with mutations in MSH2 and MSH6. *Cancer Res.*, **57**, 3949–55.

38. Goldie, J.H. and Coldman, A.J. (1979). A mathematic model for relating the drug sensitivity of tumors to their spontaneous mutation rate. *Cancer Treat. Rep.*, **63**, 1727–33.

39. Fink, D., Nebel, S., Norris, P.A. *et al.* (1998). The effect of different chemotherapeutic agents on the enrichment of DNA mismatch repair-deficient tumor cells. *Br. J. Cancer*, **77**, 703–8.

40. Brown, R., Hirst, G., Gallagher, W.M. *et al.* (1997). hMLH1 expression and cellular responses of ovarian tumour cells to treatment with cytotoxic anticancer agents. *Oncogene*, **15**, 45–52.

41. King, B.L., Carcangiu, M.L., Carter, D. *et al.* (1995). Microsatellite instability in ovarian neoplasms. *Br. J. Cancer*, **72**, 376–82.

42. Fujita, M., Enomoto, T., Yoshino, K. *et al.* (1995). Microsatellite instability and alterations in the hMSH2 gene in human ovarian cancer. *Intl J. Cancer*, **64**, 361–6.

43. Aquilina, G., Ceccotti, S., Martinelli, S. *et al.* (1999). N-(?2-Chloroethyl)-N'-cyclohexyl-N-nitrosourea sensitivity in mismatch repair-defective human cells. *Cancer Res*, **58**, 135–41.

51. Gene therapy and immunomodulation

Rosalind Graham, Michael Smith, Lukas Heukamp, Isabel Correa, Tim Plunkett, Moira Shearer, David Miles, Joy Burchell, and Joyce Taylor-Papadimitriou

Introduction

The idea of recruiting the immune system to reject tumour cells is not new, but has, in recent years, become the focus of attention of many investigators in the field of oncology. This is partly because understanding how the various components of the immune response interact to reject invading pathogens has progressed dramatically. Moreover, tumour-associated antigens have been identified which should allow the recognition of the cancer cells as non-self. However, cancer cells have developed a range of strategies to downregulate the functions of the effector cells of the immune system, so that even if these cells are activated, they may not be effective in the tumour environment. There are therefore two major challenges to be met in order to mobilize the immune system successfully to reject cancer cells, namely:

1. How to mimic the signals that are generated by invading pathogens.
2. How to combat the immunosuppressive effect of the cancer cells.

To discuss the strategies that may be used to meet these challenges, it is appropriate to consider briefly the basic components of the immune response.

Innate and adaptive immunity

In vertebrates there are two major components of the immune system: innate immunity and adaptive immunity.

Innate immunity, where the receptors recognizing pathogens are germ-line coded, is phylogenetically older than adaptive immunity.[1] Many of these receptors recognize carbohydrate-containing molecules, such as the lipopolysaccharides of bacteria or mannans of yeasts. Bacterial DNA is also recognized as foreign through the unmethylated cytosines present.[2] Innate immunity is concerned with the recognition of pathogen-associated molecular patterns (PAMPS).[1]

Adaptive immunity, which relates to the specific responses of the T and B lymphocytes, is mobilized when innate immunity is activated. This is reflected in the use of carbohydrate-containing extracts of bacterial cell walls as adjuvants in vaccines. Unlike the more general recognition of classes of molecules expressed on pathogens seen in innate immunity, the T and B cells can recognize small specific domains of antigens. In the case of T cells, antigen-derived peptides are presented by class I or class II molecules on antigen-presenting cells (APCs) to the T-cell receptor (TCR) on CD8+ and CD4+ T cells, respectively. Signals coming from the innate immune system result in the upregulation of expression of MHC molecules and co-stimulatory molecules such as B7.1 on APCs, thus rendering them functional for antigen presentation (Fig. 51.1).

A common approach to triggering innate immunity is to express, in the cancer cells themselves, genes coding for cytokines, chemokines, co-stimulatory molecules, or specific molecules from pathogens, such as the yeast mannans.[3] This changes the milieu of the tumour environment and may reverse the immunosuppressive effects of the cancer cells. We have used this approach to demonstrate, in a mouse model where the human *MUC1* gene is expressed as a transgene, that rejection of a MUC1-expressing mouse tumour is dramatically enhanced by expression of the B7.1 co-stimulatory molecule.[4] Figure 51.2 illustrates this effect, which is not seen in mice where the CD4+ and CD8+ T cells have been ablated (data not shown). This experiment demonstrates that it is possible to overcome tolerance to a self-antigen without inducing any signs of autoimmunity, and indicates that it should be safe to use MUC1 as an immunogen in patients.

The MUC1 mucin as a tumour-associated antigen

The heavily glycosylated epithelial membrane mucin, MUC1, has great potential as a cancer vaccine, being overexpressed and aberrantly glycosylated in more than 90% of breast and ovarian cancers, as well as in a proportion of other carcinomas.[5] Both humoral[6,7] and cellular[8-10] responses to MUC1 have been found in

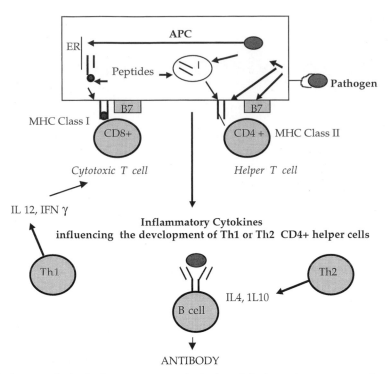

Fig. 51.1 Interaction between the innate and adaptive immune systems. Activation of the innate immune system by a pathogen mobilizes the adaptive immune system.

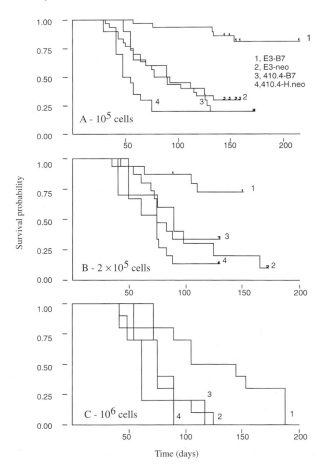

Fig. 51.2 Kaplan–Meier plots, showing survival of MUC1 transgenic mice × Balb/c F₁s after injection with a mouse mammary tumour cell line (410.4 cells) expressing *MUC1* (E3 cells) and B7.1 (E3–B7).

cancer patients, and the antigen has features that suggest that multiple components of the immune system can be activated. Figure 51.3 shows a diagrammatic representation of the mucin structure, which has an extensive extracellular domain made up largely of tandem repeats, each of which contains the sites of glycosylation (serines and threonines).

Classical class I responses

The HLA-A*0201 allele is the most common of the MHC class alleles in Caucasians, and peptide sequences (epitopes) binding to this allele have been identified in the tandem repeat domain of the MUC1 core protein[11,12] and in the flanking sequences[13]. Studies in mice transgenic for the human A*0201 allele, where the peptides identified in the flanking sequence were injected, with a helper epitope and an adjuvant, showed the induction of immune responses which protected mice from MUC1-expressing tumours, confirming that these epitopes can be presented effectively.

Non-MHC responses of cytotoxic T cells (CTLs)

An intriguing observation made by Finn and colleagues was that CTLs can be isolated from breast and ovarian cancer patients which kill MUC1-expressing cells in a non-HLA-restricted fashion.[8,10] This could be an important response, since many of the tumour cells lose expression of MHC class I molecules and thus avoid being killed by classical MHC-restricted CTLs. It has been suggested that sequences within the core protein in the tandem repeat can bind directly to the T-cell receptor, forming multiple weak interactions with the T cell, which result in its activation.

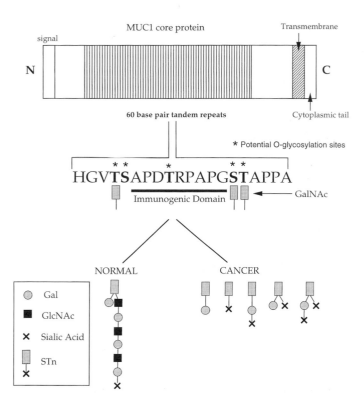

Fig. 51.3 Structure of the MUC1 core protein, illustrating the amino-acid sequence of the tandem repeat domain.

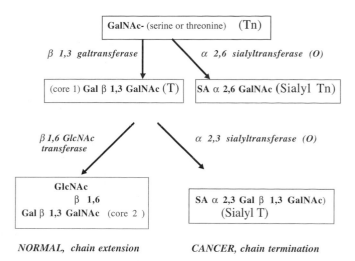

Fig. 51.4 Diagram illustrating the major O-glycosylation pathways in MUC1 expressed by normal epithelia and breast carcinoma.

Responses to the carbohydrate component of MUC1

The change to malignancy in breast cancers is accompanied by changes in the pattern of O-glycosylation of the MUC1 mucin, with the result that the O-glycans added to the serines and threonines in the tandem repeat domain of MUC1 are shorter than those added to the normal mucin. Although a detailed analysis of the O-glycans has not been done for the mucin in ovarian cancers, a similar change in glycosylation pattern is thought to occur. This is supported by the observation that the SM3 antibody, reactive with an epitope in the core protein which is exposed when short O-glycans are added, is indeed selectively exposed in ovarian cancers.[14] In radio-immunoscintigraphy, the SM3 antibody distinguishes between benign and invasive tumours, and is currently being evaluated as a second-stage screen (after CA–125 measurements) for ovarian cancer in well women.[15] Figure 51.4 summarizes diagrammatically the changes in glycosylation occurring in cancer, and it can be seen that the Tn epitope (GalNAc Ser/Thr) and the T epitope (Gal β1,3 GalNAc Ser/Thr) and their sialylated derivatives are present, with the T epitope being dominant.[16] These carbohydrate epitopes expressed on the cancer mucin have the potential to interact with lectins on the effector cells of the immune system, including the C-type lectins and sialoadhesin which are found on macrophages.[17]

To analyse the role of the cancer-associated glycoform of MUC1 in the cellular immune response, a series of glycopeptides based on the MUC1 tandem repeat carrying the T or Tn epitopes have been synthesized. A remarkable observation seen with these gly-copeptides was the induction of a polyclonal stimulation of T-cell responses of the Th1 type (Burchell *et al.* unpublished). The induction of proliferation of the CD4+ T cells depends on both the MUC1 peptide sequence and the composition and site of attachment of the O-glycan.

Preclinical studies with DNA-based immunogens expressing MUC1

The discovery that proteins could be expressed *in vivo* from DNA injected intramuscularly (IM) or intradermally (ID) is of great importance for the development of vaccines. Since both humoral and cellular immune responses are induced by the immunogen expressed from the injected nucleic acid, it means that large quantities of the actual protein or glycoprotein do not have to be produced *in vitro*. An added bonus is that the bacterial DNA is recognized as foreign by the innate immune system and the helper T cells generated in the adaptive immune response are of the Th1 type where the activation of CTL is enhanced.[18] Recombinant viruses expressing the antigen are also being developed. Again, the viral elements can be recognized as foreign and the intracellular processing ensures effective presentation of peptides by class I molecules. Both of these approaches have been shown in mouse models to elicit immune responses to MUC1 which are effective in tumour rejection.[19,20]

Should the plasmid formulation prove to be as effective in patients as the virus, then this would be preferred to the viral formulation as the production costs would be low and problems of handling viruses in the clinic would be avoided. In Fig. 51.5 the effect of three IM injections with plasmid DNA expressing MUC1 on the development of MUC1-expressing tumours is illustrated. Interestingly, although antibodies were induced, the level of induction did not relate to the ability of the mouse to reject the tumour. CTLs were generated, but only after introduction of the tumour cells following the DNA injections.[19]

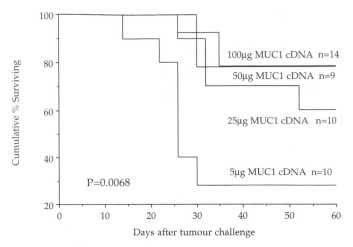

Fig. 51.5 Kaplan-Meier plot, showing survival of C57BlScSn female mice after three intramuscular immunizations with MUC1 cDNA and tumour challenge with MUC1-expressing tumour cells.

Table 51.1 Completed MUC1-based clinical trials

Immunogen	Patients	Reference
20aa MUC1 TR peptide conjugated to diphtheria toxoid	Advanced breast cancer (n = 13)	21
105aa (5 MUC1 TR) mixed with BCG	Advanced adenocarcinoma (n = 63)	22
5 TR conjugated to oxidized mannan	Advanced adenocarcinoma (n = 25)	23
32aa TR-based peptide conjugated to KLH and given with QS-21 adjuvant	Breast cancer (stages I–IV) (n = 10)	24
Recombinant vaccinia virus expressing MUC1 and IL-2	Advanced breast cancer (n = 9)	25
STn conjugated to KLH and given with DETOX adjuvant	Advanced breast cancer (n = 23)	26

aa, amino acids; TR, tandem repeats of MUC1; KLH; keyhole limpet haemocyanin.

Clinical trials with MUC1-based immunogens

Although antibodies to MUC1 have been used widely in the clinic in ovarian cancer patients, studies with the MUC1-based immunogens have been carried out largely with breast cancer patients. This is mainly because it is easier to collect larger numbers of breast cancer patients for these early studies, and companies who have taken out licences for the use of MUC1-based vaccines need to collect data for submission for approval by regulatory bodies. Although the prognosis for breast cancer patients can be much more favourable than that for ovarian cancer patients, ovarian and breast cancer cells have many similarities, including the overexpression of an aberrantly glycosylated form of MUC1. The studies in breast cancer patients which are testing the efficacy of MUC1-based vaccines will, we feel, therefore be useful for applying these formulations to ovarian cancer patients in the future.

Table 51.1 lists the clinical studies that have been, and are being, carried out using MUC1-based antigens. With the exception of the study carried out by ourselves and the Institute Curie in collaboration with TRANSGENE, using a recombinant vaccinia virus, VVMUC1,[25] the studies have focused on using tandem-repeat peptides. They therefore do not take into account either the class I epitopes flanking the tandem repeat, nor the changes in glycosylation, which may be extremely important for recruiting the innate immune response. The studies have, however, provided some data that are useful in planning strategies for applying immunotherapy. Thus the study using a multimer of the tandem repeat sequence given with BCG included analysis of parameters related to the anergic or activated state of T lymphocytes.[22] In this study, it was found that the TCR receptor on T cells showed impaired functionality, but this anergic state slowly reversed with further injections, presumably due to the general adjuvant action of BCG. It is likely that multiple injections of immunogen are required, and some component should be included for reversing the anergy of T cells. This could be done by a variety of materials.

The study by the group of McKenzie,[23] again using a multimer of the tandem repeat domain of MUC1, in this case coupled to mannan, brought home the problems of predicting from the mouse model. The preclinical mouse studies showed that the MUC1–mannan formulation showed efficacy in mice, and that this correlated with a Th1 response, with low antibody production.[27] On the contrary, in patients, the same preparation induced high antibody titres and weak or no CTL.[23]

Although the study using one of the short carbohydrates coupled to keyhole limpet haemocyanin (KLH) is not, strictly speaking, a MUC1-based vaccine, the short side-chains are carried by MUC1 on the cancer mucin. In this study an attempt was made to overcome immune suppression by the tumour by giving low-dose cyclophosphamide before administering the vaccine (Sialyl Tn–KLH) and an adjuvant.[26] Patients receiving cyclophosphamide intravenously had a stronger immune response, as measured by the production of antibodies to sialyl Tn, and the survival of these patients was extended by several months, as compared to the patients with a poor immune response. The company carrying out these studies, BIOMIRA, will now proceed to a randomized trial with 900 patients, giving intravenous cyclophosphamide followed by sialyl Tn coupled to KLH and an adjuvant in the experimental arm. The control arm will receive everything except sialyl Tn, since KLH alone may induce immune responses.

Future studies

DNA-based formulations

While clinical studies have been initiated using a recombinant vaccinia virus expressing MUC1 and interleukin–2 (IL–2), similar studies using plasmid DNA expressing MUC1 have not yet been tested in the clinic. It is envisaged that phase I trials will soon be carried out, with the plasmid DNA given IM or ID using the gene gun.

Combined vaccines

In the development of vaccines for infectious diseases, it has been observed that protocols using combinations of two different formulations of the same antigen have been found to be more effective in mouse models than either formulation used alone. In the case of the gp160 molecule of HIV, this approach has been tested in normal human adults given first a series of injections of recombinant vaccinia virus expressing the glycoprotein, followed by several boosters with the glycoprotein itself. The combination vaccine gave strong, long-lasting humoral and cellular immunity, while each formulation tested alone gave weak and transient responses.[28] This effectiveness of the combined vaccine may reflect the natural events of virus infection where the viral nucleic acid invades the cell. This is followed by the production of viral proteins and glycoproteins.

In addition to combining two formulations of the same antigen, it may be necessary to use more than one antigen to recruit an effective immune response. In this context we have recently identified a candidate antigen, PLU–1, which shows highly restricted expression in normal adult tissues.[29] It is expressed in breast and ovarian cancers. The c-*erbB2* gene, which is overexpressed in 15–30% of breast and ovarian cancers, itself is a candidate target antigen. As with chemotherapy trials, combinations of strategies will almost certainly be necessary.

Concluding remarks

Although it is early days for immunotherapeutic approaches to be included in the standard management of ovarian cancer patients, considerable effort is being applied to how these approaches might be of benefit to patients. A major advantage to the vaccine approach is the apparent lack of serious side-effects of the treatment, the main reaction being the inflammatory response at the injection site. It should be emphasized, however, that this type of therapy is most likely to be effective in patients with a low tumour burden and a functional immune system. However, the classical methods of evaluating whether a treatment may be effective, i.e. complete and partial responses based on measuring tumour size, are not necessarily appropriate, since patients appear to 'live with their tumours', i.e. the disease becomes stable, in some of the current trials. Thus there is a need for the measurement of immune responses in patients to define surrogate endpoints, which, when treatment has advanced to being used in the adjuvant setting, would involve a long time span. Patience and commitment, and collaboration between scientists and clinicians are perhaps the crucial parameters to the successful implementation of the vaccine approach to cancer treatment.

Acknowledgements

Michael Smith is supported by a fellowship provided by the Helene Harris Memorial Trust.

References

1. Medzhitov, R. and Janeway, C.A. Jr (1997). Innate immunity: impact on the adaptive immune response. *Curr. Opin. Immunol.*, **9**, 4–9.
2. Krieg, A.M., Yi, A.K., Matson, S. *et al.* (1995). CpG motifs in bacterial DNA trigger direct B-cell activation. *Nature*, **374**, 546–9.
3. Gilboa, E., Lyerly, H.K., Vieweg, J., and Saito, S. (1994). Immunotherapy of cancer using cytokine gene-modified tumour vaccines. *Semin. Cancer Biol.*, **5**, 409–17.
4. Smith, M., Burchell J.M., Graham R. *et al.* (1999). Expression of B7.1 in a MUC1 expressing mouse mammary epithelial tumour cell line inhibits tumorigenicity but does not induce autoimmunity in MUC1 transgenic mice. *Immunology*, in press.
5. Girling, A., Bartkova, J., Burchell, J. *et al.* (1989). A core protein epitope of the polymorphic epithelial mucin detected by monoclonal antibody SM3 is selectively exposed in a range of primary carcinomas. *Int. J. Cancer*, **43**, 1072–6.
6. Kotera, Y., Fontenot, J.D., Pecher, G. *et al.* (1994). Humoral immunity against a tandem repeat epitope of human mucin MUC1 in sera from breast, pancreatic and colon cancer patients. *Cancer Res.*, **54**, 2856–60.
7. Rughetti, A., Turchi, V., Ghetti, C.A. *et al.* (1993). Human B-cell immune response to the polymorphic epithelial mucin. *Cancer Res.*, **53**, 2457–9.
8. Barnd, D.L., Lan, M.S., Metzgar, R.S., and Finn, O.J. (1989). Specific, major histocompatability complex-unrestricted recognition of tumour-associated mucins by human cytotoxic T cells. *Proc. Natl Acad. Sci., USA*, **86**, 7159–64.
9. Ioannides, C.G., Fisk, B., Jerome, K.R. *et al.* (1993). Cytotoxic T cells from ovarian malignant tumours can recognise polymorphic epithelial mucin core peptides. *J. Immunol.*, **7**, 3693–703.
10. Jerome, K.R., Barnd, D.L., Bendt, K.M. *et al.* (1989) Cytotoxic T-lymphocytes derived from patients with breast adenocarcinoma recognize an epitope present on the protein core of a mucin molecule preferentially expressed by malignant cells. *Cancer Res.*, **51**, 2908–16.
11. Apostolopoulos, V., Haurum, J.S., and McKenzie, I.F. (1997). MUC1 peptide epitopes associated with 5 different H–2 class I molecules. *Eur. J. Immunol.*, **27**, 2579–87.
12. Domenech, N. and Finn, O.J. (1995). In-vitro studies of MHC-restricted recognition of a peptide from the MUC1 tandem repeat domain by CTL. *FASEB J.*, **9**, A1023.
13. Heukamp, L.C., van der Burg, S.H., Drijfhout, J.W., Melief, C.J., Taylor-Papadimitriou, J., and Offringa R. (2001). Identification of three non-VNTR MUC1-derived HLA-A*0201-restricted T-cell epitopes that induce protective anti-tumor immunity in HLA-A2/K(b)-transgenic mice. *Int. J. Cancer*, **91**, 385–92.
14. Van Dam, P.A., Lowe, D.G., Watson, J.V. *et al.* (1991). Multi-parameter flow cytometric quantitation of the expression of the tumour-associated antigen SM3 in normal and neoplastic ovarian tissues. A comparison with HMFG1 and HMFG2. *Cancer*, **68**, 160–77.
15. Granowska, M., Mether, S.J., Jobling, T. *et al.* (1990). Radiolabelled stripped mucin, SM3 monoclonal antibody for immunoscintigraphy of ovarian tumours. *Int. J. Biol. Markers*, **5**, 89–96.
16. Lloyd, K., Burchell, J., Kudryashov, V. *et al.* (1996). Comparison of O-linked carbohydrate chains in MUC1 mucin from normal breast epi-thelial cell lines and breast carcinoma cell lines. *J. Biol. Chem.*, **271**, 33325–34.
17. Nath, D., Hartnell A., Happerfield L. *et al.* (1999). Macrophage–tumour cell interactions: identification of MUC1 on breast cancer cells as a potential counter-receptor for the macrophage restricted receptor, sialoadhesin. *Immunology*, in press.
18. Roman, M., Martin-Orozco, E., Goodman, J.S. *et al.* (1997). Immunostimulatory DNA sequences function as T helper–1 promoting adjuvants. *Nature Med.*, **3**, 849–54.
19. Graham, R.A., Burchell, J.M., Beverley, P., and Taylor-Papadimitriou, J. (1996). Intramuscular immunisation with MUC1 cDNA can protect C57 mice challenged with MUC1-expressing syngeneic mouse tumour cells. *Int. J. Cancer*, **65**, 664–70.

20. Acres, R.B., Hareuveni, M., Balloul, J.-M. and Kieny, M.-P. (1993). Vaccinia virus MUC1 immunisation of mice: immune response and protection against the growth of murine tumours bearing the MUC1 antigen. *J. Immunother.*, **14**, 136–43.

21. Xing, P.-X., Michael, M., Apostolopoulos, V. *et al.* (1995). Phase I study of synthetic MUC1 peptides in breast cancer. *Int. J. Oncol.*, **6**, 1283–9.

22. Goydos, J. S., Elder, E., Whiteside, T.L. *et al.* (1996). A phase I trial of a synthetic mucin peptide vaccine. Induction of specific immune reactivity in patients with adenocarcinoma. *J. Surg. Res.*, **63**, 298–304.

23. Karanikas, V., Hwang, L.A., Pearson, J. *et al.* (1997). Antibody and T cell responses of patients with adenocarcinoma immunized with mannan–MUC1 fusion protein. *J. Clin. Invest.*, **100**, 2783–92.

24. Gilewski, T., Dickler, M., Adluri R. *et al.* (1998). Vaccination of high risk breast cancer patients (PTS) with MUC1 (32aa) keyhole limpet hemocyanin (KLH) conjugate plus QS–21: Preliminary results. *Proc. ASCO*, **17**, 433a, A1670.

25. Scholl S., Acres, B., Kieny, M.P. *et al.* (1997). The polymorphic epithelial mucin (MUC1): A phase I clinical trial testing the tolerance and immunogenicity of a vaccinia virus–MUC1–IL–2 construct in breast cancer. *Breast Cancer Treat. Res.*, **46**, 67 A268.

26. Miles D.W., Towlson K.E., Graham R. *et al.* (1996). A randomised phase II study of sialyl-Tn and DETOX-B adjuvant with or without cyclophosphamide pretreatment for the active specific immunotherapy of breast cancer. *Br. J. Cancer*, **74**, 1292–6.

27. Apostolopoulos, V., Popovski, V., and McKenzie, I. F. (1998). Cyclophosphamide enhances the CTL precursor frequency in mice immunized with MUC1–mannan fusion protein (M–FP). *J. Immunother.*, **21**, 109–13.

28. Cooney, E.L., McElrath, M.J., Corey, L. *et al.* (1993). Enhanced immunity to human immunodeficiency virus (HIV) envelope elicited by a combined vaccine regime consisting of priming with a vaccinia recombinant expressing HIV envelope and boosting with gp160 protein. *Proc. Natl Acad. Sci., USA*, **90**, 1882–6.

29. Lu, P. J., Sundquist, K., Baeckstrom, D. *et al.* (1999). A novel gene (PLU–1) containing highly conserved putative DNA/chromatin binding motifs is specifically up-regulated in breast cancer. *J. Biol. Chem.*, **274**, 15633–45.

52. Preclinical and phase I clinical studies of combinations of chemotherapy with recombinant adenovirus containing full-length, human *p53* tumor suppressor gene cDNA for p53-mutant ovarian cancer

M.D. Pegram, G. Konecny, R. Buller,
I. Runnebaum, D.J. Slamon, L.L. Nielsen,
J. Horowitz, and B.Y. Karlan

Introduction

The *p53* tumor suppressor gene encodes a 393-amino-acid nuclear phosphoprotein transcription factor which binds to sequence-specific DNA elements in the promoter regions of its target genes. These elements are involved in cell-cycle control (P21/WAF1/CIP1), DNA repair pathways (GADD45), and apoptosis (BAX).[1-3] In humans, the *p53* gene spans approximately 20 kilobases of genomic DNA and is assigned to chromosome 17p13.1.[4] In cross-species comparisons, there are five highly conserved regions (>90% sequence homology) within the gene corresponding to the amino-terminal *trans*-activation domain (amino acids 13–23) and the DNA binding domain (amino acids 102–292) of the p53 protein.[4] Expression of *p53* may be induced by a variety of stimuli (ionizing radiation, cytotoxic drugs, mutagens/carcinogens) which result in DNA damage.[5] The mechanism(s) by which p53 'senses' DNA damage are poorly understood, but the fact that the carboxy-terminal region of the p53 protein may bind to DNA ends and excision-repair damage sites, or to internal deletion loops, suggests the possibility of a direct interaction between damaged DNA and the p53 protein, with resulting initiation of p53 activation.[6,7] Activation of p53 results in tetramerization of the protein, which promotes binding of p53 to target gene sequence-specific promoter elements.[8] In epithelial ovarian cancers, mutations of the *p53* gene are the most frequently observed molecular alteration described to date, with mutations detected in 26–79% of all clinical specimens.

In an analysis of 108 consecutive, unselected ovarian cancer samples obtained from the Cedars-Sinai Medical Center, mutations in the *p53* gene were identified in 62 of 108 (57%) tumors, using the technique of complete DNA sequencing of coding exons 2 through 11 (Fig. 52.1).[9] Missense mutations accounted for 40 of 62 (65%) mutations. Mutations were found in codons 51 through 364, with 11 of 62 (18%) mutations occurring outside the 'hotspot' region in ovarian tumors. The majority of these lesions (10 of 11) were deletions, additions, or premature stop codons. The most frequent missense mutations in these ovarian tumors were G/C to A/T and A/T to G/C transitions, occurring predominantly at CpG islands, similar to findings in other studies. Thirty-six per cent (22/62) of the mutations identified were deletions, splice site, or stop codon mutations.[9] However, no mutations were identified that were ovarian cancer-specific.

Sensitivity (decreased cell proliferation/apoptosis) of *p53*-mutant ovarian cancer cells to transfection by wild-type *p53* has been demonstrated using a recombinant, replication-defective (E1a- and E1b-deleted) adenoviral vector in which *p53* expression is driven by a strong (cytomegalovirus; CMV) promoter (rAd p53).[10-12] In these experiments, an otherwise identical adenoviral vector (E1a- and E1b-deleted) lacking *p53* sequence was used as a control, thus demonstrating specificity of the observed antiproliferative effects for *p53*. The antineoplastic activity of rAd p53 against *p53*-mutant or deleted cell lines has been well-studied.[13] Indeed, rAd p53-mediated growth suppression has been demonstrated in a variety of *p53*-altered cell lines, including those

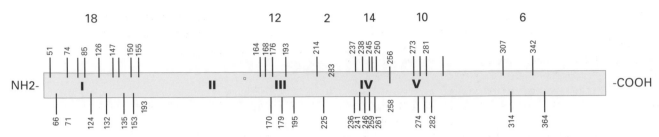

Fig. 52.1 Frequency distribution of point mutations identified in 108 consecutive ovarian cancers by DNA sequence analysis of exons 2–11. Mutations identified, 62/108 (57%); 64% point mutations; 36% frameshift, premature stop codon, or deletions; frequent occurrence of mutations outside the 'hot-spot' region. (From Casey *et al.*, 1996.[9])

of ovarian, breast, colorectal, lung, prostate, and hepatocellular origin.[13] Tumor cell lines with normal *p53*, as well as cultured nonmalignant cells, do not exhibit growth arrest/apoptosis following transfection with rAd p53; thus, the antineoplastic effect of rAd p53 is specific for cells with *p53* gene alteration.

Synergy, as it applies to drug–drug interactions, is defined as a combination of two or more drugs which achieves a therapeutic effect greater than that expected by the simple addition of the effects of the component drugs. Such synergistic interactions between drugs may improve therapeutic results in cancer treatment if the synergism is specific for tumor cells.[14] Moreover, analysis of the nature of the interaction between two drugs (synergism, addition, or antagonism) may yield insight into the biochemical mechanisms of interaction of the drugs. For example, two drugs targeting the same enzyme or biochemical pathway may compete with one another, resulting in an antagonistic interaction, whereas two drugs targeting completely independent pathways may be additive, and one drug which potentiates the action of another may result in therapeutic synergy. In order to characterize the effects of combinations of rAd p53 with cytotoxic chemotherapeutic drugs commonly used in ovarian cancer therapy, we utilized the median-effect/combination-index isobologram method of multiple drug effect analysis. With this methodology, combination index (CI) values are calculated for different dose–effect levels, based on parameters derived from median-effect plots of the chemotherapeutic drugs alone, rAd p53 alone, and the combination of the two at fixed dose ratios. CI values of less than 1 indicate synergy, CI = 1 indicates addition, and CI greater than 1 denotes antagonism.[14] We performed this analysis with rAd p53 in combination with topotecan, liposomal doxorubicin, and gemcitabine *in vitro*. Assays were performed using a cytotoxicity endpoint employing SKOV3 human ovarian cancer cells, which have deletion of both *p53* alleles and are sensitive to rAd p53.

In preclinical *in vivo* experiments using established SKOV3 human ovarian xenografts in SCID mice, intraperitoneal (IP) treatment with a combination of paclitaxel, cisplatin, and rAd p53 resulted in a significant decrease in day 20 tumor burden, compared to chemotherapy alone or vector alone controls (*P* = 0.0006).[12] Using a similar mouse model, we describe here preclinical experiments designed to evaluate potential combinations of the rAd p53 vector with other chemotherapeutic drugs used in the treatment of advanced ovarian cancer.

Despite an excellent initial response to therapy, most individuals diagnosed with advanced-stage ovarian cancer eventually die from the disease. Because this cancer generally remains confined to the peritoneal cavity throughout much of its course, it is an ideal model for the study of gene therapy strategies. Based on preclinical data, we have initiated a phase I clinical trial of intraperitoneal p53 tumor suppressor gene therapy in combination with topotecan, liposomal doxorubicin, or gemcitabine for patients with *p53*-mutant, refractory ovarian cancer. This ongoing trial is designed to measure toxicity, pharmacokinetics (in both ascites and serum), and vector-specific gene transfer in post-treatment clinical tumor material.

Materials and methods

In vitro studies: multiple-drug effect/combination index/isobologram analysis of rAd p53 in combination with chemotherapeutic drugs

Multiple drug effect/combination index analysis allows for quantitative definition of the interaction between any two antineoplastic agents (in this case, rAd p53 and cytotoxic drugs) as either additive, synergistic, or antagonistic.[14] For these experiments, aliquots of SKOV3 (*p53null*) ovarian carcinoma cells were plated in 96-well microdilution plates and treated with experimental media containing either rAd p53 or 'empty' adenoviral vector control. Chemotherapeutic drugs or drug combinations (topotecan, liposomal doxorubicin, and gemcitabine) or vehicle control solution were added to duplicate wells, and serial twofold dilutions were performed to span the dose range suitable for multiple-dose effect analysis (i.e. ~IC_{10}–IC_{90}). The dose ranges for these chemotherapeutic agents had been established previously in independent dose-finding studies in our laboratory.[15,16] Following incubation for 72 hours at 37 °C, plates were washed with phosphate-buffered saline (PBS) and stained with 0.5% *N*-hexamethylpararosaniline in methanol. Sorenson's buffer (0.025 M sodium citrate, 0.025 M citric acid in 50% ethanol) was added to each well, and the plates were analyzed in an ELISA plate reader at 540 nm wavelength. Absorbance at this wavelength correlates with cell survival.[17] Multiple-drug effect/combination index/ isobologram analysis was performed using computer software (Biosoft, Cambridge, England). Details of this methodology have been published previously.[14,18] Briefly, the $\log[(1/f) - 1]$ was plotted against $\log(D)$, where f is the fraction of cells affected by the drug dose, D. From the resulting median effect lines, the x-intercept ($\log EC_{50}$) and slope, m, were calculated for each drug. These parameters were then used to calculate doses of the component drugs (and combinations) required to produce various cytotoxicity levels, according to Equation 52.1. For each level of cytotoxicity, CI values were then calculated according to Equation 52.2, where $(D)_1$ and $(D)_2$ are the concentrations of the combination required to produce survival f, and $(Df)_1$ and $(Df)_2$ are the concentrations of the component drugs required to produce f.

$$\text{Dose I } C_{50}[1-f)/f]_{1/m} \tag{52.1}$$

$$CI=(D)_1/(Df)_1+(D)_2/(Df)_2+\alpha(D)_1)(D)_2/(Df)_1(Df)_2 \tag{52.2}$$

The CIs were calculated based on the conservative assumption of mutually nonexclusive drug interactions ($\alpha= 1$), i.e. cytotoxic drugs have unique mechanisms of action separate from rAd p53. CI values less than 1.0 are defined as synergistic, CI values equal to 1.0 are additive, and CI values greater than 1.0 are antagonistic in this model.[16]

In vivo studies: SCID mouse model of established, p53null (SKOV3) ovarian cancer xenografts

To further expand on the *in vitro* studies, we have established an experimental model of p53-altered ovarian cancer grown in the peritoneal cavity of immunodeficient (SCID) mice. This model was used for the study of rAd p53/chemotherapeutic drug combinations *in vivo*. In these studies, SKOV3 (*p53null*) ovarian cells were grown en masse, using a closed, recirculating, cell-culture system (CoStar, Cell Cube®) which provides O_2/CO_2 gas exchange for growing tumor cells. Following cell harvest and wash steps in serum-free media, cells were injected IP (5×10^6 per animal) into 4–6-week-old female SCID mice. Following tumor cell engraftment (7 days), mice were assigned randomly to treatment groups (6–10 mice/group) consisting of:

(1) control rAd (lacking p53 cDNA, 5×10^9 viral particles $\times$ 8 doses);
(2) rAd p53 vector alone (5×10^9 particles $\times$ 8 doses);
(3) chemotherapeutic drug (topotecan 10 mg/kg IP days 0, 4, and 10; gemcitabine 33.3 mg/kg IP days 0, 2, and 4; or liposomal doxorubicin 3 mg/kg IP day 0) plus control vector; or
(4) chemotherapeutic drug(s) plus rAd p53.

Animals were maintained under aseptic conditions and monitored daily for overall survival, defined as death by any cause; weight loss of 20% of the baseline body mass or more; weight gain of 20% of the body mass or more, secondary to ascites formation; immobility; or palpable tumor mass, 1500 mm³ or more. Survival data were plotted according to the methods of Kaplan and Meier,[19] and statistical tests were applied (Log Rank test) in the analysis of each data set.

Phase I clinical trial of rAd p53 in combination with cytotoxic chemotherapeutic agents with activity against ovarian cancer

Patient selection
The primary objectives of the phase I clinical trial were:

(1) to assess the safety of IP rAd p53 given alone and in combination with chemotherapy to patients with refractory, p53-mutant, advanced ovarian cancer;
(2) to measure vector-specific *p53* transgene expression in tumor tissues following treatment with rAd p53;
(3) to determine the pharmacokinetics of rAd p53 in serum and ascites fluid; and
(4) to document clinical evidence of antitumor efficacy.

Eligibility criteria included: clinical evidence of refractory ovarian carcinoma with peritoneal carcinomatosis and p53 mutation determined by IHC; free flow of radio-contrast material throughout the peritoneal cavity to assure even distribution of rAd p53 vector solutions; life expectancy of 3 months or more; preserved Karnofsky performance status; adequate end-organ function; seropositivity for type 5 adenovirus at baseline; and ability and willingness to understand and sign an IRB-approved informed consent document. Major exclusion criteria included: pregnancy or lactation; serious infection, including HIV; immunosuppressive therapy within the past 3 months (excluding chemotherapy or steroids as antiemetic therapy); and prior intraperitoneal therapy within the past 3 months.

Treatment plan
Following pretreatment with acetaminophen (650 mg orally) and metoclopromide (20 mg intravenously), rAd p53 was administered over 30 minutes via a peritoneal catheter. Intravenous chemotherapy dosing regimens were liposomal doxorubicin (50 mg/m²) and topotecan (1.5 mg/m²/day $\times$ 5 days). Chemotherapy was initiated on treatment cycle 2 following one cycle of rAd p53 alone. For each of the two chemotherapy drugs, dosing of rAd p53 was 2.5×10^{13} particles/dose $\times$ 3 days for the first three patients and 7.5×10^{13} particles/dose $\times$ 5 days for the next three patients if the combination was tolerated at the lower dose level. Dose-limiting toxicity (DLT) was defined as treatment-related death, any grade IV toxicity, or grade III toxicity lasting 1 week or longer. The maximum tolerated dose was defined as one dose level below the DLT, or 7.5×10^{13} particles/dose if DLT was not encountered. Treatment cycles were repeated at 21–28 day intervals. Patients with stable or responsive disease after cycle 3 continued treatment for a maximum of six cycles. Patients underwent clinical examinations/assessments weekly for the duration of treatment, and were followed at 1–3-month intervals thereafter.

Study endpoints
For detection of gene transfer, RNA extracted from tumor material derived from malignant ascites or from tumor biopsy specimens was analyzed for rAd p53 vector-specific transgene expression by reverse transcriptase polymerase chain reaction

(RT-PCR). Results were reported as positive or negative relative to expression of a control gene (β-actin). A two-antibody 'sandwich' ELISA assay[20] was used for detection of shed adenovirus in urine and stool samples collected pre-treatment and for 3 days post-treatment of cycle 1. If there was no evidence of viral shedding on cycle 1, the assay was not repeated on subsequent cycles. For patients with measurable disease at baseline, standard objective clinical response criteria (complete response defined as disappearance of all measurable disease with normal CA–125 level, partial response defined as 50% or greater reduction in tumor area, and disease progression defined as 25% or greater increase in tumor area) were used. CA–125 levels were measured pre-treatment and on day 28 of each treatment cycle. Clinical adverse events were defined according to the WHO grading system. Toxicity was further classified by the investigator as unrelated, possibly, probably, or definitely related to rAd p53 treatment.

Results and discussion

Multiple drug effect analysis of rAd p53 in combination with cytotoxic chemotherapy drugs on SKOV3 ovarian carcinoma cells in vitro

To extend the preclinical observation of synergy of rAd p53 in combination with cisplatin and paclitaxel,[12] rAd p53 was analyzed in combination with topotecan, liposomal doxorubicin, or gemcitabine. Dose–response curves were constructed for each drug alone, rAd p53 alone, and the combinations at fixed ratios defined by the ratio of the two agents at their maximally effective dose. In this analysis (Table 52.1), D_m is the dose required to produce the median effect (analogous to the IC_{50}), and m is the Hill coefficient used to determine whether the dose–effect relationships follow sigmoidal dose–response curves.[21] Linear regression correlation coefficients (r-values) of the median effect plots reflect that the dose–effect relationships for rAd p53, topotecan, liposomal doxorubicin, gemcitabine, and the combinations, conform to the principle of mass action (in general, r-values >0.9 confirm the validity of this methodology).[14] CI values for the combinations of rAd p53 with each of these cytotoxic drugs were significantly less than 1.0, indicating a synergistic interaction for all three drugs (Table 52.1). These results suggest that the cytotoxic activity of these drugs against SKOV3 cells is, at least in part, dependent on p53 expression. This is not surprising in light of the fact that DNA-damaging agents are known to be a potent stimulus for p53 activity, resulting in either cell cycle arrest and DNA repair, or induction of apoptosis if repair is not possible. Therefore transduction of wild-type p53 into a p53-mutant or p53-null cell might be expected to increase p53-dependent apoptotic response to chemotherapy-induced DNA damage. Another possible mechanism of synergy between rAd p53 and chemotherapy might be modulation of adenovirus infectivity of tumor cells following exposure to these drugs. Such an effect was described previously as a possible explanation for the synergistic interaction between paclitaxel and rAd p53, where pretreatment with paclitaxel increased the efficiency of adenovirus infection of tumor target cells.[10] It is also possible that adenovirus infection *per se* could influence intracellular pharmacology and/or metabolism of chemotherapeutic agents. The lack of synergy between chemotherapeutic drugs and an empty control vector argue against this explanation as an important mechanism of adenovirus/drug interaction.

Combination rAd p53 plus chemotherapy prolongs survival of SCID mice bearing SKOV3 (p53null) human ovarian carcinoma xenografts

To further evaluate the potential therapeutic effects of rAd p53/chemotherapy combinations and to extend our observations beyond a single *in vitro* preclinical model, a series of *in vivo* studies were performed using human ovarian cancer xenografts in SCID mice. Intraperitoneal engraftment of SKOV3 cells results in peritoneal carcinomatosis closely mimicking human ovarian carcinoma. Groups of 6–7 mice harboring SKOV3 xenografts were randomized to intraperitoneal treatment with:

(1) rAd p53 alone;
(2) rAd control vector devoid of *p53* sequence at an identical dose;
(3) rAd control + topotecan, gemcitabine, or liposomal doxorubicin; and
(4) rAd p53 + topotecan, gemcitabine, or liposomal doxorubicin.

All of the doses and dose intervals for the various cytotoxic drugs were based on independent dose-finding experiments for this specific strain, age, weight, and sex of SCID mouse. The cytotoxic drug doses used were at or near the maximum tolerated doses previously reported in the literature.[22–25] In these experiments, treatment with rAd p53 alone did not result in improved survival compared to rAd control vector alone ($P = 0.29$) (Figs 52.2, 52.3, and 52.4). Treatment with either topotecan + control vector, or gemcitabine + control vector resulted in significant prolongation of survival, compared to either of the vector-alone control groups ($P = 0.0002$) (Figs 52.2 and 52.3). In contrast, treatment with liposomal doxorubicin + control vector did not result in prolongation of survival, indicating relative resistance of this xenograft model

Table 52.1 Calculated values for the combination index: fractional inhibition of SKOV3 cell proliferation by a mixture of chemotherapy and rAd p53

Drug	Combination index values at:			Parameters		
	ED_{50}	ED_{75}	ED_{90}	D_m	m	r
Topotecan + rAd p53	0.93	0.78	0.68	1.10×10^5	1.60	0.94
Gemcitabine + rAd p53	0.77	0.54	0.39	7.41×10^4	1.44	0.927
Liposomal doxorubicin + rAd p53	0.61	0.43	0.50	1.22×10^6	0.86	0.98
Combined effect Synergy						

D_m is the dose of the combination (picomolar units) to achieve the median effect.

m is the slope of the median effects lines (values > 1 denote sigmoidal, and <1 inverse sigmoidal dose–effet relationships).

r is the linear correlation coefficient that determines applicability of the data to the method of analysis (should approach 1.0).

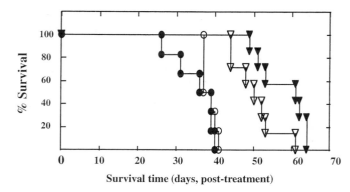

Fig. 52.2 Survival of SCID mice bearing SKOV3 xenografts following treatment with: rAd control (open circle), rAd p53 (closed circle), topotecan + rAd control (open triangle), or topotecan + rAd p53 (closed triangle).

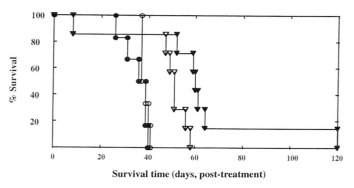

Fig. 52.3 Survival of SCID mice bearing SKOV3 xenografts following treatment with: rAd control (open circle), rAd p53 (closed circle), gemcitabine + rAd control (open triangle), or gemcitabine + rAd p53 (closed triangle).

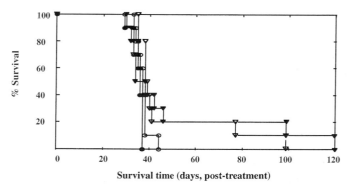

Fig. 52.4 Survival of SCID mice bearing SKOV3 xenografts following treatment with: rAd control (open circle), rAd p53 (closed circle), doxil + rAd control (open triangle), or doxil + rAd p53 (closed triangle).

to liposomal doxorubicin at the dose tested (Fig. 52.4). Combination treatment with rAd p53 + topotecan (Fig. 52.2) or rAd p53 + gemcitabine (Fig. 52.3) resulted in prolonged survival compared to the same chemotherapy treatment with control vector ($P < 0.047$). However, combination treatment with rAd p53 + liposomal doxorubicin did not significantly prolong survival

compared to either vector-alone controls, or liposomal doxorubicin + control vector ($P = NS$). These results demonstrate that the observed synergistic effects of rAd p53 in combination with topotecan and gemcitabine *in vitro* were of sufficient magnitude to translate into a survival benefit *in vivo* with these same drug/rAd p53 combinations. Furthermore, the use of a control vector devoid of *p53* sequence underscores that the improved survival was specific for rAd p53. This is in spite of the fact that we were not able to demonstrate a survival advantage for treatment with rAd p53 alone, compared to control vector alone, in these experiments. This may be due to the lower dose of rAd p53 used in these experiments as compared to previously reported results,[10,11] and the fact that the sample sizes may have been insufficient to detect a therapeutic advantage for rAd p53 alone. We were not able to confirm therapeutic synergy between liposomal doxorubicin and rAd p53 in the *in vivo* model. Notable in this experiment is the lack of activity of liposomal doxorubicin + control vector compared to vector alone at the doses tested. It is possible that higher doses of liposomal doxorubicin may be required for efficacy in the SKOV3 xenograft model.

Preliminary analysis of a phase I clinical trial of rAd p53 in combination with topotecan or liposomal doxorubicin

Characteristics of patients currently enrolled in the phase I study are shown in Table 52.2. The cohort ($N – 12$) currently consists of patients with relapsed ovarian cancer with evidence of *p53* gene mutation, demonstrated by detection of aberrant nuclear accumulation of mutant p53 protein using immunohistochemical staining techniques. The cohort was heavily pre-treated with a median number of 12 cycles of chemotherapy prior to study entry. Time from diagnosis to study entry ranged from 9 to 28 months. Six patients received topotecan + rAd p53 and six patients were treated with rAd p53 in combination with liposomal doxorubicin. Two different dose levels of rAd p53 were tested ($N = 3$ patients per dose level for each of the two drugs). Adenovirus was undetectable by ELISA in the urine or stool of patients following treatment with intraperitoneal rAd p53, suggesting that the vector remains confined to the peritoneal cavity following intraperitoneal treatment and does not pose a significant biohazard to medical personnel coming into contact with these patients.

Vector-specific transgene expression data is available from seven patients who had post-treatment tumor biopsies, or had tumor cells collected from cytospins of malignant ascites. All seven

Table 52.2 Patient characteristics

- *p53*-mutant, relapsed ovarian cancer
- Age range = 49–70 years
- KPS = 90–100
- Prior surgery: Primary tumor debulking with TAH/BSO
- Prior chemotherapy: median 12 cycles, range 6–15 cycles
- Median time from diagnosis to study entry:
23 months (range 9–28 months)

KPS,; TAH/BSO.

patients had evidence of transgene expression by RT-PCR. A majority of patients tested for transgene expression (six of seven) were treated at the lower dose of rAd p53. The high percentage of PCR-positive cases at these dose levels confirms observations made in our previous phase I clinical trial of rAd p53 as a single agent or in combination with paclitaxel + carboplatin, where transgene expression was frequently detectable at these dose levels.[26] It is important to note that tumor biopsy specimens (and ascites cytospins) are not pure populations of tumor cells. They contain variable percentages of normal stromal, vascular, and hematopoetic cell elements; thus it is possible that transduction of these nonmalignant cells could contribute, at least in part, to the positive RT-PCR results. It is interesting to note that three of the seven tumor samples were collected following the second and third cycle of rAd p53/chemotherapy treatment. This suggests that transgene expression *in vivo* is possible despite the anti-adenovirus immune responses seen uniformly following the first treatment cycle in these patients.

Clinical adverse event data are currently available on nine patients (Table 52.3). The most frequently encountered grade I/II toxicities included fever and/or chills, gastrointestinal toxicity (nausea/vomiting), and symptoms of abdominal pain, discomfort, or distention. The most frequent grade III toxicity noted was fatigue and/or malaise, which was observed in approximately half of the patients. Two grade IV adverse events (bowel obstruction necessitating surgical intervention) were noted, both at the highest dose level. One occurred in a patient treated with topotecan, and one in a patient enrolled on the liposomal doxorubicin arm. In both cases, small bowel obstruction was temporally associated

Table 52.3 Chemotherapy + gene therapy adverse events (first nine patients)

	WHO Grade:			
	1	2	3	4
Abdominal symptoms: (pain, distention, cramps)	5	3	1	0
Fever/chills	1	7	0	0
Fatigue/malaise	2	2	4	0
Nausea/vomiting/diarrhea	4	4	0	0
Small bowel obstruction	0	0	0	2

Table 52.4 Clinical response data: rAd p53 + topotecan

Patient	Dose level	CA125 screen	C1	C2	Objective response
039	2.5×10^{13}	5	5	4	SD (C6)
043	2.5×10^{13}	915	933	–	PD (C2)
044	2.5×10^{13}	14	17	8	SD (C6)
046	7.5×10^{13}	29	54	65	PD (C3)
047	7.5×10^{13}	92	46	95	SD (C3)
048	7.5×10^{13}	N/A	N/A	N/A	SD (C5)

C, cycle; PD, progressive disease; SD, stable disease, N/A, not available.

Table 52.5 Clinical response data: rAd p53 + doxil

Patient	Dose level	CA125 screen	C1	C2	Objective response
037	2.5×10^{13}	411	284	47	PD (C3)
038	2.5×10^{13}	690	1700	2060	PD (C3)
040	2.5×10^{13}	411	284	263	PR (C3)
041	7.5×10^{13}	609	ND	1190	PD (C3)
305	7.5×10^{13}	1926	–	–	PD (C2)
045	7.5×10^{13}	318	325	261	SD (C3)

C, cycle; PD, progressive disease; SD, stable disease; PR, ; ND, not determined.

with recent rAd p53 administration. Both occurred following treatment cycle 3. In both cases, dense adhesions were noted at operation, along with signs of peritoneal inflammation and exudative peritoneal fluid. In one case the adhesions and bowel obstruction occurred at the site of prior peritoneal catheter placement. It was difficult to discern whether there was a direct causal relationship between bowel obstruction and administration of rAd p53, since bowel obstruction is not an infrequent complication of underlying ovarian cancer, or adhesions from prior surgical procedures and peritoneal catheter placement. Neither of these patients had evidence of disease recurrence or progression at the time of surgery that could account for bowel obstruction.

Limited clinical response data are currently available from this cohort (Tables 52.4 and 52.5). An initial decrease in serum CA–125 was noted in three patients treated with rAd p53 + liposomal doxorubicin, and one of these patients had an objective partial response. One patient treated with rAd p53 + topotecan had a decrease in CA–125 and four patients had stable clinical responses, including three patients treated for at least five cycles. Three of the four cases with decreased CA–125 had decreases noted following the first treatment cycle in which rAd p53 was administered as a single agent, suggesting that rAd p53, even in the absence of chemotherapy, may decrease serum CA–125 levels. Pharmacokinetic data from this study are currently being analyzed and the results are forthcoming.

In summary, the available preclinical data suggest therapeutic synergy between rAd p53 and multiple cytotoxic chemotherapeutic agents used for the treatment of ovarian cancer. We have been able to document evidence of vector-encoded transcript expression *in vivo* in tumor specimens, following rAd p53 treatment using a sensitive RT-PCR assay. The toxicology of rAd p53 in combination with topotecan or liposomal doxorubicin is being further characterized. Clinical responses in terms of decreases in serum CA–125 levels or partial clinical response have been observed in this heavily pretreated patient population, including some CA–125 declines that are independent of any chemotherapy effects. A prospective, randomized clinical trial comparing chemotherapy alone versus chemotherapy plus rAd p53 for patients with *p53*-mutant ovarian cancer is currently under way and should help to define the potential future role for adding *p53* gene therapy to conventional surgery and chemotherapy for this disease.

References

1 el-Deiry, W.S., Tokino, T., Velculescu, V.E. *et al.* (1993). WAF1, a potential mediator of p53 tumor suppression. *Cell*, 75, 817–25.

2 Smith, M.L., Chen, I.T., Zhan, Q. *et al.* (1994). Interaction of the p53-regulated protein Gadd45 with proliferating cell nuclear antigen. *Science*, 266, 1376–80.

3 Miyashita, T. and Reed, J.C. (1995). Tumor suppressor p53 is a direct transcriptional activator of the human bax gene. *Cell*, 80, 293–9.

4 Soussi, T. and May, P. (1996). Structural aspects of the p53 protein in relation to gene evolution: a second look. *J. Mol. Bio.*, 260, 623–37.

5 Kastan, M.B., Onyekwere, O., Sidransky, D. *et al.* (1991). Participation of p53 protein in the cellular response to DNA damage. *Cancer Res.*, 51, 6304–11.

6 Jayaraman, J. and Prives, C. (1995). Activation of p53 sequence-specific DNA binding by short single strands of DNA requires the p53 C-terminus. *Cell*, 81, 1021–9.

7 Lee, S., Elenbaas, B., Levine, A., and Griffith, J. (1995). p53 and its 14 kDa C-terminal domain recognize primary DNA damage in the form of insertion/deletion mismatches. *Cell*, 81, 1013–20.

8 Cho, Y., Gorina, S., Jeffrey, P.D., and Pavletich, N.P. (1994). Crystal structure of a p53 tumor suppressor–DNA complex: understanding tumorigenic mutations. *Science*, 265, 346–55.

9 Casey, G., Lopez, M.E., Ramos, J.C. *et al.* (1996). DNA sequence analysis of exons 2 through 11 and immunohistochemical staining are required to detect all known p53 alterations in human malignancies. *Oncogene*, 13, 1971–81.

10. Nielsen, L.L., Lipari, P., Dell, J. *et al.* (1998). Adenovirus-mediated p53 gene therapy and paclitaxel have synergistic efficacy in models of human head and neck, ovarian, prostate, and breast cancer. *Clin. Cancer Res.*, 4, 835.

11. Nielsen, L.L., Gurnani, M., Syed, J. *et al.* (1998). Recombinant E1-deleted adenovirus-mediated gene therapy for cancer: efficacy studies with p53 tumor suppressor gene and liver histology in tumor xenograft models. *Human Gene Ther.*, 9, 681–94.

12. Gurnani, M., Lipari, P., Dell, J. *et al.* (1999). Adenovirus-mediated p53 gene therapy has greater efficacy when combined with chemotherapy against human head and neck, ovarian, prostate, and breast cancer. *Cancer Chemother. Pharmacol*, in press.

13. Nielsen, L.L. and Maneval, D.C. (1998). p53 tumor suppressor gene therapy for cancer. *Cancer Gene Ther.*, 5, 52–63.

14. Chou, T.C. and Talalay, P. (1984). Quantitation analysis of dose–effect relationships: the combined effects of multiple drugs or enzyme inhibitors. *Adv. Enz. Regu.*, 22, 27–55.

15. Pegram, M.D., Finn, R.S., Arzoo, K. *et al.* (1997). The effect of HER–2/neu overexpression on chemotherapeutic drug sensitivity in human breast and ovarian cancer cells. *Oncogene*, 15, 537–47.

16. Pegram, M.D., Hsu, S., Pietras, R.J. *et al.* (1999). Inhibitory effects of combinations of HER–2/neu antibody and chemotherapeutic agents used for treatment of human breast cancers. *Oncogene*, 18, 2241–51.

17. Gilles *et al.* (1986).

18. Bible, K.C. and Kaufmann, S.H. (1997). Cytotoxic synergy between flavopiridol (NSC 649890, L86–8275) and various antineoplastic agents: the importance of sequence of administration. *Cancer Res.*, 57, 3375–80.

19. Kaplan, E.L. and Meier, P. (1958). Nonparametric estimation from incomplete observations. *J. Am. Sts Assoc.*, 53, 457–816.

20. Cepko, C.L., Whetstone, C.A., and Sharp, P.A. (1983). Adenovirus monoclonal antibody that is group specific and potentially useful as a diagnostic reagent. *J. Clin. Microbio.*, 17, 360–4.

21. Hill, A.V. (1913). *Biochem. J.*, 7, 471–80.

22. Giovanella, B.C., Stehoin, J.S., and Shepard, R.C. (1977). *Proceedings of the Second International Workshop on Nude Mice*, (ed. T. Nomura, N. Ohsawa, N. Tamaoki, and K. Fujiwara), pp. 475–81. University of Tokyo Press.

23. Boven, E., Schipper, H., Erkelens, C.A.M. *et al.* (1993). The influence of the schedule and the dose of gemcitabine on the anti-tumor efficacy in experimental human cancer. *Br. J. Cancer*, 68, 52–6.

24. Boven and Winograd (ed.) (1991). *The nude mouse in oncologic research*. CRC Press, Boca Raton, FL.

25. Williams, S.S., Thomas, R.A., Mayhew, E. *et al.* (1993). Arrest of human lung tumor xenograft growth in severe combined immunodeficient mice using doxorubicin encapsulated in sterically stabilized liposomes. *Cancer Res.*, 53, 3964–7.

26. Buller, R.E., Pegram, M.D., Runnebaum, I. *et al.* (1998). A phase I study of gene therapy with recombinant intraperitoneal p53 in recurrent ovarian cancer. *Proceedings of the International Conference on Gene Therapy*.

53. Paclitaxel resistance in human ovarian cancer: role of apoptosis-related proteins *in vivo*

Stephen R.D. Johnston, Mansour S. Al-Moundhri, Lloyd R. Kelland, and Martin E. Gore

Introduction

Resistance to chemotherapy in ovarian cancer is a persistent clinical problem. Cisplatin and paclitaxel, the most active cytotoxic drugs against ovarian cancer, have different cellular targets, and the combination of a DNA-damaging agent together with a microtubulin-targetted drug may overcome clinical resistance to either drug alone. This may account, in part, for the improved survival advantage observed in two large phase III trials for platinum–paclitaxel chemotherapy over previous platinum-based chemotherapy regimens.[1,2] While the introduction of paclitaxel has significantly improved first-line chemotherapy for ovarian cancer, not all patients respond, as some tumours may possess innate resistance to the drug. Likewise, many patients will relapse following paclitaxel, having developed acquired resistance to the drug. Understanding the molecular pathways of response and resistance to paclitaxel has become an area of intense research.

At a cellular level, known mechanisms of resistance to paclitaxel include altered drug uptake due to overexpression of P-glycoprotein[3] and changes in microtubulin structure, resulting in either reduced drug-binding affinity or decreased intracellular levels of polymerized tubulin.[4,5] With the demonstration that most chemotherapeutic agents induce programmed cell death or apoptosis,[6] several *in vitro* studies have demonstrated that modulation of apoptosis-regulating proteins, such as the Bcl–2-related family of proteins, may induce chemoresistance to paclitaxel.[7,8] Despite these studies, evidence that modulation in expression of these proteins accounts for acquired resistance to paclitaxel *in vivo* remains limited.

We established an *in vivo* human ovarian cancer model using subcutaneous paclitaxel-sensitive (CH1/TS) and acquired-resistant (CH1/TR) xenografts. Our previous studies had shown that both cell lines contained wild-type p53 and did not overexpress P-glycoprotein, thus excluding mutant p53 or a multidrug-resistant phenotype as mechanisms for resistance.[9,10] Furthermore the CH1/TR cells retained partial sensitivity to cisplatin *in vitro*,

implying specific acquired resistance to paclitaxel. We examined the dynamic changes in cell cycle, proliferation, apoptosis, p53/p21 induction, together with expression of Bax, Bcl–2, Bcl-X_L, and Raf–1 following treatment with paclitaxel, with the specific aim of identifying any alterations in apoptosis-regulating proteins that may occur with acquired paclitaxel resistance. In subsequent experiments, we transfected CH1 paclitaxel-sensitive cells with the anti-apoptotic protein Bcl-X_L, to determine whether overexpression of this particular protein would induce resistance to paclitaxel *in vivo*.

Materials and methods

CH1 and CH1/TR cell lines for establishment of xenografts

The CH1 ovarian carcinoma cell line was derived from a moderately differentiated human ovarian carcinoma,[11] which has been shown previously to be relatively sensitive to both cisplatin and paclitaxel. The paclitaxel-resistant subline of CH1 (CH1/TR) was generated by continuous exposure to paclitaxel at escalating concentrations up to 20 nM. The 96-hour IC_{50}s of CH1 and CH1/TR to paclitaxel were 0.66 nM, and 7.93 nM, respectively, making the CH1/TR cell line twelvefold resistant to paclitaxel compared to the parent cell line.[10]

Xenograft growth experiment

A total of 60 CH1/TS and CH1/TR xenografts were established for tumour-growth studies to confirm the sensitivity and resistance to both paclitaxel and cisplatin *in vivo*. Once the tumour diameter size reached approximately 8 mm, the mice were randomized into three groups. Group A (control) received no treatment. Group B received 25 mg/kg paclitaxel by intraperitoneal (IP) injection (0.2 ml) on days 0, 4, and 8. The drug was dissolved in a vehicle containing 50% polyoxyethylated castor oil (Cremophor EL) and 50% ethanol, and further diluted in 5% glucose in water. Group C received 4 mg/kg IP cisplatin dissolved in 0.9% NaCl on days 0, 4, and 8. The tumours were measured once per week in two dimensions (length and width) using calipers. The tumour volume was calculated using formula Tv = $a \times b^2 \times \pi/6$, where a was the length measurement of longest axis, and b the width perpendicular to the length. The growth experiment was continued until either of the following endpoints was reached: tumour size greater than 20 mm in diameter, or 60 days post-treatment.

Intratumoral paclitaxel concentrations

Three tumours per time point were harvested from athymic nude mice bearing CH1/TS, and CH1/TR xenografts at 1, 3, 6, and 24 hours following administration of 25 mg/kg IP paclitaxel. Intratumoral levels of paclitaxel and pharmacokinetic parameters were measured in CH1/TS and CH1/TR xenografts by high-performance liquid chromatography (HPLC). Concentration–time curves were plotted using mean concentration of paclitaxel per time point for each tumour type.

Paclitaxel-induced pharmacodynamics

A separate group of 42 athymic nude bearing established CH1/TS tumours, together with 42 athymic nude mice bearing CH1/TR tumours, were randomized into three groups. Both CH1/TS and CH1/TR tumour-bearing mice were treated as follows:

- Group A: six mice received no treatment and were sacrificed at 24 h after start of experiment (control group);
- Group B: 18 mice received paclitaxel 25 mg/kg IP and were sacrificed in groups of six mice at 24, 48, and 72 h after treatment;
- Group C: 18 mice received cisplatin 4 mg/kg IP and were sacrificed in groups of six mice at 24, 48, and 72 h after treatment.

All mice were injected with 100 mg/kg of bromodeoxyuridine (BrdUrd) made up in 0.9% NaCl saline (10 mg/ml) 5 hours before harvesting of tumours, to facilitate the cell cycle kinetics by flow cytometry. Subsequently, the tumours were harvested and divided equally for flow cytometry (cell-cycle analysis and labelling index (LI) by BrdUrd incorporation), apoptosis (paraffin-embedded tissue for TUNEL assay), and protein extraction for Western blotting.

Flow cytometry and labelling index

Freshly prepared nuclei, which had been extracted from tumour samples, were pelleted by centrifugation at 500 g for 5 minutes and resuspended in 1 ml of 2 M HCl. After incubation at room temperature for 30 minutes the nuclei were washed twice with phosphate-buffered saline (PBS), resuspended in labelling solution, containing 1 ml of 0.5% Tween 20/1% BSA/PBS and 20 μl of anti-BrdUrd FITC-conjugated monoclonal antibody (Becton–Dickinson, UK), and incubated for 30 minutes. The suspension

was washed twice in 1 ml 0.5% Tween 20/1% BSA/PBS and resuspended in 1 ml of PBS containing 20 μg/ml propidium iodode and 100 μg/ml RNAase. Flow cytometric measurements were made on a Coulter EPICS Elite ESP (Beckman Coulter, High Wycombe, UK) using a Spectra-Physics argon-ion laser according to previously published methodology.[12] The labelling index was expressed as the percentage of tumour cells that had taken up BrdUrd.

TUNEL assay for apoptosis

From harvested tumours which had been fixed in 10% neutral buffered formalin and embedded in paraffin wax, 3 μm sections were cut onto slides coated with 3-aminopropyltriethoxysilane. The TUNEL assay was performed according to our previously published methodology for examining human tumour xenografts in mice.[13] A total of 3000 cells were counted randomly and percentage of positively labelled cells was determined to obtain the apoptotic index (AI).

Western blotting for p53/p21 and Bcl–2-related proteins

Equal amounts of protein (40 μg) were loaded onto 8–16% polyacrylamide gels, which were run under a constant current of 30 mA. Following separation of proteins, they were transferred onto nitrocellulose filters, washed with PBS containing 0.1% Tween 20 (PBST), and incubated overnight with primary antibody. All primary antibodies were polyclonal rabbit antisera (Santa Cruz Biotechnology, US) used at either 1 : 1000 dilution (Bcl–2) or 1 : 500 dilution (Bax, Bcl-X_L, p21, Raf–1), except for p53, which was the mouse monclonal antibody, DO1, used at 1 : 500 dilution. The filters were exposed to the appropriate horseradish peroxidase-labelled secondary antibody for 1 hour. Proteins were detected by enhanced chemiluminescence (ECL) with image quantification of protein bands (Molecular Dynamics). The band-density values were expressed as ratio folds increase or decrease from the respective control, untreated tumours.

Bcl-X_L transfected CH1 xenograft growth

CH1 tumour cells were transfected with Bcl-X_L using the bicistronic plasmid vector pIRES-P.[14] This vector expresses a single bicistronic mRNA driven from the human cytomegalovirus immediate early enhancer/promoter, and uses the internal ribosome entry site from encephalomyocarditis virus to direct translation of the downstream *pac* gene encoding for puromycin acetyl transferase. Xenografts of CH1 cells transfected with *bcl-xl* (CH1/bcl-xl) or with vector only (CH1/F 280) were established as above. The level of expression of Bcl-X_L protein in CH1/bcl-xl xenografts was assessed by Western blotting and expressed as fold increase from CH1/TS tumours. Subsequently, 105 athymic nude mice were divided into three equal groups and implanted with either CH1/TS, CH1/bcl-xl, or CH1/F 280 tumours, and tumour growth studies were repeated following treatment with paclitaxel or cisplatin on days 0, 4, and 8.

Results

Growth studies

The average growth rates of CH1/TS and CH1/TR tumours following paclitaxel (25 mg/kg) and cisplatin (4 mg/kg) treatment on days 0, 4, and 8 are shown in Fig. 53.1. Following either paclitaxel or cisplatin, established CH1/TS tumours demonstrated sensitivity to both drugs. The doubling time of untreated control CH1/TS tumours was 2.9 days with a growth delay of paclitaxel or cisplatin treated CH1/TS tumours of more than 60 days (Fig. 53.1a). In contrast, the CH1/TR tumours were resistant to paclitaxel, with no responses seen in any tumour, while cisplatin induced partial responses in all tumours (Fig. 53.1b). The doubling time of control, untreated CH1/TR tumours was 3 days and the growth delay of paclitaxel-treated CH1/TR tumours was only 8.7 days. In contrast, following cisplatin there was a growth delay of 32.4 days.

Paclitaxel-uptake studies

There was no significant difference in intratumoral concentration of paclitaxel between CH1/TS and CH1/TR tumours at 1, 3, 6, and

Table 53.1 The mean percentage values and standard error of the mean (SEM) of cell cycle G_2/M- and S-phases, and labelling index (LI) of CH1/TS tumours following treatment with paclitaxel or cisplatin

	Control	24 h	48 h	72 h
G_2 (%)				
paclitaxel	11.88 ± 1.03	17.54 ± 2.61	24.23 ± 3.51*	32.37 ± 5.8**
cisplatin	11.88 ± 1.03	11.30 ± 0.72	7.83 ± 0.98	18.22 ± 2.14
S phase (%)				
paclitaxel	27.4 ± 0.92	40.2 ± 3.62*	36.02 ± 2.42*	36.98 ± 2.25*
cisplatin	27.4 ± 0.92	40.7 ± 2.89*	43.37 ± 4.08**	51.98 ± 4.66**
LI (%)				
paclitaxel	26.09 ± 1.72	29.43 ± 4.55	24.15 ± 3.05	19.19 ± 2.48*
cisplatin	26.09 ± 1.72	14.28 ± 6.45*	5.18 ± 5.2**	41.36 ± 2.46

*, $P < 0.05$; **, $P < 0.01$, Mann–Whitney U-test.

24 hours following administration of 25 mg/kg of paclitaxel intrapertionally. The intratumour paclitaxel C_{max} occurred at 6 hours post-treatment, with similar values of 3.18 and 3.46 μg/ml in CH1/TS and CH1/TR tumours, respectively. The calculated AUC_{024} values for both tumours were similar.

Cell-cycle kinetics and labelling index

Flow cytometric studies confirmed that CH1/TS tumours exhibited G_2/M block following paclitaxel (32.4% cells in G_2 (72 h) versus 11.9% control, $P = 0.009$), with a significant reduction in LI (19.2% (72 h) versus 26.1% control, $P = 0.002$). Cisplatin resulted in marked retardation of cells through S phase, with a significant reduction in LI from 26% pretreatment to 5% at 48 hours (Table 53.1). In contrast, CH1/TR tumours demonstrated no alteration in cell cycle or LI after paclitaxel, yet still demonstrated partial S-phase slow-down following cisplatin, similar to CH1/TS cisplatin treated tumours (Fig. 53.2a, b).

Apoptosis

Apoptosis was significantly induced in CH1/TS tumours following both paclitaxel (9.3% (48 h) versus 0.83% control, $P = 0.002$) and cisplatin (20.4% (48 h) versus 0.83%, $P < 0.001$). Induction of apoptosis was seen in CH1/TR following cisplatin (maximum 10.4% (48 h) versus 0.99% control, $P < 0.01$), but no increase was observed following paclitaxel.

Induction of apoptosis-related proteins

The induction of p53 and p21 by Western blot analysis was compared in CH1/TS and CH1/TR tumours following paclitaxel, to determine whether any differences accounted for the failure to induce apoptosis in the paclitaxel-resistant tumour. While paclitaxel induced significant p53 and p21 protein expression in CH1/TS tumours, it failed to induce any changes in CH1/TR tumours. In contrast, cisplatin, which caused significant induction of p53 in CH1/TS tumours, was still able to induce threefold induction of p53 expression in CH1/TR tumours, despite the lack of induction seen with paclitaxel (Fig. 53.3).

There was no significant difference in the endogenous level of the pro-apoptotic protein, Bax, between sensitive and resistant

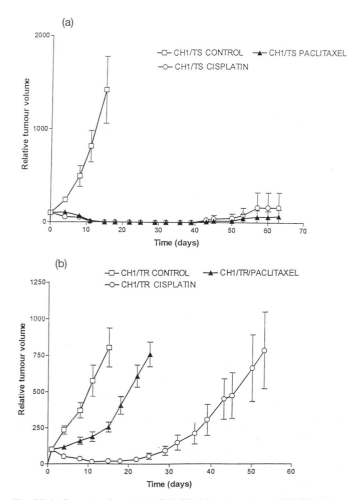

Fig. 53.1 Growth of sensitive CH1/TS (a) and resistant CH1/TR (b) ovarian cancer xenografts following intraperitoneal paclitaxel (25 mg/kg) or cisplatin (4 mg/kg given on days 0, 4, and 8.)

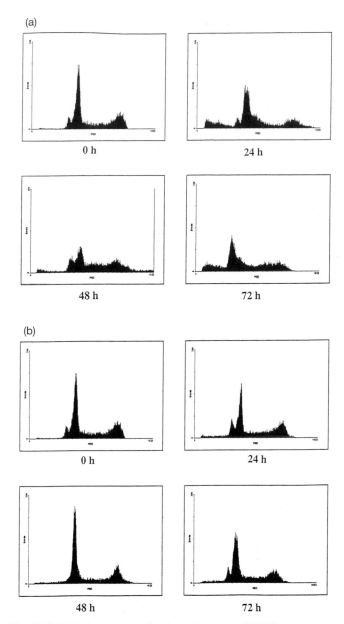

Fig. 53.2 DNA histograms of paclitaxel-resistant CH1/TR ovarian cancer xenografts harvested at 0, 24, 48, and 72 hours following either (a) cisplatin or (b) paclitaxel.

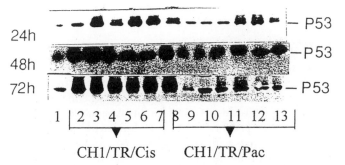

Fig. 53.3 Immunoblotting of p53 (53 kDa) in paclitaxel-resistant CH1/TR tumours following cisplatin or paclitaxel treatment. Tumours were harvested at 24, 48, and 72 hours. Lane 1, untreated CH1/TR control; lanes 2–7 cisplatin treated; lanes 8–13 paclitaxel treated.

demonstrated very little endogenous 27 kDa phosphorylated Bcl–2, and showed no induction following paclitaxel (Fig. 53.5). No changes in levels or phosphorylation status of Raf–1 were detected in either tumour type (data not shown).

bcl-xl transfected CH1 xenograft growth

Tumours established from CH1 cells transfected with either *bcl-xl* or vector control had a similar growth rate to CH1/TS tumours when established as xenografts (doubling times of 3.4, 4.6, and 2.6 days, respectively). Immunoblotting showed that there was a threefold increase in Bcl-X_L protein CH1/bcl-xl compared to CH1/TS tumours. While CH1/TS and vector control tumours displayed marked sensitivity to paclitaxel, CH1/bcl-xl tumours initially were growth delayed for 18 days, but subsequently regrew, demonstrating partial resistance to paclitaxel (Fig. 53.6). This resistance was maintained in subsequent transplanted animals.

Discussion

Over the past few years several *in vitro* studies have demonstrated the importance of apoptosis-regulating proteins in the induction and modulation of response to paclitaxel.[7,15–17] The induction of cell death by paclitaxel may involve expression of several apoptosis-related proteins, including p53, p21, the pro-apoptotic protein Bax, together with post-translational modulation by phosphorylation of the anti-apoptotic proteins Bcl–2 and Bcl-X_L.[18,19] Abnormal expression of apoptosis-regulating proteins in cancer has been associated with the development of chemoresistance.[20–22] While there is some evidence to support such a mechanism for resistance of ovarian cancer *in vitro*, little is known about changes in expression of these proteins during the development of acquired resistance *in vivo*.

Our *in vivo* model retained the phenotype of acquired resistance to paclitaxel which had been developed *in vitro*. Resistance to paclitaxel was confirmed by the growth experiments (Fig. 53.1) despite adequate intratumoral concentrations of paclitaxel. The cells were known to lack MDR–1 expression and contained wild-type p53, thus excluding either as mechanisms for resistance to

tumours, and only minimal induction of Bax was seen in CH1/TS following paclitaxel (Fig. 53.4). No phosphorylated form of the anti-apoptotic Bcl-X_L protein was detected in either tumour, although a significant 50% reduction in Bcl-X_L levels occurred following paclitaxel in CH1/TS, but not in CH1/TR tumours (Fig. 53.4). The anti-apoptotic protein, Bcl–2, was found both in its native (26 kDa) and phosphorylated (inactive) (27 kDa) form in CH1/TS tumours, a pattern further characterized by incubation of cell lysates with alkaline phosphatase, which inhibited phosphorylation and led to attentuation of the Bcl–2 27 kDa band and intensificaion of the 26 kDa band. The phosphorylated form of Bcl–2 was increased following paclitaxel in CH1/TS tumours, consistent with previous *in vitro* data. In contrast, CH1/TR tumours

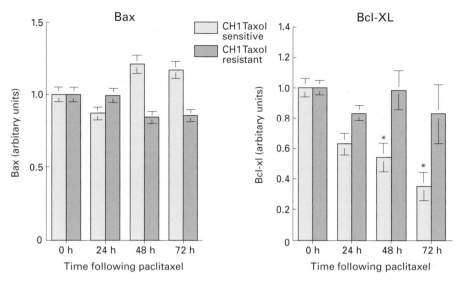

Fig. 53.4 Expression of pro-apoptotic protein Bax and anti-apoptotic protein Bcl-X$_L$ in both sensitive CH1/TS and resistant CH1/TR tumours at 24, 48 and 72 hours following paclitaxel.

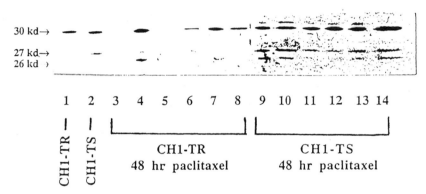

Fig. 53.5 Bcl-2 expression in resistant CH1/TR and sensitive CH1/TS tumours 48 hours following paclitaxel. Lane 1, untreated CH1/Tr; lane 2, untreated CH1/TS; lanes 3–8, six individual CH1/TR paclitaxel-treated tumours; lanes 9–14, six CH1/TS paclitaxel-treated tumours.

paclitaxel in this model. The failure of paclitaxel to induce cell-cycle changes or apoptosis was mirrored by lack of induction either of p53/p21, Bax, Bcl–2 phosphorylation, or modulation of Bcl-X$_L$ levels. The apoptotic pathway, however, was still induced by cisplatin in CH1/TR tumours. While these results imply a failure of adequate paclitaxel levels *in vivo* to trigger an apoptotic response in CH1/TR tumours with acquired resistance, they do not preclude modulation or aberrant expression of apoptosis-related proteins from playing a role in the response of resistance to paclitaxel.

p53/p21 induction by paclitaxel

Several *in vitro* studies have shown that in wild-type p53 cell lines, paclitaxel enhances p53 protein expression. This is largely due to an increase in p53 protein stability, mediated either by Raf–1 activation at high paclitaxel concentration (>9 m) or a non-Raf–1-dependent mechanism at low paclitaxel concentration.[18,23] In the present study, p53 protein induction occurred following paclitaxel in CH1/TS tumours, but not in paclitaxel-resistant CH1/TR tumours, although cisplatin was still able to induce significant p53 levels in CH1/TR (Fig. 53.3). This suggests that the p53 pathway remains intact in CH1/TR tumours, and that the lack of significant induction by paclitaxel may relate to a defect proximal to p53.

The exact role of p53 and p21 in the cellular response to mitotic spindle damage by paclitaxel remains unclear. p53 induced by paclitaxel has been shown to be involved in both G$_1$ and G$_2$ checkpoints, although in the present study, despite an induction of p53 and p21 in CH1/TS tumours treated with paclitaxel, only G$_2$/M block was observed, without any obvious G$_1$ arrest. In many *in vitro* studies involving ovarian cancer cells, the disruption of p53 resulted in no change in chemosensitivity to paclitaxel.[24,25] Recently, it was suggested that p53 may play a role during the mitotic checkpoint to ensure maintenance of diploidy, and that its induction by paclitaxel may represent a cellular response to changes in the mitotic spindle, such as abnormal chromosome segregation.[23] Murine cells devoid of a p53-dependent spindle

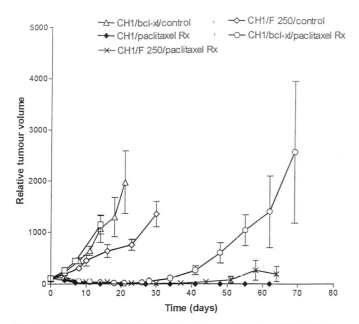

Fig. 53.6 Growth of CH1/TS, CH1/bcl-xl transfected, and CH1/F 250 (vector alone) tumours following paclitaxel on days 0, 4, and 8.

checkpoint are capable of completing subsequent cell-cycle phases, including DNA synthesis, without complete chromosome segregation.[26] However, it has been shown, in breast cancer cells treated with paclitaxel, that p21 accumulation in both p53 wild-type and p53-null situations is not involved in mitotic arrest, and may occur independently of p53 secondary to mitotic arrest.[27]

Paclitaxel and apoptosis-related protein expression

Several *in vitro* studies have demonstrated that paclitaxel in some cell types is able to induce the pro-apoptotic protein, Bax, as a consequence of transcriptional regulation by p53.[28–30] In contrast, in other cell types paclitaxel was not able to induce Bax.[7] In the present study, there was no significant increase in Bax levels in either CH1/TS or CH1/TR tumours following paclitaxel. The possibility cannot be excluded that other pro-apoptotic proteins, such as Bak or Bad, are induced. Alternatively, paclitaxel may induce cell death by post-translational hyperphosphorylation and inactivation of anti-apoptotic proteins.[31–34] The phosphorylated form of Bcl–2 is incapable of forming heterodimers with Bax, and a 50% reduction in the formation of activated Bcl–2 results in apoptotic cell death.

We showed that in our CH1/TS xenografts, in addition to the regular 26 kDa Bcl–2 band, two other bands, at 27 kDa and 30 kDa, were demonstrated (Fig. 53.5). This pattern has been described previously, both in colon and prostate cancer cell lines where, using the same Bcl–2 antibody, the 27 kDa band was shown to be the phosphorylated isoform of the 26 kDa band, although the significance of 30 kDa band was unclear.[35,36] Of note, in these studies no chemotherapy was administered, suggesting

that a proportion of Bcl–2 may be may expressed endogenously in the phosphorylated forms. In our study, it is noteworthy that, unlike the CH1/TS sensitive cells, in the untreated control CH1/TR tumours there was only faint expression of the 26 kDa Bcl–2, with no expression of the phosphorylated 27 kDa band (Fig. 53.5, lanes 1 and 2). Following paclitaxel in the resistant CH1/TR tumours, no phosphorylation of Bcl–2 occurred. In contrast, paclitaxel induced expression of the 27 kDa band in the sensitive CH1/TS tumours. It is unclear whether this difference in Bcl–2 phosphorylation, observed in the resistant tumours both prior to and following paclitaxel, accounts for the failure to induce apoptosis, and further experiments are indicated to examine this.

Recently, it has been shown that paclitaxel induces hyperphosphorylation of Bcl-X_L, abrogating its anti-apoptotic function in a manner similar to Bcl-2.[37] The reduction in Bcl-X_L level observed in this study (Fig. 53.4) has been previously shown to occur due to heterodimerization with pro-apoptotic proteins such as Bax, Bak, or Bad.[38–40] Likewise, paclitaxel treatment of the prostate cancer cell line, LNCaP, led to almost total downregulation of Bcl-X_L protein in the absence of alteration of Bax, Bak, or Bcl–2 levels.[7]

The mechanism of how phosphorylated forms of either Bcl–2 or Bcl-X_L induce cell death remains obscure. A recent report suggested that paclitaxel may induce Bcl–2 phosphorylation directly by binding to the conserved BH3 domain. Most *in vitro* work has suggested that inactivation of Bcl–2 by phosphorylation results in an alteration in the balance between the pro-apoptotic and anti-apoptotic proteins.[19] It was suggested recently that prolonged mitotic arrest itself may initiate apoptosis. It has been reported that Bcl–2 may undergo cell-cycle-dependent phosphorylation during mitosis, when there is elevated activity of the cyclin-dependent kinase (cdk2).[41] In paclitaxel-treated cells undergoing apoptosis, the phosphorylated form of Bcl–2 remained complexed with Bax, and it was suggested that, as a consequence of this, paclitaxel may function by increasing cellular susceptibility to apoptosis due to amplification of normal downstream events associated with mitotic kinase activation. However, others have reported that Bcl–2 phosphorylation by paclitaxel in cervical and ovarian cells may merely be associated with mitotic arrest, and may not be a determinant *per se* of progression into apoptosis.[42]

Signal transduction for paclitaxel-induced apoptosis

The signalling pathways linking microtubule–paclitaxel interaction and prolonged mitotic arrest with Bcl–2 phosphorylation and apoptosis remain obscure. Initially, it was suggested that paclitaxel-induced apoptosis was dependent on Raf–1 kinase activity.[19] Pharmacological depletion of Raf–1 by geldanamycin resulted in lack of Bcl–2 phosphorylation and failure to induce apoposis, suggesting that Raf–1 induction is prerequisite to Bcl–2 inactivation by phosphorylation. Subsequently, the same group showed that, in order for paclitaxel to induce Raf–1 kinase, it required the induction of tubulin polymerization.[34] Raf–1 activation was diminished markedly in paclitaxel-resistant sublines in which tubulin polymerization did not occur following paclitaxel, although other microtubule agents such as vincristine remained able to induce Raf–1 phosphorylation.

Recently, it has been demonstrated that Raf–1 activation may be paclitaxel-concentration dependent.[23] Disruption of normal microtubules occurred at low paclitaxel concentrations (1–9 nM) in the absence of Raf–1 activation. However, Raf–1 activation occurred at higher concentrations of paclitaxel and correlated with the induction of G_2/M block. The link with Bcl–2 inactivation remains unclear, as Bcl–2 phosphorylation has been demonstrated to occur in cells expressing mutant Raf–1 kinase. Thus, the role of other kinases (e.g. cdk2) in the signalling pathway between the mitotic arrest stage and Bcl–2 phosphorylation cannot be excluded.[41]

Role of the anti-apoptotic protein Bcl-X_L in paclitaxel resistance in vivo

Although, in our model of acquired paclitaxel resistance, aberrant expression of either pro-apoptotic proteins such as Bax or anti-apototic proteins such as Bcl–2 or Bcl-X$_L$ was not observed, changes in expression of these proteins may still be associated with chemoresistance to the drug. Several *in vitro* studies have shown that the overexpression of the anti-apoptotic protein Bcl-X$_L$ resulted in inhibition of apoptosis due to various stimuli, including paclitaxel.[42–44] Furthermore, Bcl-X$_L$ overexpression has been shown to inhibit paclitaxel-induced apoptosis in the A2780 ovarian cancer cell line, human acute myeloid leukaemia HL–60, and a prostate cell line.[8,15] It has been postulated that the anti-apototic effect of Bcl-X$_L$ overexpression is due to the formation of heterodimers between pro-apoptotic and anti-apoptotic proteins, which alter their balance, as discussed previously.

In our present study, we established successful xenografts of CH1 paclitaxel-sensitive cells transfected with *bcl-xl*. The growth experiments demonstrated that *bcl-xl* overexpression could modulate tumour response to paclitaxel (Fig. 53.6). There was an initial partial response to paclitaxel, but these tumours began to grow rapidly at 12 days following the last dose of treatment, whereas the sensitive CH1/TS and CH1/TS–250 (vector alone) tumours demonstrated marked persistent sensitivity to paclitaxel. An initial response to paclitaxel could be explained by the possibility of heterogeneous expression of Bcl-X$_L$ within the tumour following transfection. These results are consistent with previous *in vitro* studies and suggest that high endogenous levels of Bcl-X$_L$ may represent a distal mechanism which opposes paclitaxel-induced apoptosis.

Conclusion

Despite the abundance of *in vitro* studies, there remains a paucity of information *in vivo* regarding the mechanism of action of paclitaxel and the basis for acquired resistance. An ideal scenario would be to study xenografts established from cells of patients before and following the development resistance, to avoid cell selection pressures induced by development of acquired resistance *in vitro*.[45] However, this approach is hindered by the difficulty of obtaining adequate samples, propagation of cells from patients *in vitro*, and establishing successful xenografts *in vivo*. Nevertheless, the present *in vivo* study has provided an insight into the mechanism of action of, and resistance to, paclitaxel. While it may be concluded that the mechanism of resistance in this model could relate to a failure of paclitaxel to trigger G_2/M block and apoptosis upstream of p53/p21 and the Bcl–2-related family of proteins, the absence of endogenous levels of the 27 kDa phosphorylated form of Bcl–2 raises the possibility of an acquired defect in the apoptotic response pathway to paclitaxel. Our demonstration *in vivo* that overexpression of Bcl-X$_L$ may induce partial paclitaxel resistance supports a role for these proteins in modulating response to paclitaxel *in vivo*. Ultimately, these may represent novel molecular targets for modulation, either to overcome resistance of ovarian cancer to conventional chemotherapy, or as direct mediators of inducing an apoptotic response in the malignant cell.

References

1 McGuire, W.P., Brady, M.F., Kucera, P.R. *et al.* (1996). Cyclophosphamide and cisplatin compared with paclitaxel and cisplatin in patients with stage III and stage IV ovarian cancer. *N. Engl J. Med.*, 334, 1–6.

2. Stuart, G., Bertelsen, K., Mangioni, C. *et al.* (1998). Updated analysis shows a highly significant improved overall survival (OS) for cisplatin–paclitaxel as first-line treatment of advanced ovarian cancer. Mature results of the EORTC-GCCG, NOCOVA, NCIC CTG and Scottish intergroup trial. *Proc. Am. Soc. Clin. Oncol.*, 17, A1394.

3. Parekh, H., Wiesen, K., and Simpkins, H. (1997). Acquisition of taxol resistance via P-glycoprotein- and non-P-glycoprotein-mediated mechanisms in human ovarian carcinoma cells. *Biochem. Pharmacol.*, 53, 461–70.

4. Kavallaris, M., Bukhart, C.A., Regl, D.L. *et al.* (1997). Taxol-resistant epithelial ovarian tumors are associated with altered expression of specific beta-tubulin isotypes. *J. Clin. Invest.*, 100, 1282–93.

5. Derry, W.B., Khan, I.A., Luduena, R.F., and Jordan, M.A. (1997). Taxol differentially modulates the dynamics of microtubules assembled from unfractionated and purified beta-tubulin isotypes. *Biochemistry*, 36, 3554–62.

6. Hannun, Y.A. (1997). Apoptosis and the dilemma of cancer chemotherapy. *Blood*, 15, 1845–53.

7. Liu, Q.Y. and Stein, C.A. (1997). Taxol and estramustine-induced modulation of human prostate cancer cell apoptosis via alteration in bcl-xl and bak expression. *Clin. Cancer Res.*, 2039–2046.

8. Ibrado, A.M., Liu, L., and Bhalla, K. (1997). Bcl-xL overexpression inhibits progression of molecular events leading to paclitaxel-induced apoptosis of human acute myeloid leukemia HL–60 cells. *Cancer Res.*, 57, 1109–15.

9. Pestell, K.E., Titley, J.C., Kelland, L.R., and Walton, M.I. (1998). Characterisation of the p53 status, BCL–2 expression and radiation and platinum drug sensitivity of a panel of human ovarian cancer cell lines. *Int. J. Cancer*, 77, 913–18.

10. Rogers, P., Sharp, S.Y., and Kelland, L.R. (1996). Characterization of a non-MDR taxol resistant ovarian carcinoma cell line. *Br. J. Cancer*, 73 (Suppl. XXVI), 34 (A 33).

11. Hills, C.A., Abel, G., Siracky, J. *et al.* (1989). Biological properties of ten human ovarian carcinoma cell lines: calibration *in vitro* against four platinum complexes. *Br. J. Cancer*, 59, 527–34.

12. Ormerod, M.G. (1994). *Flow cytometry: A practical approach.* The practical approach series. Oxford University Press, New York.

13. Detre, S., Salter, J., Barnes, D.M. *et al.* (1999). Time-related effects of estrogen withdrawal on proliferation and cell-death realted events in MCF–7 xenografts. *Int. J. Cancer*, 81, 309–13.

14. Sharp, S.Y., Smith, V., Hobbs, S., and Kelland, L.R. (1998). Lack of a role for MRP1 in platinum drug resistance in human ovarian cancer cell lines. *Br. J. Cancer*, 78, 175–80.

15. Liu, J.R., Page, C., Hu, C. *et al.* (1998). Bcl-xL is expressed in ovarian carcinoma and modulates chemotherapy-induced apoptosis. *Gynecol. Oncol.*, 70, 398–403.

16. Strobel, T., Swanson, L., Korsmeyer, S., and Cannistra, S.A. (1996). BAX enhances paclitaxel-induced apoptosis through a p53-independent pathway. *Proc. Natl Acad. Sci., USA*, 93, 14094–9.

17. Wahl, A.F., Fairchild, C., Lee, F.Y. *et al.* (1996). Loss of normal p53 function confers sensitization to Taxol by increasing G2/M arrest and apoptosis. *Nature Med.*, 2, 72–9.

18. Blagosklonny, M.V., Schulte, T., Nguyen, P. *et al.* (1995). Taxol induction of p21WAF1 and p53 requires c-raf-1. *Cancer Res.*, 55, 4623–6.

19. Blagosklonny, M.V., Schulte, T., Nguyen, P. *et al.* (1996). Taxol-induced apoptosis and phosphorylation of Bcl-2 protein involves c-Raf-1 and represents a novel c-Raf-1 signal transduction pathway. *Cancer Res.*, 56, 1851–4.

20. Kromer, G. (1997). The proto-oncogene bcl-2 and its role in regulating apoptosis. *Nature Med.*, 3, 614–20.

21. Reed, J.C. (1994). Bcl-2 and the regulation of programmed cell death. *J. Cell Biol.*, 124, 1–6.

22. Reed, J.C. (1997). Double identity for proteins of Bcl-2 family. *Nature (Lond.)*, 387, 773–6.

23. Torres, K. and Horwitz, S.B. (1998). Mechanisms of Taxol-induced cell death are concentration dependent. *Cancer Res.*, 58, 3620–6.

24. Debernardis, D., De Feudis, P., Vikhanskaya, F. *et al.* (1997). p53 status does not affect sensitivity of human ovarian cancer cell lines to paclitaxel. *Cancer Res.*, 57, 870–4.

25. Wu, G.S. and EL-Deiry, W. (1996). P53 and chemosensitivity. *Nature Med.*, 2, 225–6.

26. Cross, S.M., Morgan, C.A., Schimke, M.K. *et al.* (1995). A p53-dependent mouse spindle checkpoint. *Science*, 267, 1353–6.

27. Barboule, N., Baldin, V., Vidal, S., and Valette, A. (1997). Involvement of p21 in mitotic exit after paclitaxel treatment in MCF-7 breast adenocarcinoma cell line. *Oncogene*, 15, 2867–75.

28. Miyashita, T., Krajewska, M., Wang, H.G. *et al.* (1994). Tumour suppressor p53 is a regulator of bcl-2 and bax gene expression *in vitro* and *in vivo*. *Oncogene*, 9, 1799–805.

29. Miyashita, T. and Reed, J.C. (1996). Tumour suppressor p53 is a direct transcriptional activator of the human bax gene. *Cell*, 80, 293–9.

30. Jones, N.A., McIlwrath, A.J., Brown, R., and Dive, C. (1998). Cisplatin- and paclitaxel-induced apoptosis of ovarian carcinoma cells and the relationship between bax and bak up-regulation and the functional status of p53. *Mol Pharmacol*, 53, 819–26.

31. Haldar, S., Jena, N., and Croce, C.M. (1995). Inactivation of Bcl-2 by phosphorylation. *Proc. Natl Acad. Sci., USA*, 92, 4507–11.

32. Haldar, S., Chintapalli, J., and Croce, C.M. (1996). Taxol induces bcl-2 phosphorylation and death of prostate cancer cells. *Cancer Res.*, 56, 1253–5.

33. Haldar, S., Basu, A., and Croce, C.M. (1998). Serine-70 is one of the critical sites for drug-induced Bcl-2 phosphorylation in cancer cells. *Cancer Res.*, 58, 1609–15.

34. Blagosklonny, M.V., El-Deiry, W.S., Kingston, D.G. *et al.* (1997). Raf-1/bcl-2 phosphorylation: a step from microtubule damage to cell death. *Cancer Res.*, 57, 130–5.

35. Tang, D.G., Li, L., Chopra, D.P., and Porter, A.T. (1998). Extended survivability of prostate cancer cells in the absence of trophic factors: increased proliferation, evasion of apoptosis, and the role of apoptosis proteins. *Cancer Res.*, 58, 3466–79.

36. Guan, R.J., Moss, S.F., Arber, N. *et al.* (1996). 30 KDa phosphorylated form of Bcl-2 protein in human colon. *Oncogene*, 12, 2605–9.

37. Poruchynsky, M.S., Rudin, M.R., Blagosklonny, M.V., and Fojo, T. (1998). Bcl-xl is phosphorylated in malignant cells following microtubule disruption. *Cancer Res.*, 58, 3331–8.

38. Ottilie, S., Horne, W., Chang, J. *et al.* (1997). Dimerization properties of human BAD. Identification of a BH-3 domain and analysis of its binding to mutant BCL-2 and BCL-XL proteins. *J. Biol. Chem.*, 272, 30866–72.

39. Simonian, P.L., Grillot, D.A., and Nunez, G. (1997). Bak can accelerate chemotherapy-induced cell death independently of its heterodimerization with Bcl-XL and Bcl-2. *Oncogene*, 15, 1871–5.

40. Wang, K., Gross, A., Waksman, G., and Korsmeyer, S.J. (1998). Mutagenesis of the BH3 domain of BAX identifies residues critical for dimerization and killing. *Mol. Cell. Biol.*, 18, 6083–9.

41. Scatena, C.D., Mays, D., Tang, L.J. *et al.* (1998). Mitotic phosphorylation of Bcl-2 during normal cell cycle progression and taxol-induced growth arrest. *J. Biol. Chem.*, 273, 30777–84.

42. Ling, Y.H., Tornos, C., and Perez-Soler, R. (1998). Phosphorylation of Bcl-2 is a marker of M phase events and not a determinant of apoptosis. *J. Biol. Chem.*, 24, 18984–91.

42. Minn, A.J., Rudin, C.M., Boise, L.H., and Thompson, C.B. (1995). Expression of bcl-xL can confer a multidrug resistance phenotype. *Blood*, 86, 1903–10.

43. Tang, C., Reed, J.C., Miyashita, T. *et al.* (1994). High levels of p26BCL-2 oncoprotein retard taxol-induced apoptosis in human pre-B leukemia cells. *Leukemia*, 8, 1960–9.

44. Yang, E. and Korsmeyer, S.J. (1996). Molecular thanatopsis: A discourse on the bcl-2 family and cell death. *Blood*, 88, 386–401.

45. Kaye, S.B. (1996). Ovarian cancer, from the laboratory to the clinic: challenges for the future. *Ann. Oncol.*, 7, 9–13.

54. Trials of *p53* gene therapy: rationale and preliminary studies

R.E. Buller, M. Pegram, I. Runnebaum, JoAnn Horowitz,
T.E. Buekers, Thomas P. Salko, M.E. Rybak, M.S. Shahin,
R. Kreienberg, B. Karlan, and D. Slamon

Background

Altered expression, and presumably function, of the *p53* tumor suppressor gene is one of the most fundamental changes associated with human cancers.[1–3] Mouse *p53* gene knockouts develop a variety of cancers.[4] Individuals who inherit germline mutations of the *p53* tumor suppressor gene, as with the LiFraumeni syndrome, are predisposed to multiple cancers.[5] p53 resides at an important interchange, which modifies diverse cellular functions. Wild-type p53 is a nuclear phosphoprotein containing 393 amino acids encoded at chromosome 17p13.1.[6] p53 forms homotetramers that bind to specific DNA sequences $(PuPuPuC(A/T)(A/T)GPyPy)_2$ resulting in downstream transcriptional activation or silencing of a variety of genes.[7–9] Figure 54.1 shows the spectrum and variety of important regulatory processes that are modified by p53.

Two of the most fundamental processes modified by the p53 protein include DNA repair and shunting cells with irreparably damaged DNA into apoptosis. Not only does p53 shunt cells into apoptotic pathways, but the p53 response elements both induce pro-apoptotic genes such as *bax* and suppresses anti-apoptotic genes such as *bcl–2*.[10,11] Similarly, angiogenesis is enhanced by p53 mutation via vascular endothelial growth factor (VEGF) while p53 wild type sequences are antiangiogenic via thrombospondin–1 mediated pathways [12,13]. Wild-type p53 modulates resistance to natural product chemotherapeutics by suppression of expression of the multiple-drug resistance gene, *MDR1*.[14] The normal cellular response to the delivery of either radiation or chemotherapeutics includes induction of p53. Evidence from a variety of systems has indicated that cells with altered p53 function are more resistant to the desired effects of both radiation and chemotherapy.[15]

p53 in ovarian cancer

p53 expression and mutation in ovarian cancer has been well studied.[16–23] There are currently 455 p53 mutations listed in a web site database of p53 mutations in ovarian cancer (http://perso.curie.fr/Thierry.Soussi/index.html). We have analyzed the p53 status of 198 epithelial ovarian carcinomas by immunohistochemistry using DO7 antibody, single-strand polymorphism analysis (SSCP), and directed sequencing. A summary of our results is presented in Table 54.1.

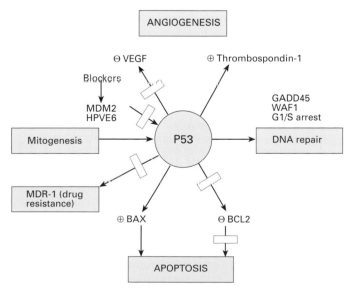

Fig. 54.1 The p53 interchange.

Table 54.1 Relationship of p53 immunoreactivity to mutation status (*n* = 198)

Immunostatus (DO7)	Mutation status	
	Mutant	**Wild type**
Positive (*n* = 99)	83 (42%)[a]	16 (8%)
Negative (*n* = 99)	32 (16%)	67 (34%)

[a] (%) is percentage distribution from the entire cohort.

Table 54.2 Correlation of p53 mutation type with distant metastasis

Mutation	Tumors analyzed	% with distant metastasis
None	36	8
Missense	62	5
Null	21	67

In this series, 53% of tumors were immunopositive. From this group, 83/99 or 84% of the DO7-antibody-positive tumors contained mutations. Most importantly, 32/99 (33%) of the immuno-negative tumors harbored mutations. Usually these mutations were null. Thus, a mutation detection strategy, which relies solely on immunohistochemistry, may result in overlooking a very important, and sizeable, subset of p53 mutations. These findings duplicate those of Saitoh *et al.* and Sjögren *et al.* in breast cancer.[24,25] Our findings have been confirmed by Casey *et al.*, both for breast and ovarian cancers, utilizing a sequencing-based approach.[26]

Ovarian cancer p53 null mutations convey a survival disadvantage (R. Buller, unpublished). This appears to relate, at least in part, to the association of null mutations with distant metastasis. In general, distant metastasis in ovarian cancer are very rare.[27] We defined distant metastasis as those found in the brain, lung, spleen, or liver parenchyma. Table 54.2 shows that this type of metastasis was found to be more commonly associated with p53 null mutations than with missense, or wild-type p53 sequence in ovarian cancers ($P < 0.001$).[28] Tumors with null mutations developed distant metastases sooner (mean 1.18 years), compared to tumors with missense or no mutations ($P = 0.015$). Even after incorporating the traditional clinical prognostic factors, multivariate analysis showed that p53 null mutation was the most significant predictor of distant metastasis. Until now, specific p53 mutations have not been correlated with clinical behavior in ovarian cancer. Evidence from other cancers also suggests aggressive tumor behavior for diseases carrying p53 with null mutations. Ruttledge *et al.* demonstrated that among patients with neurofibromatosis, individuals with protein truncating mutations (null mutations) in the *NF2* gene on chromosome 22 were significantly more likely ($P < 0.001$) to exhibit severe disease, compared to those with missense alterations.[29] Tomlinson *et al.* have reported a 16-bp deletion in exon 7 of the *p53* gene in an aggressive medulloblastoma, which developed an incision site metastasis 6 months after complete resection and radiation therapy.[30]

Only 10–25% of stage I ovarian cancers contain p53 mutations.[31–33] We have found that this percentage increases to nearly 70% in stage IV ovarian cancers (Table 54.3). Thus, the frequency of altered p53 function parallels the development of larger and

Table 54.3 Discordance between DO7-antibody staining and mutations sequenced

FIGO stage	N	DO7-positive	Mutations	Discordant
I	39	21%	18%	13%
II	12	50%	50%	0%
III	111	60%	65%	23%
IV	34	52%	68%	41%

more widely metastatic tumors. Table 54.3 relates FIGO stage of disease, DO7-antibody staining, and the frequency of actual p53 mutation. When a mutation is found in a DO7-antibody-negative tumor, or p53 wild type is overexpressed (DO7 positive, no mutation), the results are termed discordant. There is a general trend for discordance to increase with increasing stage of disease. Thus, sequencing is the gold standard for mutation detection, and antibody studies can have serious limitations.

Why gene replacement?

Despite convincing benefits of platinum-containing drugs and of taxanes on the response of ovarian cancer to treatment, the norm is that of complete clinical treatment response rates of nearly 80% followed eventually by recurrence of disease and death. The therapeutic index of most chemotherapeutics is only marginally in favor of cancer cell death. We, and others, have hypothesized (based upon an enlarging series of laboratory and *in vivo* models) that *p53* gene replacement within the cancer cell is both feasible and beneficial.[34–36] Restoration of wild-type p53 function to p53-deficient cells appears to initiate apoptosis.[34] The combination of chemotherapy with *p53* gene replacement can induce synergistic therapeutic responses.[37]

Ovarian cancer as a gene therapy model

Ovarian cancer generally remains confined to the peritoneal cavity throughout its course. This cancer tends to be a surface disease, covering intra-abdominal organs but not often burrowing deep inside organs. This is particularly true at the time of initial diagnosis and may help explain the relative ease with which widespread intra-abdominal metastases can be cytoreduced. Survival increases with optimal surgical cytoreduction, defined as residual disease no larger than 1 cm at any individual site.[38,39] Most importantly, the smaller the size of residual disease implants, the more susceptible these implants become to drug delivery by diffusion from intraperitoneally delivered drug. Instillation of large molecule therapeutics into the peritoneal cavity will bathe residual tumor in drug concentrations in excess of 1000 times the concentration attainable with intravenous delivery of the same drug.[40] These observations help to explain the survival benefits of intraperitoneal delivery, demonstrated now in three separate studies of the Gynecologic Oncology Group.[41–43] Furthermore, they have sparked interest in a number of gene replacement studies as a novel, and potentially highly specific, therapeutic approach, which may overcome the therapeutic index limitations of conventional chemotherapy. All of the usual problems associated with gene therapy must be overcome if such strategies are to become useful. These include delivery to a sufficient number of target cells, entry into these cells, selective expression within target cells, and at least no harm done to normal cells where entry is achieved simultaneously.[44] Gene delivery via adenoviral vectors has been an important initial step. These agents offer the benefit of attacking nondividing cells. This is important because a significant number of ovarian cancer cells are at rest in the G_0 phase of the cell cycle and would be refractory to infection by a retroviral vector. In addition, by utilizing adenoviral vectors, one does not need to worry about the problems of insertional mutagenesis that can occur with retroviral vectors. Recently, however, a new problem has emerged. Apparently a cell-surface receptor for the adenovirus is necessary. In the presence of the receptor, cells can be readily transfected. For both ovarian and bladder cancer cells, the absence of receptor imparts resistance to adenoviral-mediated gene transfer.[45,46]

A phase I trial of *p53* gene replacement in ovarian cancer

In February of 1997, we initiated a phase I trial of SCH58500 (Schering-Plough Corp., Kenilworth, NJ, USA) in refractory ovarian cancer. The goals of this study were:

(1) to determine a safety profile of this replication-deficient adenoviral vector containing recombinant human *p53*;
(2) to determine a maximally tolerated dose; and
(3) to demonstrate gene transfer *in vivo*.

Entry criteria are outlined in Table 54.4. Schematically, SCH58500 is shown in Fig. 54.2.

Evidence for tumor p53 mutation consisted of at least immunohistochemical evidence of p53 overexpression as determined by one of two antibodies. Only nuclear staining in a minimum of 10% of tumor cells was called positive. Alternatively, individuals with immunonegative tumors were permitted entry if a p53 mutation was sequenced from tumor DNA.

Table 54.4 Study entry criteria

Recurrent ovarian, primary peritoneal, or Fallopian tube carcinoma
Evidence of p53 mutation
Expected survival of at least 3 months
Peritoneal distribution of drug
Evidence of circulating anti-adenoviral antibodies

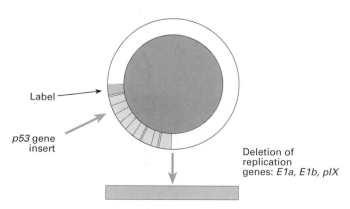

Fig. 54.2 SCH 58500 adenoviral vector.

Table 54.5 Demographic data on study cohort

Site of primary cancer	
Ovary	14
Peritoneum	1
Age at entry	61.2 years (range 41–76)
Interval from diagnosis to entry	28.9 months (range 7.8–72.5)
Prior chemotherapy regimens	3.3 (range 1–8)
Prior cycles of chemotherapy	15.7 (range 6–37)

Table 54.6 Summary of SCH58500 dosing

Dose level (particles)	Patients dosed
7.5×10^{10}	3
7.5×10^{11}	6
2.5×10^{12}	3
7.5×10^{12}	3

Demographic data on the study population is summarized in Table 54.5.

The trial design was one of escalating doses of SCH58500 delivered intraperitoneally. The agent was allowed to remain in the abdomen for 48–72 hours. At that point the fluid was removed and analyzed for transgene expression, or a laparoscopically directed biopsy obtained from those individuals who did not have ascites. Table 54.6 outlines the doses of SCH58500 delivered and the number of patients treated at each dose level.

We had planned to treat three patients at each dose level unless grade 4 WHO toxicity was obtained, or persistence of a grade 3 toxicity for more than 1 week. Nausea, vomiting, and anorexia were excluded as dose-limiting toxicities. A single grade 4 toxicity manifest by a rising alkaline phosphatase in a patient with intrahepatic metastasis was noted at dose level 2. Because of this, three additional patients (total of six) were treated at this dose level prior to escalation to level 3. A number of different toxicities were encountered in this study. Many were abdominally related, at least in part due to distension with the 2-liter infusion volume. These included bloating, swelling, pain, pressure, lack of appetite, etc. Fever was common, but rarely exceeded 39 °C. Most patients with anemia-related toxicity were anemic at the start of the study. Worsening anemia was attributed to the many blood draws required for pharmacokinetic and immunologic studies

Table 54.7 Treatment related toxicities reported by two or more subjects

Toxicity	Grade 1	Grade 2	Grade 3	Grade 4
Abdominal discomfort	3	2	1	–
Elevated alkaline phosphatase	–	–	–	1
Anemia	1	–	2	1
Edema	6	1	–	–
Fatigue	2	2	–	–
Fever	3	5	–	–
Leukopenia	–	2	–	–
Nausea	5	–	–	–
Night sweats	2	–	–	–
Vomiting	4	1	1	–

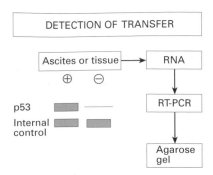

Fig. 54.3 Schematic of gene transfer detection technique.

incorporated into the trial. All WHO-graded toxicity, levels 1–4, reported by more than two patients, and their frequency distribution, are summarized in Table 54.7.

Gene transfer was measured using RT-PCR methodology on RNA prepared from tumor cells or tissue obtained at 48–72 hours following dosing with SCH58500. As an internal measure of RNA content, the level of a housekeeping gene such as β-actin was measured simultaneously. The PCR primers used were unique to a tripartite leader sequence incorporated into the recombinant *p53* sequence, thus allowing differentiation between host wild-type *p53* sequences and RNA transcribed from successfully transfected tumor cells. This is shown schematically in Fig. 54.3.

Gene transfer was seen as early as the first dose level. It was reproducible at 7.5×10^{11} particles of SCH58500. Table 54.8 summarizes the RT-PCR data. Gene transfer was demonstrated in both ascites and tissue biopsy samples.

Although only a single intraperitoneal dose of SCH58500 was delivered, baseline and 30-day follow-up CA–125 and CT scans were obtained in order to see if there was any suggestion of response. For changes in CA–125 a 20% increase or decrease was assigned as progression or response, respectively. These data are summarized in Table 54.9.

Table 54.8 Results of gene transfer measured by mimic RT-PCR

Dose of SCH58500	Patients dosed	Transfer
7.5×10^{10}	3	1
7.5×10^{11}	6	4/4[a]
2.5×10^{12}	3	3
7.5×10^{12}	3	2

[a] Internal mimic negative in 2/6 patients.

Table 54.9 Single-dose SCH58500 response measures

Disease change	CA125 change	Disease status
Stable	2	4[a]
Progression	9	11
Response	4	0

[a] Three patients subjectively noted a decrease in ascites. One patient had a 48% decrement in lesion size on CT scan.

Other potential *p53* gene therapy strategies

The *E1a* and *E1b* genes are deleted from the SCH58500 adenoviral vector.[47] Because of this, the virus can not replicate. Wild-type adenovirus relies upon these genes for lytic host cell infection. The E1a protein induces p53 and binds to the retinoblastoma gene product, pRB.[48,49] By complexing with pRB, cells enter S phase of the cell cycle, facilitating viral DNA replication within the host cell. The E1b protein binds wild-type p53, leading to a loss of p53-dependent checkpoint control, and facilitating cellular apoptosis. Blockade of p53 function is essential for efficient viral replication. ONYX–015 (Onyx Pharmaceuticals, Richmond, California, USA) is a mutated adenovirus which contains an 872-bp deletion in the *E1b* region and a nonsense point mutation at codon 2022 that generates a truncated protein from the deleted gene.[50] This agent replicates poorly in cells containing wild-type p53 sequences because it is unable to block p53 function. In contrast, when ONYX–015 is introduced into a variety of tumor cells that contain mutant p53, the virus replicates quite nicely.[51] *In vivo* modeling with human xenografts has shown potent tumor growth inhibition both with virus alone and in combination with chemotherapy.[52] Clinical trials of this agent in ovarian cancer are ongoing.

An intriguing strategy to restore wild-type p53 function to cells with mutant p53 takes advantage of the fact that p53 molecules aggregate to form homotetramers. Following DNA binding in a sequence-specific fashion by the tetramers, transcription is activated. The DNA-binding region of the p53 complex is localized to the carboxyl terminus of the molecule. In fact, DNA binding of some mutant p53 proteins can be activated by complexing with the Pab–421 monoclonal antibody which recognizes the carboxyl terminus epitope.[53] This observation has led Selivanova *et al.* to formulate a synthetic 22-mer peptide, Peptide 46, which will complex with full-length p53 to activate transcription.[54] Indeed, these investigators have shown that Peptide 46 can restore the growth suppression function to mutant p53 by treating p53 null Saos–2 cell lines which have been stably transfected with a His273 mutant vector. One advantage of a small molecule gene therapy strategy is the potential to avoid problems with the host immune response.

Summary

p53 function is altered in nearly 70% of advanced ovarian cancers. The unusual tendency of ovarian cancer to remain confined to the peritoneal cavity, coupled with the relative ease of surgical cytoreduction, makes small-volume residual disease susceptible to intraperitoneal gene replacement strategies. Extensive data from a variety of *in vitro* and *in vivo* model systems have shown that *p53* gene replacement is technically feasible and therapeutically efficacious. In a phase I trial, safety of gene therapy with SCH58500 in humans with refractory ovarian cancer has been demonstrated. Intraperitoneal delivery of SCH58500 results in readily detectable gene transfer to ovarian cancer cells. Further studies to determine the efficacy of such a strategy and the interaction of this agent with the immune system are ongoing.

References

1. Greenblatt, M., Bennett, W., Hollstein, M. *et al.* (1994). Mutations in the p53 tumor suppressor gene: Clues to cancer etiology and molecular pathogenesis. *Cancer Res*, **54**, 4855–78.

2. Soussi, T., Legros, Y., Lubin, R. *et al.* (1994). Multifactorial analysis of p53 alteration in human cancer: a review. *Int. J. Cancer*, **57**, 1–9.

3. Welsh, D., Levine, A., Perry, M. *et al.* (1994). The 1993 Walter Hubert Lecture: The role of the p53 tumour-suppressor gene in tumorigenesis. *Br. J. Cancer*, **69**, 409–16.

4. Donehower, L.A., Harvey, M., Slagle, B.L. *et al.* (1992). Mice deficient for p53 are developmentally normal but susceptible to spontaneous tumours. *Nature*, **356**, 215–21.

5. Li, F.P., Gaber, J.E., Friend, S.H. *et al.* (1992). Recommendations on predictive testing for germline p53 mutations among cancer-prone individuals. *J. Natl Cancer Inst.*, **84**(15), 1156–60.

6. Miller, C., Mohandas, T., Wolf, D. *et al.* (1986). Human p53 gene localized to short arm of chromosome 17. *Nature*, **319**, 783–84.

7. Chumakov, A., Miller, C., Chen, D. *et al.* (1998). Analysis of p53 transactivation through high-affinity binding sites. *Oncogene*, **8**, 3005–11.

8. Funk, W., Pak, D., Karas, R. *et al.* (1992). A transcriptionally active DNA-binding site for human p53 protein complexes. *Mol. Cell. Biol.*, **12**, 2866–71.

9. Kern, S., Pietenpol, J., Thiagalingam, S. *et al.* (1992). Oncogenic forms of p53 inhibit p53-regulated gene expression. *Science*, **256**, 827–30.

10. Miyashita, T. and Reed, J.C. (1995). Tumor suppressor p53 is a direct transcriptional activator of the human bax gene. *Cell*, **80**, 293–9.

11. Miyashita, T., Harigai, M., Hanada, M., and Reed, J.C. (1994). Identification of a p53-dependent negative response element in the bcl–2 gene. *Cancer Res.*, **54**, 3131–5.

12. Mukhopadyay, D., Tsiokas, L., and Sukhatme, V. (1995). Wild-type p53 and v-Sre opposing influence on human vascular endothelial growth factor gene expression. *Cancer Res.*, **57**, 6161–5.

13. Dameron, K.M., Volpert, O.V., Tainsky, M.A., and Bouck, N.P. (1994). Control of angiogenesis in fibroblasts by p53 regulation of thrombospondin–1. *Science*, **265**, 1582–4.

14. Zastawny, R.L., Salvino, R., Chen, J. *et al.* (1993). The core promoter region of the P-glycoprotein gene is sufficient to confer differential responsiveness to wild-type and mutant p53. *Oncogene* **8**(6), 1529–35.

15. Lowe, S.W, Bodis, S., McClatchey, A. *et al.* (1994). p53 status and the efficacy of cancer therapy *in vivo*. *Science*, **266**, 807–10.

16. Skilling, J., Sood, A., Niemann, T. *et al.* (1996). An abundance of p53 null mutations in ovarian carcinoma. *Oncogene*, **13**, 117–23.

17. Kim, J., Cho, Y., Kwon, D. *et al.* (1995). Aberrations of the *p53* tumor suppressor gene in human epithelial ovarian carcinoma. *Gynecol.Oncol.*, **57**, 199–204.

18. Klemi, P., Pylkkanen, L., Killholma, P. *et al.* (1995). p53 protein detected by immunochemistry as a prognostic factor in patients with epithelial ovarian carcinoma. *Cancer*, **76**, 1201–8

19. Kohler, M., Marks, J., Wiseman, R. *et al.* (1993). Spectrum of mutation and frequency of allelic deletion of the p53 gene in ovarian cancer. *J. Natl Cancer Inst.*, **85**, 1513–19.

20. Kupryjanczyk, J., Thor, A., Beauchamp, R. *et al.* (1993). p53 gene mutations and protein accumulation in human ovarian cancer. *Proc. Natl Acad. Sci. USA*, **90**, 4961–5.

21. Marks, J., Davidoff, A., Kerns, B. *et al.* (1991). Overexpression and mutation of p53 in epithelial ovarian cancer. *Cancer Res.*, **51**, 2979–84.

22. Mazars, R., Pujol, P., Maudelonde, T. *et al.* (1991). *p53* mutations in ovarian cancer: a late event? *Oncogene*, **6**, 1685–90.

23. Teneriello, M., Ebina, M., Linnoila, R. *et al.* (1993). p53 and Ki-*ras* gene mutations in epithelial ovarian neoplasms. *Cancer Res.*, **53**, 3103–8.

24. Saitoh, S., Cunningham, J., De Vries, *et al.* (1994). P53 gene mutations in breast cancers in midwestern US women: Null as well as missense-type mutations are associated with poor prognosis. *Oncogene*, **9**, 2869–75.

25. Sjögren, S., Inganäs, M., Norberg, T. *et al.* (1996). The p53 gene in breast cancer: Prognostic value of complementary DNA sequencing versus immunohistochemistry. *J. Natl Cancer Inst.*, **88**, 173–82.

26. Casey, G., Lopez, M.E., Ramos, J.C. *et al.* (1996). DNA sequence analysis of exons 2 through 11 and immunohistochemical staining are required to detect all known p53 alterations in human malignancies. *Oncogene*, **13**, 1971–81.

27. Geisler, J. and Geisler, H. (1995). Brain metastases in epithelial ovarian carcinoma. *Gynecol. Oncol.*, **57**, 246–49.

28. Sood, A.K., Sorosky, J.I., Dolan, M. *et al.* (2000) Distant metastases in ovarian cancer: Why do they occur? *Clin. Cancer Res.*, submitted.

29. Ruttledge M., Andermann A., Phelan C. *et al.* (1996). Type of mutation in the neurofibromatosis type 2 gene (NF2) frequently determines severity of disease. *Am. J. Hum. Genet.*, **59**, 331–42.

30. Tomlinson, F., Jenkins, R., Scheithauer, B. *et al.* (1994). Aggressive medulloblastoma with high-level N-myc amplification. *Mayo Clinc. Proc.*, **69**, 359–65.

31. Kohler, M., Kerns, B.-J., Humphrey, P. *et al.* (1993). Mutation and overexpression of p53 in early-stage epithelial ovarian cancer. *Obstet. Gynecol.*, **81**, 643–50.

32. Milner, B., Allan, L., Eccles, D. *et al.* (1993). p53 mutation is a common genetic event in ovarian carcinoma. *Cancer Res.*, **53**, 2128–32.

33. Sheridan, E., Hancock, B., and Goyns, M. (1993). High incidence of mutations of the p53 gene detected in ovarian tumours by the use of chemical mismatch cleavage. *Cancer Lett.*, **68**, 83–9.

34. Nielsen, L.L. and Maneval, D.C. (1998). p53 tumor suppressor gene therapy for cancer. *Cancer Gene Ther.*, **5**(1), 52–63.

35. Nielsen, L.L., Dell, J., Maxwell, E. *et al.* (1997). Efficacy of p53 adenovirus-mediated gene therapy against human breast cancer xenografts. *Cancer Gene Ther.*, **4**(2), 129–38.

36. Roth, J.A., Nguyen, D., Lawrence, D.D. *et al.* (1996). Retrovirus-mediated wild-type *p53* gene transfer to tumors of patients with lung cancer. *Nature Med.*, **2**(9), 985–91.

37. Nielsen, L.L., Lipari, P., Dell, J. G. *et al.* (1998). Adenovirus-mediated p53 gene therapy and paclitaxel have synergistic efficacy in models of human head and neck, ovarian, prostate, and breast cancer. *Clin. Cancer Res.*, **4**, 835–46.

38. Hoskins, W.J., McGuire, W.P., Brady, M.F. *et al.* (1994). The effect of diameter of largest residual disease on survival after primary cytoreduction surgery in patients with suboptimal residual epithelial ovarian carcinoma. *Am. J. Obstet. Gynecol.*, **170**, 924.

39. Hoskins, W.J., Bundy, B.N., Thigpen, J.T., and Omura, G.A. (1992). The influence of cytoreductive surgery on recurrence free interval and survival in small volume stage III epithelial ovarian cancer: a Gynecologic Oncology Group Study. *Gynecol. Oncol.*, **47**, 159.

40. Dedrick, R., Myers, C.E., Bungay, P.M., and DeVita, V.T. Jr (1978). Pharmacokinetic rationale for peritoneal drug administration in the treatment of ovarian cancer. *Cancer Treat. Rep.*, **62**, 1–9.

41. Berek, J.S., Stonbraker, B., Lentz, S.S. *et al.* (1998). Intraperitoneal alpha-interferon in residual ovarian carcinoma: A phase II Gynecologic Oncology Group study. Thirty-Fourth Annual Meeting, **17**, 358.

42. Markman, M., Bundy, B., Benda, J. *et al.* (1999). Randomized trial of standard dose intravenous (iv) cisplatin/paclitaxel versus moderately high-dose carboplatin followed by intravenous paclitaxel and intraperitoneal (ip) cisplatin. Thirtieth Annual Meeting of the Society of Gynecologic Oncologists, **72**, 446.

43. Alberts, D.S., Liu, P.Y., Hannigan, E.V. *et al.* (1996). Intraperitoneal cis-platin plus intravenous cyclophosphamide versus intravenous cisplatin plus intravenous cyclophosphamide for stage III ovarian cancer. *N. Engl. J. Med.*, **335**(26), 1950–5.

44. Hwu, P. (1995) The gene therapy of cancer. *Princ. Pract. Oncology*, **9**(4), 1–13.

45. Pegram, M., Tseng, Yiou, Baldwin, R.A. *et al.* (1999). Expression of Coxsackie and adenovirus receptor (CAR) correlates with efficiency of adenovirus transduction of human ovarian carcinoma cells. Thirtieth Annual Meeting of the Society of Gynecologic Oncologists, **72**, 452.

46. Li, Y., Pong, R.-C., Bergelson, J.M. *et al.* (1999). Loss of adenoviral receptor expression in human bladder cancer cells: A potential impact on the efficacy of gene therapy. *Cancer Res.*, **59**,325–30.

47. Wills, K.N., Maneval, D.C., Menzel, P. *et al.* (1994). Development and characterization of recombinant adenoviruses encoding human p53 for gene therapy of cancer. *Hum. Gene Ther.*, **5**,1079–88.

48. Yew, P.R. and Berk, A.J. (1992). Inhibition of p53 transactivation required for transformation by adenovirus early 1B protein. *Nature*, **357**(6373), 82–5.

49. Land, H., Parada, L.F., and Weinberg, R.A. (1983). Tumorigenic conversion of primary embryo fibroblasts requires at least two cooperating oncogenes. *Nature*, **304**(5927), 596–602.

50. Barker, D.D. and Berk, A.J. (1987). Adenovirus proteins from both E1B reading frames are required for transformation of rodent cells by viral infection and DNA transfection. [Published erratum appears in *Virology*, **158**(1), 263.]

51. Bischoff, J.R., Kirn, D.H., Williams, A. *et al.* (1996). An adenovirus mutant that replicates selectively in p53-deficient human tumor cells. *Science*, **274**, 373–76.

52. Heise, C., Sampson-Johannes, A., Williams, A. *et al.* (1997). ONYX–015, an E1B gene-attenuated adenovirus, causes tumor-specific cytolysis and antitumoral efficacy that can be augmented by standard chemotherapeutic agents. *Nature Med.*, **3**(6), 639–45.

53. Hupp, T.R. and Lane, D.P. (1994). Allosteric activation of latent p53 tetramers. *Curr. Biol.*, **4**, 865–75.

54. Selivanova, G., Iotsova, V., Okan, I. *et al.* (1997). Restoration of the growth suppression function of mutant *p53* by a synthetic peptide derived from the p53 C-terminal domain. *Nature Med.*, **3**(6), 632–8.

55. Shahin, M.S., Sood, A.K., Hughes, J.H., Buller, R.E. (2000). The prognostic significance of p53 tumor suppressor gene alternations in ovarian cancer. *Cancer*, **89**(9), 2006–17.

55. Phosphatidylinositol 3′-kinase in ovarian cancer: from genomics to therapeutics

Yiling Lu, Laleh Shayestri, Ruth Lapushin, Shuangxing Yu, Bruce Cuevas, Xianjun Fang, Astrid Eder, Tatsuro Furui, Daniel Plikoff, Wen-Lin Kuo, Russ Baldocchi, Bart Vanhaesebroeck, Robert C. Bast, Dan Pinkel, Kathy Siminovitch, Robert Jaffe, Joe Gray, and Gordon B. Mills

Background

Overview

In the United States, ovarian cancer is the leading cause of death from gynecological malignancies and is the fifth most common female malignancy.[1] In 1999 approximately 26 800 women will be newly diagnosed and 14 500 will die from ovarian cancer.[1] Epithelial ovarian cancers are classified histologically as serous (60%), endometrioid (20%), mucinous (15%), and clear cell (5%). Clear cell tumors exhibit a particularly poor prognosis. Prognosis is also closely linked to stage and grade or degree of differentiation, as well as to clinical factors. Unfortunately, the majority of patients are diagnosed with advanced epithelial ovarian cancer with disease spread throughout the abdomen. The dismal prognosis results from an inability to detect ovarian cancer at an early, treatable stage, as well as from lack of effective therapies for advanced disease. Although current therapy, consisting of radical surgery, radiation therapy, and chemotherapy, has resulted in improved survival times, there has been no significant improvement in cure rates in the past 30 years.[2] The most likely way to develop new, effective therapies for ovarian cancer, and perhaps to identify disease at an early stage, is to improve our understanding of the genetic changes leading to the initiation and progression of ovarian cancer.

Phosphatidylinositol 3-kinase in growth regulation

Phosphatidylinositol 3-kinase (PI3K) is a member of a superfamily of proteins that also includes the p70S6 regulatory kinase FRAP/TOR, the ataxia telangiectasia mutated gene (ATM) and the related ATR protein, the PAF400 and TRRAP components of the histone acetylase complex, and the DNA-dependent protein kinase (DNA-PK) involved in DNA repair.[3–5] Several, but not all, of the members of the PI3K superfamily have the ability to phosphorylate proteins on serine and threonine residues.[3–5] PI3K has the unique additional ability to also phosphorylate membrane phosphatidylinositols (PtdIns), thus activating and recruiting specific intracellular proteins to the membrane (Figs. 55.1, 55.2).

Phosphorylation of membrane PtdIns by PI3K plays a pivotal role in the control of cell proliferation, differentiation, senescence, cytoskeletal organization, motility, metastases, invasion, angiogenesis, and cell survival,[3–5] suggesting that PI3K plays a critical role in cell growth regulation and, potentially, tumorigenesis. Indeed, several lines of evidence have directly linked the PI3K pathway to oncogenesis. For example, the avian PI3K p110 homolog is a potent transforming gene in avian embryonic fibroblasts,[6] increased PI3K activity is associated with transformation by v-src, polyoma middle T antigen, v-abl, and v-ros,[7] and a mutant form of PI3K p85 is directly transforming.[8] In addition, functional PI3K is required for Ras-mediated transformation.[9] Further, the PTEN tumor suppressor gene that dephosphorylates the D3 hydroxyl on the inositol ring of phosphorylated PtdIns, which is phosphorylated by PI3K (Fig. 55.1), is frequently mutated in endometrioid ovarian cancer, advanced prostate cancer, glioma, endometrial cancer, and breast cancer.[10–17] Germline mutations in PTEN are the cause of the Cowden's tumor susceptibility syndrome,[14–16] further implicating the PI3K cascade in tumorigenesis. The AKT1 downstream target of PI3K (Fig. 55.2) is implicated in tumorigenesis by being incorporated into a transforming retrovirus.[18] In contrast, AKT2 is implicated in tumorigenesis by being amplified in ovarian and pancreatic cancers,[19,20] and exhibiting transforming activity,[21] respectively.

PI3K may also play a critical role in metastases. PI3K is necessary for Ras-induced production of the angiogenic factor, vascular endothelial growth factor (VEGF).[22] PI3K also plays a role in the

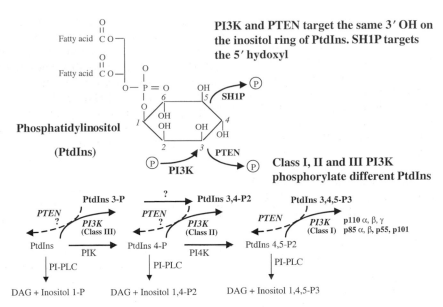

Fig. 55.1 Phosphatidylinositol targets of PI3K, PTEN, and SHIP.

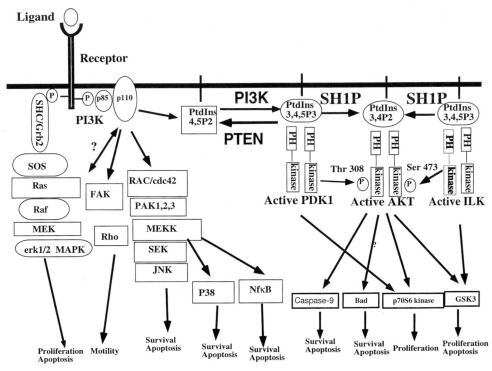

Fig. 55.2 Growth factor signaling through the phosphatidylinositol cascade.

production of the proteases that degrade the extracellular matrix.[3-5] Furthermore, PI3K regulates cytoskeletal reorganization and motility.[3-5] PI3K is a critical regulator of apoptosis and anoikis,[3-5] a form of apoptosis that occurs when cells are dissociated from their extracellular matrix.[23,24] Anoikis must be bypassed for a cell to survive following detachment from the extracellular matrix and particularly to survive in the circulation, where the majority of shed tumor cells die.[23-27] Integrin-mediated activation of PI3K and AKT appear to be critical in preventing anoikis, as

does activation of the focal adhesion protein–tyrosine kinase (FAK).[24-27] The integrin-linked kinase (ILK) is recruited to the membrane by binding to β-integrins as well as by the PI3K product, PtdIns 3,4,5P3, where it can phosphorylate Ser473 of AKT (Fig. 55.2).[28] Overexpression of ILK increases fibronectin matrix assembly, decreases E-cadherin expression, and increases tumorigenicity, at least in part, through its ability to phosphorylate AKT and to protect cells from anoikis.[29] FAK, along with many other intracellular proteins, interacts with PI3K.[3-5,30]

PI3K signaling cascade in ovarian cancer

Several previous observations have implicated the P13K pathway in ovarian epithelial cell growth and, potentially, tumorigenesis. Receptors known to signal through P13K and to be present on ovarian cancer cells include those for lysophosphatidic acid (LPA), epidermal growth factor (EGF), transforming growth factor-α (TGF-α), heparin-binding EGF (HB-EGF), heregulin, betacellulin, amphiregulin, kit ligand (KITL), keratinocyte growth factor (KGF), hepatocyte growth factor (HGF), basic fibroblast growth factor (FGF), platelet-derived growth factor (PDGF), interleukin-1, -6 and -8 (IL-1, IL-6, and IL-8), insulin, insulin-like growth factor I (IGF-I), and colony-stimulating growth factor 1 (CSF-1, mCSF).[31] We have demonstrated that Ras, which interacts functionally with P13K,[32] is activated constitutively in ovarian cancer[33] despite infrequent mutations.[31] The AKT2 downstream target of PI3K, which is amplified in a subset of ovarian cancers,[19] is activated by EGF, IGF-I, PDGF, insulin, and basic FGF through P13K in ovarian cancer cells.[34] Further, activated Ras and src stimulate AKT2 through a P13K-dependent mechanism in ovarian cancer cells.[34] In addition, we have demonstrated that inhibition of the p70S6 kinase, which is a downstream target of P13K, increases apoptosis in a number of model systems, including apoptosis induced by cisplatin.[35] Both phosphatidylinositol kinase (PI kinase; PIk) and phosphatidylinositol 4-kinase (PI4-kinase; PI4K) activity, which are critical for the production of substrates for PI3K (see Fig. 55.1), have been reported to be markedly increased in ovarian cancer cell lines (32- and 11-fold, respectively) and in primary ovarian cancers (4.4- and 2.9-fold).[36] Indeed, effective but non-specific inhibitors of PI and PI4 kinases (quercetin and genestein, respectively) have been reported to inhibit synergistically the growth of the OVCAR-5 ovarian cancer cell line under anchorage-dependent and -independent conditions.[36] Thus the PI3K pathway is likely to contribute to ovarian epithelial tumorigenesis.

PI3K signaling

The catalytic subunits of PI3K all phosphorylate the 3' hydroxyl group of the inositol ring of membrane phosphatidylinositols (Fig. 55.1).[3–5] Of the identified PI3Ks, class I PI3Ks are most closely linked to tumorigenesis, cell growth, and viability in mammalian cells.[3–5] Class I PI3Ks preferentially phosphorylate PtdIns 4,5P2, producing PtdIns 3,4,5P3; class II P13Ks phosphorylate PtdIns 4P, producing PtdIns 3,4P2; and class III P13K phosphorylate PtdIns, producing PtdIns 3P.[3–5] The production of the substrates for class II and class I PI3Ks is catalyzed by the sequential action of PI and PI4 kinases (Fig. 55.1). The SH2 domain containing lipid phosphatase SH1P dephosphorylates the 5' position of PtdIns 3,4,5P3, producing PtdIns 3,4P2.[37] Thus PtdIns 3,4P2 can be produced by the sequential action of PI kinase and class II PI3Ks, or through the SH1P-catalyzed dephosphorylation of PtdIns pleckstrin 3,4,5P3 produced by class I PI3Ks.

Although 3'-phosphorylated PtdIns have been demonstrated to bind to a number of different proteins with low affinity, they bind to pleckstrin homology (PH) domains (an approximately 120-amino-acid protein interaction motif) with relatively high affinities.[3–5,38–40] PtdIns 3,4,5P3 and PtdIns 3,4P2 bind *to a differ-ent subset* of PH domains, thus recruiting to the membrane and frequently activating specific PH-domain-containing proteins.[38–40] PH domains are found in over a hundred proteins, including the ILK, PDK1, AKT1, and AKT2 serine–threonine kinases, all phospholipase-C isoforms, the TEC family of tyrosine kinases (of which we have cloned ITK[41] and demonstrated its regulation by PI3K[42]), the plectstrin and spectrin structural proteins, and the VAV, GAP and SOS G-protein-regulating proteins.[38] PH domains can also bind, and are regulated by specific isoforms of protein kinase C (as we have demonstrated for ITK[43]) and by $\beta\gamma$-subunits of G proteins.[38]

Class I P13Ks consist of a p110 catalytic subunit constitutively complexed to a p50–101 regulatory subunit.[3–5] Class IA P13K consists of p110α, β or δ interacting with p85α, β, or δ, whereas class IB P13K consists of p110γ interacting with p50 or p101.[3–5] p110α and β are pan-expressed whereas p110δ appears restricted to hematopoietic cells under normal conditions,[3–5,44] but may be expressed by ovarian cancer cells (not presented). p110α, β or δ complexes are regulated primarily by binding of the p85 regulatory subunit to tyrosine-phosphorylated receptors, kinases, or linking proteins, whereas p110γ complexes are regulated primarily by binding of p50 or p101 $\beta\gamma$-subunits of heterotrimeric G proteins.[3–5] Each of the p85 subunits appears to be able to interact with each of the p110α, β, or δ subunits but not with p110γ. The p85 subunits of P13K contain one SH3 and two SH2 protein–protein interaction motifs. In addition, they contain an inter-SH2 domain responsible for binding to p110. Tyrosine phosphorylation of transmembrane receptors or linker molecules thus recruits P13K through SH2 domains in p85 to the context of the membrane and its PtdIns substrates.[3–5,45] Further binding of the p85 SH2 domains to tyrosine phosphorylated targets appears to remove constraints to P13K p110 activity.[46] The SH2 domains of p85 bind to a tyrosine-phosphorylated motif, pYxxM, with a high affinity. The presence of the YxxM motif in multiple cell-surface receptors, and phosphorylation of the tyrosine in this motif in response to different extracellular ligands, leads to the recruitment of P13K to the membrane, placing it in the context of its PtdIns substrates.[3–5] The SH2 domains of p85 also appear to bind to a number of other tyrosine-phosphorylated motifs, such as YVxV, albeit with a lower affinity.[3–5] p85 can also stabilize the p110 protein,[46] thus increasing P13K enzyme levels and likely responsiveness to ligand.

AKT

AKT1 and AKT2 are both downstream targets of P13K.[18,34] AKT1 (aka protein kinase B (PKB); see Fig. 55.2) is the cellular homolog of the v-*akt* oncogene,[18] and has been shown to deliver cell-survival signals induced by growth factors in neurons, fibroblasts, and lymphoid cells.[18,23]. AKT2 exhibits transforming activity on its own[21] and is overexpressed[19] and regulated[34] in ovarian cancer. Both AKT homologs appear to be regulated in a similar manner. As shown in Fig. 55.2, AKT is distinguished by the presence of a pleckstrin homology (PH) domain, which mediates high-affinity interactions of AKT with the P13K lipid product, PtdIns 3,4P2, resulting in AKT recruitment to the cell membrane.[23,40] At the membrane, phosphorylation of Ser473 and Thr308 of AKT (residue numbers represent AKT1) by the PtdIns 3,4,5P3-regulated integrin-linked kinase (ILK aka PDK2),[28] and PDK1[40] respectively, complete activation of AKT. Following binding and dimerization by PtdIns 3,4P2, AKT may also autophosphorylate on Ser473.[23] Thus both PtdIns 3,4,5P3 produced by P13K and PtdIns 3,4P2 produced by SHIP play critical roles in AKT activation. Phosphorylation of Ser473 appears to be strictly dependent on the action of P13K,[23,40] making assessment of phosphorylation of Ser473 an excellent surrogate for activity of P13K in intact cells. AKT can, however, be activated through non-P13K-dependent pathways, presumably involving phosphorylation of Thr308.[18]

Sequestration model of apoptosis

The anti-apoptotic effect of activated AKT is realized, at least in part, by AKT-mediated phosphorylation and inactivation of the Bcl-2 family member, Bad (Ser136),[18,23] and of caspase-9 (Ser196) (Fig. 55.3).[47] Dephosphorylated Bad is thought to induce cell death by heterodimerizing with Bcl-X or Bcl-2 in the mitochondrial membrane, leading to an increase in the amount of free Bax and Bak, thereby inducing a death-promoting protease cascade through release of cytochrome C from the mitochondria (Fig. 55.3).[48,49] Cytochrome C binds to APAF-1, leading to activation of caspase-9 and caspase-3 and subsequently other caspases.[48,49] Phosphorylated Bad, in contrast, binds to 14-3-3, sequestering Bad in the cytosol away from its Bcl-X$_L$ or Bcl-2 targets (Fig. 55.3).[48,49] AKT also has other potential downstream substrates (e.g. glycogen synthase kinase 3 and p70 ribosomal S6 kinase), which may also be relevant to its anti-apoptotic affects (Fig. 55.2).[18,50] Indeed, we have demonstrated that inhibition of p70S6 kinase by rapamycin increases cell death by apoptosis in a number of cellular models.[35]

PTEN

The PTEN (aka MMAC1/TEP) tumor suppressor on 10q23 is mutated in advanced sporadic endometrial cancers (30–50%),

breast cancers (20–30%), glioblastomas (20–30%), prostate cancers (15%), head and neck tumors (10%), and melanomas (10%).[10–12,51–53] Strikingly, PTEN does not appear to be mutated in a significant portion of serous epithelial ovarian cancers,[51,54–56] but it is mutated in 30–50% of endometrioid epithelial ovarian cancers.[56] This is intriguing given that the 3q amplicon, which contains PI3K, is frequently observed in serous epithelial ovarian cancers, but is not observed in endometrioid ovarian cancers.[57,58] A similar observation has been made in serous and endometrioid tumors of the uterus, with 50% of uterine serous tumors versus 8% of uterine endometrioid tumors demonstrating amplification at 3q26.[59] The observation that germline mutations in PTEN cause the Cowden's and Bannayan–Zonana cancer predisposition syndromes,[14–16] and are found in endometrial hyperplasia[52,53,60,61] as well as in advanced cancer,[10–12,51] indicates that PTEN plays a role at multiple stages of tumorigenesis. This further suggests that the PI3K pathway may be important for the development of both serous and endometrioid ovarian cancers, but that these tumors may be targeted by different genetic changes, resulting in the same outcome.

The PTEN 55 kDa multifunctional phosphatase can dephosphorylate Ser, Thr and Tyr residues in proteins,[20] as well as the same D3 hydroxyl in PtdIns which is phosphorylated by PI3K (Figs 55.1, 55.2).[17] Thus PI3K and PTEN catalyze opposing reactions (Figs 55.1, 55.2). As yet, focal adhesion kinase (FAK) is the only identified protein substrate and binding partner for PTEN.[57] PTEN, either directly or indirectly, induces dephosphorylation of a downstream target of FAK, p130 Cas, without altering phosphorylation of paxillin, c-Src, or tensin.[62,63] Dephosphorylation of FAK by PTEN is associated with a decrease in migration, cell spreading, adhesion, and focal adhesion formation.[62]

Introduction of PTEN into breast, prostate, and glioma cancer cell lines lacking PTEN decreases their anchorage-dependent and-independent proliferation and *in vivo* growth,[64–66] a process that requires a functional PTEN lipid phosphatase but not protein

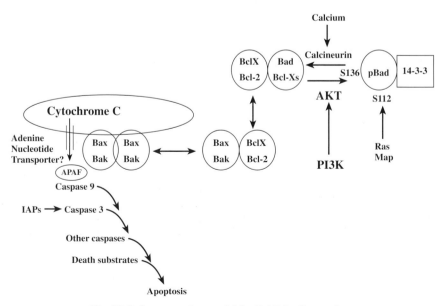

Fig. 55.3 Sequestration model for Bcl-2 family members.

phosphatase activity.[64,67] Thus protein phosphatase activity is not sufficient for the growth-regulatory activity of PTEN. PTEN can introduce growth arrest, apoptosis, or anoikis, dependent on culture conditions and cellular lineage.[64–68] Introduction of PTEN into cell lines expressing PTEN has limited effects on cellular proliferation, suggesting that PTEN is not a rate-limiting enzyme in normal cells and that PTEN may thus be a good target for gene therapy.[64,65,68]

Current studies

P13K p110α is increased in copy number in the majority of ovarian cancers

Using comparative genomic amplification, we have demonstrated that chromosome 3q25–26 is amplified in a significant proportion of freshly isolated ovarian cancer samples as well as ovarian cancer cell lines,[57] and is one of the most common defects seen in early grade and late-stage tumors (not presented). Fine mapping, using fluorescent *in situ* hybridization (FISH) with a BAC contig across this region[57] demonstrated amplification of 3q25–26 (with the smallest region at 3q26.3) or of the whole chromosome 3 in more than 80% of late-stage primary ovarian cancer specimens, but not in breast cancers or melanomas, implicating this region in ovarian tumorigenesis. The gene, *PIK3CA*, that encodes the p110α catalytic subunit of P13K maps to the center of the genomic amplicon present in ovarian cancer.[57] Increased copy number of *PIK3CA* was found in 8 of 9 ovarian cancer cell lines, 7 of 12 primary ovarian cancers, and 5 of 5 ascites tumors. In addition, as assessed by FISH, *PIK3CA* copy number was increased two- to fourfold relative to 3p25 in 8 of 17 primary ovarian cancers and 7 of 9 ovarian cancer cell lines. Compatible with the genomic amplification, we have demonstrated that the amount of P13K mRNA, protein, and enzyme activity are also consistently increased in ovarian cancer cell lines with increased *PIK3CA* copy number[57] and in ovarian cancer cells freshly isolated from ascites fluid.[57] The consistent genomic amplification and overexpression of P13K in ovarian, but not several other cancers strongly implicates P13K in the genesis of ovarian cancer.

Multiple components of the P13K signaling cascade are amplified in ovarian cancer

As indicated in Table 55.1, several components of the P13K family are coordinately amplified in ovarian cancer cell lines with P13K

Table 55.1 Copy number changes in components of the P13K signaling pathway

	p110α	p110β	p85α	p85β	PTEN	AKT1	AKT2
Location:	3q26.3	3q22	5q12–13	19q13	10q23	14q32	19q13
Lymphs	2	2	2	2	2	2	1
Dov13	2	2	2		2	2	2
OVCA433	6	5	2		1.4	3	3
OVCAR3	4	5	2	High	4	5	13
CAOV3	4	6	1.2		2	2.6	4
SKOV3	3	3	2		1	2	2

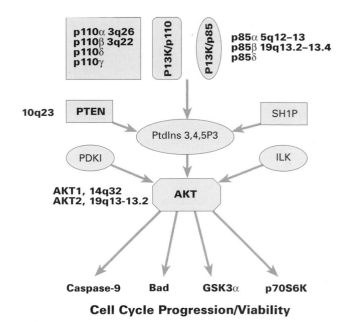

Fig. 55.4 Chromosome location of components of the P13K cascade.

p110α (Fig. 55.4). The 3q26 amplicon in ovarian cancer appears to include p110β, which is located at 3q22 (Fig. 55.4). Intriguingly, both p85β and AKT2 colocalize to 19q13 and appear to be part of the same amplicon (Table 55.1). AKT2 is frequently amplified (6 of 6 tumors; not presented) in primary tumors, as assessed by FISH analysis. AKT1 copy number appears to be modestly elevated in ovarian cancer cell lines, despite previous reports failing to detect AKT1 amplification in tumors by Southern blot analysis (Fig. 55.4, Table 55.1). p85α gene copy number does not appear to be altered in ovarian cancers. RNA expression array analysis indicates that P13K p110δ, primarily found in hematopoietic cells, is present at high levels in the OVCAR3 ovarian cancer cell line. We have demonstrated elevated levels of p85β and AKT2 protein in OVCAR3 cells as compared to normal ovarian epithelial cells or Dov13 cells, confirming that the genomic amplification translates into increased protein levels.[57] Taken together, the data suggest that ovarian cancers likely contain elevated amounts of p85β/p110α, p85β/p110β and potentially p85β/p110δ dimers. These dimers may link selectively to AKT2. Given that recent studies have suggested that different P13K heterodimeric complexes mediate signaling downstream of specific cell-surface receptors,[69] the presence of specific P13K dimers may link to the signaling pathways particularly important for tumorigenesis in ovarian cancer. In particular, a p110β complex has been reported to mediate LPA signaling.[69] We have confirmed that LPA increases p110β specific activity without significantly increasing p110α specific activity.

Dov13 was the only ovarian cancer cell line identified without amplification of p110α in our previous studies.[57] Strikingly, Dov13 also does not demonstrate amplification to any significant level of other components of the P13K pathway. Further, the data also suggest that Dov13 utilizes a P13K-amplification-independent pathway for tumorigenesis.

Consequences of amplification to the PI3K signaling cascade in ovarian cancer

Ovarian cancer cell lines with amplification of 3q26.3 and increased PI3K p110α levels demonstrate increased sensitivity to extracellular ligands, including fetal calf serum, LPA, and EGF, as assessed by the ability to induce phosphorylation of AKT (not presented), which is a surrogate for PI3K activity in intact cells.[3–5] This effect is seen most clearly with weak mitogens or with limiting concentrations of ligand. Furthermore, the most clear effect is an increase in duration of signaling by ligands (not presented). The effects are reversed by LY294002 and wortmannin, demonstrating a role for PI3K in the process. Thus amplification of multiple components of the PI3K signaling cascade contribute to an increased sensitivity of ovarian cancer cells to their extracellular environment. Given the effects of the PI3K signaling pathway on cellular proliferation, neovascularization, viability, and senescence, amplification of signaling through the PI3K pathway could contribute to ovarian tumorigenesis by multiple mechanisms.

Regulation of gene expression by PI3K

We have begun to evaluate the effect of altered signaling through the PI3K pathway on gene expression, using RNA expression arrays. From the arrays, we have identified over 100 genes and a similar number of anonymous ESTs, the expression of which is altered more than twofold by inhibition of PI3K signaling by treatment of SKOV3 or OVCAR3 ovarian cancer cells with LY294002. The most prominent changes in expression involve genes associated with cell-cycle progression (cyclin *A*, *B1*, *D2*, *cdk2*, *p15*, *wee1*, *PCNA*, *cdc20*, *cdc25*), signal transduction (*ILK*, *EAR2*, *myb*, *APC*, stk kinase, kap phosphatase, *MKK6*, *IGFRII*, *pim-1*, *IGFBP*), growth factors (heregulin, VEGF, teratocarcinoma-derived growth factor) and apoptosis (*apol*, *bak*, *bax*), multiple genes associated with ubiquitination, and multiple forms of tubulin.

PTEN specifically targets the PI3K signaling pathway

The following results represent our studies with glioma and breast cancer cells lacking PTEN. However, these results likely apply to the significant portion of endometrioid ovarian cancers that lack PTEN.[56] They also likely apply to the majority of endometrial cancers which lack PTEN.[52,53,60,61] Introduction of wild-type PTEN into breast or glioma cancer cell lines lacking PTEN decreases signaling through the PI3K pathway, as indicated by a decrease in PtdIns 3,4,5P3, AKT, and PDKI activity; phosphorylation of AKT, p70S6 kinase, GSK3α, and Bad, as well as increased expression of the p27Kip1 cyclin-dependent kinase inhibitor.[64,66–68,70–72] Each of these proteins plays a role in the regulation of cell-cycle progression or apoptosis.[3–5,18,24,50,73] The lipid phosphatase activity of PTEN is critical for its regulation of AKT phosphorylation, as wild-type but not a mutant (C124S), which inactivates the protein and lipid phosphatase activity of PTEN, or a mutant (G129E), which inactivates the lipid phosphatase activity of PTEN while leaving the protein phosphatase activity intact, decreased AKT phosphorylation.[68] PTEN appears primarily to

regulate the duration of activation of the PI3K pathway, having minimal effects on the magnitude of PI3K signaling.[68] This also suggests that PTEN activity is regulated during growth factor-dependent signaling. The effects of expression of PTEN on phosphorylation of AKT, p70S6 kinase, GSK3α, and Bad were similar to that of wortmannin or LY294002,[68] which inhibit PI3K, further implicating the PI3K pathway as a specific target for PTEN. Enforced expression of exogenous PTEN in cells that contain PTEN (SKBR3 and MCF7) did not result in a change in phosphorylation of AKT (not presented). Thus effects of PTEN are most clearly manifest in cells lacking PTEN, and PTEN enzymatic activity is not rate limiting in normal cells.

Strikingly, PTEN expression did not alter basal or ligand-induced phosphorylation of the Erk1 and Erk2 mitogen-associated protein kinases,[66,68] indicating that PTEN does not target the Ras/MAPK pathway. Further, there was no effect of expression of PTEN on phosphorylation of either P38 Hog or JNK,[66] indicating that these MAP kinases are also not affected by PTEN. Together, these data strongly suggest that PTEN specifically inhibits the PI3K signaling pathway without altering the Ras/MAPK pathway, and identify modulation of the PI3K pathway as a potentially key mechanism whereby PTEN realizes its tumor suppressor properties.

PTEN regulates cell-cycle progression, apoptosis, and anoikis, dependent on signals transmitted through growth factor receptors and integrins

We and others have demonstrated that the PI3K pathway, as well as activation of FAK, is critical to the regulation of cell death through apoptosis and anoikis.[3–5,18,23,25–27,35,66,68] Since PTEN regulates AKT phosphorylation and activity, as well as Bad phosphorylation,[64,66–68,71,72] and has been reported to alter integrin-mediated FAK activation,[62,63] PTEN may potentially regulate apoptosis and anoikis.

Expression of PTEN or inhibition of PI3K with LY294002 in breast cancer cells lacking PTEN decreases cellular proliferation.[68] PTEN did not decrease proliferation of the MDA-MB-435 cell line, which expresses normal PTEN. Indeed, expression of PTEN in breast cancer,[68] Cos, or 293 cells (not presented), which express normal PTEN, does not detectably alter AKT phosphorylation. The effects of PTEN on proliferation of breast cancer cells lacking PTEN could be due to decreased cell-cycle progression or increased apoptosis. In the presence of high concentrations of serum, enforced expression of PTEN induces a predominant G_1 arrest, compatible with the effects of PTEN on expression of the p27 cell-cycle regulator (Table 55.2). In the presence of low concentrations of serum, enforced expression of PTEN induces apoptosis compatible with effects of PTEN on phosphorylation of the Bad, p70S6 kinase, and GSK3α apoptosis regulators.[68] Under anchorage-independent conditions, where integrins are not ligated, PTEN induces anoikis, which is exacerbated by culture in low serum conditions.[68] Thus, dependent on the level of activation of the PI3K signaling cascade by growth factors in serum or by ligation of integrins under anchorage-dependent conditions, expression of PTEN can induce cell-cycle arrest, apoptosis, or anoikis in breast cancer cells lacking PTEN. Similar effects are

Table 55.2 Effect of PTEN on growth arrest, apoptosis, and anoikis

	Culture conditions			
Serum:	+	−	+	−
Adhesion:	+	+	−	−
Effect of PTEN	Growth arrest	Apoptosis, 10–20%	Anoikis, low level 10–20%	Anoikis, high level 60–80%

likely to occur in endometrioid ovarian cancer and endometrial uterine cancers.

Phosphorylation of specific residues in bad as a consequence of activation of the PI3K and MAPK signaling cascades

As indicated above, PI3K and PTEN play a critical role in the phosphorylation of Bad, a critical apoptotic regulator. Phosphorylation of Bad at serine 112 or serine 136 abrogates its ability to bind to Bcl-X and instead results in binding to 14–3–3 (see Fig. 55.3).[48,49,73] This is in contrast to AKT, where phosphorylation of both sites is required for optimal activation.[23,28,40] Thus phosphorylation of either site of Bad leads to increased levels of free Bcl-X and decreases apoptosis. We have demonstrated that, in contrast to phosphorylation of serine 136 in Bad, which is a consequence of PI3K activity,[23,28,40] phosphorylation of serine 112 in Bad is regulated by the Ras/Raf/MEK/MAPK cascade.[74] Indeed, activated Ras, Raf, or MEK is sufficient to induce phosphorylation of serine 112 but not serine 136 in Bad, and inhibition of the Ras/Raf/MEK cascade (Fig. 55.2) abrogates phosphorylation of serine 112 but not serine 136 in Bad. Thus Bad appears to provide a convergence point for the anti-apoptotic activities of the PI3K and Ras pathways.

Mutations in PTEN and amplification of PI3K generate a similar sensitivity to LY294002

To begin to determine whether the abnormalities in the PI3K cascade observed in ovarian cancer could potentially be a target for novel therapeutics, we have assessed the effect of inhibition of PI3K with the relatively specific PI3K inhibitor, LY294002, on the

Table 55.3 Sensitivity to PI3K inhibitor LY294002 is determined by status of PI3K pathway in breast and ovarian cancer (as assessed by MTT dye conversion at 96 hours)

Breast cell line	IC$_{50}$(μM)	Ovarian cell line	IC$_{50}$ (μM)
Mutant PTEN		**Overexpressed PI3K**	
BT-549	3	OCC1	4
MDA-MB 468	2	OVCAR3	3
Normal PTEN		SKOV3	2
MDA-MB-231	15	**Normal PI3K**	
MDA-MB-453	15	Dov13	16
MCF7	10	IOSE	15
		(2 independent lines)	
SKBR3	17	NOE	16
		(2 independent lines)	

proliferation and viability of normal and malignant ovarian epithelium under anchorage-dependent conditions. Strikingly, ovarian cancer cell lines with amplified PI3K, or breast cancer cells with mutated PTEN, are consistently more sensitive to growth inhibition by LY294002 than are normal ovarian epithelial cells or ovarian cancer cells where PI3K is not amplified (Table 55.3). This appears counterintuitive, as cells with increased PI3K levels or with decreased PTEN levels would be expected to be resistant to pharmacological inhibition of PI3K, due to increased amounts of target present. This growth inhibition is associated with the induction of programmed cell death by apoptosis.[57] These data suggest that the PI3K pathway is particularly critical to the survival or proliferation of breast and ovarian cancer cells with mutations in PTEN or amplification of PI3K, respectively. Further, the differential sensitivity to LY294002 between ovarian cancer cells and normal ovarian epithelium and breast cancer cells with and without mutations in PTEN suggests that the PI3K signaling cascade should be evaluated as an indicator of prognosis and as a target for therapy in ovarian cancers.

As noted above, lung cancers demonstrate amplification of 3q26.3. Similar to our studies of ovarian cancer cells, they exhibit increased PI3K activity as well as increased sensitivity to wortmannin, a relatively specific inhibitor of PI3K,[75] providing additional support to the concept that cells with amplifications of the PI3K pathway are particularly dependent on functionality of the pathway and thus sensitive to the effects of inhibitors of the pathway.

Effects of LY294002 in vivo

In preliminary experiments with 24 mice over a 1-month period, we have demonstrated that treatment of the human ovarian cancer cell line OVCAR3, established in the peritoneal cavity of nude mice, for 14 days with the PI3K inhibitor LY294002 (2 mg/mouse intraperitoneally daily for 2 weeks) results in a marked decrease in tumor burden (65%, $P < 0.05$) and in the production of ascites (3 ml in control versus undetected in treated mice). The response to LY294002 is associated with morphologic changes compatible with apoptosis. Thus, at doses of LY294002 which are well tolerated by the normal tissues of mice, growth of ovarian cancer cells is markedly inhibited.

We have demonstrated previously that inhibition of p70S6 kinase, which is downstream of PI3K (Fig. 55.2), increases the sensitivity of a number of different cell lineages to apoptosis induced by multiple mechanisms.[35] Importantly, inhibition of p70S6 kinase increases the sensitivity of ovarian cancer cell lines to apoptosis induced by cisplatin, the primary drug used in the therapy of ovarian cancer. This suggests that p70S6 kinase may, at least in part, mediate the prevention of apoptosis induced by activation of PI3K.

SHP1 regulates PI3K

me and *mev* autoimmune mice have a spontaneous mutation or 'knockout' of the *SHP1/PTP1C* tyrosine phosphatase gene.[76] We have demonstrated that heterozygous mice with this syndrome have a high incidence of tumors and that these tumors have lost function of the normal *SHP1* allele, implicating *SHP1* as a tumor suppressor gene.[77] We have demonstrated that SHP1 co-immunoprecipitates with the p85 regulatory subunit of PI3K, and that this association is inducibly increased by ligation of cell-surface receptors.[78] The carboxyl terminal SH2 domain of PI3K inducibly associates with a phosphorylated tyrosine (Tyr564) in the carboxyl terminus of SHP1. Wild-type SHP1 dephosphorylates p85 and alters PI3K lipid kinase activity and phosphorylation of AKT.[79] These results indicate the presence of a functional interaction between PI3K and SHP1, and suggest that PI3K signaling can be regulated by SHP1.

Conclusions

We have demonstrated that the p110α subunit of PI3K, located at 3q26.3, is consistently amplified in ovarian cancer cell lines and tumors but not in breast cancer or melanoma, implicating PI3K in ovarian carcinogenesis. p110α expression and PI3K activity, as well as sensitivity to the specific PI3K inhibitor, LY294002, are consistently increased in ovarian cancer cell lines with amplified p110α copy number, compared to normal ovarian epithelium and cell lines with normal copy number. In addition to increased expression of p110α, ovarian cancer cells also demonstrate increased expression of multiple components of the PI3K signaling pathway. PTEN mutations, which are functionally similar to amplification of PI3K, are frequently observed in endometrioid ovarian cancers. This implies that PI3K may function as an oncogene in ovarian cancer and should be evaluated as an indicator of prognosis and as a target for therapy in ovarian cancer.

References

1. American Cancer Society (1998). *Cancer facts and figures – 1997*. American Cancer Society, Inc., Atlanta, GA.
2. Teeriello, M. *et al.* (1995). Early detection of ovarian cancer. *CA Cancer J. Clin.*, **45**, 71–87.
3. Wymann, M.P. and Pirola, L. (1998). Structure and function of phosphoinositide 3-kinases. *Biochim. Biophys. Acta*, **1436**, 127–50.
4. Toker, A. and Cantley, L.C. (1997). Signaling through the lipid products of phosphoinositide-3-OH kinase. *Nature*, **387**, 673–6.
5. Vanhaesebroeck, B., Leevers, S.J., Panayotou, G., and Waterfield, M.D. (1997). Phosphoinositide 3-kinases: a conserved family of signal transducers. *Trends Biochem. Sci.*, **22** (7), 267–72.
6. Chang, H.W., Aoki, M., Fruman, D. *et al.* (1997). Transformation of chicken cells by the gene encoding the catalytic subunit of P13 kinase. *Science*, **276**, 1848–50.
7. Cantley, L.C., Auger, K., Carpenter, R. *et al.* (1991). Oncogenes and signal transduction. *Cell*, **64**, 281–302.
8. Jimenez, C., Jones, D.R., Rodriguez-Viciana, P. *et al.* (1998). Identification and characterization of a new oncogene derived from the regulatory subunit of phosphoinositide 3-kinase. *EMBO J.*, **17**, 743–53.
9. Downward, J. (1997). Role of phosphoinositide-3-OH kinase in Ras signaling. *Adv. Second Messenger Phosphoprot. Res.*, **31**, 1–10.
10. Li, J., Yen, C., Liaw, D. *et al.* (1997). PTEN, a putative protein tyr phosphatase gene mutated in human brain, breast and prostate cancer. *Science*, **275**, 1943–7.
11. Steck, P., Pershouse, M.A., Jasser, S.A. *et al.* (1997). Identification of a candidate tumor suppressor gene, MMAC1, at chromosome 10q23.3 that is mutated in multiple advanced cancers. *Nature Genet.*, **15**, 256–362.
12. Li, D.M. and Sun, H. (1997). TEP1, encoded by a candidate tumor suppressor locus, is a novel protein tyr phosphatase regulated by transforming growth factor b. *Cancer Res.*, **57**, 2124–9.
13. Starink, T.M., van der Veen, J.P., Arwert, F. *et al.* (1986). The Cowden syndrome: a clinical and genetic study in 21 patients. *Clin. Genet.*, **29**, 222–3.
14. Nelen, M.R., van Staveren, M.C.G., Peeters, E.A.J. *et al.* (1997). Germline mutations in the PTEN/MMAC1 gene in patients with Cowden disease. *Hum. Mol. Genet.*, **6**, 1383–7.
15. Marsh, D.J., Dahia, P.L.M., Zheng, Z. *et al.* (1997). Germline mutations in PTEN are present in Bannayan–Zonana syndrome. *Nature Genet.*, **16**, 333–4.
16. Liaw, D., Marsh, D.J., L.I.J. *et al.* (1997). Germline mutations of the PTEN gene in Cowden's disease, an inherited breast and thyroid cancer syndrome. *Nature Genet.*, **16**, 64–7.
17. Maichama, T., and Dixion, J.E. (1998). The tumor suppressor, PTEN/MMAC1, dephosphorylates the lipid second messenger, phospatidylinositol 3,4,5-trisphosphate. *J. Biol. Chem.*, **273**, 13375–8.
18. Coffer, P.J., Jin, J. and Woodgett, J.R. (1998). Protein kinase B (c-Akt): a multifunctional mediator of phosphatidylinositol 3-kinase activation. *Biochem. J.*, **335**, 1–13.
19. Bellacosa, A., de Feo, D., Godwin, A.K. *et al.* (1995). Molecular alterations of the AKT2 oncogene in ovarian and breast carcinomas. *Int. J. Cancer*, **64** (4), 280–5.
20. Cheng, J.Q., Ruggeri, B., Klein, W.M. *et al.* (1996). Amplification of AKT2 in human pancreatic cells and inhibition of AKT2 expression and tumorigenicity by antisense RNA. *Proc. Natl Acad. Sci., USA*, **93** (8), 3636–41.
21. Cheng, J.Q., Altomare, D.A., Klein, M.A. *et al.* (1997). Transforming activity and mitosis-related expression of the AKT2 oncogene: evidence suggesting a link between cell cycle regulation and oncogenesis. *Oncogene*, **14** (23), 2793–801.
22. Arbiser, J.E., Moses, M.A., Fernandez, C.A. *et al.* (1997). Oncogenic H-ras stimulates tumor angiogenesis by two distinct pathways. *Proc. Natl Acad. Sci., USA*, **94** (3), 861–6.
23. Datta, S.R., Dudek, H., Tao, X. *et al.* (1997). AKT phosphorylation of BAD couples survival signals to the cell-intrinsic death machinery. *Cell*, **91**, 231–41.
24. Frisch, S.M. and Ruoslahti, E. (1997). Integrins and anoikis. *Curr. Opin. Cell Biol.*, **9**, 701–6.
25. Valentinis, B., Reiss, K. and Baserga, R. (1998). Insulin-like growth factor-I-mediated survival from anoikis: role of cell aggregation and focal adhesion kinase. *J. Cell Physiol.*, **176** (3), 648–57.
26. Frisch, S.M. and Francis, H. (1994). Disruption of epithelial cell–matrix interactions induces apoptosis. *J. Cell Biol.*, **124** (4), 619–26.
27. Frisch, S.M., Vuori, K., Ruoslahti, E. and Chan-Hui, P.Y. (1996). Control of adhesion-dependent cell survival by focal adhesion kinase. *J. Cell Biol.*, **134** (3), 793–9.
28. Delcommenne, M., Tan, C., Gray, V. *et al.* (1998). Phosphoinositide-3-OH kinase-dependent regulation of glycogen synthase kinase 3 and protein kinase B/AKT by the integrin-linked kinase. *Proc. Natl Acad. Sci., USA*, **95** (19), 11211–16.
29. Wu, C., Keightley, S.Y., Leung-Hagesteijn, C. *et al.* (1998). Integrin-linked protein kinase regulates fibronectin matrix assembly, E-cadherin expression, and tumorigenicity. *J. Biol. Chem.*, **273** (1), 528–36.

30. Plopper, G.E., McNamee, H.P., Dike, L.E. *et al.* (1995). Convergence of integrin and growth factor receptor signaling pathways within the focal adhesion complex. *Mol. Biol. Cell*, **6** (10), 1349–65.

31. Bast, R.C. and Mills, G.B. (2001). The molecular pathogenesis of ovarian cancer: In *The molecular basis of cancer*, (eds J., Mendelsohn, P., Howley, M., Isreal, and L. Liotta), in press.

32. Rodriguez-Viciana, P., Warne, P.H., Vanhaesebroeck, B. *et al.* (1996). Activation of phosphoinositide 3-kinase by interaction with Ras and by point mutation. *EMBO J.*, **15** (10), 2442–51.

33. Patton, S.E., Martin, M.L., Nelson, L.L. *et al.* (1998). Activation of the RAS-MAP kinase pathway and phosphorylation of Ets-2 at position threonine 72 in human ovarian cancer cell lines. *Cancer Res.*, **58** (10), 2253–9.

34. Liu, A.X., Testa, J.R., Hamilton, T.C. *et al.* (1998). AKT2, a member of the protein kinase B family, is activated by growth factors, v-Ha-ras, and v-src through phosphatidylinositol 3-kinase in human ovarian epithelial cancer cells. *Cancer Res.*, **58** (14), 2973–7.

35. Shi, Y., Frankel, F., Radvanyi, L. *et al.* (1995). Rapamycin enhances apoptosis and increases sensitivity to cisplatin *in vitro*. *Cancer Res.*, **55**, 1982–8.

36. Shen, F. and Weber, G. (1997). Synergistic action of quercetin and genistein in human ovarian carcinoma cells. *Oncol. Res.*, **9**, 597–602.

37. Liu, L., Damen, J.E., Ware, M. *et al.* (1997). SHIP, a new player in cytokine-induced signaling. *Leukemia*, **11**, 181–4.

38. Rebecchi, M.J. and Scarlata, S. (1998). Pleckstrin homology domains: a common fold with diverse functions. *Annu. Rev. Biophys. Biomol. Struct.*, **27**, 503–28.

39. Klippel, A., Kavanaugh, M., Pot, D. *et al.* (1997). A specific product of phosphatidylinositol 3-kinase directly activates the protein kinase AKT through its pleckstrin homology domain. *Mol. Cell. Biol.*, **17**, 338–44.

40. Stokoe, D., Stephens, L.R., Copeland, T. *et al.* (1997). Dual role of phosphatidylinositol-3,4,5-triphosphate in the activation of protein kinase B. *Science*, **277**, 567–70.

41. Gibson, S., Leung, B., Squire, J.A. *et al.* (1993). Identification, cloning, and characterization of a novel human T cell specific tyrosine kinase located at the hematopoietin complex on chromosome 5q. *Blood*, **82**, 1561–72.

42. Lu, Y., Cuevas, B., Gibson, S. *et al.* (1998). Phosphatidylinositol 3-kinase is required for optimal CD28 but not CD3 regulation of the Tec family Tyrosine kinase EMT/ITK/TSK. *J. Immunol.*, **161**, 5404–12.

43. Kawakami, Y., Yao, L., Tashiro, M. *et al.* (1995). Activation and interaction with protein kinase C of a cytoplasmic tyrosine kinase, Itk/Tsk/Emt, on FceR1 cross-linking on mast cells. *J. Immunol.*, **155**, 3556–62.

44. Vanhaesebroeck, B., Welham, M.J., Kotani, K. *et al.* (1997). P110delta, a novel phosphoinositide 3-kinase in leukocytes. *Proc. Natl Acad. Sci., USA*, **94** (9), 4330–5.

45. Rordorf-Nikolic, T., Van Horn, D.J., Chen, D. *et al.* (1995). Regulation of phosphatidylinositol 3' kinase by tyrosyl phosphoproteins. *J. Biol. Chem.*, **270** (8), 3662–6.

46. Yu, J., Zhang, Y., McIlroy, J. *et al.* (1998). Regulation of the p85/p110 phosphatidylinositol 3'-kinase: stabilization and inhibition of the p110alpha catalytic subunit by the p85 regulatory subunit. *Mol. Cell. Biol.*, **18** (3), 1379–87.

47. Cardone, M.H., Roy, N., Stennicke, H.R. *et al.* (1998). Regulation of cell death protease caspase-9 by phosphorylation. *Science*, **282** (5392), 1318–21.

48. Green, D.R. and Reed, J.C. (1998). Mitochondria and apoptosis. *Science*, **281** (5381), 1309–12.

49. Nunez, G., Benedict, M.A., Hu, Y. and Inohara, N. (1998). Caspases: the proteases of the apoptotic pathway. *Oncogene*, **17** (25), 3237–45.

50. Pap, M. and Cooper, G.M. (1998). Role of glycogen synthase kinase-3 in the phosphatidylinositol 3-kinase/Akt cell survival pathway. *J. Biol. Chem.*, **273** (32), 19929–32.

51. Teng, D.H.F., Hu, R., Lin, H. *et al.* (1997). MMAC1/PTEN: Mutations in primary tumor specimens and tumor cell lines. *Cancer Res.*, **57**, 5221–5.

52. Risinger, J.I., Hayes, K., Maxwell, G.L. *et al.* (1998). PTEN mutation in endometrial cancers is associated with favorable clinical and pathologic characteristics. *Clin. Cancer Res.*, **4** (12), 3005–10.

53. Risinger, J.I., Hayes, A.K., Berchuck, A. and Barrett, J.C. (1997). PTEN/MMAC1 mutations in endometrial cancers. *Cancer Res.*, **57** (21), 4736–8.

54. Yokomizo, A., Tindall, D.J., Hartmann, L. *et al.* (1998). Mutation analysis of the putative tumor suppressor PTEN/MMAC1 in human ovarian cancer. *Intl J. Oncol.*, **13**, 101–5.

55. Tashiro, H., Blazes, M.S., Wu, R. *et al.* (1997). Mutations in PTEN are frequent in endometrial carcinoma but rare in other common gynecological malignancies. *Cancer Res.*, **57**, 3935–40.

56. Obata, K., Morland, S.J., Watson, R.H. *et al.* (1998). Frequent PTEN/MMAC mutations in endometrioid but not serous or mucinous epithelial ovarian tumors. *Cancer Res.*, **58**, 2095–7.

57. Shayesteh, L., Lu, Y., Kuo, W.L. *et al.* (1999). PIK3CA is implicated as an oncogene in ovarian cancer. *Nature Genet.*, **21**, 99–102.

58. Tapper, J., Butzow, R., Wahlstrom, T. *et al.* (1997). Evidence for divergence of DNA copy number changes in serous, mucinous and endometrioid ovarian carcinomas. *Br. J. Cancer*, **75** (12), 1782–7.

59. Pere, H., Tapper, J., Wahlstrom, T. *et al.* (1998). Distinct chromosomal imbalances in uterine serous and endometrioid carcinomas. *Cancer Res.*, **58**, 892–5.

60. Maxwell, G.L., Risinger, J.I., Gumbs, C. *et al.* (1998). Mutation of the PTEN tumor suppressor gene in endometrial hyperplasias. *Cancer Res.*, **58**, 2500–3.

61. Levine, R.L., Cargile, C.B., Blazes, M.S. *et al.* (1998). PTEN mutations and microsatellite instability in complex atypical hyperplasia, a precursor lesion to uterine endometrioid carcinoma. *Cancer Res.*, **58**, 3254–8.

62. Gu, J., Tamura, M. and Yamada, K.M. (1998). Tumor suppressor PTEN inhibits integrin- and growth factor-mediated mitogen-activated protein (MAP) kinase signaling pathways. *J. Cell Biol.*, **143** (5), 1375–83.

63. Tamura, M., Gu, J., Takino, T. and Tamada, K.M. (1999). Tumor suppressor PTEN inhibition of cell invasion, migration, and growth: differential involvement of focal adhesion kinase and p130Cas. *Cancer Res.*, **59** (2), 442–9.

64. Furnari, F.B., Lin, H., Huang, H.J. *et al.* (1997). Growth suppression of glioma cells by PTEN requires a functional phosphatase catalytic domain. *Proc. Natl Acad. Sci., USA*, **94**, 12479–84.

65. Cheney, I.W., Johnson, D.E., Vaillancourt, M.T. *et al.* (1998). Suppression of tumorigenicity of glioblastoma cells by adenovirus-mediated MMAC1/PTEN gene transfer. *Cancer Res.*, **58**, 2331–4.

66. Davies, M.A., Lu, Y., Sano, T. *et al.* (1998). Adenoviral transgene expression of MMAC/PTEN in human glioma cells inhibits AKT activation and induces anoikis. *Cancer* **58**, 5285–90.

67. Myers, M.P., Pass, I., Batty, I.H. *et al.* (1998). The lipid phosphatase activity of PTEN is critical for its tumor suppressor function. *Proc. Natl Acad. Sci. USA*, **95** (23), 13513–18.

68. Lu, Y., Lin, Y., Lapushin, R. *et al.* (1999). The PTEN/MMAC1/TEP tumour suppressor gene decreases cell growth and induces apoptosis and anoikis in breast cancer cells. *Oncogene*, **18**, 7034–45.

69. Roche, S., Downward, J., Raynal, P., and Courtneidge, S.A. (1998). A function of phosphatidylinositol 3-kinase β (p85α–p110β) in fibroblasts during mitogenesis: requirement for insulin- and lysophosphatidic acid-mediated signal transduction. *Mol. Cell. Biol.*, **18** (12), 7119–29.

70. Hass-Kogan, D., Shalev, N., Wong, M. *et al.* (1998). PKB/akt activity is elevated in glioblastoma cells due to mutation of PTEN/MMAC1. *Curr. Biol.*, **8**, 1195–8.

71. Stambolic, V., Suzuki, A., de la Pompa, J.L. *et al.* (1998). Negative regulation of PKB/Akt-dependent cell survival by the tumor suppressor PTEN. *Cell*, **95** (1), 29–39.

72. Li, J., Simpson, L., Takahashi, M., *et al.* (1998). The PTEN/MMAC1 tumor suppressor induces cell death that is rescued by the AKT/protein kinase B oncogene. *Cancer Res.*, **58** (24), 5667–72.

73. Katayose, Y., Kim, M., Rakkar, A.N. *et al.* (1997). Promoting apoptosis: a novel activity associated with the cyclin-dependent kinase inhibitor p27. *Cancer Res.*, **57** (24), 5441–5.

74. Zha, J., Harada, H., Yang, E. *et al.* (1996). Serine phosphorylation of death agonist BAD in response to survival factor results in binding to 14–3–3 not BCL-X. *Cell* **84** (4), 6619–28.

75. Fang, X., Yu., S., Eder, A. *et al.* (1999). Regulation of BAD phosphorylation at serine 112 by the Ras-Mitogen-activated protein kinase pathway. *Oncogene*, **18**, 6635–40.

76. Moore, S.M., Rintoul, R.C., Walker, T.R. *et al.* (1998). The presence of a constitutively active phosphoinositide 3-kinase in small cell lung cancer cells mediates anchorage-independent proliferation via a protein kinase B and p70s6k-dependent pathway. *Cancer Res.*, **58** (22), 5239–47.

77. Tsui, H.W., Siminovitch, K.A., de Souza, L., and Tsui, F.W. (1993). Motheaten and viable motheaten mice have mutations in the haematopoietic cell phosphatase gene. *Nature Genet.*, **4** (2), 124–9.

78. Siminovitch, K.A., Lamhonwah, A.M., Somani, A.K. *et al.* (1999). Involvement of the SHP-1 tyrosine phosphatase in regulating B lymphocyte antigen receptor signaling, proliferation and transformation. *Curr. Top. Microbiol. Immunol.*, **246**, 291–7.

79. Cuevas, B., Lu, Y., Watt, S. *et al.* (1999). SHP-1 regulates LCK-induced phosphatidylinositol 3′ kinase phosphorylation and activity, *J. Biol. Chem.*, **274**, 27583–89.

Index

426　INDEX

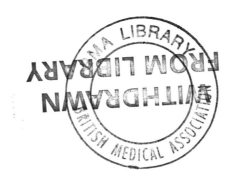